DEVELOPMENTAL NEUROBIOLOGY

DEVELOPMENTAL NEUROBIOLOGY
Second Edition

Marcus Jacobson
The University of Utah College of Medicine
Salt Lake City, Utah

Springer Science+Business Media, LLC

Library of Congress Cataloging in Publication Data

Jacobson, Marcus, 1930-
Developmental neurobiology.

Bibliography: p.
Includes index.
1. Developmental neurology. I. Title. [DNLM: 1. Nervous system–Embryology. 2. Nervous system–Growth and development. WL01 J17d]
QP363.5.J3 1978 599'.01'88 77-26068

DOI 10.1007/978-1-4757-4951-9

First Printing – March 1978
Second Printing – July 1979

Originally published by Plenum Press, New York in 1978.
MyCopy version of the original edition 1978

Preface to the Second Edition

When the first edition of this book was completed in 1969, most aspects of neural ontogeny could be surveyed at a glance. Such an overview is more difficult now that mountains of research reports have newly risen on all sides. It is not my intention in this book to explore every pathway through that literature. Rather, my purposes are to find the main avenues leading to an understanding of how the nervous system develops and to point out some of the obstacles I can see on the way.

There were errors of fact and judgment in the first edition that I have corrected in this one. As I have added much that is new, this edition has been virtually rewritten, but mistakes must surely have entered this book as easily as they were removed from the other. My most constant unwritten concern in writing this book is that I may be helping to preserve conventional forms of thought which might be injurious to the neophyte who trusts any guide other than his own intelligence. Books such as this may prove injurious to minds that are not open to direct experience of a more vital work, the book of nature. This book will prove useful only to the extent that it serves as an aid to direct observation.

My appraisal of facts and concepts, partly positive and partly negative, is determined not only by an understanding of the facts as they are now known but also by a sense of their historical evolution. Our training to think of organisms in terms of their evolution and development should prepare our minds to think about the historical evolution of our ideas. R. G. Collingwood has eloquently made the point in *The Idea of History* (1946) that "progress . . . happens only in one way: by the retention in the mind, at one phase, of what was achieved in the preceding phase. The two phases are related not merely by way of succession, but by way of continuity, and continuity of a peculiar kind. If Einstein makes an advance on Newton, he does it by knowing Newton's thought and retaining it within his own, in the sense that he knows what Newton's problems were, and how he solved them, and, disentangling the truth in those solutions from whatever errors prevented Newton from going further. . . . Newton thus lives in Einstein in the way in which any past experience lives in the mind of the historian, as a past experience known as past—as the point from which the development with which he is concerned started—but re-enacted here and now together with a development of itself that is partly constructive or positive and partly critical or negative." Thus my occasional criticisms of those who have helped to make my own ideas possible are always done in the spirit of Collingwood's dictum that "progress is not the replacement of the bad by the good but of the good by the better."

I am uncomfortably aware of my limitations in writing this book. I have done so now because I have something to say and because the problems with which I am concerned are enlarging exponentially while my grasp of them increases at a much slower rate. Each successive advance in knowledge of how the brain develops gives rise to new problems that make the ideal of complete understanding seem even further from attainment. Therefore, I write from a conviction that I can make new arrangements of some old ideas and advance some new ones, and not from any belief in the final certitude of what I have to offer. I admit that there are many subtle points which the blunt instrument of my understanding has failed to touch accurately. However, I have been sustained by the thought that as one cannot hope to attain complete knowledge of the information available to date, one should not be afraid to say something before one has mastered the last jot and tittle on the subject.

M. J.

Salt Lake City, Utah
January 1978

Preface to the First Edition

It would be better to have no Book of History *than to believe all of it.*

Mencius (371?–289? B.C.), Mêng Tzu 7B:3

Socrates: Then anyone who leaves behind him a written manual, and likewise anyone who takes it over from him, on the supposition that such writing will provide something reliable and permanent, must be exceedingly simple minded. . . .

Plato (424?–347 B.C.), Phaedrus 275C

In the writing of this book my main aim has been to understand nature and to communicate my measure of understanding. I have also tried to convey the sense of wonder that studying the developing nervous system always evokes. Other preoccupations, whether with techniques, theory, or the history of the subject, have not been permitted to obscure the main aim.

Our knowledge of the development of the nervous system has been gained almost entirely in the past century. As I have reviewed a large part of the literature, this book may be of help in placing our present understanding of the subject in historical perspective. History not only illuminates the present state of our knowledge but also gives us a kind of foresight. I have chosen some examples from the work of Ramón y Cajal to make this clearer, for few men have anticipated the future as he did.

While most of this book is merely an attempt at a selective assembly and arrangement of the great mass of data in the literature dealing with development of the nervous system, it has been augmented by occasional historical and speculative excursions. These are fragmentary and unsystematic, and I have not made the procrustean attempt to fit all the evidence into a single theory. The main speculative sally is at the end of the book, where it can easily be passed over by those without a taste for more surmises and conjectures. I have tried to give fair warning wherever the discussion veers perilously close to speculation. In the present state of the subject, a mixture of skepticism and willingness not to persist in error is an essential defense against the hazards encountered by author and readers alike. "I would, therefore, have you, gentle reader, take nothing on trust from me. . . ."*

M. J.

Baltimore
September 1970

*William Harvey, *Preface to Anatomical Exercises on the Generation of Animals,* London, 1651.

Contents

9. Neuronal Specificity and Development of Neuronal Circuits

Introduction

In our attempts to interrogate Nature about the development of the nervous system, we ask such questions as "How do the nerve cells originate and how do the correct types of cells differentiate at their correct positions; how do the neurons link together to form circuits whose functions are properly coordinated; and how are the functions of nerve cells related to behavior, to thought, and to consciousness?" Those problems are intellectually challenging, not only because solving them would give us practical advantages but also because while they remain unsolved they stimulate the imagination and challenge the intelligence. It is precisely because they are difficult and controversial and have defied complete solution that such problems continue to attract subtle minds.

The understanding that we now have of neural ontogeny seems to me to be farther from complete knowledge than from total ignorance. Nonetheless, it gives us a slightly elevated position from which to survey the vicissitudes of the past, to appraise our present understanding, and to consider ways in which our knowledge might develop in the future. The history of this subject affords a particularly piquant illustration of Arthur Lovejoy's comment that the "adequate record of even the confusions of our forebears may help, not only to clarify those confusions, but to engender a salutary doubt whether we are wholly immune from different but equally great confusions. For though we have more empirical information at our disposal, we have not different or better minds; and it is, after all, the action of the mind upon the facts that makes both philosophy and science—and, indeed largely makes the 'facts'. . . . Yet—as many historic examples show—the utility of a belief and its validity are independent variables; and erroneous hypotheses are often avenues to the truth" (*The Great Chain of Being,* 1936).

The cardinal problems of developmental neurobiology are persistent; although they have been reworked by each generation using new tools, they remain incompletely solved. The central question of developmental biology—how organized systems composed of many different types of cells arise from a single cell—is posed acutely by the nervous system, in which cellular diversification is greater and multicellular organization is more complex than in any other system.

The central nervous system of vertebrates is composed of millions of cells and hundreds of distinct cell types which all originate from an embryonic rudiment, the neural plate, composed of a few thousand cells. One of the problems to be considered here is how those stem cells, all quite similar in appearance, give rise to the different types of neurons and glial cells found in the mature nervous system. We want to know where and when the neurons and glial cells originate; we want to trace their lineage and to discover the programs resulting in the differentiation of the many types of cells found in the mature nervous system. How do the newly born nerve cells move to their final positions, and what mechanisms control their assembly in the correct spatial order? How are the total number of cells and the size of individual cells in each part of the nervous system regulated to achieve constancy of size and proportions? What are the mechanisms of outgrowth of axons and dendrites, and what factors regulate their direction of growth toward their postsynaptic targets? How do connections develop between neurons within sets and between sets in different parts of the nervous system? What are the roles of glial cells in the development of the nervous system? How and when do the activities of functional sets of neurons become expressed as behavior, and how is the development of behavior controlled?

Should the complexity of the nervous system make one despair of ever arriving at any understanding of its development? Not if one conceives of the organization and development of the nervous system in terms of a few hundred neuronal sets each composed of about five different types of cells. Development of the neuronal set, then, presents no more complex a problem than development of a limb or the kidney. It is probably better to oversimplify than to overcomplicate a problem such as that of development of the nervous system, whose full dimensions are not known at present. Therefore, we might conceive of the organization of the developing nervous system in the following way. Each neuronal set is composed of one principal neuron which links its set with other sets of different kinds, another type of neuron which connects its set with other sets of the same kind, and three or four local circuit neurons which connect neurons within a set. The complexity of organization arises from the interconnections between sets rather than from connections within sets or from diversification of a very large number of neuronal types. Consider also that the brain is assembled at a more leisurely tempo and reaches maturity more slowly than any other organ. The final product is not merely the result of a program initiated and sustained by the genes but is also regulated by a network of positive and negative controls which constrain the production of nerve cells, their migration, the differentiation of neuronal phenotypes, their assembly into neuronal sets, the development of circuits within and between sets, and their functional expression.

In considering the development of the nervous system, our dilemma is that, while the organization of neuronal sets and their development are easily comprehended, the entire program of development is beyond our intellectual grasp. Therefore, while in principle we should think in terms of organizing relations within a spatial and temporal continuum, in practice we have to particularize and thus to reduce the scope of our apprehension. Thus we recognize five morphogenetic processes: cellular proliferation, migration, differentiation, growth, and death. They are vectorial; that is, they have directions in space and time as well as magnitude. These processes are coordinated as a developmental program, and it is only for convenience that they are treated separately in this book; not because of any predilection for separating the organically interrelated processes of development but rather because of the impossibility of simultaneously grasping them all in a complete synthesis. Nevertheless, **to arrive at any understanding of neural ontogeny as an integrated whole, it is essential to cultivate an awareness of the interdependence of the parts, and of the subtle balance of their relations in space and time.**

It is essential to cultivate the flexibility of thought that gives us the freedom to move easily between a holistic and a reductionistic approach to the subject—to try to consider the development of the entire nervous system while adducing the development of each of its individual elements. We may try to conceive of the organism as a network of interrelated elements, but because complexity makes the whole organism virtually incomprehensible we have to attend to the elements, and their diverse properties and functions, one at a time. But in concentrating on one particular part the rest of the organism goes out of focus. The scientist, like the artist, is in the predicament of having to remain acutely aware of the entire composition while maintaining an intense concentration on a particular element. The difficulty, as Henry James recognized it, is that "Really, universally, relations stop nowhere and the exquisite problem of the artist is eternally but to draw, by a geometry of his own, the circle within which they shall *happily* appear to do so. He is in the perpetual predicament that the continuity of things is the whole matter. . . . That this continuity is never by the space of an instant or an inch, broken, and that to do anything at all, he has at once intensely to consult and intensely to ignore it" (preface to *Roderick Hudson,* 1876).

1

Beginnings of the Nervous System

1.1. Neural Induction and Determination

This brief account is intended merely to serve as an introduction to the phases of neural development that follow primary neural induction. The subject of primary embryonic induction has been reviewed by Saxén and Toivonen (1962) and the classical studies have been dealt with magisterially by Spemann (1938).

Hilde Mangold and Spemann, in the 1920s, first showed that neural determination resulted from contact of the prospective neuroectoderm with the roof of the archenteron—that is, with the tissue that moves from the dorsal lip of the blastopore forward beneath the region of ectoderm that later differentiates as neural tissue. Close proximity between the archenteron roof (which later forms the notochord, somites, and prechordal plate) and the overlying ectoderm is the essential normal condition for development of the nervous system from that ectoderm. This effect is known as *primary neural induction.* The ectoderm is called the *induced tissue,* while the prospective chordomesoderm (tissue arising from the dorsal lip of the blastopore in amphibians and from the primitive streak in birds and mammals) is the *inducer* or *inductor* from which the inducing stimulus arises.

The capacity of a tissue to react to the influence of the inducer is known as its *competence.* Competence for neural induction is uniquely limited to the ectoderm of the gastrula—ectoderm from the blastula or from the neurula cannot respond to the primary inductive stimulus. Conversely, the ectoderm of the early gastrula has the ability under the appropriate conditions to differentiate along many different lines. The *prospective potency* of the ectoderm is its ability to differentiate into a variety of tissues under different conditions. The *prospective significance* of a tissue is its fate if left undisturbed during normal development. Prospective neuroectoderm is that part of the ectoderm that will differentiate as neural tissue during normal development. The prospective neuroectoderm gradually undergoes a progressive restriction of prospective potency. Pieces of prospective neuroectoderm from the early gastrula, if grafted elsewhere in the embryo, can become epidermis, endoderm, or mesoderm, but toward the end of the period of gastrulation the prospective neuroectoderm will differentiate only as neural tissue when translocated or when isolated *in vitro*. This restriction of prospective potency is known as *determination*. By the end of gastrulation the nervous system as a whole and the major part of the nervous system—forebrain, midbrain, hindbrain, and spinal cord—have been determined. Some specific neuronal types, for example, the Rohon-Beard cells of the spinal cord and Mauthner's neurons of the medulla, are already determined by the end of gastrulation, and the progressive restriction of the prospective potency of parts of the neural plate continues throughout neurulation.

The first phase of neural determination consists initially of repression of genes that support differentiation of nonneural tissue. No specific histological or ultrastructural changes can be seen in the prospective neural cells at this stage. The second phase of neural determination consists of the expression of the activity of genes that support differentiation of specific types of neurons. We may think of neural determination as a process that becomes progressively more restrictive during development. At first, the general relationship between parts of the nervous system is determined; later in development, particular relationships such as the synaptic connections between nerve cells are determined.

As the archenteron roof moves forward from the dorsal lip of the blastopore, it exerts its inductive effect on progressively more anterior regions of the overlying ectoderm. This temporospatial progression of primary neural induction is one of the causes of the regional diversification of the neuroectoderm. The more posterior regions of the neuroectoderm are subject to the inductive stimulus for the longest time and, moreover, have a greater contact with the somitic mesoderm than the anterior part of the neuroectoderm, which comes into contact with the prechordal mesoderm only for a relatively short time. In the newt *Triturus* the entire prospective neuroectodermal area is determined in less than 14 hours after first contact with the archenteron roof, but while the posterior part is in contact with the inducer for that entire period, the anterior part is subject to induction only for 3 or 4 hours before it loses its competence to respond (Suzuki and Kuwabara, 1974). The time of contact with the inducer tissue that is required to produce neural determination in competent ectoderm has been studied by sandwiching inducing tissue between pieces of competent ectoderm and then separating the tissues after varying periods of contact. Using ectoderm of *Triturus,* weak induction is found after 1 hour of contact, while strong induction requires 3–4 hours (Johnen, 1964; Suzuki *et al.,* 1975). Gebhardt and Nieuwkoop (1963) have shown that the dorsal lip of the blastopore can act as a primary inducer upon the ectoderm for a period of less than 24 hours in *Ambystoma mexicanum.*

How the regional determination of the neuroectoderm occurs seems to have been resolved into two phases that overlap but are spatially and temporally almost separate at their extreme limits. One of the definitions of these two phases has been given by Nieuwkoop (1962, 1967*a,b*): first, *activation* of the ectoderm by the underlying chordomesoderm determines the size and form of the neural plate and results in the development of forebrain structures only; second, *transformation* of the already activated neuroectoderm is brought about by interaction with mesoderm and results in development of more caudal structures of the nervous system. Both activation and transformation are distributed as morphogenetic fields; that is, they have continuous, quantitative variation in space and time which, because the thickness of the neuroepithelium is negligible compared with its length and width, results in mediolateral and anteroposterior (rostrocaudal) differences in morphological development. From the point of view of the substances involved in these gradients, regional determination is seen as the result of at least two different agents acting on the neuroectoderm: the neuralizing agent emanating from the anterior part of the archenteron roof and prechordal plate induces rostral structures in the nervous system such as forebrain and eyes, while increasing ratios of mesodermalizing agent arising from the notochord and somites induce more caudal neural structures. These agents or other similar substances with the same effects, which have been identified as protein, have been isolated from various sources, the neuralizing agent from alcohol-treated liver and the mesodermalizing agent from alcohol-treated guinea pig bone marrow (Toivonen and Saxén, 1955*a,b;* T. Yamada, 1958; H. Tiedemann, 1968).

The quantitative effect of mesoderm on competent neuroectoderm has been elegantly assayed by Saxén and Toivonen (1961) and Toivonen and Saxén (1968). They disaggregated neuroectodermal cells of the forebrain region, mixed them in different ratios with trunk mesoderm cells, and reaggregated the mixtures. The aggregates were cultured for 14 days and then examined histologically. Only forebrain structures with nasal and optic rudiments developed in aggregates composed mostly of neuroectodermal cells (ratio of neural to mesodermal cells 10:1 or 5:1). Increasing the ratio of mesodermal cells in the aggregates resulted in corresponding increases in caudal structures of the nervous system. Hindbrain and ear rudiments developed when the ratio of neural to mesodermal cells was 5:2, and spinal cord developed when the ratio was 5:5 or less (Fig. 1.1). Toivonen and Saxén (1968) concluded: "During the initial stage of induction the cells are determined to become neural, but they acquire no stable regional character. This is subsequently controlled by the mesodermal cells and apparently in a quantitative way, since an increasing amount of mesoderm surrounding the neural cells

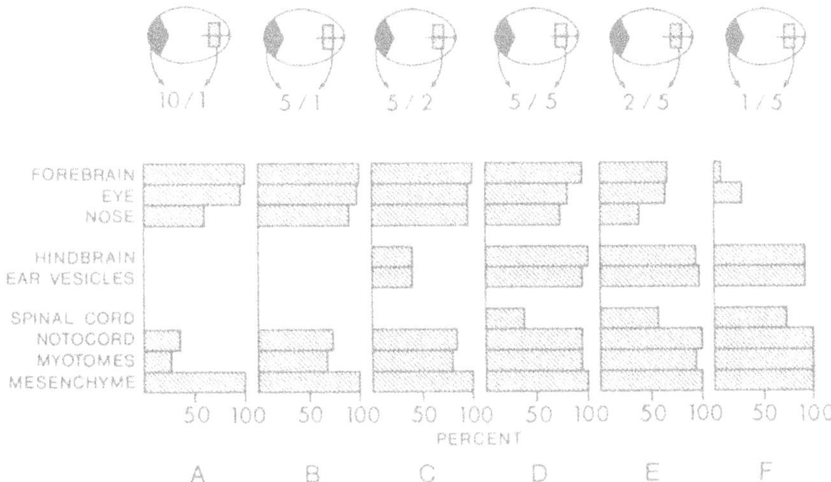

Figure 1.1. Percentages of different structures that developed in reaggregates consisting of different ratios of presumptive neural and mesodermal cells cultivated *in vitro* for 14 days. The diagram shows the ratios of presumptive neural tissue (black) and presumptive mesodermal tissue (stippled) that were explanted in different series of experiments. From S. Toivonen and L. Saxén, *Science 159:*539–540 (1968), copyright 1968 by the American Association for the Advancement of Science.

shifts segregation in the caudal direction." This effect may also be seen by grafting a fold of competent ectoderm onto the presumptive neural ectoderm of the preneurula (Nieuwkoop, 1952). The basal portion of such grafts differentiates into nervous structures like those in the host brain at the point of attachment of the graft, whereas the apical region of the graft always develops into prosencephalic structures.

A variety of physical and chemical agents may induce neural differentiation in competent ectoderm. Holtfreter (1944, 1945) and T. Yamada (1950) found that neural induction is quite unspecific. Isolated pieces of early gastrula ectoderm from *Ambystoma* and *Triturus* differentiate into neural structures when treated with a variety of chemicals or even when subjected to changes in pH or to transient exposure to high concentrations of cations (Barth and Barth, 1969). It is generally believed that these multifarious inductive agents produce their effects indirectly, either by release of the normal inducers by sublethal cytolysis or else by means of the second messenger cyclic AMP. Neural transformation of cultured cells derived from ectoderm of amphibian gastrulae is obtained after treating the explanted cells with cyclic nucleotides (Wahn *et al.,* 1975). These results suggest that the inductor acts via the second messenger cyclic AMP, a hypothesis that has been considered in detail by D. McMahon (1974).

From the time of discovery of the induction phenomena, it has been tacitly implied that liberation of an inducer substance or substances occurs and that the site of origin, rate of diffusion, and stability will determine the "field" of action of the inducer. Holtzer (1968) has suggested that transfer of a specific instructive molecule does not occur during induction but rather that interaction of the tissues produces conditions that permit a particular kind of developmental process. However, in the case of primary neural induction, direct contact of the interactants is not necessary, since embryonic induction occurs when direct contact between the interacting tissues is prevented by a nucleopore filter (Toivonen *et al.,* 1975). Moreover, at the time when neural induction occurs in the chick embryo, at Stage 4 of the Hamburger and Hamilton (1951) series (Waddington, 1952; Abercrombie, 1950; Abercrombie and Bellairs, 1954), the neural ectoderm and chordomesoderm are not in direct contact but are separated by a basement membrane and extracellular matrix about 200–500 Å wide (Bellairs, 1959).

There is some evidence of transfer of materials between the tissues that interact during embryonic induction (C. Grobstein, 1953, 1957, 1959; Lash *et al.,* 1957; Auerbach, 1960; Saxén and Toivonen, 1962; Golosow and Grobstein, 1962; Nyholm *et al.,* 1962; Koch and Grobstein, 1963; Muthukkaruppan, 1966; Koch, 1967; Gallera, 1967; Gallera *et al.,* 1968). Primary embryonic induction in amphibians can occur across a membrane filter (Saxén, 1961; Toivonen *et al.,* 1975); so can neural induction in the chick embryo (Gallera, 1967; Gallera *et al.,* 1968); and so can induction of salivary rudiment or kidney rudiment (C. Grobstein, 1953, 1957). C. Grobstein (1957) found that induction between dorsal spinal cord and metanephrogenic mesenchyme occurs through a millipore filter. The interaction between the tissues is maximal when the filter has an average pore diameter of 0.5 μm or more, but occurs with a reduced range and intensity through a filter with an average pore diameter of 0.1 μm. No interaction occurs through cellophane, but when a small hole is made in it the inductive reaction is localized to the region of the hole. After labeling the dorsal spinal cord with tritiated amino acids, Koch and Grobstein (1963) showed that labeled material of high molecular weight is produced by the spinal cord *in vitro:* this material has the same mobility as the inductor material. Mesenchyme can interact with pancreatic epithelium or with thymus epithelium across a millipore filter (Auerbach, 1950; Golosow and Grobstein, 1962). Spinal cord or notochord can interact across a millipore filter with somites to form cartilage (Lash *et al.,* 1957; G. W. Cooper, 1965; Flower and Grobstein, 1967). Induction through a membrane filter has also been shown in the case of lens induction (Muthukkaruppan, 1966) and induction of tooth rudiments (Koch, 1967).

Whether embryonic morphogenetic tissue interactions in general, and neural inductions in particular, are mediated by direct contact between the interacting cells or by diffusion of materials from one to the other has been a controversial topic for many years but is now being resolved with better techniques. The earlier studies of kidney tubule induction across a millipore filter led to the conclusion that a diffusible substance was involved (C. Grobstein, 1959; Koch and Grobstein, 1963). The first evidence to throw strong doubt on this was provided by Nordling *et al.* (1971), who found that a second millipore filter interposed between the spinal cord and metanephric mesenchyme increases the time for kidney tubule induction by about 12 hours. This is far too long for the increased diffusion time across the additional filter but is consistent with the increased time required for growth of fine cytoplasmic processes across the additional filter. The use of a filter interposed between the interacting tissues had been used since 1961 to study neural induction, but there are limitations in the use of millipore filters for such studies: the millipore filter is an irregular mesh, and it is not possible to completely exclude the possibility that very fine cytoplasmic processes penetrate the filter by a tortuous path that cannot be seen with the electron microscope. Recently a new type of filter has become available with pores passing directly through, and studies using such nucleopore filters have given different results, depending on the tissues that were used. Thus it now seems certain that induction of metanephric kidney tubules through a nucleopore filter requires direct cell contact (Wartiovaara *et al.,* 1974; Saxén *et al.,* 1976). It is known that metanephric tubules can be induced by direct contact with a number of embryonic tissues, including spinal cord and salivary mesenchyme. However, when a nucleopore filter with pore diameter 0.1 μm is interposed, only the spinal cord is effective, whereas either tissue is effective through a filter of 0.6 μm pore diameter. This correlates with the fact that spinal cord is able to send processes through 0.1 μm pores, whereas salivary mesenchyme requires a minimum pore diameter of 0.6 μm. Induction of kidney tubules is never seen when the interposed filter does not permit penetration of cytoplasmic processes between inductor cells and the responding mesenchyme. By contrast, the conclusion that the signal in neural induction is carried by diffusible substances was reached by Toivonen *et al.* (1975). They separated newt gastrula dorsal lip mesoderm from competent surface ectoderm by means of nucleopore filters with pore diameters from 0.1 to 0.8 μm. Neural induction occurred in all cases, although electron microscopic examination did not reveal any cytoplasmic processes in the pores.

The evidence now shows that while intercellular contact is required for induction of kidney tubules in mouse metanephrogenic mesenchyme, the inductive signal can be transmitted by diffusion in primary neural induction in amphibians. Extracellular materials on the cell surfaces between the interacting tissues have been shown to play an important role during induction in mouse salivary gland (C. Grobstein, 1967; Bernfield and Wessells, 1970), while small vesicles in the intercellular matrix appear to convey the inductive signal between mesenchyme and epithelium during induction of the tooth rudiment in the rabbit (Slavkin, 1972).

From this mass of observations it now becomes clearer that **inductive tissue interactions have evolved in several ways in different tissues and in different species. The tissues may interact by direct contact, or the interaction may be mediated by a diffusible agent or even by an agent packaged in vesicles.** In all cases, the essence of the interaction is the transmission of a signal or signals from one tissue and the reception of the signal and its transduction as a change in the other tissue. Inductive interactions are not limited to the embryo but, as discussed in Chapter 8, are also essential for the initial differentiation and stability of the differentiated state of muscle and other tissues that have an obligatory dependence on the nervous system.

1.2. Development of Polarity and Pattern in the Neural Plate and Neural Tube

Polarization is already evident in the neuroepithelial cells of the neural plate. The outer surface of the neuroepithelium is covered by a basement membrane, but the inner surface is not. The cells round up toward the basement membrane during metaphase and extend the full thickness of the epithelium after division while their nuclei undergo the interkinetic migration first described by F. C. Sauer (1935*a,b,* 1936). The changes in shape of the neuroepithelial cells during neurulation are also indicative of their morphological and functional polarity. The basal–apical polarity of the neuroepithelial cells is not altered by reversal of the inner–outer relationships of the neuroepithelium that occurs during neurulation. The outer or basal surface of the neural plate becomes the surface lining the lumen of the neural tube, and the inner surface of the neural plate comes to lie on the outside of the neural tube. This polarization of the cytoplasm of the neuroepithelial cells may be of great importance in the regulation of gene expression by cytoplasmic factors, for, as the nucleus moves away from the basal region of the cytoplasm during telophase, it is subjected to the effects of the apical cytoplasm during interphase and finally returns to the base of the cell in preparation for mitosis. These interkinetic nuclear movements are dealt with in some detail in Section 2.2, but here attention is directed to the possibility that polarization of the cell from base to apex may allow regionally different cytoplasmic factors to enter the nucleus in order to promote differential gene activation (Britten and Davidson, 1969, 1971; Stebbins, 1973). As each region of the neural plate has a different prospective significance, that is, will give rise to different brain regions if left undisturbed, regional specificity of gene activation would seem to be essential, but it is not known how that might be controlled.

One may think of the neural plate as a morphogenetic field of the central nervous system in the sense that it is the smallest unit of tissue that alone can form the entire central nervous system *in situ* or in isolation. This definition can be extended to include the fact that the embryo cannot regulate after removal of an entire morphogenetic field, but removal of parts of the field can be restored by regulation of the residual cells. This capacity for partial regulation becomes progressively restricted topographically within the neural plate, so that, as neurulation advances, separate fields emerge for the eyes, forebrain, midbrain, and hindbrain, and these regional or secondary fields contain elements which are uniquely determined as regards prospective cellular phenotypes. The first such phenotype determination occurs for Mauthner's neurons in the hindbrain and for Rohon-Beard cells in the neural folds, as discussed later in this section and in Section 4.6.

Detailed maps of the prospective brain regions in the neural plate have been made by the vital staining method invented by Vogt (1925). In this method, small regions of the neural plate have been stained with Nile blue sulfate or neutral red, and the stained parts of the nervous system have been identified at later stages of development (Fig. 1.2). Maps have been made in this way of the presumptive eye region (Petersen, 1923; Woerdeman, 1929; Manchot, 1929), of the neural crest (R. C. Baker and Graves, 1939; Fautrez, 1942; Hörstadius, 1950), and of the entire neural plate of amphibian embryos (Nieuwkoop, 1955; C.-O. Jacobson, 1959; von Woellwarth, 1960) as shown in Fig. 1.3. Prospective brain regions in the

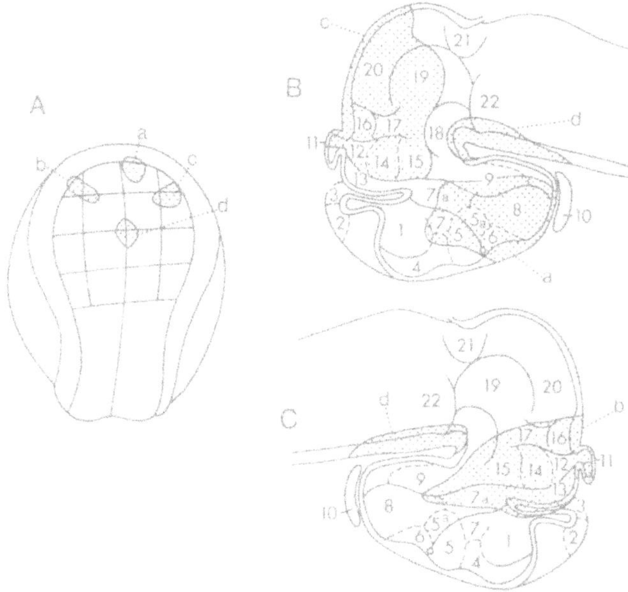

Figure 1.2. Mapping the presumptive brain regions on the neural plate of the axolotl neurula. A: The positions of marks placed on the neural plate which gave rise to the marked regions shown by stipple in the brain of the embryo at Stage 38 as shown in B and C. The following is the key to the numerals indicating the different regions of the brain: 1, area olfactoria primitiva; 2, primordium piriforme; 3, primordium hippocampi; 4, septum (primordium); 4a, septum ependymale; 5, nucleus praeopticus, pars anterior; 5a, nucleus praeopticus, pars posterior; 6, chiasma ridge; 7, area strioamygdaloidea; 7a, cranial parts of pars ventralis thalami; 8, pars ventralis hypothalami; 9, pars dorsalis hypothalami; 10, pars buccalis of the hypophysis; 11, primordium epiphyse; 12, pars intercalaris diencephali; 13, primordium habenulae; 14, pars dorsalis thalami; 15, pars ventralis thalami; 16, commissura posterior (eminentia); 17, commissura posterior (nucleus); 18, tuberculum posterius (pedunculus); 19, tegmentum dorsale; 20, tectum mesencephali; 21, regio cerebellaris; 22, tegmentum isthmi. From C.-O. Jacobson, *J. Embryol. Exp. Morphol.* 7:1–21 (1959).

neural plate of the chick embryo have been mapped by marking cells with carbon particles (Spratt, 1952). The vital staining method has the advantages of leaving the neurula intact and of not interfering seriously with normal development. Its main disadvantage is that it does not give any information about the degree of determination at the time of staining but shows only the potential fate of different regions of the neural plate. The surgical methods of excision and transplantation interfere more or less with normal development but give information about the regulative capacity and the extent to which each region of the neuroepithelium is committed to the formation of specific parts of the nervous system.

Several experimental methods have been used to map the prospective fate of different parts of the neuroepithelium and to discover the time at which its axes of symmetry are fixed. The degree of restitution that is possible after surgical excision of various parts of the neuroepithelium at different stages of development provides clues to the time of determination of the parts that are not reconstituted and to the regulative capacity of the remaining parts (Du Shane, 1938; Aufsess, 1941; Detwiler, 1947; Piatt, 1949; Holtzer, 1951; Stefanelli, 1951; Watterson and Fowler, 1953; Corner, 1963, 1964).

Other investigators have studied the capacity of isolated pieces of neural epithelium to differentiate into parts of the central nervous system when transplanted to other parts of the embryo (Mangold, 1931, 1933; Aufsess, 1941; Ter Horst, 1947; von Woellwarth, 1952; Waechter, 1953; Källén, 1958; Corner, 1964). These studies have shown the remarkable capacity of isolated pieces of the neural plate and neural tube to develop as if they had been left *in situ*. Excised pieces of neural plate or neural tube are replaced by regeneration from the sides or, in the case of unilateral excision, from the intact half and never from the rostral or caudal margin of the wound. Regeneration from the contralateral tissue has been

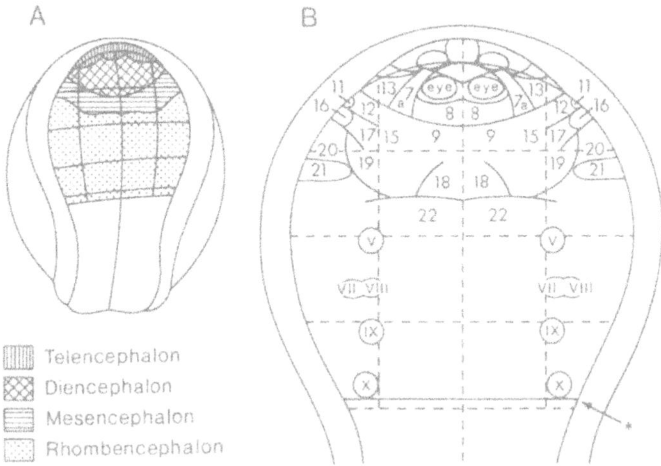

Figure 1.3. Positions of the main presumptive brain regions in the neural plate of the axolotl, mapped by the method of dye marking. The whole neurula is shown in A and the more detailed map on the neural plate in B. The asterisk marks the limit between the presumptive brain and the presumptive spinal cord. The key to the numbers is given in caption of Fig. 1.2. From C.-O. Jacobson, *J. Embryol. Exp. Morphol.* 7:1–21 (1959).

observed after unilateral excision of the neural plate (W. H. Lewis, 1910; Harrison, 1947; Corner, 1963), of the forebrain (Burr, 1916), of the midbrain (Detwiler, 1944; Harrison, 1947), and of the spinal cord (Detwiler, 1947; Holtzer, 1951).

Another strategy has been to excise and transpose pieces of neural plate or neural tube. Reversal of the axes of the graft has given information about the time of axial polarization of the neural epithelium (Spemann, 1906, 1912; Detwiler, 1940, 1943, 1949, 1951; Roach, 1945; Sládeček, 1952, 1955; C.-O. Jacobson, 1964). The time of axial polarization and the regulative capacity of the neural retina have been determined by transplantation and inversion of the eye rudiment (L. S. Stone, 1944, 1948, 1953, 1960; Székely, 1954, 1957; M. Jacobson, 1967, 1968*a*). In summary, these experiments show that axial polarization of the neuroepithelium of the neural plate and optic retina occurs in the anteroposterior and mediolateral (dorsoventral) axes, sequentially and independently in the two axes, within a relatively short period of several hours (see Section 9.7).

The effects of reversing the axes of the neural plate were first tested in amphibians by Spemann (1906, 1912). He excised a large piece of the anterior part of the neural plate with the underlying mesoderm and reimplanted it with its anteroposterior axis reversed. The rotated piece of neuroepithelium develops according to its original position; that is, it is inverted in the rostrocaudal axis. This was confirmed by Roach (1945), who showed that bilateral or unilateral anteroposterior inversion of the neuroepithelium, with or without underlying mesoderm in the preneurula (Stages 13 and 14) of *Ambystoma,* results in anteroposterior inversion of the parts of the nervous system formed from the graft (see Fig. 1.4). This shows that the anteroposterior polarity of the neuroepithelium is already determined in the preneurula. However, different results were obtained by Sládeček (1955). He excised the anterior part of one side of the neural plate in *Ambystoma* neurula (Stages 14–16), rotated the piece 180 degrees, and reimplanted it with anteroposterior and mediolateral axes inverted. Complete regulation occurs in grafts made at Stage 14 and almost complete regulation in grafts made at Stages 15 and 16, resulting in development of a normal brain. Sládeček suggested that this occurs because his grafts are entirely within the neural folds, whereas grafts such as those made by Roach (1945) do not regulate because part of the neural fold is included in the graft. Most likely, the differences are related to the size of the grafts. The tendency of small grafts of rotated neuroepithelium to regulate and larger grafts not to regulate was observed by Alderman (1935), Nicholas (1957), and C.-O. Jacobson (1964).

Inversion of the mediolateral axis only of the anterior part of the neural plate can be achieved by interchanging the left half of the neural plate of one *Ambystoma* embryo with the right half of another (Roach, 1945; Sládeček, 1952), as is shown in Fig. 1.4. In Roach's experiments the grafts were made at Stage 14, and they subsequently developed according to their inverted position; that is, almost complete regulation occurred, resulting in a normal brain. This shows that the mediolateral polarity is not fixed in the neuroepithelium at Stage 14. Sládeček (1952) found that the mediolateral axis is already fixed at Stage 15, since a separate neural tube develops from a piece of neural plate inverted in the mediolateral axis at Stages 15 and 16. That there may be regional differences in the time of polarization of the neuroepithelium is shown by the results of inverting pieces of the presumptive hindbrain. Detwiler (1940, 1943, 1949, 1951) found that almost complete regulation occurs after anteroposterior inversion of the presumptive hindbrain of *Ambystoma* at Stages 19–26, and evidence of failure of regulation is seen only after inversion at Stage 27.

In the experiments described so far, attention is given only to the external morphology of the brain or to the large internal structures of the parts of the brain that develop from the grafts. When the gross morphology of the brain is normal, the graft is considered to have regulated; abnormalities of gross morphology are taken as evidence of determination of various brain structures. More convincing evidence of determination of neural connectivity may be obtained from detailed anatomical studies (Holtzer, 1951; C.-O. Jacobson, 1964), studies of motor function (Székely, 1963; Straznicky, 1963; Straznicky and Székely, 1967) and electrophysiological mapping of connections (M. Jacobson, 1967, 1968*a;* R. Levine and Jacobson, 1974).

Holtzer (1951) found that after unilateral excision of the spinal cord of *Ambystoma* at Stages 18–24 the regeneration that occurs from the intact side is less complete when the excision is made at later rather than earlier stages. The cells that are not reconstituted at later stages are assumed to have been determined at earlier stages. Similar conclusions about the early determination of specific neurons were reached by Stefanelli (1951). He showed that Mauthner's neurons,

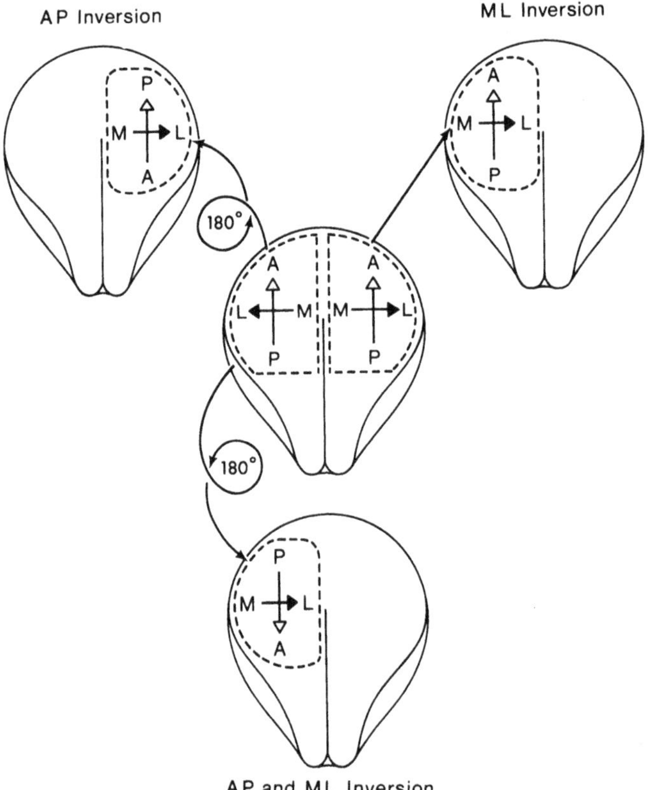

Figure 1.4. Method of producing axial inversion of the neural plate by unilateral grafts of neural ectoderm, either with or without underlying mesoderm, in the early neurula of *Ambystoma.* By this method, Roach (1945) and Sládeček (1952, 1955) showed that the anteroposterior axis of the neural plate is determined before the mediolateral axis.

which differentiate in the medulla, are already determined in the neural plate at Stages 15–16 in *Ambystoma*. If the region of the neural plate containing the prospective Mauthner's cells is excised after Stage 16, Mauthner's neurons fail to develop at later stages. Extirpation of parts of the neural fold has shown that the Rohon-Beard cells, which are the primary sensory neurons of the spinal cord of early larval amphibians, are already determined in the early neurula. Bilateral removal of the neural fold of the prospective trunk region of Stage 13 *Ambystoma* embryos results in absence of Rohon-Beard cells from spinal segments 3–19, whereas from 10 to 20 Rohon-Beard cells normally develop in each spinal segment (Du Shane, 1938).

C.-O. Jacobson (1964) made a detailed histological study of the brain that develops after anteroposterior inversion of the prospective hindbrain region of the neural plate without underlying mesoderm, using *Ambystoma* at Stages 15 and 16. Although the external morphology of the brain at Stages 43–46 appears normal, there are significant deviations from normal histology which indicate that the structures in the graft develop in accordance with their origin. The most obvious abnormality is the development of primary motor nuclei in ectopic positions in reversed order in the rostrocaudal axis of the hindbrain. The motor roots emerge at the level of the nucleus and innervate adjacent muscles nonselectively. For example, eye muscles are innervated by cranial nerve VII, and hyoid muscles by cranial nerve V. This is in agreement with other evidence of nonselective innervation of muscles such as limb muscles innervated by cranial nerves (Braus, 1905; Detwiler, 1930*a,b;* Nicholas, 1933; Hibbard, 1965*b*), the nonselective reinnervation of skeletal muscles after cross union of motor nerves (Sperry, 1948, review), and the innervation of skeletal muscle by implanted foreign motor nerves (Aitken, 1950; H. Hoffman, 1951*b*). C.-O. Jacobson (1964) also reported that the sensory roots enter the rotated hindbrain nonselectively at the points of emergence of the motor roots. However, their central fibers form apparently normal longitudinal fiber tracts in the medulla regardless of the abnormal positions of entry of sensory roots. This was assumed to be the result of selective affinity between the sensory nerve fibers. The central connections of sensory nerves in the rotated hindbrain were not studied. It would be of great value to determine whether sensory nerves grow into inverted hindbrain to form connections congruent with their peripheral sense organs, as they appear to do after inversion of their peripheral sensory fields (Weiss, 1942; Kollros, 1943*b;* Sperry and Miner, 1949; Miner, 1956; Eccles *et al.*, 1962*b;* M. Jacobson and Baker, 1968, 1969; R. E. Baker and M. Jacobson, 1970). Evidence of the polarizing influences of the graft on the course of cranial nerve VIII was obtained by C.-O. Jacobson (1964). In five of eight cases in which nerve VIII entered the inverted medulla, the course of the ascending and descending branches of nerve VIII was appropriate to the polarity of the graft; in one case both normal and repolarized branching occurred, and in two cases the branches grew according to their original polarity and contrary to that of the graft. In general, it appears that the motor neurons must already have developed stable position-dependent properties before the surgical inversion of the hindbrain anlage, and that these properties, or locus specificities, are later expressed according to the original position of the cells. This precocious determination is apparently characteristic of large neurons with long axons (Type I neurons of M. Jacobson, 1970*a*).

This rule that Type I neurons are programmed at a very early stage is best illustrated by Mauthner's neuron, which comes into existence as a postmitotic cell in the late gastrula stage in amphibians (Stefanelli, 1951). Vargas-Lizardi and Lyser (1974) have shown that the stem cell that gives rise to the Mauthner's neuron in *Xenopus* undergoes its final DNA synthesis in the late gastrula (Stage 12, i.e., 12–14 hours after fertilization). Thus the mitosis that gives rise to the Mauthner's neuron occurs 1–2 hours later, at Stage 13. Stefanelli (1951) showed that extirpation of the medulla before Stage 13 can result in restoration of the missing part, including Mauthner's neuron, while after Stage 13 the Mauthner's neuron is missing, although the medulla may be largely or completely restored. Although the program for differentiation of Mauthner's neuron is initiated at Stage 13, the Mauthner's cell cannot be recognized histologically until Stages 29–30, about 20 hours later.

The polarity of Mauthner's neuron and the course of its axon were studied in inverted hindbrain grafts by C.-O. Jacobson (1964). The polarity of Mauthner's neuron accords with that of the rostrocaudally inverted medulla if the graft includes the presumptive Mauthner's neuron, which lies at the lateral margin of the neural plate. In 25 animals in which Mauthner's axons initially grew toward the head instead of toward the tail, 16 ultimately reached the spinal cord, either by making a hairpin bend within the graft or by following a tortuous course through graft and normal brain. In cases where Mauthner's cell body is not included in the graft and is normally polarized, the majority of cases in which Mauthner's axon runs through the graft follow a course that accords with the inverted polarity of the graft. Although C.-O. Jacobson (1964) reached somewhat different conclusions, I am of the opinion that his results show that the initial direction of outgrowth of Mauthner's axon is determined by the polarity of the cell body, but that the subsequent direction of axonal growth is highly influenced by the polarity of the medium through which the axon grows. A discussion of whether the controlling factors are mechanical, chemical, or electrical, or a combination of several factors, appears in Chapter 4. This interpretation is in agreement with conclusions reached by Stefanelli (1951) and Hibbard (1965*a*) from their observations of the growth adjustments of Mauthner's nerve fibers, which are discussed more fully in Section 4.6.

1.3. Formation of the Neural Tube

The process of folding of the neural plate to form the neural tube is called *neurulation* (reviewed by Karfunkel, 1974). The margins of the neural plate become raised to form the neural folds, and the midline region of the neural plate is depressed to form the neural groove. The neural folds meet dorsally and fuse, forming a tube first at one point in the region of the future hindbrain, and fusion of the neural folds progresses rostrally and caudally from that point. The lateral ectoderm, which is pulled medially by the process of neurulation, fuses dorsally over the neural tube. The cells at the margin of the neural folds and the lateral ectoderm move into the space between the dorsal part of the neural tube and the overlying ectoderm, where they form the neural crest, which is discussed in Section 1.4.

The cells of the neural epithelium migrate toward the midline of the embryo during formation of the neural plate. This displacement has been shown by observing the movement of groups of cells that had been marked by a supravital stain (Goerttler, 1925; Vogt, 1929; Manchot, 1929; C.-O. Jacobson, 1962). Displacement of cells in the neural plate is not due to differential cell proliferation. Very few mitotic figures are seen in the neural epithelial cells during formation of the neural plate and during neurulation, and Gillette (1944) has shown that the number of cells in the neural plate of *Ambystoma* does not increase significantly during this period. The number of cells increases from 113,000 at Stage 13, just before formation of the neural plate, to 139,000 at Stage 19, after closure of the neural tube. In the chick embryo, there is a higher mitotic index in the neural plate than in the surrounding nonneural ectoderm, and within the neural plate the mitotic index is highest in the part where the neural folds are coming together (Derrick, 1937). The significance of this for the mechanism of neurulation is hard to see, and the mitotic index alone is not a reliable assay of cell proliferation unless the duration of the cycle is also known (see Section 2.3.).

Time-lapse cinematography of the movement of vitally stained cells (C.-O. Jacobson, 1962) or of naturally pigmented cells (Burnside and A. G. Jacobson, 1968) in the neural plate of amphibian embryos has shown (Fig. 1.5) that the cells

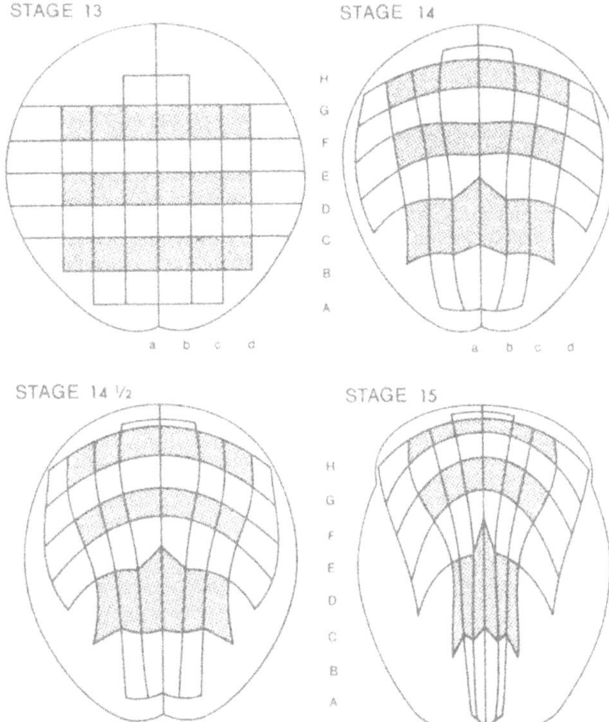

Figure 1.5. Displacement of pigmented cells, observed by time-lapse cinematography, at the intersections of the lines of the grid projected on the neural epithelium of a newt embryo. The transformation of the grid is shown from Stage 13 to Stage 15. Each square at Stage 13 was 0.69 mm^2 in area. From B. Burnside and A. G. Jacobson, *Dev. Biol. 18:*537–552 (1968), copyright Academic Press, Inc.

do not move independently of each other. The neural epithelium moves as a whole, with different parts moving at different speeds. Cells retain their contacts with their neighbors while they are migrating at speeds ranging from 4 to 95 μm per hour for distances up to 896 μm in the neural plate of a 2.5-mm newt embryo (Burnside and A. G. Jacobson, 1968), as shown in Fig. 1.6. Independent movement of cells is not possible because the cells of the neural plate (P. C. Baker and Schroeder, 1967) and neural tube (Duncan, 1957; Bellairs, 1959) are bound together at their apices by intercellular junctions.

Characteristic changes in the shape of the neuroepithelial cells occur during neurulation (Fig. 1.7). The cells of the early neural plate are cuboidal, and they become progressively more elongated and narrower at the apex and ultimately become flask shaped. In the newt (Burnside, 1971, 1973, 1975) and the chick (Karfunkel, 1971, 1972, 1974), the elongation occurs before apical construction of the cells and thus cell elongation precedes the folding of the neural plate to form a tube. The neural plate of urodeles and the chick embryo is a single layer of columnar cells forming a pseudostratified epithelium, whereas that of anurans is already two cells thick before neurulation starts (Schroeder, 1970). This results in a reduction in the area and an increase in the thickness of the neural plate. Burnside and A. G. Jacobson (1968) observed that displacement of cells in the neural plate can be correlated with changes in the area of regions of the neural plate, which in turn are inversely correlated with changes in thickness of the neural epithelium. They concluded that migration of cells is due to regional differences in the change of shape of the cells composing the neural plate and not due to free migration of cells to their proper sites (Figs. 1.5 and 1.6). The cause of these regional differences is unknown.

Closure of the neural tube has been shown to occur as the result of changes in the shape of the cells of the neural plate. Formation of the neural tube does not depend on external forces, since the neural plate, or parts of it, isolated or transplanted to the belly of another embryo can close to form a neural tube (Boerema, 1929; Holtfreter, 1939; Aufsess, 1941). Wilhelm His anticipated mod-

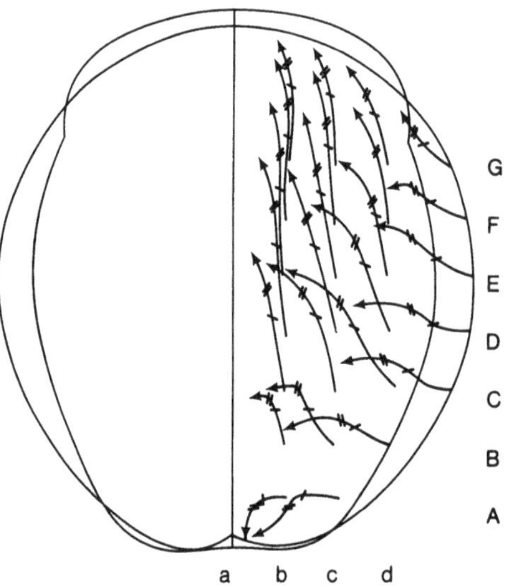

Figure 1.6. Trajectories of cells displaced in the neural plate of the newt followed with time-lapse cinematography. The cells were at the origin of the arrows at embryonic Stage 13; had reached the position of the single transverse bar at Stage 14; were at the position of the double transverse bar at Stage 14½; and had arrived at the points of the arrows at Stage 15. Meanwhile, the embryo had changed its shape from the wider outline at Stage 13 to the narrower outline at Stage 15. From B. Burnside and A. G. Jacobson, *Dev. Biol. 18*:537–552 (1968), copyright Academic Press, Inc.

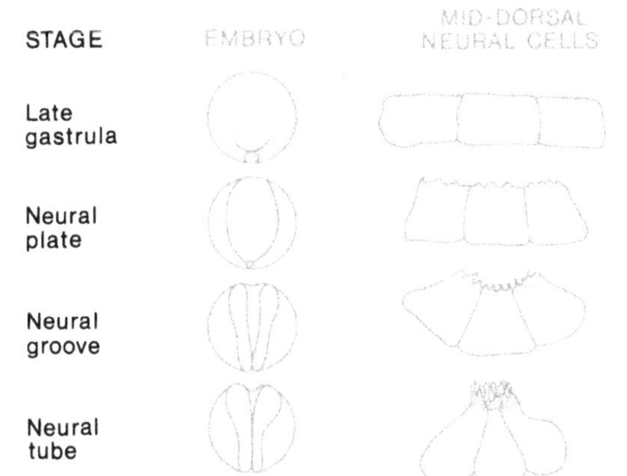

Figure 1.7. Correlation between the apical contraction of the neural plate cells and the formation of the neural tube in the frog embryo. From P. C. Baker and T. E. Schroeder, *Dev. Biol. 15*:432–450 (1967), copyright Academic Press, Inc.

ern conceptions of neural plate folding when he wrote in 1894: "Suppose we have a sheet of cells, the elements of which are as wide at their bases as they are at the free surface. If now, as a result of internal forces, the cells are all induced to become thicker at their bases and thinner at their free ends, the result will be that the sheet bends and folds together to form a hollow structure."

It is now safe to conclude that changes in shape of neural epithelial cells during neurulation are due to intracellular microtubules which produce cell elongation and to intracellular microfilaments which produce apical constriction of the neuroectodermal cells. The first direct evidence implicating microtubules in the mechanism of neurulation came from Waddington and Perry (1966), who noticed that vertically oriented microtubules are present in the neural fold cells of the newt and inferred that elongation of the cells might be due to elongation of microtubules. This has been confirmed in the newt (Burnside, 1971) and also supported by the finding of microtubules oriented in the long axis of the neural fold cells in the chick (Karfunkel, 1972) and in *Xenopus* (Schroeder, 1970; Karfunkel, 1971). Additional confirmation has come from observing the effects of alkaloids that disrupt microtubules. Thus treatment of the *Xenopus* neurula with vinblastine sulfate results in inhibition of neurulation and in rounding up of neural epithelial cells that have already elongated (Karfunkel, 1971). The same result is observed in the neural epithelial cells of the chick embryo after treatment with colchicine (Karfunkel, 1972). By counting the number of microtubules at different cross-sectional levels in neuroectodermal cells of the newt, Burnside (1971) observed no changes in the number of microtubules at different levels that would be predicted if the microtubules produced cell elongation by sliding past one another. Therefore, Burnside suggested that the microtubules produce cell elongation by displacing cytoplasm toward the base of the cell.

P. C. Baker and Schroeder (1967) have shown that during the closure of the neural tube in *Xenopus* embryos the neuroepithelial cells become narrower at their apices and that the deformation of the cells is accompanied by the appearance of microfilaments oriented parallel to the outer surface in the apical cytoplasm of the cells (Fig. 1.7). They suggested that the changes in cell shape are due to shortening of microfilaments, and supported their suggestion by citing evidence of the presence of microfilaments in ameboid cells, where they have been assumed to play a role in cell locomotion (Wohlfarth-Bottermann, 1964, review). The role of microfilaments in changes of cell shape and in cell locomotion is discussed in Section 4.2. It has been suggested (Linville and Shepard, 1972) that anencephaly and meningomyelocele, two of the most common severe congenital defects in humans, may be due to a substance, possibly dietary, that inhibits the action of microfilaments. This suggestion seems reasonable in view of the finding by Linville and Shepard (1972) that neural tube closure in chick embryos is inhibited by cytochalasin B, a substance known to inhibit a large number of cell processes that involve contractile microfilaments (Wessells *et al.*, 1971*a,b*).

It is to be expected that changes in cell shape may play a role in morphogenetic cell movements in the nervous system—for example, in the formation of the optic vesicle and otic vesicle. However, migration of cells, differential cellular proliferation, and differential cell death are other factors of importance in the morphogenesis of the nervous system. Of course, from the time of outgrowth of axons and dendrites from the neurons, changes in the shapes of the nerve cells become of the greatest importance.

1.4. Ontogenesis of Neural Crest Derivatives

During closure of the neural tube, which is described in Section 1.3, some cells at the margins of the neural plate separate dorsally from the neural tube to form the neural crest. Cells migrate from the neural crest to populate the entire embryo, and the challenging questions posed by the neural crest are how the crest cells are set apart, in the first instance, from neural plate and from lateral ectoderm, what determines their migration routes and sites of distribution, and what are the factors that determine the cytodifferentiation of specific cellular phenotypes stemming from neural crest precursors (Holmdahl, 1928; Raven, 1936; Hörstadius, 1950; Weston, 1970, review).

Various experimental methods have been used to study the migration and fate of neural crest cells. They are, first, ablation of the crest or neural folds, second, grafting crest to other sites or explantation into culture systems, and, third, grafting marked crest cells from one level to another in the neural axis. Others have grafted parts of the neural crest to abnormal sites and have studied the tissues that originated from the grafts (L. S. Stone, 1929; Du Shane, 1935; Dorris, 1939; Koeke, 1960). Some of the difficulties with this strategy are that the residual crest may regulate or regenerate, thus replacing the ablated region, or that the ablation might have been done after the migration of some crest cells had occurred. This technique has the disadvantages that it may not show *all* the derivatives of the crest: specific tissue interactions required for differentiation of some or all crest derivatives may not be possible in the graft site or *in vitro.* Vital staining of neural crest cells has also been used to trace the fate of the cells (Detwiler, 1937*a;* Yntema, 1943). Another strategy for marking the neural crest cells has been to graft to an unlabeled host the neural crest from a chick embryo labeled with tritiated thymidine. The labeled cells can subsequently be identified by means of autoradiography (Weston, 1963; Weston and Butler, 1966; Johnston, 1966; Chibon, 1967).

The use of a natural cell marker which is stable and can be seen in all the cells that originate from a transplant has great advantages over an artificially introduced marker such as [^{3}H]thymidine, which becomes diluted as a result of cell division. Raven (1937) grafted neural crest between two species of amphibians with different sizes of nuclei (xenoplastic grafting) and was able to identify the cells that originated from the graft. More recently, some very elegant studies have been done by reciprocal grafting of neural tube and crest between quail and chick. The grafts can be exchanged between different levels of the neural axis (heterotopic grafting) or between different stages of development (heterochronic grafting), and the types of cells derived from the grafts, their migration routes, and their final positions can be determined (Le Douarin and Teillet, 1973, 1974). Identification of the cells derived from chick or quail grafts is possible because of characteristic differences between the interphase nuclei stained with the Feulgen technique: the nucleolar heterochromatin is dispersed in the chick but forms large clumps in the quail (Le Douarin, 1973).

These studies have shown that a variety of cell types distributed throughout the animal are derived from the neural crest. The cranial neural crest gives rise to the visceral skeleton, odontoblasts, the carotid body and catecholamine-containing cells of the carotid artery, part of the trigeminal ganglion (the other part is derived from cranial placodes), facial ganglion, glossopharyngeal and vagus ganglia, enteric ganglia of the entire digestive tract, ciliary ganglion, Schwann cells, melanocytes, and the leptomeninges of the diencephalon and telencephalon. The leptomeninges (pia-arachnoid) are entirely derived from neural crest, while the dura mater is of mesodermal origin (Harvey and Burr, 1926; Harvey *et al.*, 1933). Thus, if the telencephalic region of the neural tube is transplanted to another part of the body in larval *Ambystoma,* the transplanted brain develops without pia-arachnoid, while the leptomeninges develop with the brain if neural crest is transplanted with neural tube. The origin of the trigeminal, facial, glossopharyngeal, and vagus ganglia from the cranial neural crest is well established, but the origin of the acoustic ganglion is uncertain. Much evidence shows it to be derived entirely from the otic placode (Halley, 1955; Batten, 1958), but there is other evidence that the part of the acoustic ganglion innervating the cochlea and saccule originates from the cranial neural crest in mice (Deol, 1967, 1970). The trunk neural crest gives rise to the spinal sensory ganglia, the primary and secondary sympathetic ganglia, chromaffin cells of the adrenal medulla, enteric ganglia of the postumbilical intestinal tract, Schwann cells, and melanocytes. In this book, only the neural derivatives of the neural crest will be discussed.

Because of the diversity of cell types and the wide distribution of neural crest derivatives, the neural crest is an excellent system in which to study differential cell migration. The mechanisms involved in the release of cells from the neural crest are unknown. Perhaps some kind of contact inhibition (Abercrombie and Heaysman, 1954) or differential changes in adhesiveness (Steinberg, 1964) may play a part in releasing cells from the neural crest. Differential distribution of neural crest cells could, *a priori,* occur as a result of one of the following:

1. Random migration and selective trapping of cells.
2. Random release of cells followed by selective migration.
3. Sequential origin and programmed release of cells destined for different locations.

The first possibility is that neural crest cells originate and are released at random but are trapped selectively in favorable environments. Although crest cells are not disseminated by the vascular route, the experiments dealing with the fate of intravenously injected cells are tangentially relevant to the problem of trapping of cells in various tissues. The results of experiments by Weiss and Andres (1952) and G. Andres (1953) suggest that melanoblasts settle preferentially in specific locations. Cell suspensions containing melanoblasts were prepared from early chick embryos of a pigmented breed and were injected intravenously into 3- to 5-day chick embryos of a nonpigmented breed. In about 8 percent of the cases the recipient embryos developed patches of pigment in sites that were normally pigmented in the donors. The interpretation of this result was that injected melanoblasts tend to settle preferentially in "a location that offers the appropriate specific conditions and associations for a cell of that particular type" (Weiss and Andres, 1952). However, the frequency of occurrence of pigmented patches was not high enough to exclude the alternative possibility that melanoblasts might have been trapped at random and not selectively. Similar experiments by Burdick (1968) gave negative results. He injected dissociated cells—from mesonephros, limb, or heart of 5¼-day check embryos labeled with tritiated thymidine—intravenously into unlabeled hosts of the same age. The injected cells were traced by autoradiography in tissues of the hosts killed 6 and 24 hours after receiving the injection of labeled cells. No evidence of selective lodging of cells was obtained: "The distribution of cells among the three organs was found to be almost identical for the three types of cells" (Burdick, 1968). Essentially the same conclusion, that intravenously injected cells as well as polystyrene particles are trapped nonselectively in different organs, was reached by Hollyfield and Adler (1970).

The possibility that the neural crest cells originate at random but are guided selectively to their appropriate destinations has been tested by Weston (1963). He grafted a segment of neural crest from a chick embryo labeled with tritiated thymidine in place of a segment of neural crest in an unlabeled host of the same age. Labeled neural crest cells could be seen migrating in two streams, one leaving the neural tube dorsolaterally and the other ventrally. These streams of cells entered the host's superficial ectoderm and the mesenchyme between the neural tube and somites. The same two streams migrated from a graft that was dorsoventrally inverted, but the migrating cells entered different tissues of the host. This shows that the initial direction of migration is determined by factors within the neural crest and is not in response to a chemical gradient or other cues in the host's tissues through which the cells migrate.

Weston and Butler (1966) tested the third alternative, that localization of neural crest cells is determined by the temporal order of their release from the neural crest. Radioactive neural crest cells from old chick embryos were grafted in place of neural crest of unlabeled young embryos. All the normal neural crest derivatives developed from the old grafts. This shows that they had retained their full developmental capacity even though a large percentage of neural crest cells had migrated from the graft before it was transplanted. This rules out the possibility that neural crest cells of different types are dispatched in a programmed sequence to different locations. Weston and Butler (1966) also tested the hypothesis that a sequence of changes in the host's tissues exert a selective action on neural crest cells. They grafted radioactive neural crest cells from young chick embryos to progressively older, unlabeled hosts. The result was an increasing failure of formation of sympathetic ganglia, and of spinal ganglia to a lesser extent, in progressively older hosts. This might mean that, with increasing developmental age, some changes occur in the host tissues that restrict migration and localization of neural crest cells. This result is not conclusive because, as the investigators realized, the same result might be due to saturation of the host's tissues with neural crest cells that migrate before the grafts are made. The inadequacy of the evidence does not yet permit an analysis of the factors that control the production, release, migration, and settling down of neural crest cells. We have a plethora of descriptions of stages in the development of structures derived from the neural crest, but we have only a rudimentary understanding of the cellular mechanisms, for example, that play a role in the morphogenesis of the sensory ganglia and autonomic nervous system.

That the spinal sensory ganglia originate solely from the neural crest is shown by their absence after adequate extirpation of the neural crest at an early stage of development (Harrison, 1924*a;* Detwiler, 1937*a*). Detwiler (1934, 1937*a*) concluded that the neurons of the sensory ganglia form compact aggregates under the influence of the somites (Fig. 1.8). Removing somites results in loss of the corresponding ganglia, whereas additional ganglia develop in juxtaposition to supernumerary somites. Weston (1963) also showed an enhanced rate and duration of migration of neural crest cells in somite mesenchyme and an attenuation of migration between the somites. The factors that result in segmental aggregation of

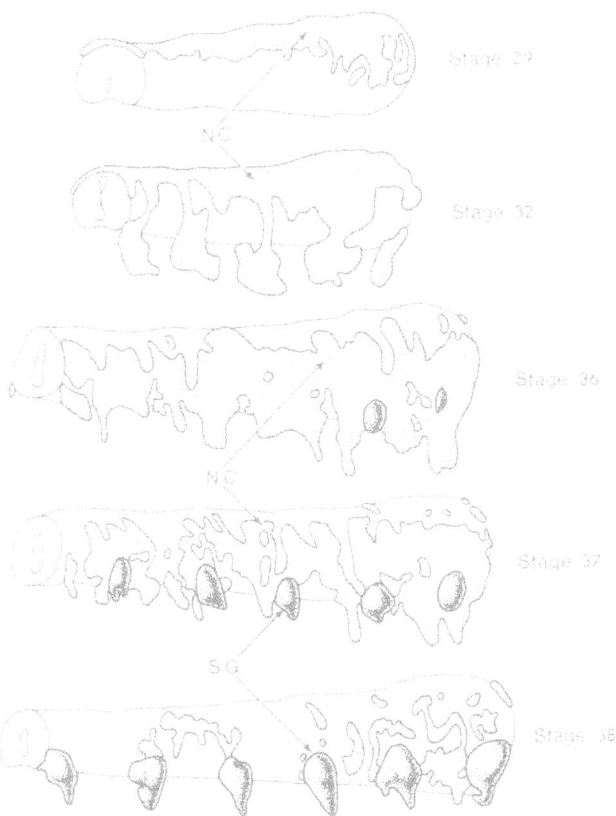

Figure 1.8. Reconstructions of the spinal cord of *Ambystoma* at different embryonic stages to show the migrating neural crest (NC) and the development of the spinal ganglia (SG). 75×. From S. R. Detwiler, *Am. J. Anat. 61*:63–94 (1937*a*).

cells to form spinal ganglia, as is shown in Fig. 1.8, are poorly understood. Further development of the spinal ganglia of the chick embryo is described in Chapter 7 in connection with the effects on the ganglion of changing the size of its peripheral sensory innervation zone.

The postganglionic neurons of the autonomic nervous system are derived from cells that have migrated out of the neural crest (W. His, Jr., 1897; Van Campenhout, 1930*b*, 1931; Detwiler, 1937*a;* Detwiler and Kehoe, 1939; E. Müller and Ingvar, 1923; Yntema and Hammond, 1947; Nawar, 1956). The sympathetic neurons migrate from the neural crest to form a primary sympathetic chain along the dorsolateral surface of the aorta. Many of the sympathetic neurons reach their prevertebral positions considerably before the aggregation of neurons to form the spinal ganglia (Detwiler, 1937*a*). Some neurons of the primary sympathetic chain persist as the prevertebral sympathetic ganglia, but the majority migrate laterally, using the segmental branches of the aorta as routes of migration, to form the secondary chain of paravertebral sympathetic ganglia (Tello, 1925; Van Campenhout, 1931). Van Campenhout (1930*b,* 1931) showed that the neurons in the walls of the thoracic and abdominal viscera migrate into the viscera from the neural crest and do not differentiate from mesodermal or endodermal cells. The history of the debate as to whether any neurons of the autonomic nervous system differentiate locally from mesodermal or endodermal cells or whether they are all derived from the neural crest has been reviewed by Yntema and Hammond (1947). They concluded that a neural crest origin for all autonomic neurons is most probable. The glia (satellite cells) of the spinal and sympathetic ganglia are probably entirely derived from the neural crest, although there may be some that originate from the neural tube (Brizzee, 1949).

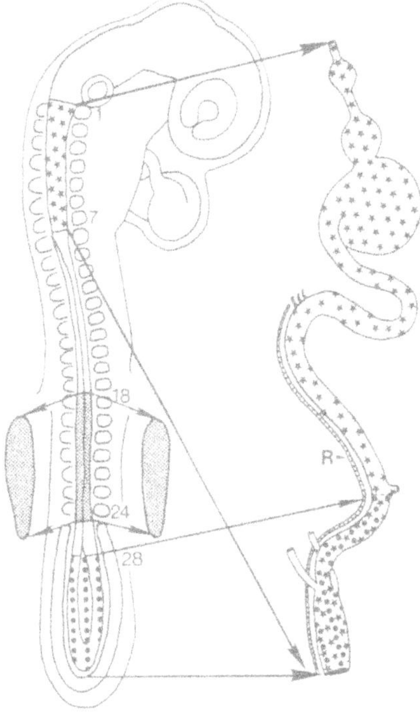

Figure 1.9. Anterior and posterior levels of the embryonic neural axis from which the enteric ganglion cells originate as demonstrated by isotopic and isochronic transplantations of quail neural tube into chick embryo (Le Douarin and Teillet, 1973). The neurons arising from the anterior level (between the levels of somites 1 and 7) colonize the whole gut. Those which come from the posterior level located behind somite 28 contribute only to the formation of the ganglia of the postumbilical gut. The neural crest of the cervical and dorsal region (from 8 to 28 somites) does not participate in the formation of enteric ganglia but gives rise to adrenergic orthosympathetic neurons and to adrenomedullary cells which come from the precise level of somites 18–24. R, nerve of Remak originating from the lumbosacral level of the neural axis (behind somite 28). From N. M. Le Douarin and M.-A. M. Teillet, *Dev. Biol. 41:*162–184 (1974).

The origin of the intramural ganglion cells has finally been analyzed by using the technique of transplanting quail neural tube into chick, and this method of analysis has also helped solve the problems of the prospective potency of neural crest cells, the selectivity of their migration routes, and the factors involved in control of their differentiation. Le Douarin and Teillet (1973) showed that the ganglion cells in the intestinal wall in the plexuses of Auerbach and Meissner arise from two different levels of the neural crest. In the chick embryo, ganglion cells for the entire length of the digestive tract are derived from neural crest of the caudal rhombencephalon at the level of somites 1–7, while lumbosacral neural crest caudal to somite 28 gives rise to some enteric ganglion cells of the intestine below the umbilicus and is the main source of neurons of the ganglion of Remak (see Fig. 1.9.). These two sources of origin thus correspond to the vagal and lumbosacral divisions of the parasympathetic nervous system, while the sympathetic ganglia develop from an entirely different region of trunk neural crest at the level of somites 8–28. The chromaffin cells of the adrenal medulla originate only from neural crest at somites 8–24.

There is thus a regional origin of different derivatives of the neural crest, and the question arises whether the neural crest cells from each region are fully or partially determined or whether cells from one level retain the potency to differentiate into the cell types normally originating from other levels. The various alternatives are, first, that the different cell types are determined before they migrate out of the neural crest, although they may only differentiate later; second, that the cells are pluripotent and that determination of cell type occurs only in response to conditions along the route of migration and/or at the terminal site. This question has been answered by grafting quail neural tube to a different level of the neural axis in chick embryos (Le Douarin and Teillet, 1974). In all cases the neural crest cells migrated along the usual route from the graft to the appropriate tissues, showing that there are constraints on the route of migration which lead the cells to the proper terminal sites at each level. On the other hand, the neural crest cells differentiated according to the sites in which they settled, regardless of their origin, showing that the cells are pluripotent, that they are not fully determined at the beginning of their migration, and that their terminal differentiation is controlled by local factors along the route and at the end of their migration. Only the nonneural mesenchymal derivatives of the cephalic neural crest are determined early as they differentiate into connective tissue regardless of their final location.

The importance of conditions along the route of migration is shown by the work of A. M. Cohen (1972) and Norr (1973). The differentiation of sympathetic neurons containing norepinephrine depends on an inductive action of the somitic mesenchyme on the neural crest cells during their migration (A. M. Cohen, 1972). The somitic mesenchyme has this inductive action only if it has previously been in contact with ventral neural tube and notochord (Norr, 1973). When neural crest cells are obtained and cultured clonally before any contact with somitic mesenchyme has occurred, only melanocytes but no neural cells differentiate (A. M. Cohen and Konigsberg, 1975).

2

The Germinal Cell and Histogenesis of the Nervous System

2.1. Introduction

One of the most enduring concepts of developmental neurobiology is that of the *germinal cells* situated in well-defined *germinal zones* located in characteristic places in the developing nervous system. Identification of these specialized cells, from which all neurons originate, was made almost a century ago, and hundreds of publications have appeared dealing with their identification and location and with many aspects of their proliferation. Nevertheless, we still do not know how the different types of neurons and glia are generated from the apparently homogeneous population of germinal cells, and how their proliferation is controlled so as to produce the correct numbers of different cells in each part of the nervous system.

From about 1870 an increasing number of observations were published on the histology of the developing nervous system. As the result of great improvements in histological techniques, these observations were reliable and relatively free of artifacts in comparison to older observations. There was a consensus, founded on confidence in the new histological methods, that mitotic figures are confined to the layer of cells lining the lumen of the neural epithelium during the early stages of development (see Ramón y Cajal, 1901–1911, Vol. l, p. 590, for references).However, even at that early time, an exception to the rule was reported by Rauber (1886*a,b*), who observed extraventricular mitotic figures in the neural tube of the frog embryo; this was confirmed by McKeehan (1966). This may be a peculiarity of the amphibians, since in the neural tube of the early chick embryo and mammalian embryo, mitotic figures occur only in the cells lining the lumen. Wilhelm His (1887, 1888*a,b,* 1889, 1890*a,b*) proposed that these mitotically active cells are the germinal cells (Keimzellen) that give rise to all neurons; in contrast, the remaining cells, which he could not identify as neurons, were termed "spongioblasts," and he suggested that they give rise to glia. His, and many others after him, believed that the spongioblasts form a syncytium, called the "neurospongium."

In every epoch, histologists have overestimated the reliability of their methods. At present we observe the same confidence—which can persist only as a result of a lack of hindsight—that structures are so well preserved in histological preparations that they show neither more nor less than in the living tissue. The neurospongium, that fictitious tissue composed of spongioblasts (the presumed precursors of neuroglia), provides an interesting example. It took later generations of histologists to appreciate that the neural epithelium appeared to be a syncytium because the tissue was poorly preserved by the histological methods available to His and his contemporaries. With the advent of electron microscopy it became clear that the cells of the neural epithelium are separated by intercellular clefts, although the width of the clefts and the amount of extracellular space are still controversial topics (Van Harreveld, 1972). However, the syncytial theory held a grain of truth, albeit for the wrong reasons. There are restricted intercellular junctions which may serve as channels for transfer of materials and as a means of communication between embryonic cells, including the cells of the neural tube. Indeed, the intercellular pathways for ionic current flow have been demonstrated most often in embryonic tissues that are actively proliferating, including the germinal cells of the neural tube (Warner, 1970, 1973). Intercellular flow of ions and molecules up to about 1000 daltons has been demonstrated by injection of a recognizable substance into one cell and observation of its spread to neighboring cells, and by measurement of a low electrical resistance between the cells, as shown in Fig. 2.1 (D. D. Potter *et al.*, 1966; J. D. Sheridan, 1966, 1968, 1973; Loewenstein, 1968*a,b,* 1970, 1973, 1975). Such low-resistance pathways may also indicate that the cells are coupled in a way which allows intercellular flow of signals that are significant for cell differentiation (see comments on cell interactions in Section 7.1).

The dogmatists, both for and against the syncytial theory, were wrong, but for some it remained an open question whether neurons that are merely in contact might not also have direct intercellular connections, especially at some stages of their development. Even the supreme exponent of the neuron doctrine—which states that the nervous system is composed of discrete nerve cells, in close contiguity at synapses but never or rarely in cytoplasmic continuity—was willing to admit that "Perhaps technology will in time discover some staining procedure capable of revealing new and more intimate connections between neurons which we suppose to be in contact. One cannot reject *a priori* the possibility that the tangled forest of the brain, of which we imagine we have discovered the last leaves and branches, may still possess some bewildering system of filaments binding together the neuronal mass as lianas bind the trees of tropical forests" (Ramón y Cajal, Nobel Prize Lecture, 12 December 1906).

According to His (1887, 1888*a,b,* 1889), the germinal cell divides repeatedly: one daughter cell remains close to the lumen of the neural tube and reenters the mitotic cycle, while the other daughter cell becomes a neuroblast. Then the neuroblast, which is incapable of further division, migrates away from the germinal layer and eventually develops into a neuron. Only the latter part of His's theory has been upheld by subsequent research. In the past few years, the advent of radioactive isotope techniques has made it possible, by means of autoradiography, to show that neuroblasts do not incorporate [^{3}H]thymidine, which indicates that they have ceased DNA synthesis and mitosis (Fujita, 1962, 1963, 1965*a*). Since the suffix "blast," derived from the Greek word for a germ or a bud, indicates that the cell is capable of mitosis, it would be better to refer to the neuroblast as a young or immature neuron, and henceforth in this book it is referred to as a *young neuron* or simply as a *neuron*.

Another theory of neuronal and glial histogenesis, in almost total disagreement with the theory of His, was proposed by Schaper (1897*a,b*). Both His and Schaper based their theories on the same histological observations, but they

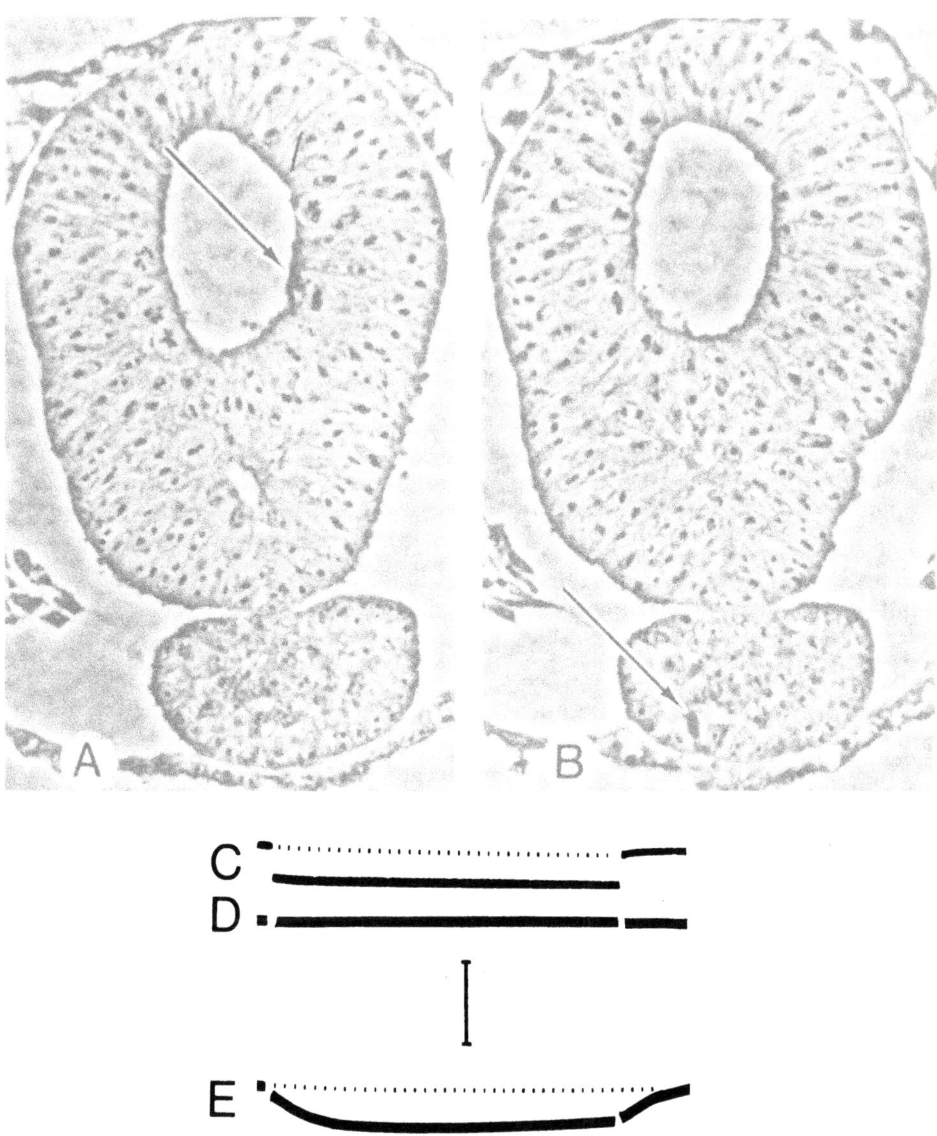

Figure 2.1. Transverse sections through the neural tube of a 16-somite chick embryo (A, B). The arrows indicate the marks made by release of a small quantity of dye from the tip of the microelectrodes used to record the electrical potentials shown below. In A the arrow points to the position of the microelectrode tip in the neural tube, and in B the arrow points to the position of the tip of the microelelectrode in the notochord. Both microelectrodes were inside cells, as is shown by the electrical records C, D, and E. Current pulse in the neural tube cell (2×10^{-8} amp for 0.98 sec) shown in C produced electrotonic potential change (E) in the notochord cell, but no potential change just outside the notochord cell, as is shown in record D. Voltage calibration for D and E, 20 mV. From J. D. Sheridan, *J. Cell Biol.* *37*:650–659 (1968).

interpreted them in different ways. The observation that mitotic figures occur only in the cells lining the lumen of the early neural tube had been interpreted by His to mean that the mitotic figures belong to germinal cells (Keimzellen), while the other cell nuclei of the neural tube belong to different classes of cells, one of which is the neuroblast, while others are spongioblasts which give rise to neuroglia. Schaper recognized that there was an alternative interpretation of the histological picture. He suggested that "the so-called 'Keimzellen' of His lying near the central cavity of the neural tube, along the membrana limitans interna, are not to be considered as a special type of cell in contrast to the main epithelial cells in process of continuous proliferation" (Schaper, 1897*b*). According to Schaper, the so-called germinal cells and spongioblasts are really cells of the same type which move to different levels in the neural tube during different phases of the mitotic cycle. The "Keimzellen" of His are therefore the neuroepithelial cells during metaphase that have moved closer to the lumen of the neural tube.

Schaper also showed that the young neuron, with large clear, oval nucleus and abundant cytoplasm, could be distinguished from the glial precursors. Some of the glial precursors have a small, round, densely chromatic nucleus and very scanty cytoplasm, but others may have different appearances (see Section 2.6). We would now call these cells *glioblasts.* Schaper showed that the young neurons and glioblasts migrate away from the lumen and form the mantle layer outside the germinal zone. Some of the cells in the mantle layer undergo mitosis. According to Schaper (1897*a,* p. 100), these are "indifferent cells," which he thought are capable of differentiating either into neurons or into neuroglia. Schaper's scheme has been supported by the evidence accumulated since his time, except as regards to "indifferent cells." Such indifferent cells have not been identified histologically. However, this does not rule out their existence, because the "indifference" or multipotentiality refers to their developmental potential and not necessarily to any aspect of their morphology. The possibility that there are multipotential glial cells, capable of giving rise to different types of neuroglia depending on circumstances, has again been mooted by Vaughn and Peters (1968, 1971) as discussed in Section 2.6.

All types of neurons as well as glia are generally presumed to arise from a common stem cell, which has been termed the *germinal cell* (His, 1889), *ependymal cell* (Schaper, 1897*a,b*), *primitive ependymal cell* (Sidman *et al.*, 1959), and *matrix cell* (S. Fujita, 1963). In this discussion the common precursor cell will be called the *neuroepithelial germinal cell,* or simply *germinal cell,* since that term has priority and adequately describes the cell. This does not mean that the concept of germinal-cell totipotency can be accepted uncritically. In the neural plate the germinal cells already form a mosaic of cells with different prospective fates, as the experimental transplantation and extirpation of pieces of neural plate have shown (C.-O. Jacobson, 1959, 1964; Corner, 1963, 1964). Thus fragments of neural plate, composed entirely of neuroepithelial germinal cells, when cultured *in vitro* or when transplanted to other parts of amphibian embryos, develop into nervous tissue containing types of nerve cells that would normally have developed from the part of the neural plate from which each explant was derived.

One of the questions that has not yet been answered is whether and how the germinal cells at any particular position are programmed to produce specific types of nerve cells. It is not known when differential gene expression occurs in the germinal cells, which is thought to result in divergent differentiation of the various types of neurons on the one hand and various types of neuroglia on the other.

The origins of the glial cells and the mechanisms that control their differentiation are unsolved problems that will be discussed in Section 2.6. Evidence of programmed production of different types of neurons by the germinal cells and of progressive restriction of their developmental potential has been found in the retina. The evidence comes from experiments reported by Hicks and his collaborators on the repair of radiation damage to the retina (Hicks *et al.*, 1959, 1961; Hicks and D'Amato, 1963, 1966). After exposure to X-rays, many cells in the developing retina are destroyed, and the survivors roll up into tubes or vesicles called *rosettes.* As development progresses, the neuroepithelial germinal cells in the rosettes show a reduction in their potential to produce different retinal cells. Exposure of the retina to X-rays before day 15 of gestation in the rat fetus results in extensive destruction of cells, but the surviving germinal cells produce all types of retinal cells, resulting in the development of a small but otherwise normal retina (Rugh and Wolff, 1955*a,b;* Hicks *et al.*, 1959). The germinal cells that survive after irradiation between days 15 and 19 are able to produce ganglion cells, amacrine cells, bipolar cells, horizontal cells, and photoreceptors, but after irradiation on day 23 just before birth they generate only photoreceptors and some horizontal cells and bipolar cells. By the time the rat is 4 or 5 days old, the retinal germinal cells can make only photoreceptors. These results indicate that the retinal germinal cells undergo a progressive restriction in their capacity to give rise to different types of retinal cells.

From this digression on the subject of the developmental potential of the germinal cells, we return to the historical sketch of the theories of neurogenesis and find that the great authority of Ramón y Cajal was cast in favor of the theory of His and in opposition to that of Schaper. The misconception that nerve cells originate from a separate class of stem cells located at the lumen of the neural tube persisted until 1935, and even after the accumulation of much evidence to the contrary the old theory survived in textbooks for another 20 years, thus supporting Goethe's comment that "phrases oft repeated finally ossify to conviction and utterly dull the organs of intuitive perception" (*On the Intermaxillary Bone,* Jena, 1786).

Schaper's theory was consigned to obscurity until new evidence in its favor was adduced by F. C. Sauer (1935*a,b*). He confirmed that the neural epithelium, until the time of closure of the neural tube, consists of a single type of epithelial cell in various stages of the mitotic cycle. In addition, Sauer showed that the appearance of the cell changes and its nucleus moves to different positions in the cytoplasm during the different phases of the mitotic cycle. The "Keimzellen" of His are merely cells that have rounded up close to the lumen in preparation for mitosis, after which the nuclei of the daughter cells move away from the lumen during interphase and return inward during prophase.

2.2. Neuroepithelial Germinal Cells during the Mitotic Cycle

F. C. Sauer (1935*a,b*, 1936, 1937) correlated the size and histological appearance of nuclei with their distance from the lumen of the neural plate and neural tube of pig and chick embryos. He showed that the cells are separate, each bounded by a distinct plasma membrane, and that they do not form a syncytium, as was widely believed at that time. Sauer observed that the cells of the neural epithelium are columnar, extend from the inner to the outer surface of the neural tube, and are joined to each other by terminal bars at the lumen. These observations have since been confirmed by electron microscopy (Duncan, 1957; Bellairs, 1959; Tennyson and Pappas, 1962; Brightman and Palay, 1963, H. Fujita and Fujita, 1963; E. Robbins and Gonatas, 1964*a;* S. Fujita, 1966; Wechsler, 1967; P. C. Baker and Schroeder, 1967; Fisher and M. Jacobson, 1970; Hinds and Ruffett, 1971).

During the early stages of development of the neural tube, metaphase nuclei occur only close to the lumen or ventricle, whereas nuclei of different sizes and staining characteristics are seen at all levels between the ventricle and outer surface of the neural tube (Fig. 2.2). Sauer identified telophase and early interphase nuclei as the smaller nuclei that form a series, gradually becoming larger and more basophilic as they are situated at increasing distances from the ventricle of the neural tube. He concluded that these nuclei are moving away from the ventricle following mitosis (Fig. 2.2). The late interphase and prophase nuclei form a series leading to mitosis as they approach the lumen. They are intensely basophilic and ovoid, with the sharper end pointing toward the lumen, and have 6–9 times the volume of the early postmitotic nuclei. Interphase is very short or nonexistent in rapidly dividing cells—the synthesis of chromosomal DNA recommences immediately after telophase. During interphase and prophase the neuroepithelium germinal cells are attached to the internal and external limiting membranes. During metaphase the cells lose their external attachment and round up toward the ventricle of the neural tube where cell division occurs.

The orientation of the mitotic spindle may be important, not only in determining whether a daughter cell is released or remains attached to the luminal

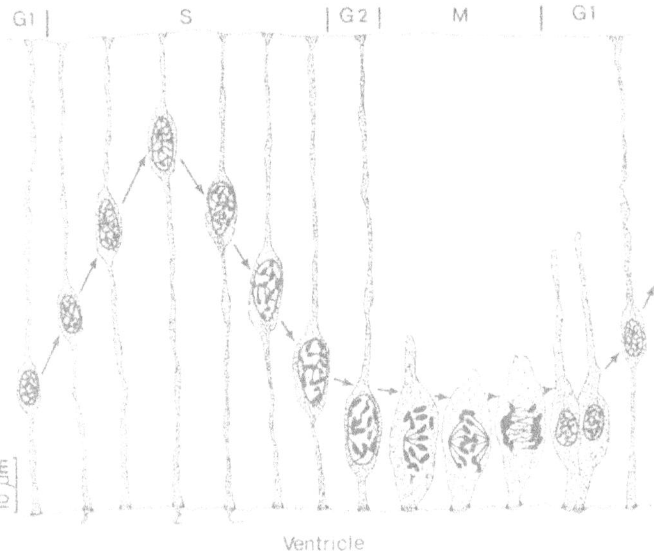

Figure 2.2. Section of neural tube of the chick embryo showing the intermitotic migration of the nucleus of a single neuroepithelial germinal cell at approximately half-hour intervals throughout the mitotic cycle. Adapted from F. C. Sauer, *J. Comp. Neurol. 62:*377–405 (1935).

surface of the neural tube but probably also in determining the spatial arrangement of cells. A simple case is seen in the division of Schwann cells, which normally occurs with the axis of the mitotic spindle transverse to the long axis of the nerve (see Section 4.14). According to F. C. Sauer (1935*a,b*), during mitosis in the neural plate and tube the spindle axis is always tangential and the plane of cleavage is always radial so that the daughter cells lie side by side and retain their basal attachment at the lumen of the neural tube and both cells reenter the mitotic cycle. In the neural plate and early neural tube the daughter cells reenter the mitotic cycle, but at later stages of development an increasing number of dividing neuroepithelial germinal cells are seen with the plane of cleavage tangential, so that one daughter cell loses its basal attachment and does not reenter the mitotic cycle but migrates into the mantle layer (A. H. Martin and Langman, 1965; A. H. Martin, 1967). In the ganglionic eminences of the newborn mouse, over 90 percent of mitotic figures near the lateral ventricle cleave at right angles to the ventricular wall, whereas the plane of cleavage is random in mitotic figures in the subventricular zone of the lateral ventrical (Smart, 1976).

The phenomena just described raise many unanswered questions about the mechanism of the to-and-fro movement of the nucleus and about the functions of such movement. Interkinetic nuclear migration is not peculiar to neuroepithelial germinal cells but is seen in a wide variety of embryonic tissues that are in the form of a pseudostratified epithelium (F. C. Sauer, 1936, 1937; Zwaan *et al.*, 1969). It seems likely that movement of the nucleus might allow regionally different cytoplasmic factors to enter the nucleus to promote differential gene activity.

The changes in cell shape that occur during the cell cycle are probably due to contractile microfilaments whose presence has been correlated with cell movements in many different types of cells (Wohlfarth-Bottermann, 1964; P. C. Baker and Schroeder, 1967; Schroeder, 1969; Wessells *et al.*, 1971*a,b*). The involvement of microfilaments in interkinetic nuclear migration is suggested by the observation that cytochalasin B, a drug that is believed to inhibit the action of intracellular microfilaments, totally inhibits interkinetic nuclear migration in the neural tube of chick embryos (P. E. Messier and Auclair, 1974).

It is not known how the duration of the cell cycle and the rate of proliferation of germinal cells are controlled. Sauer (1935*b*) pointed out that as the wall of the neural tube thickens during development, the distance the nuclei may have to travel is increased. This may be a cause of the progressive increase in intermitotic time that occurs during development (Table 2.1) if it is assumed that the rate of nuclear migration remains the same throughout development. The rate of nuclear migration in the neural tube of the 11-day mouse embryo is about 10 μm per hour (Atlas and Bond, 1965). How this compares with rates in other stages in the mouse or in other species is unknown. F. C. Sauer says that the movement of the nucleus away from the lumen occupies most of the intermitotic period and is much slower than the return movement in the premitotic period. According to Sauer (1935*b*), the volume of the nucleus doubles on the outward journey (from 98.7 to 127.5 μm^3 in pig; from 46 to 80 μm^3 in chick) and doubles again on the inward journey (from 157.5 to 280 μm^3 in pig; from 90 to 135 μm^3 in chick). Subsequent work has confirmed that nuclear size is related to nuclear DNA content (Szarski, 1976, review).

Additional evidence of intermitotic nuclear migration in the neural tube was obtained by Watterson *et al.* (1956), who used colchicine to inhibit mitosis in the

Table 2.1. Cell Cycle of Neuroepithelial Germinal Cells (hours)

Tissue	Species	Age	Cycle time	S	G_2	M	G_1	Reference
Neural tube	Chick	E1	5	—	—	—	—	Fujita (1962)
	Mouse	E10	8.5	4.6	0.6	1.3	2	Kauffman (1968)
	Mouse	E11	10.5	5.4	1.2	1.3	2.7	same
	Mouse	E11	11	5.5	1	1	3.5	Atlas and Bond (1965)
Telencephalon	Mouse	E10	7	5.1	1	0.8	0.1	Hoshino *et al.* (1973)
	Mouse	E13	15.5	6.9	1	0.8	6.8	same
	Mouse	E17	26	10.4	1	0.8	13.8	same
Cerebral cortex	Mouse	E15	11	7.5	2	2	—	Langman and Welch (1967)
	Rat	E12	11	6–8	2	—	3.7	Waechter and Jaensch (1972)
	Rat	E18	19	6–8	2	—	11.2	same
Cerebral sub-ependymal zone	Rat	E18	19	6–7	—	—	10	same
	Rat	P1	18.3	10	3.7	—	3.1	same
	Rat	P6	17.2	10.8	2.5	—	2.5	same
	Rat	P21	20.1	12.4	2.1	—	5.2	Lewis and Lai (1974)
			—	9.4	3	—	—	Korr *et al.* (1973)
Neural retina	Chick	E6	10	—	—	—	—	Fujita (1962)
	Mouse	P2	28	12.5	1.5	0.8	13	Denham (1967)
Optic tectum	Chick	E3	8	4	1.5	0.3	2.2	Wilson (1973, 1974)
	Chick	E4	9	5	1.5	0.4	2.1	same
	Chick	E5	13	4	1.5	0.8	6.7	same
	Chick	E6	15	5	1.5	1.4	7.1	same
	Mouse	E10	8.5	5	1	1	1.5	Wilson (1974)
	Mouse	E11	11	6	0.9	1.2	2.9	same
Rhombic lip	Rat	E14	12	—	—	—	—	Ellenberger *et al.* (1969)
Cerebellum ext.	Mouse	P1–10	21.5	7	2	0.6	11.9	Fujita *et al.* (1966)
Granule cells	Mouse	P7–14	24	—	5	—	—	Miale and Sidman (1961)
	Mouse	P2–10	18	8.3	2	—	7.8	Mareš *et al.* (1970)

chick neural tube. Three hours after the chick embryo has been treated with colchicine, several layers of cells arrested in metaphase are seen close to the lumen of the neural tube. An increasing number of cells are affected until, after about 7½ hours of colchicine treatment, almost all cells of the neural tube are arrested in metaphase. These observations of the effect of colchicine have been confirmed by Källén (1961, 1962), and by Langman *et al.* (1966), who used vincristine sulfate to inhibit mitosis. These experiments show that cells at all levels in the neural epithelium, and not just the cells close to the lumen, can undergo mitosis. It is assumed that colchicine blocks only cell division and that nuclear migration is unaffected, so that the nuclei are unable to reach the lumen because their migration is obstructed by layers of cells arrested in metaphase.

Intermitotic migration of the nuclei of neuroepithelial germinal cells has also been confirmed independently by two other methods: by cytophotometric measurements of the DNA content of nuclei at different depths in the neural epithelium (M. E. Sauer and Chittenden, 1959) and by observation of the position of labeled nuclei in the neural epithelium at progressively longer intervals after administration of a pulse of [^{3}H]thymidine (M. E. Sauer and Walker, 1959; Sidman *et al.*, 1959; S. Fujita, 1962, 1963, 1965*a,* 1966; Atlas and Bond, 1965; A. H. Martin and Langman, 1965).

The amount of DNA in nuclei at various levels in the neural epithelium should provide a crucial test of whether nuclear migration occurs, since the DNA content of the telophase and early interphase nucleus is constant and characteristic of the species (Vendrely and Vendrely, 1956, review), and the DNA content of the nucleus is doubled during cell division before visible prophase (Alfert, 1950; Swift, 1950). M. E. Sauer and Chittenden (1959) cytophotometrically measured the DNA content of the nuclei of the neural tube in the chick embryo neural tube stained for DNA by the Feulgen method (Feulgen and Rossenbeck, 1924; Hale, 1966; also see Section 3.4.2). They showed that the DNA content of the nuclei is approximately proportional to their size (M. E. Sauer and Chittenden, 1959; Meek and Harbison, 1967). This is consistent with other observations showing that nuclear volume is a fairly reliable index of DNA content (Szarski, 1976, review), although some exceptions have been recorded (Billings and Swartz, 1969; C. J. Herman and Lapham, 1969). In the early neural tube the small nuclei close to the lumen contain more than the diploid value of DNA. This shows that the postmitotic gap (G_1) is very short, and DNA synthesis starts soon after mitosis while the nucleus is beginning its outward migration. Visible prophases are seen in the inner third of the neural epithelium, and the prophase nuclei contain the tetraploid amount of DNA, showing that they are in the postsynthetic (G_2) phase of the cell cycle. Therefore, while DNA replication is initiated during the outward migration of the nucleus, it continues during the movement of the nucleus toward the lumen (Fig. 2.2).

Additional evidence that DNA synthesis occurs mainly in nuclei in the outer half of the neural tube comes from the results of [^{3}H]thymidine autoradiography. One hour after a single injection of tritiated thymidine, labeled nuclei appear only in the external half of the germinal cell layer of the cerebral vesicle of the 11-day mouse fetus (Sidman *et al.*, 1959), indicating that this is the site of DNA synthesis. A single injection of [^{3}H]thymidine is available for DNA synthesis for less than 1 hour in mammals, and only a single generation of cells takes up the label. These labeled nuclei migrate at approximately the same rate and divide synchronously

(Sidman *et al.*, 1959; Atlas and Bond, 1965). Six hours after the injection, the labeled cells have arrived at the inner half of the germinal layer and numerous mitotic figures are labeled. Some of the labeled daughter nuclei migrate out into the mantle layer by 48 hours after the label has been given, and these cells remain labeled for their lifetime. Most labeled nuclei repeat the cycle of migration and mitosis in the germinal layer. With each cell division the radioactivity per daughter cell is halved. Similar results have been obtained after [^{3}H]thymidine labeling of the nuclei of the neural groove, neural tube, and spinal cord of the chick embryo (S. Fujita, 1962, 1963; H. Fujita and Fujita, 1964, Martin and Langman, 1965). One hour after a single injection of [^{3}H]thymidine, only nuclei in the outer half of the wall of the neural groove are labeled. Three hours later, labeled nuclei are seen mainly in the inner half of the wall, but 10 hours after injection of the label they have returned to the outer half of the wall (A. H. Martin and Langman, 1965), and the density of labeling is reduced to half that at the beginning. This shows that, within 13 hours, the labeled nuclei move from the outer to the inner margin of the neural tube, complete mitosis, and return to the outer half of the neural tube.

The rate of cell production is a function of the duration of the cell cycle and of the number of germinal cells. The duration of the cell cycle lengthens approximately linearly (S. L. Kauffman, 1968; Hoshino *et al.*, 1973) as development progresses (Fib. 2.3). The number of germinal cells first increases, then reaches a steady state, and finally declines as histogenesis ceases. Cumulative labeling experiments, in which repeated injections are given to make the [^{3}H]thymidine continuously available for DNA synthesis, show that during the early phases of neurogenesis all the daughter cells reenter the mitotic cycle and thus the number of germinal cells increases. This period of logarithmic increase in the number of germinal cells is followed by a period in which only one postmitotic daughter cell is produced at each division of a germinal cell, so that the population of germinal cells remains constant while the population of postmitotic cells increases arithmetically. Such a linear increase in the number of neurons, apparently as the result of asymmetrical mitosis of a constant number of germinal cells, is seen in the retina of the frog tadpole (Jacobson, 1975*b*, 1976*a*). Finally, some germinal cells enter their

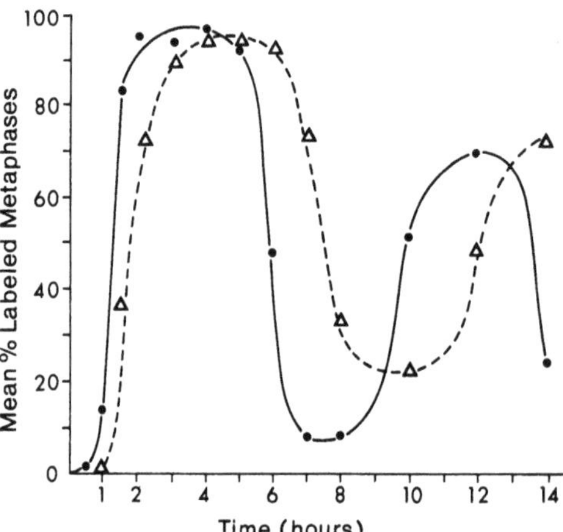

Figure 2.3. Comparison of the generation cycle of neuroepithelial germinal cells in the mouse fetus at 10 days of gestation (solid line) and 11 days of gestation (broken line). The mean percentage of labeled mitotic figures in the neural tube at different times after an injection of tritiated thymidine (1 μCi/g) to pregnant mice. From S. L. Kauffman, *Exp. Cell Res.* *49:*420–424 (1968), copyright Academic Press, Inc.

terminal cell cycle and produce two postmitotic cells. The rate of cell production gradually declines as the cell cycle increases in length and as germinal cells withdraw from the mitotic cycle.

2.3. Kinetics of the Cell Cycle of Neuroepithelial Germinal Cells

In a proliferating cell population such as the neuroepithelial germinal cells, the cells pass through a cycle of DNA synthesis and mitosis. The mitotic cycle has several phases—M, G_1, S, and G_2—as defined by A. Howard and Pelc (1953). They showed that S, the period of DNA synthesis (which can be recognized by observing the incorporation of tritiated thymidine into DNA), is separated from mitosis by a period of several hours, which is called G_2; the period between the end of mitosis and the beginning of DNA synthesis is called G_1. During mitosis (M phase), the maternal cell divides into two daughter cells, each with the diploid ($2n$) quantity of DNA. The duration of the M phase is usually 40–70 minutes. Jelínek (1959) has shown that the M phase becomes progressively more prolonged during development of the chick embryo neural tube. At 3 days of incubation (E3), the M phase is 0.7 hour; at 4 days, 1.1 hours; and at 6 days, 2.5 hours. A similar increase in the duration of the M phase has been found in the chick optic tectum, the M phase increasing from 0.3 hour at E3 to 1.4 hours at E6 (D. B. Wilson, 1973, 1974). In the telencephalon of the mouse embryo, the duration of the M phase is constant at 0.8 hour from E10 to E17 (Hoshino *et al.*, 1973).

Following mitosis the cell enters the G_1 phase or postmitotic gap. Different cell populations show a wide range in the duration of G_1. It may be entirely absent in very rapidly proliferating cells, or it may last for hours, for days, or for the duration of the animal's life. There is a progressive increase in the duration of G_1 during development, and the gradual slowing of the cell cycle is largely due to lengthening of G_1 with each successive cycle. For example, in the telencephalon of the mouse, G_1 increases from 0.1 hour at E10 to 13.8 hours at E17 (Hoshino *et al.*, 1973). Most types of neurons are permanently arrested in the G_1 phase and are therefore diploid.

After mitosis the daughter cells may remain in the G_1 phase and commence cytodifferentiation, or one or both daughter cells may start DNA synthesis. In the early neural tube stages all the cells probably reenter the mitotic cycle; the cycle is short, G_1 is very short, and DNA synthesis starts immediately after mitosis during the initial stage of outward migration of the nucleus. The period of DNA synthesis is termed the S phase, which usually lasts for 6–8 hours and occupies about half of the total cell cycle in rapidly dividing cells. The rate of DNA synthesis is approximately constant during the S phase. Replication of the chromosomal DNA occurs during this time. DNA synthesis is usually completed before the onset of morphological prophase (Fig. 2.2).

The S phase is followed by a premitotic gap, or G_2 phase, which has a duration from 1 to 4 hours in various types of cells. The cell may be permanently arrested in the G_2 phase and retain the tetraploid amount of DNA. This occurs in some types of neurons. As a rule, the cell passes from G_2 into the M phase.

In neuroepithelial germinal cells, as well as glioblasts, the duration of mitosis is very short when compared with the duration of the cell cycle. This is reflected in the paucity of metaphase figures seen at all stages of development of the nervous system. Usually the total fraction of mitotic figures seen in histological preparations of the developing neural tube does not exceed 2–5 percent. One method of determining the duration of the cell cycle is to count the proportions of labeled and unlabeled mitotic figures in autoradiographs made after administration of [^{3}H]thymidine. However, this method is subject to large counting errors and to random variations in the distribution of mitoses because, in a rapidly proliferating population of cells, small changes in the duration of mitosis or in the intermitotic period may result in relatively large changes in the percentage of mitotic figures (Hughes, 1952; Saetersdal, 1958). Counts of mitotic figures should be interpreted very critically, regardless of the way in which they are expressed. The methods of expressing mitotic activity are briefly as follows:

1. The average number of mitotic figures per section (Hamburger and Keefe, 1944; Hamburger, 1948)
2. The number of mitotic figures per 100 cells capable of mitosis, i.e., the mitotic rate or mitotic index (Coghill, 1924, 1933; Derrick, 1937; Fujita, 1964, 1967)
3. The average number of mitoses per unit area, i.e. the mitotic density (Hamburger, 1948)

These expressions of mitotic activity are of very limited value unless the duration of the phases of the mitotic cycle is also taken into account, which seldom is the case. For example, the condition termed "neural overgrowth," which can be induced experimentally in chick embryos and which has been likened to neoplasia (Källén, 1962), is not due to increased proliferation, as was once thought; rather, the increased number of mitotic figures is due to lengthening of the M phase of the cell cycle (D. B. Wilson, 1972, 1974). The progressive lengthening of the duration of mitosis and particularly of the intermitotic period that generally occurs during development (Table 2.1) should always be taken into account when comparisons are made between mitotic activity measured at different stages of development.

Two main experimental methods have been used to study cell population kinetics in the developing nervous system and other tissues. In one method, colchicine (or another drug such as vinblastine, vincristine, or mitomycin C) is used to inhibit mitosis (Deysson, 1968, review); in the other method, tritiated thymidine is used to label the DNA; or both methods may be used in combination. Direct measurement of the time between mitoses may be obtained by the use of time-lapse cinephotomicrography, but this is applicable only to cells in tissue culture.

Both the colchicine and thymidine methods of studying cell population dynamics have shortcomings which ought to be widely appreciated. Colchicine inhibits mitosis by binding to tubulin, the subunit of the microtubules of the mitotic spindle, and so preventing their assembly (E. Robbins and Gonatas, 1964*b;* Borisy and Taylor, 1967*b*). Colchicine has no effect on the rates of synthesis of DNA, RNA, or protein (E. W. Taylor, 1965; J. O. Karlsson *et al.*, 1971), or on the duration of G_1, S, or G_2 phase (Puck and Steffen, 1963). The minimal effective dose of colchicine that inhibits all mitoses is close to the toxic dose.

Insufficient colchicine does not inhibit all the mitoses, but higher doses may be fatal and therefore the effective dose has to be determined by trial and error for every species. Colchicine also binds with high affinity to the tubulin of other types of cytoplasmic microtubules—for example, to neurotubules (Borisy and Taylor, 1967*a;* Wisniewski and Terry, 1968; Wisniewski *et al.*, 1968). Colchicine inhibits the elongation of axons and blocks the proximodistal transport of proteins in the axon (see Section 4.8.4). The half-life of the colchicine–tubulin complex is 36 hours (Garland and Teller, 1973), and so the recovery from colchicine is slowed. Colcemid has a similar but more rapidly reversible effect on mitosis (Kleinfeld and Sisken, 1966). When administered in the correct dose, colchicine or colcemid arrests the cells in metaphase. The rate of proliferation can be obtained from the rate of increase of metaphase cells (Fig. 2.4).

Other drugs that block mitosis are more liable than colchicine to produce irreversible damage (L. Wilson *et al.*, 1974). Thus the vinca alkaloids, vinblastine sulfate and vincristine sulfate, bind to microfilaments as well as to microtubules, and also inhibit protein synthesis when given in doses sufficient to block mitosis (Creasey, 1968). The vinca alkaloids also have the disadvantage that they are insoluble in water. Mitomycin C, which is water soluble, inhibits mitosis by cross-linking the chromatids within the chromosomes. A dose of 20–40 μg/ml has been found to be effective in blocking mitosis (Kiehlman, 1966).

Other drugs have been used to inhibit cell proliferation in the developing nervous system. 5-Fluorodeoxyuridine (FUdR or FdUR) is not incorporated into DNA but stops mitosis by inhibiting thymidylate synthetase, resulting in a deficiency of thymidylic acid. DNA synthesis stops when thymidylic acid is no longer available, and this occurs rapidly within hours of administration of FUdR. At low doses (10^{-8}–10^{-6} M for 1–4 hours) this is the only action of FUdR, and recovery

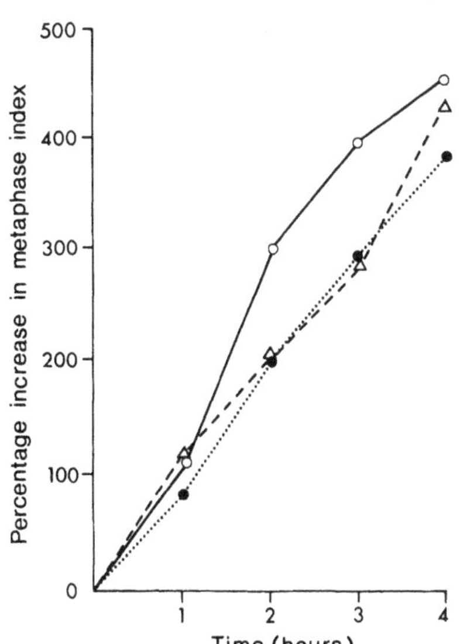

Figure 2.4. Percentage increases in metaphases in the retina of the newborn rat after administration of colcemid at 2 days after birth. Results of three experiments are shown. The average duration of mitosis was approximately 1 hr. From S. Denham, *J. Embryol. Exp. Morphol. 18:*53–66 (1967).

can occur. The inhibitory effect of FUdR on mitosis can be reversed by thymidine in concentrations 100 time higher than that of FUdR. At high doses FUdR results in chromosome breakage and cell death.

Cytotoxic agents which have a specific effect on cultured nonneuronal cells may not show the same effect on neurons or on neuronal stem cells *in vivo*. This is strikingly demonstrated by the drug 5-bromodeoxyuridine (BUdR, BrdU, or BrUdR), an analogue of thymidine, which is incorporated into DNA instead of thymidine in cells that are engaged in DNA synthesis (Wilt and Anderson, 1972, reveiw). BrdU is effective only if it is available during the S phase, and its effects may be prevented or reversed by equimolar concentrations of thymidine. BrdU has been reported to have little or no effect on cell viability or growth of mammalian or chick cells *in vitro*. However, the drug may cause chromosome breakage (Hsu and Somer, 1961) and may inhibit cell differentiation in chondrocytes *in vitro* (Abbott and Holtzer, 1968; Lasher and Cahn, 1969) and in myoblasts *in vitro* (Holtzer, 1972, review). Whether it can prevent or delay nerve cell differentiation remains to be shown. There is good evidence that retinal ganglion cell precursor cells terminate their DNA synthesis shortly before differentiation of retinal ganglion cells occurs in the *Xenopus* embryo (M. Jacobson, 1968*b*) and chick embryo (Kahn, 1973, 1974), and in Mauthner's neuron of *Xenopus* (Vargas-Lizardi and Lyser, 1974). Therefore, it seemed that the neural retina and Mauthner's neuron might be promising systems in which to use BrdU to inhibit cell differentiation without affecting cell viability. Initial reports suggested that it might be possible to achieve such a "chemical dissection" of the program of differentiation of retinal ganglion cells in *Xenopus* (Bergey *et al.*, 1973; R. K. Hunt *et al.*, 1977). In a more extensive study of the effects of BrdU injected in *Xenopus* embryos at different stages from 9 to 27, at different doses ranging from ineffective to lethal, we found that at maximum doses that permit further development the drug has little or no effect on the differentiation of Mauthner's neuron, and that it has a predominantly cytotoxic effect on the neural retina proportional to the dose, at all doses (Dribin and Jacobson, 1978). We were unable to see a specific effect on nerve cell differentiation *in vivo*. Because of the difficulty of interpreting the effects of the drug on nerve cell differentiation in the presence of cytotoxic effects resulting in cell death, BrdU cannot be expected to provide a clear-cut method of analyzing the developmental programs of nerve cells.

Tritiated thymidine becomes incorporated specifically into DNA during its synthesis, and, once incorporated, it remains permanently in the DNA. The incorporation of thymidine into DNA proceeds by phosphorylation to its nucleotides: first to thymidine monophosphate, then to thymidine diphosphate, and finally to thymidine triphosphate, which is assembled, with other nucleoside triphosphates, into DNA (Cleaver, 1967). It should be noted that thymidine monophosphate is also synthesized from simple precursors such as aspartic acid. Thus the exogenously administered labeled thymidine is diluted by the endogenous pool of unlabeled thymidine monophosphate. Since the size of the pool cannot be known, it is not possible to calculate rates of DNA synthesis from the time course of incorporation of labeled thymidine. However, the endogenous pool of thymidine can be reduced by inhibiting endogenous synthesis of thymidine monophosphate by means of amethopterin (Siegers *et al.*, 1974).

Because of the low energy of β-particles emitted from tritium, an autoradiograph may be obtained with a resolution of 0.2–0.3 μm using light microscopy (Salpeter *et al.*, 1974). By combining autoradiography with electron microscopy, a resolution as high as 600 Å may be achieved (Salpeter *et al.*, 1969; Stevens, 1966) so that it is possible not only to identify the cell that has incorporated the [^{3}H]thymidine into its DNA but also to localize the site of DNA synthesis to the chromosomes, nucleolus, or mitochondria. Spurious results may be obtained as a result of the breakdown of [^{3}H]thymidine (for example, due to self-radiolysis) and the incorporation of the radioactive breakdown products into macromolecules other than DNA (Wand *et al.*, 1967).

The danger of radiation damage to the cells after incorporation of [^{3}H]thymidine should be kept in mind (Samuels and Kisielski, 1963; Cleaver *et al.*, 1972). There is less danger of chromosomal damage from [^{14}C]thymidine than from [^{3}H]thymidine because the greater energy of the β-particle emitted from ^{14}C is mainly absorbed outside the nucleus. For example, abnormalities of cell proliferation in the subependymal layer of the rat brain have been observed after the cells had incorporated [^{3}H]thymidine, and were attributed to endogenous irradiation of the cells by radioactive DNA (P. D. Lewis, 1968*a*). An excess of thymidine, whether radioactive or not, can inhibit DNA synthesis (Xeros, 1962; Blenkinsopp, 1967). A dose of 10 μCi/g body weight is usually used in mammals, and doses larger than 20 μCi/g body weight cause radiation damage to various tissues (Cronkite *et al.*, 1962).

Labeled DNA can be detected by autoradiography in the developing nervous system within 5–10 minutes after injecting a single dose of tritiated thymidine directly into the egg or embryo, or injecting intraperitoneally or intravenously into the pregnant mammal. Injection of [^{3}H]thymidine directly into the brain (Altman, 1962*a*) has the advantages of low cost and of localizing the highest uptake of the label to a specific brain region or to the brain rather than other organs. Intracisternal injection of [^{3}H]thymidine directly into the cerebrospinal fluid has very limited application because the nucleotide is unevenly distributed to the brain, with the result that labeling is capricious (Altman, 1963; Altman and Chorover, 1963). Another method, exposure of brain tissue to tritiated thymidine *in vitro,* is the only way in which human brain histogenesis can be studied autoradiographically. In this so-called *supravital labeling,* pieces of freshly excised human fetal brain are exposed to [^{3}H]TdR for 1 hour in a suitable culture medium, then fixed and processed for autoradiography (Rakic and Sidman, 1968, 1970). This method is also applicable to the study of cellular kinetics in excised brain tumors.

After a single injection the thymidine is available for DNA synthesis for only 30–60 minutes and is metabolized and excreted after 2 hours in mammals. Since the duration of labeling is short relative to the S phase, only cells of one generation, which are in the process of DNA synthesis while the [^{3}H]thymidine is available, are labeled. This method is called *pulse labeling.* With each subsequent division, the label is halved, and this is measured by counting the number of silver grains over each cell in the autoradiograph. The labeled DNA is predominantly nuclear because the total quantity of mitochondrial DNA in the cell is only a small fraction of 1 percent of the nuclear DNA (Nass, 1969).

Interspecies differences in the availability of tritiated thymidine may have to be taken into account in planning experiments. For example, the clearance of the label from the plasma is about 10 times more rapid in monkeys than in rats (Nowakowski and Rakic, 1974). In monkeys, a shorter pulse of label can be achieved, but to obtain the same level of labeling, the dose of [^{3}H]TdR has to be greater and the exposure time has to be longer for autoradiographs of monkeys than of rats. As the thymidine is cleared very slowly after injection into the chorioallantois of chick embryos, it is not possible to label the chick embryo with a short pulse. In poikilothermic animals, the rate of DNA synthesis and the duration of the cell cycle are temperature dependent, so it is essential to record the temperature at which the experiments are done (Brugal, 1971).

Thymidine autoradiography provides a relatively easy means of determining the duration of phases of the cell cycle. The time for the average grain count to decrease to half is approximately the generation time. The generation time can also be determined from the percentage of labeled mitoses. The time taken for 100 percent of the mitotic figures to become labeled is approximately the duration of G_2 + M + ½S. The percentage of labeled mitoses stays close to 100 for several hours and then decreases to almost zero. When the generation of labeled cells again enters the cell cycle, a new wave of labeled mitoses appears, each mitotic figure carrying half the label of the maternal cells; then the cycle repeats itself. The generation time can be obtained by measuring the time interval between two identical points (for example, the time at which the percentage of labéled mitoses reaches a maximum on two succeeding waves of labeled mitoses) (Fig. 2.5). The duration of the S phase is approximately the time interval between the midpoints of the ascending and descending limbs of a wave of labeled mitoses. A useful discussion of the percent labeled mitosis curve is given by Shackney (1974).

The duration of the S phase and the generation time may also be obtained by cumulative labeling with [^{3}H]thymidine. In this method, injections of

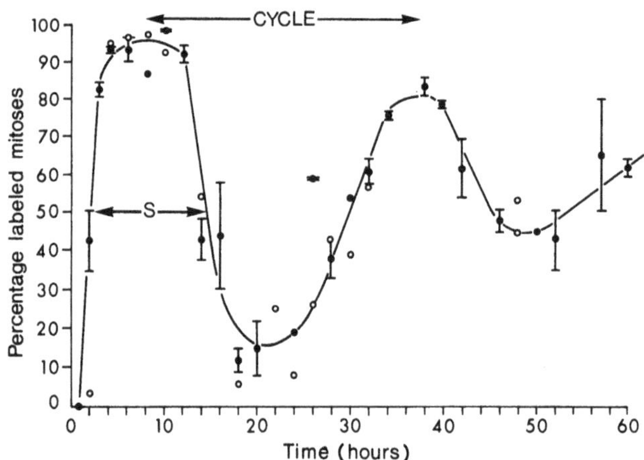

Figure 2.5. Percentage of labeled mitotic figures in the retina of the newborn rat at different times after an injection of tritiated thymidine at 2 days after birth. Circles indicate a dose of 3 μCi/g of body weight, dots a dose of 1 μCi/g body weight. The duration of the cell cycle was 28 hr, and the duration of its phases was S = 12.5 hr, G_2 = 1.5 hr, M = 1 hr, G_1 = 13 hr. From S. Denham, *J. Embryol. Exp. Morphol. 18:*53–66 (1967).

[^{3}H]thymidine are given at frequent intervals in order to make the nucleotide continuously available for DNA synthesis for hours or days. The following pattern of labeling is observed when [^{3}H]thymidine is made available continuously to a population of proliferating cells at random phases of the cycle. The first cells to take up the label are those in the S phase, and therefore the percentage of cells labeled shortly after the injection will equal the percentage duration of the S phase relative to the generation time (G). If S = 50 percent of G, 50 percent of the cells start to incorporate the label immediately after it becomes available. Thereafter, the rate of labeling will be linear until 100 percent of the cells have become labeled in a period approximately equal to $\frac{1}{2}S + G_2 + M + G_1$ (that is, when the cells that have just completed DNA synthesis at the start of labeling have passed through $G_2 + M + G_1$ and entered the S phase). If, instead of counting every cell that is lightly labeled, only heavily labeled cells are counted, a different result is obtained because the cell must complete a considerable part of its DNA synthesis in order to become heavily labeled. The time for 100 percent of the cells to become heavily labeled will be close to the generation time. In practice, an intermediate result is obtained.

Methods have also been devised for determining the durations of all phases of the cell cycle in a single experiment in which colchicine and [^{3}H]thymidine are administered simultaneously at the start of the experiment and then by repeated injections in order to sustain their action for at least the time of the cell cycle. The durations of the phases of the cycle can be calculated from determinations of the percentages of labeled and unlabeled mitoses and interphase cells at progressive intervals after the beginning of the experiment (Puck and Steffen, 1963; Maekawa and Tsuchiya, 1968). In such an experiment the percentage of unlabeled interphase cells decreases linearly, in a time equal to G_1, to a minimum which represents the percentage of nonproliferating cells. The percentage of labeled metaphases increases linearly to a maximum in a time equal to the cell cycle. The percentage of metaphases that remain permanently unlabeled represents the percentage of the total cycle occupied by G_2. The ratio of unlabeled to labeled cells declines to a minimum in a time equal to S. The combination of colchicine and [^{3}H]thymidine probably makes possible the analysis of the cell cycle with a high degree of resolution that is unobtainable by the use of either method alone.

The data available in the literature on the proliferation kinetics of neuron and glia precursors have been assembled in Table 2.1. It can be seen that the evidence is as yet too fragmentary to show clearly whether there are consistent changes in the mean durations of the phases of the cell cycle of the precursors of neurons and glia. There is some indication that the cell cycle of germinal cells gradually becomes more prolonged during development of the chick neural tube (Jelínek, 1959; Fujita, 1962; Wilson, 1973, 1974) and neural tube of the mouse fetus (S. L. Kauffman, 1968; Hoshino *et al.*, 1973; Wilson, 1974). If the neuroepithelial germinal cells behave like other dividing cells, their generation time would be expected to become progressively longer as development proceeds (Fig. 2.3). In mammalian cells this is due to progressive lengthening of the G_1 phase, whereas the S and G_2 phases remain relatively constant (Defendi and Manson, 1963; Cameron, 1964; Prescott, 1964; Wegener *et al.*, 1963, 1964). In amphibians all phases of the cycle increase progressively in duration from blastula to late tailbud stages (C. F. Graham and Morgan, 1966; Flickinger *et al.*, 1967). In the telencephalon of the mouse fetus the lengthening of the cell cycle is the result of an increase in the duration of G_1 and S phases, while the G_2 and M phases remain the same from the 10th to the 17th day of gestation (Hoshino *et al.*, 1973). In the chick embryo optic tectum the cell cycle lengthens at later stages of development because of increases in the G_1 and M phases, while G_2 and S remain constant (D. B. Wilson, 1973, 1974).

Much more information is needed before any conclusions can be drawn from the data in Table 2.1. However, the evidence should be noted that the cell cycle of glioblasts is much longer than that of the germinal cells that produce neurons. In the neonatal mouse, the generation time of the external granule cells of the cerebellum is about 24 hours (Miale and Sidman, 1961; S. Fujita *et al.*, 1966), whereas that of cerebellar glioblasts lasts 5 days (S. Fujita *et al.*, 1966). Neuroepithelial germinal cells of the cerebrum of the 15-day mouse fetus have a generation time of 11 hours (Langman and Welch, 1967), which may be compared with the 65-hour generation time of subpial glioblasts in the cerebrum of the newborn mouse (Fujita *et al.*, 1966).

The relative roles of chromosomal and cytoplasmic factors in regulating the rate of DNA synthesis and mitosis have been reviewed by Gurdon and Woodland (1968). They concluded that "DNA synthesis in multicellular organisms appears to be subject to two kinds of control. First, cytoplasmic components are responsible for the initiation of DNA synthesis, the S-phase. Secondly, there are nuclear components which typically prevent a second round of replication taking place until the chromosomes have passed through mitosis." After reviewing the experiments showing that the duration of the S phase lengthens progressively during development but that gastrula nuclei transplanted to eggs revert to the short S phase typical of the first divisions after fertilization, Gurdon and Woodland (1968) conclude that the duration of the S phase is controlled by cytoplasmic as well as nuclear components, as yet unidentified.

2.4. Germinal Zones Producing Neurons and Glial Cells

During development the neural tube is at first composed only of neuroepithelial germinal cells at asynchronous phases of the mitotic cycle. At this state of development, cumulative administration of tritiated thymidine results in labeling of 100 percent of the cells composing the neural tube, with a linear increase in the percentage of labeled cells (S. Fujita, 1963, 1964, 1966; M. Jacobson, 1968*b*). At a later stage of development some cells remain unlabeled regardless of the duration of cumulative exposure to tritiated thymidine (Fig. 9.19.).

The absence of label shows that these cells are postmitotic, and they have been shown to migrate out of the ventricular germinal zone and to differentiate into neurons (S. Fujita, 1966; M. Jacobson, 1968*b*). By definition, these unlabeled cells are young neurons, because after they have completed their final division these cells are already committed to a developmental program leading to the differentiation of specific types of neurons. After their terminal cell cycle some kinds of neurons are programmed to develop position-dependent properties determined by the position that each cell occupies in its cellular set, which specifies the position of the synaptic connections made with nerve cells in other neuronal sets (M. Jacobson, 1968*a,b,* 1973; M. Jacobson and Hunt, 1973; R. K. Hunt and Jacobson, 1974*c*).

The young neurons migrate out to form a mantle zone of differentiating neurons surrounding the ventricular germinal zone. At this stage the neural tube consists of an inner zone of germinal cells bound together by terminal bars at their ventricular margins, an intermediate or mantle zone consisting of young neurons at various positions in the course of their outward migration, and an outer marginal zone composed of the external cytoplasmic processes of the neuroepithelial germinal cells (Fig. 3.3). Glial cells are probably also produced at this stage by division of neuroepithelial germinal cells. It is not known whether the same germinal cells can produce both neurons and neuroglia, or whether different neuroepithelial cells, histologically indistinguishable, give origin to glial cells and neurons. It has been reported that the neuroepithelial germinal cells are homogeneous as regards DNA synthesis and proliferation kinetics (H. Fujita and Fujita, 1963, 1964; S. Fujita, 1966), and electron microscopic examination has failed to disclose ultrastructural differences between germinal cells that might indicate differences in their developmental potential (S. Fujita, 1966; Wechsler, 1966*b;* Meller *et al.*, 1968*a;* W. F. Blakemore, 1969; Fisher and M. Jacobson, 1970).

It is not known when the differential gene expression occurring in neuroepithelial germinal cells results in divergent cytodifferentiation of their progeny. However, it is very likely that some germinal cells in the early neural tube are committed to producing neurons only, and others are committed to producing neuroglia exclusively. Another possibility, favored by S. Fujita (1965*b,* 1966), is that the neurons and neuroglia may arise consecutively from the same cell line. It has also been proposed that oligodendrocytes and astrocytes are different stages of a single cell line in which transitional forms may be seen (Ramón-Moliner, 1958; Smart and Leblond, 1961). However, there is no evidence that neurons and glial cells may arise from a common "indifferent cell," as has often been suggested (Schaper, 1897*a;* J. H. Globus and Kuhlenbeck, 1944; Vaughn, 1969). The absence of labeled glial cells following the injection of tritiated thymidine in early embryonic stages is not convincing evidence against the early origin of neuroglia. Labeled glial cells might easily be overlooked because any label taken up by glial cells in the early embryo will be greatly diluted by many cell divisions before the animal is killed after birth and examined by autoradiography. The label taken up in the final round of DNA synthesis is retained undiluted for the remaining life of the neuron.

2.5. Development of Neuroglia

The notion that glial cells are relatively idle bystanders of the activities of the neurons tended to persist for as long as the functions of the neuroglia remained almost unknown. Not long ago the neuroglia were considered to play no more than a passive supporting function; as their name implies, they were supposed to act as the cement between the neuronal bricks (*neuroglia,* "nerve cement" in Greek, was the term introduced by Virchow in 1859). This misconception has been replaced by the concept of a functional interdependence of neurons and glial cells.

The functions of glial cells during development, once considered important only during myelination, are slowly becoming more fully apparent. For example, the importance of microglial response to death of neurons has assumed greater significance since the ubiquity of nerve cell death during normal development has become known (see Section 7.6). The role of astrocytes is still enigmatic, but it is now thought that one of their specialized functions during development is to guide some neurons during their outward migrations from the germinal zones to their final resting positions in the cerebral cortex and cerebellar cortex (see Sections 3.2 and 3.5). It is very likely that glial cells function in a similar way in other places where young neurons have to migrate through complex terrain. Recent evidence that glial cells are a source of nerve growth factor (see Section 6.9) brings to mind the classical hypothesis of the nutritive functions of glia.

The morphology of glia is also being interpreted in more dynamic terms. Thus one expects to see morphological reflections of the varied functions of glial cells during development as well as in the mature nervous system. For example, one sees differences between microglia at rest and during reaction to trauma, differences between astrocytes that reflect their interactions with neurons at different stages of development and in different functional states, and differences between resting oligodendrocytes and those that are engaged in myelination. In brief, **one has to interpret the morphology of neuroglia as well as of neurons in relation to the functional roles of the neurons or glial cells at the particular times and places at which they are observed,** and one should expect the morphology to change under different conditions at different stages of development. Such changes can range from relatively slight ultrastructural alterations to complete transformation of the cell's morphology. A dramatic example of such a transformation occurs in the radial neuroglial cells of the mammalian telencephalon. They are extremely elongated and span the full thickness of the telencephalon at early stages while they function as guides for migrating neurons, but later, after neurogenesis has ceased, the radial neuroglia are transformed into astrocytes whose functions are different from those of the radial neuroglia (Ramón y Cajal, 1909–1911; Bignami and Dahl, 1974*a,b;* Rakic, 1975*a*).

Since the advent of the electron microscope, new criteria have been established for identifying the astrocytes and oligodendrocytes (Farquhar and Hartmann, 1957; R. L. Schultz *et al.*, 1957; Luse, 1958, 1960; De Robertis and Gershenfeld, 1961; R. L. Schultz, 1964; Mugnaini and Walberg, 1964; Wendell-Smith *et al.*, 1966; Kruger and Maxwell, 1967) and for identifying the microglia (Mori and Leblond, 1969). The use of autoradiography has resulted in rapid progress in documenting the sites of origin and time of origin of glial cells. The history of this problem, then, has largely been written in terms of technical advances in the methods of recognizing glial cells. Yet solutions to the problems of glial development could not have been arrived at while the functions of glial cells remained largely unknown, so that it was not possible, until very recently, to arrive at functional interpretations of glial cell histogenesis.

The very existence of microglia as a type of cell intrinsic to the nervous system remained in doubt until quite recently, but these doubts have now been dispelled and clear descriptions of microglia should enable us to identify them with the light microscope (Ling *et al.*, 1973) or with the electron microscope (Mori and Leblond, 1969; Phillips, 1973). The distinguishing morphological features of microglia are a small nucleus containing dense chromatin clumps and light nucleoplasm, scant cytoplasm containing lipid inclusions, lysosomes, and abundant vesicles but sparse endoplasmic reticulum, scattered ribosomes, and few or no microfilaments or microtubules. The presence of microglia containing abundant inclusion bodies and what appears to be phagocytosed debris, in the normal developing central nervous system, indicates that the microglia play a role as macrophages which remove the debris of cells that die during normal development. These macrophages are especially numerous in those regions where massive cell death occurs during a short period of development, for example, in the lateral motor column of the spinal cord of the chick embryo (see Sections 7.6 and 7.9).

By contrast with microglia, there is little difficulty in recognizing the two types of macroglia, namely, astrocytes and oligodendrocytes, when they are mature, although immature forms are more difficult to distinguish from one another. Mature astrocytes have a lucent cytoplasm, sparse cytoplasmic organelles, and bundles of microfilaments 70–100 Å in diameter, may contain glycogen granules, and may be attached to a capillary. Oligodendrocytes have fewer cytoplasmic processes than astrocytes, have abundant endoplasmic reticulum and ribosomes, have a high density of cytoplasmic organelles, and contain prominent Golgi apparatus and vesicles and many cytoplasmic microtubules. A wide spectrum of cytoplasmic densities in developing oligodendrocytes has been seen. This may make it difficult to distinguish between young astrocytes and young oligodendrocytes. To add to the difficulty, the appearance of glial cells changes with their functional states. For example, the oligodendrocyte active in myelination has more extensive cytoplasmic processes, more abundant cytoplasmic organelles, and more dispersed nuclear chromatin than the mature, resting oligodendrocyte.

This précis of the ultrastructural characteristics of different types of glial cells barely does justice to the diversity of structures that are actually seen. This polymorphism is due to regional variations in cell structure and especially to differences that reflect various functional states. For those reasons, one has to be particularly critical of attempts to deduce glial cell lineage from electron microscopic pictures of small areas of fixed tissue. It is best to be skeptical of any interpretation such as that of Vaughn and Peters (1968) and Vaughn (1969) that "small glioblasts which resemble microglia very closely, are multipotential cells capable of producing macroglia as well as microglia." Ideally, careful evaluation of cell types and transitional forms can provide circumstantial evidence of the lineal relationships between the forms. In practice, it is extremely difficult to deduce cell lineages from morphology. The fact that one type of cell can be recognized earlier in development than another is very poor evidence that the first gave rise to the second. Nevertheless, many authors have been victims of such *post hoc ergo propter hoc* reasoning.

A historical perspective is useful when trying to appreciate the difficulties that are now having to be overcome in discovering the developmental origins of glial cells and their functions during development. The early workers in this field made slow progress in understanding the origin and development of neuroglia because they were hampered by inadequacies of their histological techniques. As a result, a diversity of opinions held sway about the origin and morphology of glial cells until more selective histological methods were invented. The Golgi method and the silver methods are not selective for neuroglia, but the Golgi technique nevertheless shows some of the morphological differences between neurons and glial cells, as well as between the types of glial cells. In 1913, Ramón y Cajal introduced his gold chloride sublimate method, which selectively stains the astrocytes. The silver carbonate method of del Rio-Hortega (1919, 1921), which selectively stains microglia, allows those cells to be distinguished from the macroglia, namely astrocytes and oligodendrocytes. However, the silver method used to study the oligodendrocytes is not completely selective and cannot always be depended on to show those glial cells (Penfield and Cone, 1929).

Although the existence of glial cells was guessed at before 1850 and the term *neuroglia* was coined by Virchow in 1859, it was not until the introduction of the Golgi technique in 1875 that nerve cells could confidently be distinguished from glial cells (E. Clarke and O'Malley, 1968). The precursors of the glial cells were then thought to be the epithelial cells of the neural tube, which withdraw from their pial and ventricular attachments to become glial cells. These radially arranged columnar epithelial cells were called "spongioblasts" by His (1887) and "radiate neuroglial cells" by Magini (1888). The spongioblasts were considered to be the precursors of all the nonneuronal cells, which were thus derived from the ectoderm. Ramón y Cajal (1909–1911, Vol. 2, p. 860) dismissed the hypothesis which was held by many at the end of the nineteenth century (see Hatai, 1902*b*) that glial cells have dual origins—some originating from neuroectodermal cells and some arising from mesodermal cells. Instead, he concluded that "the neuroglial cells are all of ectodermal origin, because they are derived from elements of the primitive medullary canal" (Ramón y Cajal, 1909–1911, Vol. 1, p. 635). Later research has confirmed the ectodermal origin of the macroglia (astrocytes and oligodendrocytes in mammals and their equivalents in submammalian vertebrates), but the microglia have been shown to have a mesodermal origin since they are macrophages that invade the nervous system from the blood.

His (1889, p. 336) realized that, unless proliferation of spongioblasts occurs, the theory that the germinal cells (Keimzellen) give rise exclusively to nerve cells while the "spongioblasts" give rise to glial cells cannot account for the origin of all the glial cells from a relatively small number of precursors. This difficulty was never fully overcome, although Ramón y Cajal showed "spongioblasts" in the process of cell division.

An explanation that was more consistent with the evidence was proposed by Schaper (1897*a,b*). He postulated that the germinal cells give rise to "indifferent cells," which migrate out into the marginal or mantle zone and divide there one or more times before their progeny differentiate into neurons or glial cells. More recently, S. Fujita (1965*a,b*) has proposed that neuroglia originate from precursor cells called "glioblasts," which arise from neuroepithelial germinal cells (which he terms "matrix cells") after the latter have ceased to produce neurons.

The reader should be acutely aware that the neurocytologist selects his facts according to the prevailing prejudices—in this he is no different from other scientists and nonscientists. The only difference between them is that the scientist, more often than the nonscientist, submits his prejudices for refutation. The microglia provide an ideal case to illustrate this point. For del Rio-Hortega (1919,

1932) they are mesodermal cells, derived, he thought, from the pia mater; for J. H. Globus and Kuhlenbeck (1944) and for Vaughn (1969) the microglial cells arise from the same "indifferent" precursor cell as the macroglial cells; for Konigsmark and Sidman (1963*a,b*) the microglial cells originate mainly from the blood, but these authors leave open the possibility that some arise from within the central nervous system; others question the very concept of microglia (Kruger and Maxwell, 1966), while yet others would have microglia arise from small glioblasts which also give rise to macroglia (Vaughn and Peters, 1968; Vaughn, 1969; S. Fujita and Kitamura, 1975). In short, the microglial cell is an obliging fellow who always does whatever is necessary for the neurocytologist's theories.

2.6. Histogenesis of Glial Cells

It is clear that very few mitotic figures are seen in the periventricular germinal zone during the period when glial cells are being produced—for example, after day 8 of embryonic development in the chick embryo hindbrain (Harkmark, 1954) or spinal cord (Bensted *et al.*, 1957; H. Fujita and Fujita, 1964; S. Fujita, 1965*a,b*), as shown in Fig. 2.6. The neuroglia are formed by cells that have migrated away from the ventricular germinal zone at an earlier stage. Therefore, the precursors of glial cells, which are aptly termed *glioblasts,* must originate from the neuroepithelial germinal cells at the same time as they give origin to neurons, but the glioblasts migrate into the intermediate or mantle zone and into fiber tract and commissures, and continue proliferating in those extraventricular sites. These glioblasts appear to be very susceptible to chemical carcinogens, while neurons and their stem cells are greatly resistant to the same agents. As a result, vulnerability of

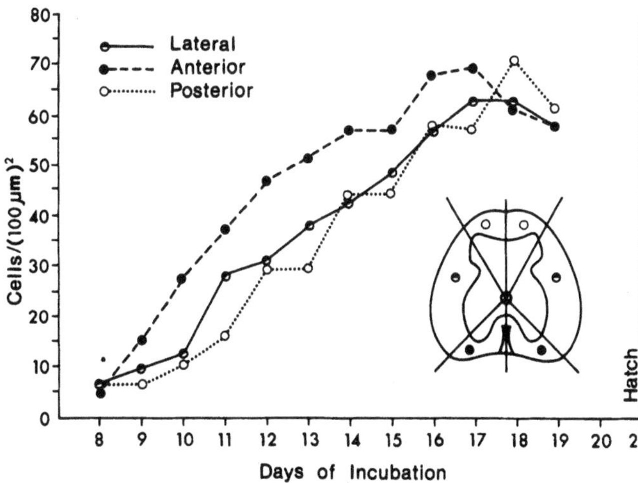

Figure 2.6. Neuroglial cell density (number of cells per 100 μm^2) in the anterior, lateral, and posterior column of the spinal cord of the chick embryo on successive days from the 8th to the 19th day of incubation. From J. P. M. Bensted *et al.*, *J. Embryol. Exp. Morphol.* 5:428–437 (1957).

the nervous system to chemical carcinogens is virtually nil in the rat before 11 days of gestation, during the period of maximal production of neurons. The susceptibility to carcinogens increases after day 11 of gestation, reaches a peak toward the end of gestation, and declines to a low level after the first postnatal month. Virtually all tumors induced by carcinogens are gliomas (Kleihues *et al.*, 1976, review).

It is a general rule that neurons are produced before their associated glial cells in each region and that the proliferation of glial cells occurs in relation to the differentiation and growth of neurons. This may be obscured in those regions where production of several types of neurons occurs over an extended period, in the cerebral cortex and cerebellar cortex, for example. However, the first neurons always appear to originate before the first glial cells. It may be assumed that this apparent sequence of neurons first and glial cells afterwards is not merely due to the delayed differentiation of glial cells that are produced at the same time or before neurons. This possibility, although unlikely, cannot be excluded because there are no certain criteria for identifying glial cells at the earliest stage of their existence. One has to appeal to indirect evidence which shows that neurons stimulate proliferation of glial cells. Thus failure of production of glial cells occurs after death of the associated neurons. This has been observed in the superior colliculus of the newborn mouse after removal of an eye (DeLong and Sidman, 1962), in the optic tectum of the frog tadpole after eye removal (Cowan *et al.*, 1968), and in the spinal ganglia after removal of a limb (Carr, 1975, 1976). More direct evidence that neurons stimulate glial cell proliferation has been obtained in tissue culture. A pure culture of glial cells is nonproliferative, but addition of neurons stimulates mitosis in the glial cells in proportion to the number of added neurons (McCarthy and Partlow, 1976*a,b*).

Ascertaining the time of origin of astrocytes and oligodendrocytes, and whether they arise simultaneously or consecutively, may help in deciding whether they arise from the same or different precursors. Unfortunately, there is conflicting evidence on this point. Smart and Leblond (1961), using light microscopic autoradiography after administration of tritiated thymidine, reported that oligodendrocytes originate before astrocytes in the corpus callosum of the mouse. They suggested that the two types of macroglia might arise independently from different precursors or that oligodendrocytes might become transformed into astrocytes. On the other hand (Vaughn (1969), using electron microscopy to identify the types of glial cells in the optic nerve of the rat, found that astrocytes appear first during development. Oligodendrocytes can be recognized only in later development, just before the time at which myelination begins (Fig. 2.7). There seems to be no problem in distinguishing between the two types of macroglia, and Vaughn (1969) reported that intermediate types between astrocytes and oligodendrocytes are not seen. However, Ramón-Moliner (1958) recognized a number of intermediate types with the light microscope. This suggested that one type might transform into another type at an early stage of their differentiation or that an intermediate type might be the common precursor of both astrocytes and oligodendrocytes. In the light of the present evidence, it seems most likely that astrocytes and oligodendrocytes arise separately from different precursors and that the mistaken notion of transitional forms has arisen because they are rather similar in appearance during early stages of differentiation, because they are polymorphic at later stages, and because they alter their appearance under different functional conditions.

Another difficulty is that microglia and small glioblasts may sometimes be very similar in their histological appearance, even in electron micrographs. Seen with the light microscope, both are small cells with dark nuclei and sparse cytoplasm with irregular, short processes. According to Mori and Leblond (1969), numerous authors have identified these cells incorrectly. Mori and Leblond (1969) used the electron microscope to identify microglia in the rat corpus callosum in sections stained with del Rio-Hortega's weak silver carbonate method. The microglia have a small nucleus with dark chromatin contrasting strongly with the light nucleoplasm. Young oligodendrocytes have dispersed chromatin, which probably indicates active synthesis of messenger RNA. In addition, the microglial cells contain little endoplasmic reticulum, few ribosomes, and many dense bodies presumed to be lysosomes. After injection of tritiated thymidine followed by autoradiography, no microglial cells are labeled, indicating that they do not proliferate. Glioblasts are capable of proliferation but may remain temporarily arrested in the G_1 phase of the cell cycle; they may proliferate very slowly, with a generation time as long as 120 hours in the cerebellar glioblasts of the mouse, 1–3 days after birth (S. Fujita *et al.*, 1966), or 65 hours in the case of the subependymal glioblasts of the newborn mouse (S. Fujita *et al.*, 1966). However, the rate of glioblast proliferation may also be quite rapid: generation times between 19 and 20 hours were measured in the subependymal zone of the rat between E18 and P21, and these dividing subependymal cells are probably all glioblasts (P. D. Lewis and Lai, 1974).

Production of glial cells in the central nervous system of adult mammals is well established (F. Allen, 1912; Smart, 1961; Smart and Leblond, 1961; Altman, 1962*a,* 1966*a;* Hommes and Leblond, 1967), but the significance of gliogenesis in adults is not clear. New glial cells may be produced to replace those that have degenerated, but there is no evidence of death of glial cells in the normal nervous system of young mammals. On the other hand, there may be a turnover of glial cells in various pathological conditions and states of increased function. Reactive

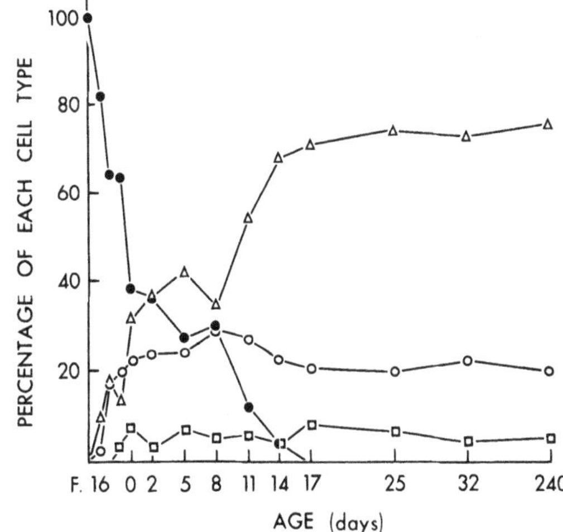

Figure 2.7. Percentage of glial cell types in the anterior limb of the anterior commissure of the mouse brain from fetal day 16 to 240 days after birth. ●, Glioblasts; Δ, oligodendroblasts and oligodendrocytes; ○, astroblasts and astrocytes; □, microglia (pericytal and interstitial); F16, days after conception; 0, birth, normally 20 days after conception. From R. R. Sturrock, *J. Anat.* *117:*37–53 (1974).

hypertrophy without obvious hyperplasia of astrocytes occurs in many pathological conditions—for example, in slow loss of neurons in man and in hypoglycemia—and has been most fully described and investigated in liver failure, so-called hepatocerebral disease (Cavanagh and Kyu, 1971; Cavanagh, 1974). In these conditions in which the astrocytes increase in size, the number of astrocytes of both fibrous and protoplasmic varieties may also increase, but such reactive hyperplasia is most often the result of acute or subacute loss of neurons (R. D. Adams and Foley, 1953). The possibility, erroneous as it now seems, that in response to brain injury astrocytes might increase by "amitosis" or division of the nucleus without the formation of a mitotic figure was proposed by Penfield (1932) and reviewed later by Lapham (1962). It has been shown that there is a duplication of the chromosomes, which fail to separate at metaphase, finally resulting in a polyploid cell, which may later repeat the former process or may undergo normal mitosis (Cavanagh, 1974). Lapham (1962) reported that reactive astrocytes may continue to synthesize nuclear DNA without undergoing mitosis and may thus become polyploid. Normal glia, however, are diploid, and, with the exception of a report of tetraploidy in an unidentified type of glial cell in the human cerebellum (Lapham and Johnstone, 1963; Mann and Yates, 1973*b*), glial cells in several species have been shown to be diploid.

Several other conditions are associated with an increase in the number of glial cells. Proliferation of glial cells has been observed around neurons undergoing chromatolysis after their axons have been cut (Cammermeyer, 1963, 1965*a,b;* J. Sjöstrand, 1965, 1966*a,b;* W. E. Watson, 1965, 1974*c;* Chow and Dewson, 1966, as is discussed in Section 7.4. An increase in the number of glial cells around motor neurons in the spinal cord of the mouse has been reported after greatly increased motor activity (Kuhlenkampf, 1952). Dehydration of rats results in an increase in the proliferation of glial cells in the hypothalamus (M. Murray, 1968). Autoradiography has also shown proliferation of glial cells in the brains of mice reared in an "enriched environment" (Altman and Das, 1964; Diamond *et al.*, 1964, 1966). The factors in these experiments that might have stimulated the production of glial cells are not known. Any of a variety of factors such as increased sensory and motor activity, increased nutrition, or hormonal stimulation and metabolic changes, independently or in combination, might have stimulated proliferation of glial cells. The reports do not show whether the glial cells originate from stem cells that remain quiescent under normal conditions or whether DNA synthesis can be reinitiated in fully differentiated glial cells.

Death and replacement of neuroglia in the adult human brain were first proposed long ago (F. Allen, 1912). This proposal remained a subject of debate and disagreement until autoradiography enabled Smart and Leblond (1961) to confirm that glial cells are formed in the adult mouse brain. Postnatal gliogenesis has since been repeatedly confirmed in mice and rats (Altman, 1962*a*, 1966*a,b;* Hommes and Leblond, 1967; Dalton *et al.*, 1968; P. D. Lewis, 1968*a,b;* Hinds, 1968*a,b;* Gilmore, 1971; H. Korr *et al.*, 1973; Sturrock, 1974*a,b*). While almost all such evidence comes from mice and rats, there are some studies indicating that postnatal turnover of glial cells occurs in the rabbit (Robain, 1970) and cat (Fleischauer, 1966, 1968; Haug, 1972). From these studies it is clear that glial cells are produced throughout life in mice and rats, and probably in other mammals.

There have been conflicting reports about the response of glial cells to injury of the central nervous system. Cavanaugh (1970) reported astrocytic proliferation around a needle stab wound in the adult rat brain, whereas Murray and Walker (1973) found no evidence of glial proliferation following brain injury, but concluded that all the cells labeled with [^{3}H]thymidine after brain injury are leukocytes. One reason for the disagreement is that it is difficult to identify radioactively labeled glial cells in autoradiographs because the heavy metal stains for glial cells are incompatible with autoradiography (Sidman, 1970). The present evidence is overwhelmingly in favor of the classical view that the microglia are derived from the blood (del Rio-Hortega, 1919, 1932) and that the cells that appear at the site of a brain injury are leukocytes or are derived from cells connected with blood vessels, or so-called pericytes. The appearance of glial cells around the cell body of neurons whose axons have been cut as a well-known phenomenon Sjöstrand, 1965, 1966*a,b;* Blinzinger and Kreutzberg, 1968; Torvik and Skjörten, 1971*b;* W. E. Watson, 1974*b;* Davidoff, 1973). In such cases, where peripheral nerves have been cut or crushed, there is no direct injury to the brain, and the labeled glial cells appear around the perikarya of the neurons far from the site of injury to the axons. The problem of the origin of these brain macrophages, as of the origin of the microglia in general, is controversial. Adrian and Smothermon (1970) concluded that the cells that enter the hypoglossal nucleus after injury to the hypoglossal nerve are leukocytes. Other have concluded that the microglia that appear around axotomized neurons originate from perivascular cells, the so-called pericytes.

The classical view of del Rio-Hortega (1919, 1932) was that microglia enter the brain from connective tissue of blood during the prenatal period and remain quiescent until activated and transformed into macrophages by trauma or infection. Later authors distinguished between the microglia that enter the brain from the blood and those that arise by mitosis in the brain (Maxwell and Kruger, 1965, 1966; Cammermeyer, 1965*a,b,c;* Sjöstrand, 1965, 1966*a,b*). Konigsmark and Sidman (1963*a,b*) found that after injection of [^{3}H]TdR into adult mice many labeled leukocytes appear in the blood but few labeled cells are found in the uninjured brain. However, after a stab wound has been made in the brain the previously labeled blood cells appear in the brain. They concluded that leukocytes are a major source of brain macrophages but left open the possibility that up to one-third of the labeled macrophages might originate in the brain. The same conclusion was reached by Adrian and Williams (1973*a,b*) and Matthews (1974).

One of the difficulties in accepting the hematogenous origin of microglia in normal central nervous system is that microglia appear much later than the vasculature. For example, the capillaries are present in chick embryo spinal cord at 4 days of incubation (Feeney and Watterson, 1946) while the glial cells cannot be recognized until the 8th day (S. Fujita, 1965*b*). Finding a complete series of transitional forms leading to microglia either from the blood vessels or from other elements in the central nervous system, including the subventricular zone, would help to settle the origin of these cells, but no intermediates have been found.

The uncertainty about the origin of microglia is due to several factors: microglia are difficult to identify and to distinguish from immature forms of macroglia; the silver carbonate method of impregnating microglia is incompatible with autoradiography; the microglia have different appearances in different functional states. Perhaps that is why microglia were not found in two recent studies of gliogenesis (Caley and Maxwell, 1968*b;* Blunt *et al.*, 1972), whereas they have been found in other electron microscopic studies of developing mammalian central nervous system (Bodian, 1966*a;* Hildebrand, 1971; Stensaas and Reichert, 1971; Phillips, 1973).

To a large extent the problem of the ontogeny of neuroglia has been bedeviled by the fact that there is a long delay between the time of origin of glial cells and the time at which they reach their final state of differentiation. During this interval there are several ways in which glial cell differentiation may occur. The glial cell may remain dormant, or it may undergo slow but continuous differentiation to one or other type of glial cell. These alternative modes of development make the study of glial development even more difficult than that of neuronal development. The problem of the origin and differentiation of glial cells is rendered particularly difficult because reliable criteria for recognizing newly formed, immature, or transitional forms of glial cells have yet to be established. It is here that immunological methods of detecting young neuroglia may prove to be of great value. For example, fluorescent labeled antibodies to glia-specific proteins, such as the S 100 protein localized in oligodendrocytes (Gombos *et al.*, 1971), may prove to be useful to label immature oligodendrocytes. The glial fibrillary protein (Bignami and Dahl, 1973, 1974*a,b,* 1975) localized in astrocytes may be detected in immature astrocytes by means of labeled antibodies. To this date, however, the immunofluorescent methods have not demonstrated the presence of glial cells before they can be detected by conventional techniques of light and electron micrsocopy. Thus, in the cerebellum, the Bergmann glial cells are known to be present from before birth in the mouse and are active in guiding migrating granule cells before the immunofluorescent method first shows the presence of glial–fibrillary protein in the Bergmann glial cells on the 3rd postnatal day (Bignami and Dahl, 1973, 1974*b*). In the spinal cord of the chick embryo, the glial cells are present several days before the fibrillary astrocytes become detectable by their immunofluorescence with antiserum to glial–fibrillary protein (Bignami and Dahl, 1975).

The advent of tritiated thymidine autoradiography has mitigated the problem to some extent by making it possible to determine the time of the final cell cycle in neurons and neuroglia. This technique has revealed great differences between neurons and glial cells in the programming of the final cell cycle: the neuron precursors enter their final cell cycle in a distinct germinal zone which contains proliferating cells and some postmitotic cells that are migrating out, while the glial cell precursors may be in any position, and are usually extraventricular, when they enter their final cell cycle. The glial precursors may divide and migrate repeatedly. The result of these differences is that while neurons exposed to $[^3H]$TdR in their final cell cycle remain permanently and heavily labeled and can be easily identified in autoradiographs, glial cells that are labeled at the same time usually undergo further divisions which dilute the label to below detectable levels.

The most important concept that has emerged from the autoradiographic studies is that each distinct set of neurons originates in a fairly invariant timetable. Thus in any one neuronal set (which may contain several neuronal types) the entire population of each type of neuron completes the final cell cycle and becomes permanently postmitotic within a relatively short period, usually in less than 1 day in rodents. **By contrast, glial cells in any region withdraw from the mitotic cycle over a much longer time than the neurons in the same region.** This applies to astrocytes as well as to oligodendrocytes, but it is particularly applicable to the latter, which continue to divide in the fiber tracts and commissures long after all the neurons have become postmitotic.

The problem of the ontogeny of neuroglia shows how difficult it is to determine their origins and birthdates, and these matters are as yet far from being settled. Indeed, the problem of control of glial histogenesis remains a *tabula rasa* not merely awaiting adequate techniques but also severely limited by the lack of understanding of glial cell functions.

3

Histogenesis and Morphogenesis of the Central Nervous System

3.1. Time and Sequence of Origin of Neurons and Glial Cells

Evidence of temporal and spatial regularities in the origin of neurons and glia was extremely difficult to obtain before the advent of the technique of autoradiography following the administration of tritiated thymidine. Information about the time of origin of neurons in the developing nervous system is now obtained with relative ease by injecting pregnant mammals with tritiated thymidine (1–5 μCi per gram body weight) intravenously or into the amniotic fluid, killing the fetuses at various intervals after the injection, and examining their brains autoradiographically.

Since, in mammals, the nucleotide is available for less than an hour after injection, the presence of the label in a cell is an indication that the cell must have been engaged in DNA synthesis during the hour following the injection. Thymidine is cleared more slowly in cold-blood animals and may remain available for hours or even days after administration. Heavy labeling of cell nuclei is an indication that tritiated thymidine has been incorporated during the final period of DNA synthesis in preparation for the terminal mitosis of the heavily labeled cell. The label is then retained for the remainder of the life of the cell. Light labeling is an indication that the label has been diluted by several divisions of the cell after it has taken up the label. Absence of label is of little significance following a single injection of tritiated thymidine. However, cells that remain unlabeled after several injections of the nucleotide (cumulative labeling) may be regarded as postmitotic provided that there is no reason to suspect that the injected nucleotide was not able to enter the unlabeled cells.

There is great consistency in the pattern of labeling of cell nuclei with tritiated thymidine. According to Angevine (1965), "plots made from littermates injected and processed in identical fashion could be superimposed to show remarkable similarity in number and placement of labelled neurons. The origin of neurons in the various regions [of the hippocampal formation of the mouse] follows a precise timetable; thus speciments injected at the same time yield identical patterns and specimens injected serially display an orderly succession of patterns."

Autoradiographic studies of the time of origin and migration of neurons and glial cells in the mammalian central nervous system have been made in the retina (Sidman, 1961; S. Fujita and Horii, 1963; M. Jacobson, 1968*b,* 1976*a;* Hollyfield, 1968), anterior olfactory nucleus and nucleus of the lateral olfactory tract (Creps, 1974*a*), olfactory bulb (Hinds, 1968*a,b*), hippocampus (Angevine, 1965; Altman and Das, 1965*b,* 1966, 1967), cerebral neocortex (Angevine and Sidman, 1961; Berry and Eayrs, 1963, 1966; Berry and Rogers, 1965, 1966; Berry *et al.,* 1964*a,b;* Caviness and Sidman, 1973; Bisconte and Marty, 1975), preoptic and septal areas (Creps, 1974*b*), diencephalon (Angevine, 1970*b*), mesencephalic nuclei (Hanaway *et al.,* 1971), hypothalamus (Ifft, 1972; Shimada and Nakamura, 1973), cerebellum (L. L. Uzman, 1960; Miale and Sidman, 1961; S. Fujita, 1967; S. Fujita *et al.,* 1966; Altman, 1969; Rakic, 1973), brain stem (Taber Pierce, 1966, 1967*a,b,* 1973; Ellenberger *et al.,* 1969), and spinal cord (S. Fujita, 1964; Langman and Haden, 1970; Nornes and Das, 1974).

These studies have revealed several features that are common to all regions of the brain:

1. Spatial and temporal gradients of proliferation in the neuroepithelial germinal zone
2. Separate origin of neighboring regions that are different cytoarchitectonically
3. An orderly sequence of production of large neurons first, then intermediate-sized neurons, and finally small neurons
4. A tendency for glial cells to originate after neurons in any particular region of the brain
5. A predisposition for phylogenetically older parts of the brain to arise earlier in ontogenesis

These general features will be discussed below, before reviewing the development of parts of the brain from a topographical point of view.

Spatial gradients of proliferative activity in the neuroepithelial germinal zone are of great importance in programming the time of origin of neurons and number of neurons that are produced at any time. The spatiotemporal pattern of origin of neurons, revealed by [^{3}H]thymidine labeling of cells during their terminal phase of DNA synthesis, shows that neurons assemble either by stacking in laminar structures or by packing into nuclear regions in regular spatiotemporal gradients. Such gradients are described as "inside-out" when the neurons that originate at successively later times migrate past those formed earlier and take up successively more external positions, that is, successively farther from the ventricular germinal zone from which they originate. This "inside-out" pattern of assembly or stacking is generally characteristic of laminar structures, especially the cerebral cortex, optic tectum, hippocampal formation, and substantia nigra. There are apparently some exceptions such as the granular layer of the hippocampal dentate gyrus and the granular layer of the cerebellar cortex, but in such cases the granule cells arise from displaced germinal zones and not directly from the ventricular germinal zone. These cases of apparent "outside-in" assembly should be contrasted with those cases in which the neurons assemble in a true "outside-in" sequence which is characteristic of nuclear regions such as the thalamus and hypothalamus. Such lateral-to-medial gradients of time of origin of neurons have been reported in the isthmo-optic nucleus of the chick (P. G. H. Clarke *et al.*, 1976), the hypothalamus of the mouse (Shimada and Nakamura, 1973) and rat (Ifft, 1972), the anterior thalamus of the rabbit (V. Fernandez, 1969), and the dorsal thalamus of the mouse (Angevine, 1970*a,b*) as shown in Fig. 3.1.

Differences in the time of origin of different types of neurons are superimposed on the spatiotemporal gradients. Large neurons are produced before small ones in any part of the nervous system, and the neurons produced last are invariably local circuit neurons such as granule cells or Golgi type II neurons. In the retina the ganglion cells are formed first and differentiate before the receptors, bipolar cells, and the amacrine cells in the same region of retina, although not necessarily before those cells in other parts of the retina that originated earlier (Sidman, 1961; S. Fujita and Horii, 1963; M. Jacobson, 1968*b;* Hollyfield, 1968). In the cerebellar cortex the Purkinje cells are formed first and then the Golgi type II cells, followed by basket and stellate cells, and finally the granule cells. (Nineteenth-century work culminated in that of Ramón y Cajal, 1909–1911. Other references are given in Section 3.7) The large neurons are formed before the small neurons in the cerebellar roof nuclei (Miale and Sidman, 1961; Taber

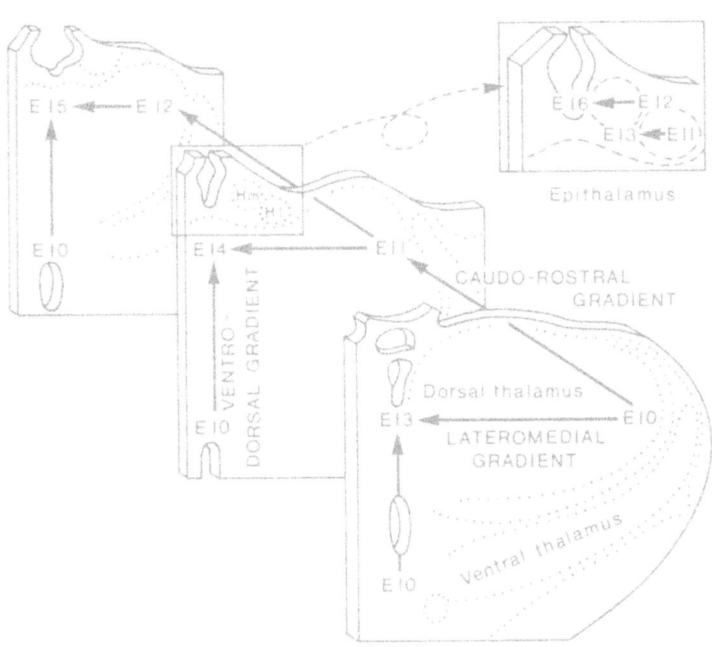

Figure 3.1. Gradients of time of origin of neurons determined autoradiographically in the diencephalon of the mouse embryo from the 10th to the 16th day of gestation (E10–E16). Hm and Hl are the medial and lateral habenular nuclei shown in the rectangle. From J. B. Angevine, Jr., in *The Neurosciences: Second Study Program,* F. O. Schmitt (ed.), Rockefeller University Press, New York, 1970.

Pierce, 1967*b*). In the cerebral cortex the pyramidal cells are formed first and the granule cells last (Angevine, 1965; Hinds and Angevine, 1965). In the olfactory bulb the mitral cells are formed before the tufted cells and the granule cells are formed last (Hinds, 1968*a,b;* Creps, 1974*a*). The large neurons are formed first in the spinal cord (H. Fujita and Fujita, 1963), in the diencephalon (Angevine, 1968, 1970*a*), and in the cochlear nuclei (Taber Pierce, 1967*a*). There is also a **tendency for motor nuclei to commence their histogenesis and complete their cell populations before the sensory nuclei at the same level of the neuraxis, and for the histogenesis of the motor systems to have a shorter duration than that of the sensory systems.**

In some respects the ontogeny of the brain recapitulates its phylogeny. The "biogenetic law" that ontogeny recapitulates phylogeny should be regarded only as a parallelism, not as a necessary causal relationship, and always with the reservation that ontogenetic–phylogenetic parallelism may merely be the fortuitous result of the operation of circumstances and of principles of efficiency that are similar in evolution and in development. Bearing these reservations in mind, the parallels between ontogeny of the nervous system and its presumed phylogeny are often so striking as to demand explanations. It is the general rule that parts of the nervous system that appeared first in phylogeny have a tendency to appear early in ontogeny, and structures that arose later in evolution also often arise late in ontogeny. For example, neurons in the phylogenetically older accessory olfactory bulb develop before their counterparts in the more recently evolved olfactory bulb (Hinds, 1968*a*). The late origin of the hippocampal granule cells reflects the phylogenetic increase in granule cells in the hippocampus of placental mammals as compared with nonplacental mammals (Angevine, 1965). The early origin of the ventral thalamus in mammals reflects the early evolution of the homologous thalamic structures in submammalian vertebrates (Angevine, 1970*a*). The phylogenetically older accessory olive develops first ontogenetically (Harkmark, 1954; Ellenberger *et al.*, 1969). Finally, in the cerebral isocortex, the neurons of the outer layers (except I) originate last and are the most recent to have appeared in evolution. Layers I and VI appear to have evolved first and are the first cortical layers to develop. In the cat, Marin-Padilla (1972) has shown that the first intracortical circuits are developed between layers I and VI: the Martinotti neurons of layer VI connecting with layer I and the horizontal neurons (Cajal-Retzius cells) of layer I projecting to layer VI (Fig. 3.2). These neurons, together with the pyramidal neurons of layer VI, are the first to form in the mammalian cortex, and intially form an organization that, according to Marin-Padilla (1972), resembles the reptilian neocortex.* This precocious organization is completely transformed during late prenatal development, and its interconnections apparently disappear completely by the time of birth in the cat.

What is the purpose of preserving the genetic information and developmental processes for such transient structures that seem to have no nervous

*The dangers of reading profound meaning into such resembances can be illustrated by Gaskell's (1889) theory of the origin of the nervous system. According to this theory, the central nervous system of vertebrates has evolved from the alimentary canal of invertebrates. Analogies are drawn from the resemblance between the ventricular system of the brain and the lumen of the gut, with the infundibulum being derived from the mouth, and, among the absurd conclusions that follow, the substantia nigra of the vertebrate brain is thought to be derived from the invertebrate stomatogastric ganglion.

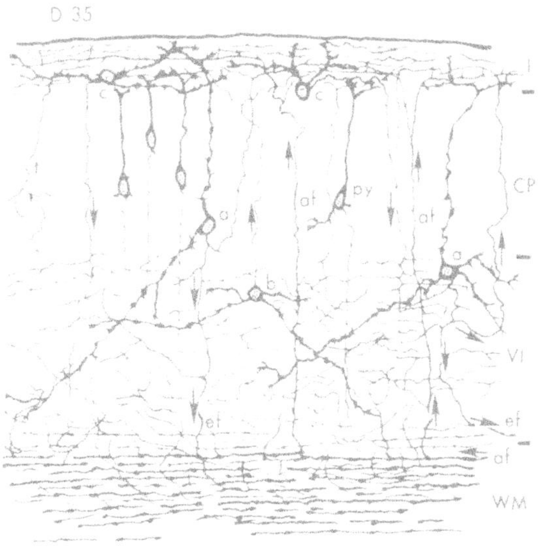

Figure 3.2. Organization of the cat neocortex at 35 days of gestation, illustrating its structure and basic neuronal types. The fibrillar structure of the cat neocortex during early gestation (25th–45th days of gestation) is characterized by a superficial (layer I) and a deep (layer VI) plexiform layer composed predominantly of ascending collaterals from the afferent fibers of the white matter. Three types of neurons are recognized in the neocortex of the cat during this gestational period: the horizontal neurons (c) with descending axons terminating in layer VI; the Martinotti neurons (b) with ascending axons terminating in layer I; and the pyramidal-like stellate neurons (a) with recurrent axonic collaterals to layer I and terminal efferent fibers. The cortical plate (CP) is composed of immature pyramidal neurons (py) at a bipolar stage of development. The dendrites of the three types of neurons of the primordial neocortical organization are covered by a few spinelike projections suggesting the presence of a postsynaptic apparatus. This, in addition to the obvious fibrillar and neuronal interactions between layers I and VI, supports the idea that the primordial neocortical organization of the cat is a functionally active structure. Layer I (superficial plexiform layer) seems to be predominantly an associative layer of the neocortex, while layer VI (deep plexiform layer) has associative and projective characteristics. Analogies between the reptillian cortex (see Fig. 534 in Ramón y Cajal, 1911) and the primordial neocortical organization of the cat are suggested. Rapid Golgi method. Camera lucida drawing. From M. Marin-Padilla, *Z. Anat. Entwicklungsgesch. 134:*117–145 (1971).

function in the embryo or fetus? Are such primitive structures truly vestiges of the state of organization reached by the ancestral forms? We should question whether such apparently vestigial neural circuits give a true indication of the neural circuitry of ancestral forms or whether they are so greatly modified and specialized that they cannot give more than a vague indication of the ancestral forms from which they might have evolved. Do the times of origin of neurons give a reliable indication of their phylogeny, or do the gradients of time of origin reflect a purely developmental adaptation to achieve an efficient assembly of complex structures?

These examples show that **the time of neuron origin depends on a complex set of factors, including the type of neuron, its position in the gradients of mitotic activity, and probably its phylogenetic status.** It is important to recognize that the time of cell origin is not necessarily correlated simply with the time of any single aspect of cytodifferentiation, such as the formation of synapses. Cells may be "dormant" for relatively long times—months in the mammalian cerebral cortex—in their final positions, before they become connected in their definitive neural circuits. One cannot simply deduce the subsequent timetable of neuron differentiation from a knowledge of the time of neuron origin; one has to take other factors into consideration, such as the type of neuron, the region in which it is situated, and especially the time of arrival of the axons, usually from several sources, that are destined to synapse on the neuron in question.

3.2. Development of the Cerebral Cortex

Four zones can be distinguished at different depths in the developing telencephalon (Boulder Committee, 1970). The zones, shown in Fig. 3.3, are as follows, from the external surface to the ventricle. The *marginal zone* initially contains only cytoplasmic processes of cells whose nuclei are at deeper levels, but later it becomes sparsely populated by neurons that form layer I of the cerebral cortex, which is the first cortical layer to develop. The *intermediate zone* develops as a result of ingrowth of afferent axons and migration of cells to form the cortical plate. As cells and fibers continue to invade this zone, the cortical plate undergoes progressive differentiation to form the definitive layers of the cerebral cortex. The *subventricular zone* contains proliferating cells that mainly give rise to macroglia.

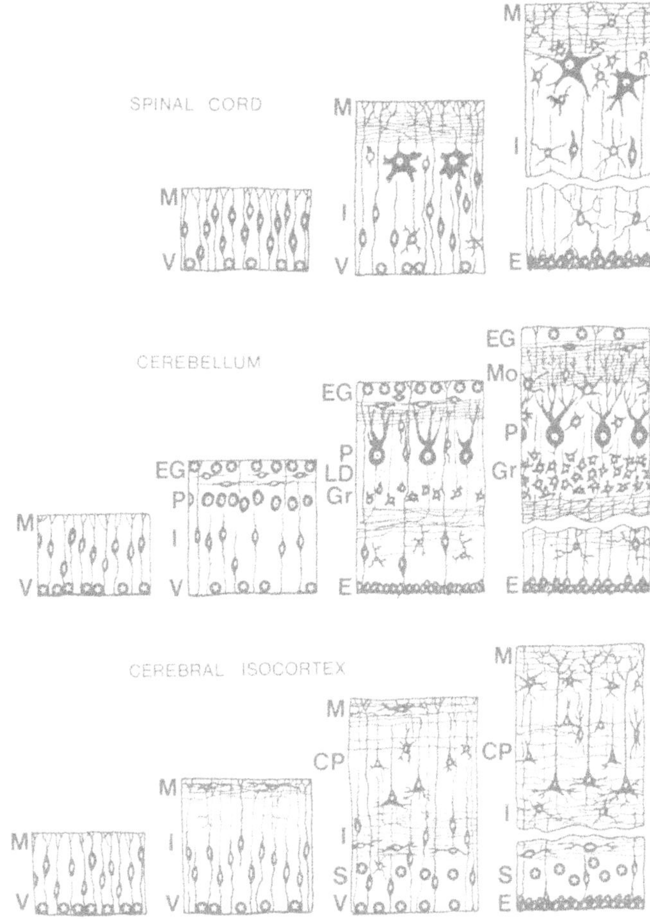

Figure 3.3. Germinal and other cellular zones and layers in the developing cerebral isocortex, spinal cord, and cerebellum of mammals. Progressively later stages of development are shown from left to right. CP, Cortical plate; E, ependymal layer; EG, external granule layer; Gr, granule layer; I, intermediate zone; LD, lamina dissecans; M, marginal zone; Mo, molecular layer; P, Purkinje cell layer; S, subventricular zone (also called subependymal zone); V, ventricular germinal zone. Mitotic figures are denoted by stars.

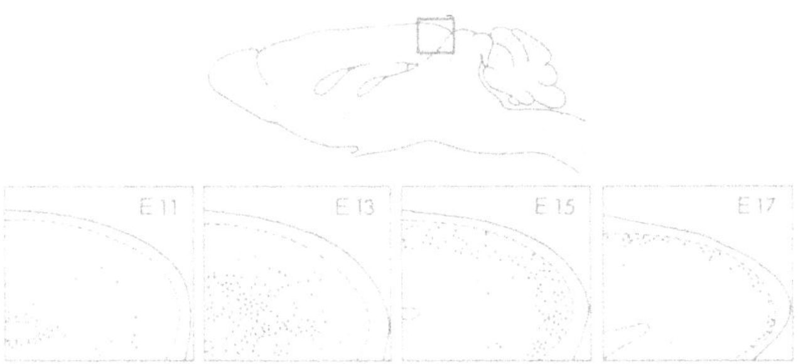

Figure 3.4. "Inside-out" sequence of time of origin of neurons in the cerebral isocortex of the mouse. Four different mice each received a single injection of tritiated thymidine on either the 11th, 13th, 15th, or 17th day of gestation (E11–E17). All were killed 10 days after birth when the neurons of the cerebral cortex had reached their final positions. The positions of labeled cells are shown by dots in the autoradiographs of sections of the region of cerebral cortex outlined by the rectangle. From J. B. Angevine, Jr., and R. L. Sidman, *Nature 192:*766–768 (1961).

This zone persists after birth, and in some mammals its functions continue into adulthood. The *ventricular zone,* which contains the ventricular germinal cells, is the first zone to develop, gives origin to the other zones, and then disappears at an early stage of development.

The time of origin of neurons in the mammalian cerebral cortex has been determined by injecting the gravid female with tritiated thymidine, killing the fetuses at intervals after the injection, and determining the pattern of labeled neurons in autoradiographs of histological sections of their brains.

Angevine and Sidman (1961) showed that 1 hour after an injection of tritiated thymidine to the pregnant mouse at 11, 13, 15, and 17 days of gestation (E11, E13, E15, E17), the label is present only in cells close to the ventricle, in the forebrain of the fetus. If the injection is given on the same day of gestation but the mice are killed 10 days after birth, the labeled cells are found only in the gray matter of the cerebral cortex. Angevine and Sidman found that young neurons labeled on day 11 *in utero* migrate from the ventricular germinal zone to the deep layer of the occipital cortex, and cells labeled on subsequent days migrate to more superficial levels of the cortex (Fig. 3.4). The "inside-out" sequence of arrival of neurons in the cerebral isocortex is also seen in the rat fetus (Berry and Rogers, 1965; Berry *et al.,* 1964*a,b*). Young neurons that are generated on intrauterine day 16 in the cerebral cortex of the rat fetus migrate out to the subpial level and differentiate there. Neurons formed on days 17–22 of gestation migrate between the cells of the previously formed layers to form new layers superficial to them. Thus the cells of the deepest cellular layer of the isocortex (layer VI) originate on day 16, and cells that form layer II originate last on day 21 of gestation. No waves of cell migration are seen, but young neurons are generated continuously by mitosis of germinal cells close to the ventricle and move outward as a continuous stream. The neurons that arrive in the cortex first are displaced to deeper levels by those that arrive later (Fig. 3.5). Note that this does not apply to the Cajal-Retzius cells of layer I, which are the first cells to appear in the mammalian cerebral cortex.

The cells of Cajal-Retzius are an exception to the rule that the pyramidal cells in the deeper layers of the cortex mature first. The Cajal-Retzius cells are the first neurons to mature in all regions of the cerebral cortex of mammals, and cells of similar appearance and position also occur in the cerebral cortex of submammals. The Cajal-Retzius cell has a large stellate cell body in the marginal zone which becomes the molecular layer of the cerebral cortex. It has an axon running for a long distance in the molecular layer, with short branches running vertically down into cortical layer II. It has two dendrites 500 μm to 1 mm long running parallel to the surface of the cortex and sending branches to make contact with the pia. The Cajal-Retzius cells have the morphology of neurons, as seen in Golgi preparations (Marin-Padilla, 1970*a*) and in electron micrographs (Raedler and Sievers, 1976), and they contain cholinesterase as well as aerobic enzymes found in adult neurons (Duckett and Pearse, 1968). Their functions remain an enigma.

Cajal-Retzius cells were discovered by Ramón y Cajal (1891) and later described by Retzius (1893, 1894), who called them "Cajal's cells"; Ramón y Cajal later jokingly referred to them as "Cajal's cells of Retzius" (see E. Clarke and O'Malley, 1968, p. 443). They have already arrived in the marginal zone of the rat occipital cortex on day 13 of gestation before any other neurons of the isocortex have been born, and differentiate rapidly to reach maturity before the rat's birth (Raedler and Sievers, 1976). They appear during the intrauterine period in man and have been said to atrophy and disappear shortly after birth (Noback and Purpura, 1961; Duckett and Pearse, 1968). In the human fetus during the last months of gestation and early postnatal period, the Cajal-Retzius cells lose their dendritic attachments to the pia and move more deeply into the molecular layer, and shortly after birth they seem to disappear (Conel, 1939–1963: Vol. I, p. 103; Vol. II, p. 9; Vol. III, p. 9; Vol. IV, p. 7). In the adult, there are horizontal cells in layer I which are called the "horizontal cells of Cajal." Ramón y Cajal (1909–1911) distinguished between the fetal and adult forms of horizontal cells in layer I, and suggested that the fetal type matures and persists as the adult type of horizontal cell.

There is some controversy regarding the fate of Cajal-Retzius cells and whether they atrophy and disappear or merely become altered in position and

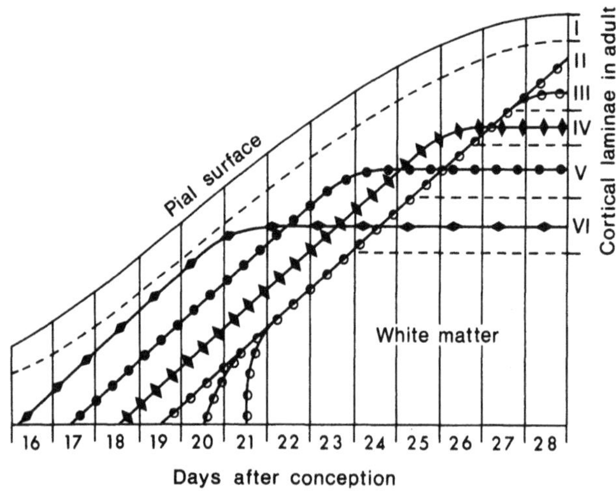

Figure 3.5. Time of origin and pattern of migration of young neurons in the cerebral isocortex of the rat as revealed by labeling of the cells with tritiated thymidine injected on the 16th, 17th, 18th, and 19th–21st days of gestation. From M. Berry, A. W. Rogers, and J. T. Eayrs, *Nature 203*:591–593 (1964).

morphology after birth. For example, Molliver and Van der Loos (1970) reported that Cajal-Retzius cells can be found only until 12 days after birth in the dog, but similar cells have been reported in the adult dog brain (M. W. Fox *et al.*, 1966). According to Marin-Padilla (1970*a*), the Cajal-Retzius cells of the human motor cortex are preceded by the arrival of afferent fibers in layer I of the cortex. He suggests that these afferents connect with the Cajal-Retzius cells to form the first neuronal circuits to be found in the motor cortex, and that these persist through life.

There is still some uncertainty about the **mode of migration of newly formed neurons** from the ventricular germinal zone to the cerebral cortex. The word "migrate" is often used loosely to describe movement of the nucleus, in autoradiographs, for example, where the disposition of the cytoplasm is not completely known. It is not entirely clear whether the young migrating neurons retain an attachment to the ventricular or pial surfaces of the cerebrum or whether they lose their attachments and migrate freely as unattached cells. F. C. Sauer (1935*a,b*, 1936) has shown that neuroepithelial cells lose their external (pial) attachment and round up toward the ventricle before mitosis. This may also occur in the telencephalon during the early stages of its development before a thick mantle layer has developed. Neurons formed at that stage might lose attachments to internal and external surfaces of the telencephalon and therefore migrate into the mantle layer free of attachments, as Angevine and Sidman (1961) and Stensaas (1967*b*) suggest. The germinal cells of the telencephalon have numerous branching cytoplasmic processes that are attached to the pial surface, and it is improbable that these external connections break down during every mitotic cycle as the nucleus moves toward the ventricle during metaphase. In the Golgi and silver preparations of the developing cerebral cortex of the rat, Berry and Rogers (1965) found that the germinal cells retain their attachment to the pial and ventricular surfaces, and they did not find cells that detach from the pia and round up toward the ventricle during mitosis. They proposed that the cytoplasm of the germinal cell may not divide immediately after mitosis, but that the daughter nucleus may migrate within the cytoplasm of the maternal cell toward the pial surface where cytoplasmic division may occur. This proposal was founded on the evidence that neuroepithelial cells occasionally appear to have two nuclei, but Berry and Rogers (1965) do not seem to have excluded the possibility that this appearance might have been due to superimposition.

Golgi studies of neurogenesis in the forebrain of the opossum (Morest, 1969*a*, 1970*a*) do not reveal any evidence of free, ameboid migration of young neurons. According to Morest, the young neuron remains attached by a cytoplasmic process to the germinal zone and extends a cytoplasmic process to the external surface of the forebrain. The nucleus and perikaryon then move into the cytoplasmic process toward the external surface. Next, the primitive processes disappear and the axon and dendrites differentiate. In many cases, the axon and dendrites begin to form before the primitive process entirely disappears. It thus seems likely that at least some neurons remain attached to the pial surface, and their migration from the ventricular germinal zone to the cortex may be the result of shortening of the external cytoplasmic process that is anchored at the pial surface.

The rate of migration of young neurons from the ventricular zone to the cortical plate is initially fairly uniform, but later becomes spread over a longer time. In the rat, Hicks and D'Amato (1968) reported that young neurons labeled at E14–E18 migrate to the cortical plate in about 2 days, almost synchronously, whereas cells labeled at E19–E21 take from 3 to 10 days to arrive at the superficial layer of the cortex. This lag in the migration of neurons formed late in development has been confirmed by Rakic (1974) in the rhesus monkey visual cortex. Young neurons labeled at early stages (E46–E53) move about 200 μm from the ventricular zone to the cortical plate in about 3 days (5.5 μm per hour; compare rates on p. 87) and almost all arrive at their destinations in less than 7 days. But with advancing age, as the cortical plate thickens, the spatial dispersion is found to be much greater. In a fetus injected at E92 and killed 5 days later, only a few labeled neurons have migrated the full distance, about 1.2 mm, to the superficial layers of the cortex, and the majority of cells are still *en route,* either in the deep cortical layers or in the subventricular and intermediate zones.

It seems likely that the ripid and almost synchronous migration of neurons born together at early stages occurs because all the cells span the full thickness of the cortical plate in a simple radial alignment. At late stages of histogenesis of the cortex, the cells have to migrate a longer distance and to traverse a more complex terrain. At those stages, Rakic (1971*a*) has demonstrated that the migrating neurons use radial glial cells as guides (Fig. 3.6). However, it is not known whether those neurons originate from the ventricular zone or from the subventricular zone. The ventricular germinal cells probably maintain their full span from pial to ventricular surfaces, but the cells of the subventricular zone do not appear to be attached to the inner and outer surfaces of the brain. It is very likely that neurons originating in the ventricular zone migrate independently, because they span the full thickness of the telencephalon whereas neurons originating in the subventricular zone migrate with the assistance of radial neuroglia.

Prenatal ontogenesis of the human cerebral cortex follows the same program as homologous regions of the cerebral cortex in other mammals, taking into consideration the prolonged period of human gestation, the altricial state of the human newborn, and the vastly increased numbers of neurons in the human cerebral cortex (Poliakov 1953, 1956, 1959, 1961, 1965; Sarkisov and Preobrazhenskaya, 1959; Marin-Padilla, 1970*a*). In the motor cortex (precentral gyrus, Area 4) the arrival of afferent fibers follows a regular sequence, occurring in each layer before and during the time of arrival of neurons in that layer (Marin-Padilla, 1970*a*). The first fibers arrive in layer I and are followed by the Cajal-Retzius cells, which are the first neurons to originate and to differentiate in the human motor cortex. Thereafter, the pyramidal cells of layer VI and layer V can be seen at 5 months of gestation (Fig. 3.7.) These are followed by the interneurons of layer IV (cortical basket cells) about the 7th prenatal month. Then follow the pyramidal cells of layer III, and finally those of layer II can be readily recognized at 7.5 months of gestation. Various types of Golgi type II neurons and small neurons of diverse forms appear in all cortical layers during the late prenatal period.

The time of origin of neurons in the allocortex of the hippocampal formation has been elucidated in considerable detail by Angevine (1965) and Altman (1966*b,* 1967). Angevine (1965) has shown that there is a very close correspondence between developmental patterns and cytoarchitectonic divisions

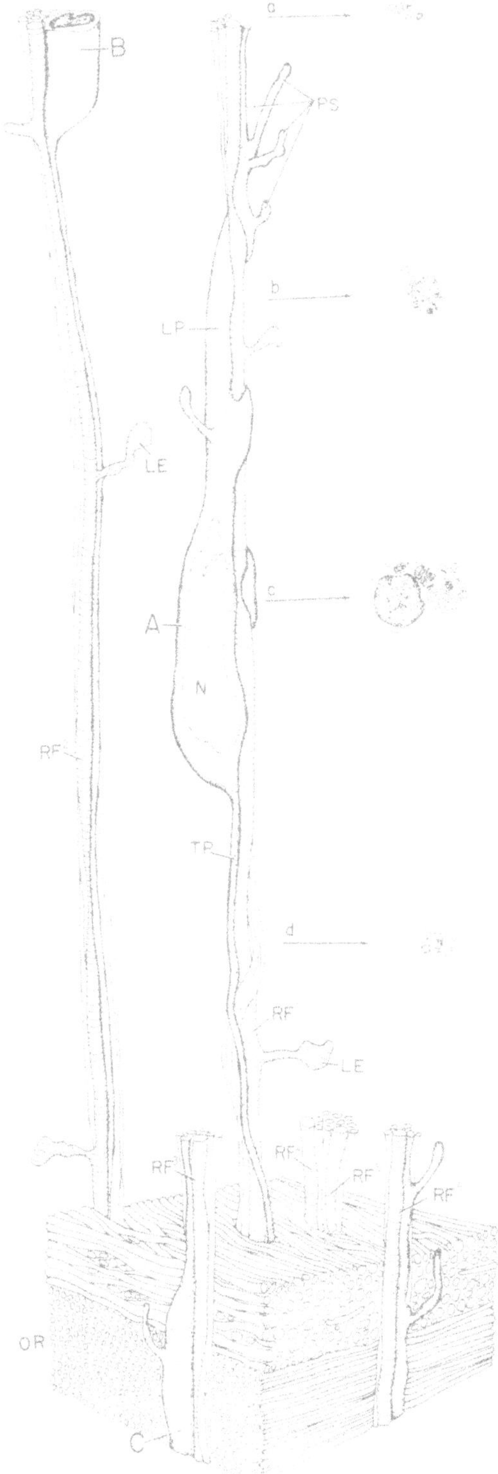

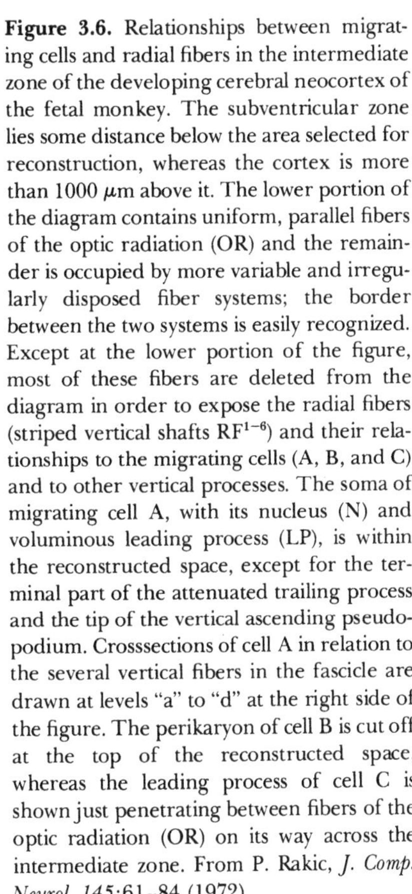

Figure 3.6. Relationships between migrating cells and radial fibers in the intermediate zone of the developing cerebral neocortex of the fetal monkey. The subventricular zone lies some distance below the area selected for reconstruction, whereas the cortex is more than 1000 μm above it. The lower portion of the diagram contains uniform, parallel fibers of the optic radiation (OR) and the remainder is occupied by more variable and irregularly disposed fiber systems; the border between the two systems is easily recognized. Except at the lower portion of the figure, most of these fibers are deleted from the diagram in order to expose the radial fibers (striped vertical shafts RF^{1-6}) and their relationships to the migrating cells (A, B, and C) and to other vertical processes. The soma of migrating cell A, with its nucleus (N) and voluminous leading process (LP), is within the reconstructed space, except for the terminal part of the attenuated trailing process and the tip of the vertical ascending pseudopodium. Crosssections of cell A in relation to the several vertical fibers in the fascicle are drawn at levels "a" to "d" at the right side of the figure. The perikaryon of cell B is cut off at the top of the reconstructed space, whereas the leading process of cell C is shown just penetrating between fibers of the optic radiation (OR) on its way across the intermediate zone. From P. Rakic, *J. Comp. Neurol. 145:*61–84 (1972).

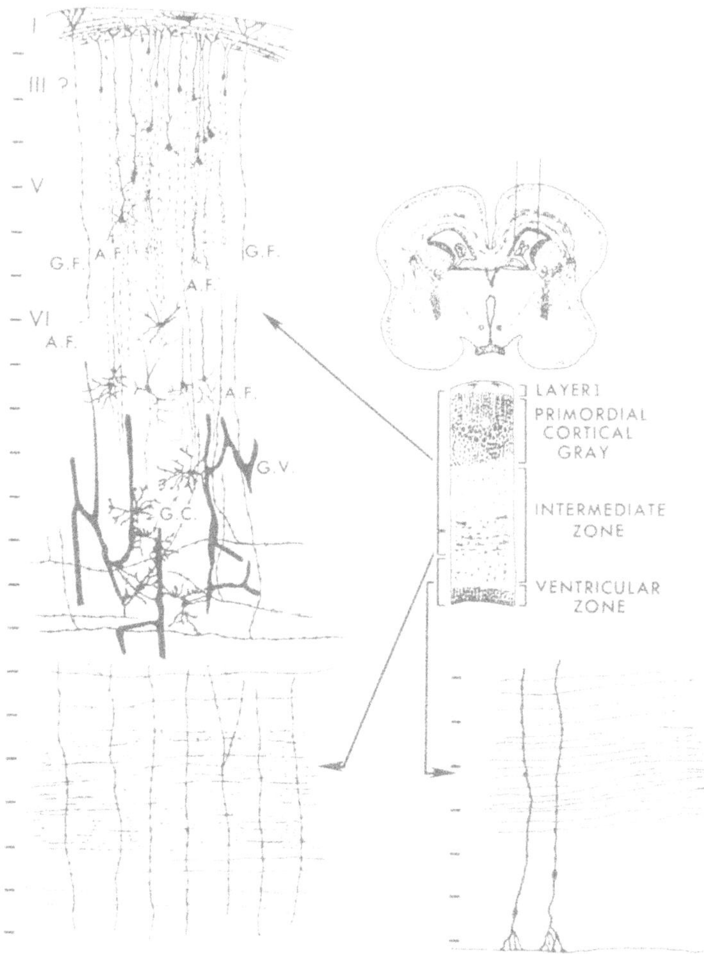

Figure 3.7. Composite of camera lucida drawings made from Golgi preparations of the cerebral cortex of the 5-month human fetus. Included are a diagram of a cross section of the brain of this infant reconstructed from Golgi and H-E sections to illustrate the general disposition of the horizontal systems of fibers of the intermediate zone of the cortex, and an enlargement of the cortical region between the vertical bars to illustrate the general structure and the different zones of the cerebral cortex at this age. The general structure of the cerebral cortex of this infant and the stage of development of its neurons, systems of fibers, and cortical layers as seen in Golgi preparations are illustrated. Only layers I, V, and VI, and possibly the beginning of the formation of layer III are recognizable here. Layer I appears more advanced in development than the rest of the cortical gray matter. The two systems of horizontal fibers of the intermediate zone are prominent structures of the cortex at this age. The fibers of these systems come from the region of the internal capsule and cross in the corpus callosum to the other cerebral hemisphere. From these two systems of fibers, two ascending types penetrate the developing coritcal gray matter. Some of these ascending fibers terminate in the inner region of the marginal zone (layer I), in which region they become horizontal (tangential fibers of layer I). Other fibers terminate around and below the developing pyramidal cells of layer V (internal band of Baillarger). Glial fibers are abundant at this age, and they are easily recognizable by their peculiar types of termination under the pial membrane. AF, Afferent fiber; GC, glial cell; BV, blood vessel; GF, glial fiber. Rapid Golgi method. Scale 100 μm. From M. Marin-Padilla, *Brain Res.* *23:*167–183 (1970).

of the hippocampal formation (Fig. 3.8). **The pattern of histogenesis may thus be of considerable value in helping to delimit cytoarchitectonic regions of the cerebral cortex.** The first neurons of the hippocampus are generated from the ventricular germinal zone on day 10 of gestation in the mouse fetus (Fig. 3.8). The hippocampus displays the "inside-out" sequence of time of origin similar to that described in other regions of the cortex. The younger neurons migrate through previously formed layers to form more superficial layers. Neuron formation in the hippocampus, area retrospelenialis, and area enterorhinalis is completed before birth in the fetal mouse. However, neurons in the area dentata continue to be formed until postnatal day 20.

In the stratum granulosum of the fascia dentata there is an "outside-in" order of formation. The primary germinal zone for these cells is in the wall of the lateral ventricle, whence cells migrate along the fibers of the hippocampal fimbria to the

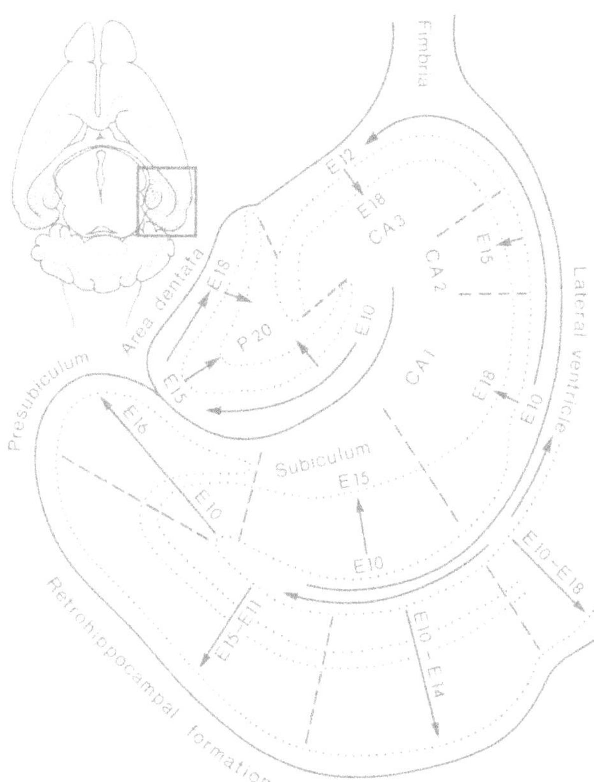

Figure 3.8. Top left: A horizontal section of mouse brain, illustrating the position of the hippocampal region (rectangle), which is shown in greater detail below. The time of origin of neurons in the allocortex of the hippocampus was determined autoradiographically. A series of pregnant mice were each given a single injection of tritiated thymidine on different days of gestation (E10–E18), resulting in labeling of the fetuses. These were killed after birth, when the neurons had arrived at their final positions, and autoradiographs were made of their brains. Note the gradients of time of neuron origin, indicated by arrows. From J. B. Angevine, Jr., in *The Neurosciences: Second Study Program,* F. O. Schmitt (ed.), Rockefeller University Press, New York, 1970.

area dentata. These cells continue to divide to produce glia and granule cells. The granule cells that originate first migrate to the outer edge of the stratum granulosum, and the stratum granulosum grows simply by addition of new neurons to its inner edge. The "outside-in" addition of neurons to the stratum granulosum occurs from E10 to P20 in the mouse.

Angevine (1965) has provided evidence that the granular neurons of the fascia dentata that are formed postnatally originate locally and are derived from germinal cells within the cortex. This has been confirmed by Altman and Das (1967), who injected tritiated thymidine into a newborn guinea pig and found labeling of granular neurons in the inner layer of the stratum granulosum of the fascia dentata 6 hours after injection. Clearly, these labeled granular neurons must have originated locally, for they could not have migrated from the wall of the lateral ventricle in the short period of 6 hours. This is the only example known at present of a germinal zone within the cortex itself giving rise to neurons of the cerebral cortex, and it should be noted that only granule cells originate in that way. The external granular layer of the cerebellum is rather similar in that it consists of germinal cells that have migrated from the rhombic lip (ventricular germinal zone in the alar plate of the medulla) over the surface of the cerebellum, where they give rise to the local circuit neurons of the cerebellum. This cerebellar external granular layer is continuous with the germinal zone in the lateral wall of the fourth ventricle and with the pontobulbar body caudally. This extensive germinal zone gives origin to the granule cells of the cerebellum, cochlear nuclei, and the pontobulbar nuclei (Essick, 1907, 1909, 1912; Harkmark, 1954; Taber Pierce, 1966, 1967*a,b*). In the mouse, granule cells originate from this extensive germinal zone until at least 20 days after birth.

In the later stages of embryonic development of the central nervous system of mammals, a second zone of proliferating cells forms between the ventricular germinal zone and the mantle or intermediate zone. This proliferative zone has been called the *subependymal zone* (Kershmann, 1938; Smart, 1961), the *subependymal cell plate* (J. H. Globus and Kuhlenbeck, 1944), or the *subventricular zone* (Boulder Committee, 1970). This zone has been described only in the mammalian forebrain, but may be present in other parts of the central nervous system at some stage of development. The subventricular zone progressively diminishes during development. It persists in a vestigial manner in the lateral ventricles of the forebrain into adult life (Fig. 3.9) in mice (B. Messier *et al.,* 1958; Smart, 1961), rats (Bryans, 1959; Altman, 1963; P. D. Lewis, 1968*a;* Privat and Leblond, 1972), cats (Altman, 1963), dogs (K. Fischer, 1967; W. F. Blakemore and Jolly, 1972), and primates (Opalski, 1933; J. H. Globus and Kuhlenbeck, 1944; Noetzel and Rox, 1964; P. D. Lewis, 1968*a*). The subventricular zone is "limited to those parts of the ventricles underlying the neocortex and paleocortex and is not found in relation to the phylogenetically older archicortex or other parts of the brain stem" (Smart, 1961).

The subventricular cells have been considered to be a potential source of gliomas (Globus and Kuhlenbeck, 1944; K. Fischer, 1967; P. D. Lewis, 1968*a*). The subventricular zone is one of the commonest sites of brain tumors induced by chemical carcinogens, and it is significant in relation to the origin of glia that the induced neoplasms are almost all gliomas. This is in marked contrast to the great rarity of neoplastic transformations of neurons, either spontaneous or induced by carcinogens (Kleihues *et al.,* 1976, review).

According to Rakic (1974), the subventricular zone can be recognized in the rhesus monkey's telencephalon as early as 45 days of gestation (E45) and its thickness increases markedly during the next 10 days. The ventricular zone coexists with the subventricular zone for the next 5 weeks, both zones giving rise to cells that migrate into the overlying cortical plate. It is usually assumed that the subventricular zone gives rise to neurons as well as glia during this period, while glia only are produced in the subventricular zone after birth. During the period from E50 in the rhesus monkey, the ventricular zone gradually diminishes and has disappeared by E90, while at the same time the subventricular zone increases in width and continues to provide glial cells to the cortex until the end of gestation (about 165 days after conception) and probably for a short time postnatally.

The presence of mitotic figures shows that the subventricular zone retains its capacity to generate new cells in the adult. The germinal cells of the subventricular zone divide *in situ* and do not exhibit interkinetic nuclear migration. The generation time of subventricular cells in the adult rat is 18 hours (P. D. Lewis, 1968*a*), which is considerably longer than the generation times of 8.5–12 hours found in the ventricular zone of the mouse and rat (Table 2.1). Some of the cells that arise in the subventricular zone are destined never again to divide, as is shown by their presistent heavy labeling after exposure to tritiated thymidine during their final round of DNA synthesis. These cells may differentiate into small neurons. Other

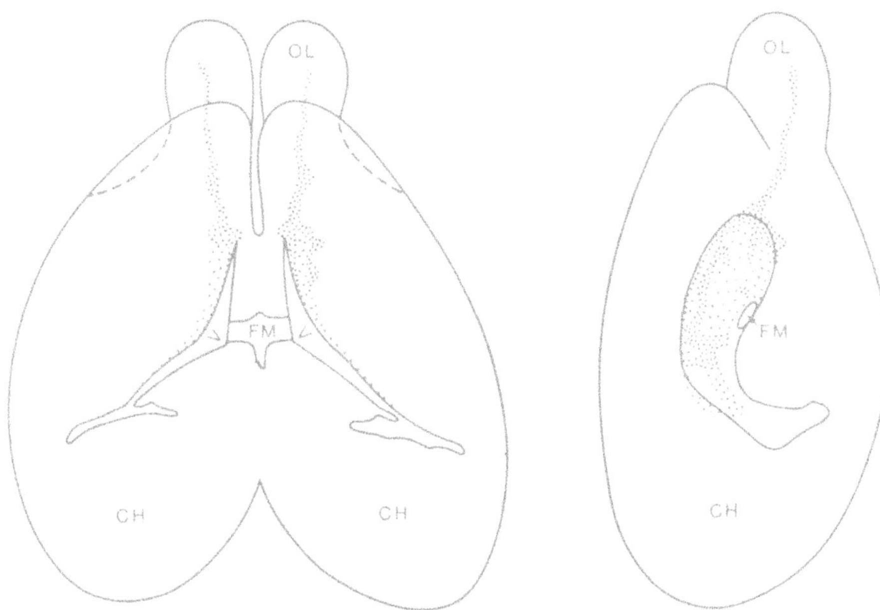

Figure 3.9. Cerebral hemisphere of the adult mouse shown in dorsal view (left) and in right lateral view (right) to show the extent of the subventricular zone (stipple). The denser stipple shows where the subventricular zone is thicker. CH, Cerebral hemisphere; FM, foramen of Monro; V, lateral ventricle; OL, olfactory lobe. From I. Smart, *J. Comp. Neurol. 116:*325–347 (1961).

cells continue to divide and to dilute their label after migrating from the subventricular zone into the overlying mantle zone. Some of these cells may give rise to neurons, others to glia. There is no reason to believe that an indifferent cell is formed that could give rise by division to both glia and neurons, as J. H. Globus and Kuhlenbeck (1944) proposed. The neurons and glia originating in the subventricular zone migrate out through the white matter to the overlying gray matter. Smart (1961) and Altman (1963) have emphasized the role that fiber tracts such as the corpus callosum play in guiding the migrating cells to their destinations. The role of radial glial cells in guiding these cells to their destinations in the telencephalon has been stressed by Rakic (1971*a,b,* 1972*a*).

Two types of cells are seen in the subventricular zone at all stages (Smart, 1961; K. Fischer, 1967; W. F. Blakemore and Jolly, 1972). One has a small, deeply stained nucleus (dark-nucleated type) and the other has a lighter, larger nucleus (light-nucleated type). Smart (1961) found a series of transitional forms from the light-nucleated cells leading to immature neurons, and considered the dark-nucleated type to be precursors of glia. Mitotic figures are present in both types. The subventricular germinal cells have the ultrastructural characteristics of immature cells: they have a high nuclear–cytoplasmic ratio, many free ribosomes and polysomes, and little endoplasmic reticulum (W. F. Blakemore, 1969). In adult mice the two types are uniformly dispersed and present in equal numbers, but at earlier stages the dark-nucleated cells predominate (Smart, 1961). Cumulative labeling with tritiated thymidine in adult mice results in labeling of only 1.5–6 percent of the light nuclei, and a maximum of 41 percent of the dark nuclei are labeled (Smart, 1961). Smart concluded that the subventricular zone produces microneurons and macroglia for a postnatal period that varies in different species; thereafter, a gradual reduction in the production of neurons occurs, but macroglia continue to be produced into adult life. Privat and Leblond (1972) found that in young rats the subventricular layer is composed of a few microglia and a single cell type, which they term the "subependymal cell," which gives rise to astrocytes and oligodendrocytes. Macrophages invade the subventricular zone from the blood, are found in large numbers (Cammermeyer, 1965*b;* W. F. Blakemore, 1969), and are probably concerned with removal of the debris of degenerating cells. Many degenerating cells with pyknotic nuclei are found in the subventricular zone of the adult brain. Because the number of pyknotic nuclei seen in the adult subventricular zone is approximately equal to the number of metaphase figures, Smart (1961) concluded that the majority of cells formed in the subventricular zone of the mouse are destined to degenerate and that the subventricular zone does not add significantly to the cell population of the adult brain. However, P. D. Lewis and Lai (1974) found that there are twice as many mitoses as degenerating nuclei in the subventricular zone of postnatal rats up to 21 days of age, and estimated that only 18 percent of the newly formed cells degenerate.

The functions of the subventricular zone in adult mammals is not known. While its role in gliogenesis during the early postnatal period is well established, its only role in adult life may be to replace glial cells. This role is consistent with the fact that the incidence of glial tumors in different species is directly related to the size of the residual subventricular zone in the adult brain of that species. There is no evidence showing that neurons are formed in the subventricular zone in adult mammals, although granule cells continue to be formed in various other germinal zones for a relatively short period after birth. For example, **postnatal neurogenesis occurs in the following sites in the mouse:**

1. In the olfactory bulb, granule cells originate from day 18 of gestation to day 20 after birth (Hinds, 1968*a,b*).
2. In the hippocampus, granule cells of the fascia dentata originate from day 10 of gestation to postnatal day 20 (Altman, 1966*b;* Altman and Das, 1965*b,* 1967; Angevine, 1965).
3. In the brain stem nuclei, granule cells originate from the rhombic lip from intrauterine day 10 to day 15 after birth (Taber Pierce, 1966, 1967*a,* 1973); granule cells of the cerebellar cortex originate from intrauterine day 17 to day 15 after birth (Miale and Sidman, 1961).

Formation of synaptic connections in the cerebral isocortex occurs some time after the migration of cortical neurons. The stream of young neurons from the periventricular germinal zone into the cortex meets a contingent of thalamocortical nerve fibers that grow into the cerebral cortex in advance of the cells upon which they will eventually synapse (Poliakov, 1961; Marin-Padilla, 1970*a*). It is believed that interactions between these afferent nerve fibers and the cortical neurons may occur which finally result in the formation of synapses between them. Angevine and Sidman (1961) and Morest (1970*a*) have suggested that the neurons may form synapses as a result of intercellular contacts that they make with thalamocortical axons and with previously formed neurons that lie in their path of migration. This interesting suggestion is discussed in Chapter 5 in connection with the development of dendrites and the formation of axodendritic synapses.

The maximum increase in connectivity in the rat isocortex occurs between days 12 and 20 after birth as evidenced by the increase in density of cortical axons (Eayrs and Goodhead, 1959) and by the increase in synapses in the cortex (Aghajanian and Bloom, 1967). Rapid increase in the number of synapses in the cortex during the early postnatal period has also been reported in mouse (Meller *et al.,* 1968*b*), rabbit (Gruner and Zahnd, 1967), and cat (Voeller *et al.,* 1963). Only axodendritic synapses form initially, while the axosomatic synapses develop afterwards (Voeller *et al.,* 1963; Meller *et al.,* 1968*b*). The precocious development of the human brain is shown by the fact that synaptogenesis in the cerebral cortex starts during the second month of gestation and is advanced by the time of birth (Molliver *et al.,* 1973), whereas in subprimates there are very few synapses in the cortex before birth.

Lamination of the mature cerebral cortex is already reflected in the orderly succession of arrival of young neurons in an "inside-out" sequence. However, the organization of the developing cerebral cortex is at first radial: the main axis of the cell bodies of the pyramidal cells is radial and their axons and apical dendritic shafts are oriented radially and develop before the lateral dendritic branches. The *maturation* of cortical neurons also occurs in a radial inside-out sequence starting in layer V and subsequently progressing through layers IV, III, and II, as first noted by Vignal (1888) and confirmed later by others (Koelliker, 1896; Stefanowska, 1898; Ramón y Cajal, 1906; Lorentí de Nó, 1933*b*). The general validity of this principle of inside-out maturation has been criticized by Molliver and Van der Loos (1970) in that it applies only to the differentiation of basal dendrites of pyramidal cells, which starts earlier in the deeper than in the more superficial pyramidal cells, whereas they note that the apical dendritic bouquets of superficial pyramidal neurons mature earlier than those of deep pyramids. This radial arrangement presages the columnar functional organization of the mature isocortex (Mountcastle, 1957; Hubel and Wiesel, 1968). The tangential organization of dendrites develops only during the postnatal period—for example, during the first 3 postnatal weeks in the mouse (Kobayashi *et al.*, 1964; Meller *et al.*, 1968*b*) and kitten (Noback and Purpura, 1961), during the first month in the dog (M. W. Fox *et al.*, 1966), and during the first 24 months after birth in man (Conel, 1939–1963; Schadé *et al.*, 1962). An important part of this tangential connectivity of the cerebral cortex is provided by the Golgi type II neurons, whose dendrites develop much later than those of the pyramidal neurons (Morest, 1969*a,b*).

The normal pattern of lamination of the cerebral cortex is not essential for the development of normal connectivity, as is shown by the studies on the reeler mouse. In the reeler mutant mouse (see section 3.4.5), the cortical neurons are conspicuously malpositioned in the retrohippocampal and olfactory cortical structures (Caviness and Sidman, 1972, 1973; Devor *et al.*, 1975). The defect in this mutant appears to be in the mechanism of migration of the young neurons from the ventricular zone to a subpial position. The various types of neurons are produced at the normal times and apparently in normal numbers, but the cells fail to migrate outward past those that were formed earlier. Thus the polymorphic neurons, which originate earliest in the retrohippocampal cortex, normally lie in the deepest stratum, but in the reeler mutant they lie in an immediately subpial position. A class of large cells is generated next. These cells fail to migrate past the polymorphic cells as they normally do, but take up positions deep to the polymorphic cells. The granule cells originate last and also fail to complete their migration to a subpial position, but instead come to lie deepest in the reeler cortex. The "inside-out" order is thus reversed in the reeler. One result of this malpositioning of cortical neurons is that the neurons in the isocortex receiving input from vibrissae do not assemble into the usual "barrel" formations (Cragg, 1975*b*).

Despite the malposition of all neuron somata of the olfactory cortex in the reeler mouse, their connections develop normally (Devor *et al.*, 1975). These anatomical observations of normal connectivity despite disordered positioning and orientation of cell bodies are in agreement with the electrophysiological evidence showing normal connectivity in the hippocampus of the reeler mouse despite gross cell malpositioning (Bliss and Chung, 1974). To this conservation of the connectivity should be added the preservation of the characteristic morphology of the pyramidal cells despite their malpositioning and disorientation in the reeler mouse cerebral cortes (Devor *et al.*, 1975). The characteristic phenotype of cerebral cortical pyramidal cells is also conserved in the few percent of pyramidal cells that have improper orientations, including totally inverted cells, in the otherwise normal cerebral cortex (Van der Loos, 1965). That the malpositioned pyramidal cells project their axons via the corpus callosum to form connections at the proper positions in the opposite hemisphere (Caviness, 1976; Caviness and Yorke, 1976) shows that the cellular recognition mechanisms can easily overcome large extracellular perturbations in order to link neurons according to their intrinsic specificities (also see R. Levine and Jacobson, 1974). These observations show that the principal neurons of the cerebral cortex, namely the pyramidal cells, have considerable autonomy in expressing their phenotypes. It is well to emphasize this aspect of the neuron's differentiation while also pointing out that although the main features of the principal cell's morphology can develop independently there are some structures, such as the dendritic spines, that tend to be fewer and smaller in the absence of their afferent axons, and complete maturation of the dendrites may require adequate functional stimulation. This topic is discussed more fully in section 5.6.

3.3. Comments on Assembly of Complex Neuronal Systems

Morphogenesis of the cerebellar cortex illustrates the main phases of neuromorphogenesis: first, consecutive production of different types of neurons and their migration to characteristic levels; second, a period of growth which sometimes includes production of redundant dendritic and axonal branches and the formation of transient connections; and, finally, pruning of the excessive growth and death of redundant neurons. **The establishment of the final definitive pattern of cellular relationships is thus the resultant of several processes that are patterened in space and time, namely histogenesis, cell migration, cell differentiation, and cell death.**

First, concerning the order of genesis of various types of neurons, the cerebellar cortex nicely illustrates the differences between the two main classes of neurons. In most regions of the central nervous system there is one type of neuron, termed the *principal neuron* or Type I neuron or macroneuron, which is surrounded by a constellation of *local circuit neurons,* also called Type II neurons or microneurons. The principal neuron is usually the largest neuron in its neuronal set, is the first neuron to originate and to differentiate in that set, and is usually the only neuron to project its axon outside its neuronal set. All these criteria of a principal neuron are met by the cerebellar Purkinje cell. All inputs converge, either directly or indirectly, on the Purkinje cell, and it is the sole pathway for outflow of information from the cerebellar cortex. The local circuit neurons, namely Golgi type II, stellate, basket, and granule cells, all originate later than the Purkinje cell, and all make their axonal connections entirely within the cerebellar cortex. The cerebellum also illustrates the rule that **neuronal sets are composed of a small number, usually about five, of different types of neurons and the complexity arises from the patterns of connections between the neurons, not from the variety of neuronal types.**

The Purkinje cells have already lined up in an orderly layer before the local circuit neurons originate or migrate to their final positions. We do not know how these cells assemble in their correct spatial relationships, but it is a plausible hypothesis that, in each system, the principal neuron, being the first in the field, serves as the main organizing influence on the assembly of the local circuit neurons. The principal neuron has greater autonomy than the local circuit neurons, and this is shown by the fact that the program of development of principal neurons is relatively insensitive to changes in the external conditions. For example, although the granule cells and their parallel fibers are destroyed by panleukopenia virus or by X-rays, the Purkinje cells retain their dendritic spines, which are normally connected to the parallel fibers, showing that the spines are generated by factors within the Purkinje cell itself (Llinás *et al.,* 1973). The Purkinje cell dendritic spines persist in the complete absence of both climbing fibers and parallel fibers when fragments of cerebellum are cultured *in vitro* and stellate and basket cells synapse normally on the smooth fragments of the Purkinje cell dendrites in such cultures (Privat and Drian, 1976). In spite of the absence of most granule, basket, and stellate interneurons as a result of X-irradiation, the Purkinje cells exhibit essentially normal physiological characteristics such as spontaneous discharge and chemosensitivity (Woodward *et al.,* 1974).

The complexity of the mammalian brain has prompted a search for "simple" nervous systems in which the analysis of neuromorphogenesis might be accomplished more easily. While such simple systems as are found in some worms and some molluscs may provide the advantages of large neurons and relatively small total numbers of cells, the complexity in such nervous systems is no less than it is in the basic set of five neurons in the mammalian cerebellum. Indeed, there are no more than a few hundred different types of neurons in the entire mammalian brain, and each part of brain can be reduced to a neuronal set that contains about five types of neurons, as in the neuronal set that is the basic circuit module of the cerebellar cortex. Therefore, it is not the variety of cell types that makes the cerebellum more complex than the kidney, for example. Rather, complexity arises from the variety of interconnections between the different cell types belonging to a neuronal set, from the combinations of connections between similar neuronal sets within the cerebellar cortex, and from the connections of neuronal sets in the cerebellar cortex with different sets in other parts of the central nervous system.

The complexity of connectivity poses a considerable obstacle, but that can sometimes be overcome by looking at the development of connectivity. Organization of fearsome intricacy, when it is fully developed, may arise gradually by simple stages. In favorable cases, especially in systems in which development is protracted over a long time relative to the formation of individual components, it is not difficult to see the separate stages of development leading to the final complex organization. The cerebellar cortex provides such a favorable arena in which the genesis of each component can be mapped in time and space, and in which the components can be followed during their migrations and as they enter into synaptic associations. The way in which the five neuronal types are assembled in the cerebellar cortex may serve as a model of neuromorphogenesis that may help us to understand the morphogenesis of other systems that do not have the protracted developmental timetable and pristine geometry of the cerebellum.

3.4. Development of the Cerebellum

This section deals mainly with the development of the cerebellar cortex, which is similar in all vertebrates (Nieuwenhuys, 1964; Larsell, 1967). The adult cerebellum has three cortical layers—named in order from the outer surface: the molecular layer, the Purkinje cell layer, and the granular layer. The relationships of the cells in these layers are shown diagrammatically in Fig. 3.10. The connectivity of the cerebellum and the functions of the five types of neurons of which it is constructed are known in considerable detail (Eccles *et al.,* 1967).

The Purkinje cell is the principal neuron and the sole pathway out of the cerebellar cortex. Impulses are conducted into the cortex by the climbing fibers, which originate in the inferior olive, and by the mossy fibers, which are mostly the terminals of spinocerebellar and pontocerebellar fibers. There are also axons containing monoamines that originate in the locus coeruleus, raphe nuclei, and substantia nigra that enter the cortex and target on Purkinje cells. The afferent mossy and climbing fibers synapse with unerring precision on their postsynaptic targets: the climbing fibers terminate on thorns on the large dendritic branches of Purkinje cells and the mossy fibers terminate in structures called glomeruli in which they form synapses with dendrites of granule cells and the axons of Golgi type II cells. The local circuit neurons of the cerebellar cortex, so called because all their connections are within the cortex itself, are the Golgi, basket, stellate, and granule cells. The granule cell receives input from the mossy fiber. The granule cell axon, called the parallel fiber because it has a trajectory parallel with the axis of the folium, forms synaptic connections on dendritic spines of a row of Purkinje cells (Fig. 3.11). The parallel fibers also synapse on the dendrites of stellate, basket, and Golgi cells. The stellate cell forms synapses on Purkinje cell dendritic shafts, while the basket cell makes synapses with the soma of the Purkinje cell. The Golgi cell forms a local circuit that does not directly include Purkinje cells: the Golgi cell dendrites receive inputs from parallel fibers, while the Golgi cell axon synapses with granule cell dendrites within the glomerulus.

The geometrical organization of the cerebellum poses special problems of how such precisely specified interneuronal relationships develop. For these rea-

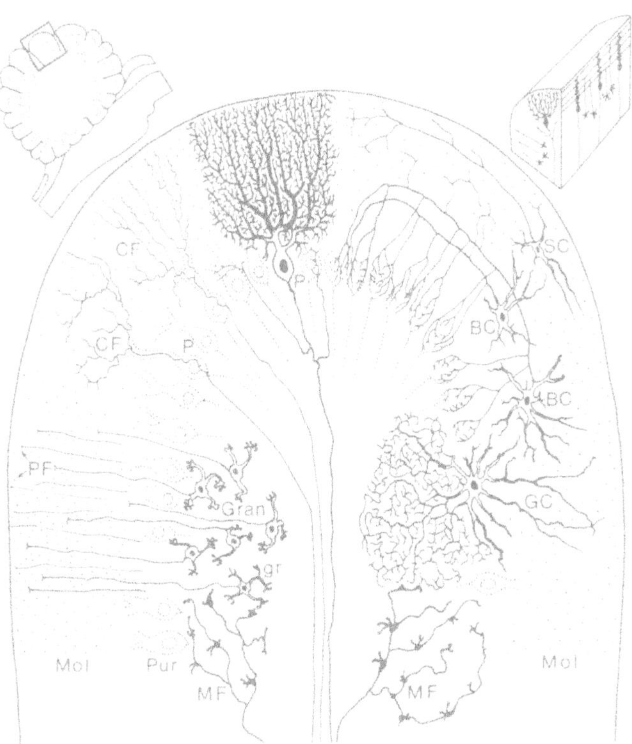

Figure 3.10. Folium of the mammalian cerebellum (a magnified section of the region shown in the rectangle). BC, Basket cell; CF, climbing fiber; Gran, granular layer; GC, Golgi II cell; gr, granule cells; MF, mossy fiber; Mol, molecular layer; P, Purkinje cells; Pur, Purkinje cell layer; PF, parallel fibers; SC, stellate cell.

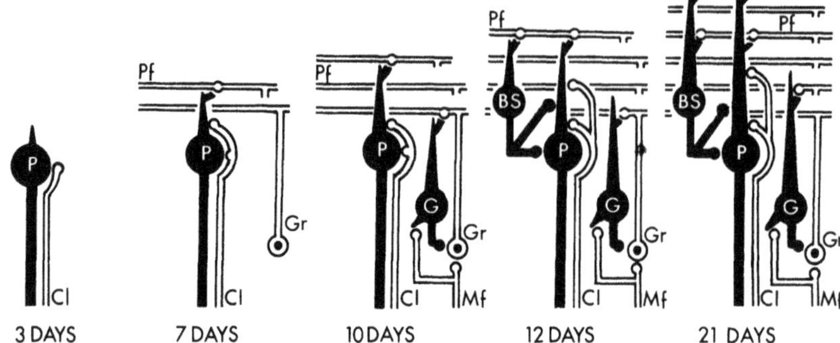

Figure 3.11. Diagram of the assembly of functional cerebellar cortical circuits during development in the white rat at 3–21 days after birth, assayed electrophysiologically. The dark cells are inhibitory, the light cells are excitatory. BS, Basket and stellate cells; Cl, climbing fiber; G, Golgi cell; Gr, granule cell; Mf, mossy fiber; P, Purkinje cell; Pf, parallel fiber. From T. Shimono, S. Nosaka, and K. Sasaki, *Brain Res. 108:*279–294 (1976).

sons, the cerebellum may well be the main battlefield upon which the conflict between various theories of neurogenesis may be decided.

The development of the cerebellar cortex proceeds in a similar order but at different rates in different vertebrates (Figs. 3.12 and 3.13). An extreme example is the bullfrog *Rana catesbeiana,* during the premetamorphic stages lasting about 2 years, the cerebellum remains in the form of a cerebellar plate containing undifferentiated Purkinje cells but no external granular layer. Only with the onset of metamorphosis does the external granular layer form and do the Purkinje cell dendrites grow and branch. These events occur rapidly at the same time as growth of the limbs (Gona, 1972, 1973, 1975, 1976). Other structural changes related to changes of function also occur after metamorphosis in the frog; the lateral line input to the auricular lobe (homologous with flocculus in mammals) disappears, and spinal and vestibular inputs develop as the frog emerges onto land (Larsell, 1923, 1925). The stage of development of the cerebellum at birth can be corre-

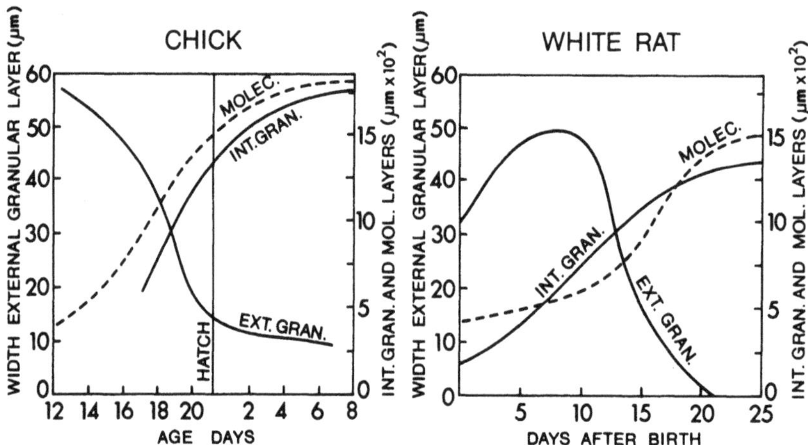

Figure 3.12. Changes in the average widths of layers of the cerebellar cortex of the chick and rat at various stages of development. Plotted from data in Saetersdal (1956); and Addison (1911).

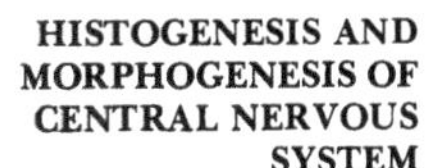

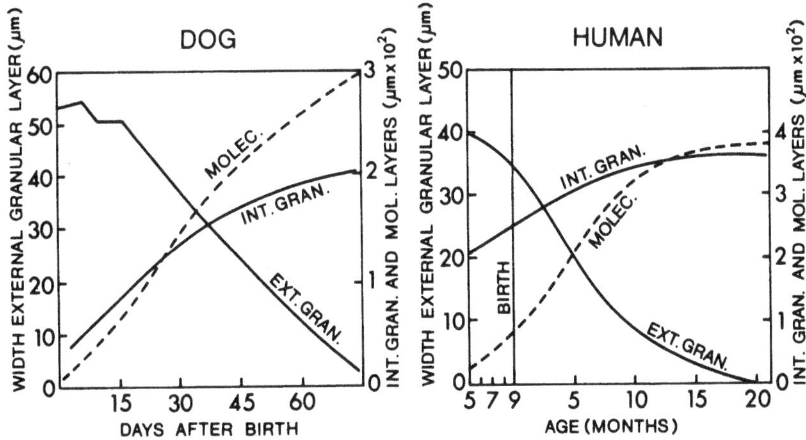

Figure 3.13. Changes in the average widths of layers of the cerebellar cortex of the dog and human at various stages of development. Plotted from data in Phemister and Young (1968) and Raaf and Kernohan (1944).

lated with the newborn animal's powers of locomotion and motor coordination. In precocial animals that are able to walk soon after birth (such as the chick, guinea pig, and ungulates), the cerebellum is well developed at birth, whereas in altricial animals (such as the mouse, rat, and man) that are helpless at birth, the cerebellum is in a corresponding state of immaturity, and its histogenesis and morphogenesis mainly occur after birth. That birth itself does not trigger the postnatal events of cerebellar neurogenesis and morphogenesis is shown by the fact that those events occur at the normal time but before birth in rat fetuses in which gestation is prolonged for 3 days beyond its normal duration (Zagon, 1975).

3.4.1. Histogenesis of the Cerebellar Cortex

The times and sites of origin of the Purkinje cell and of the four types of cerebellar local circuit neurons, as well as their migration routes to specific positions in the cortex, their distinctive patterns of differentiation and growth, and their synaptogenesis, have been described in several species. These observations show that assembly of such a complex system is in no way random but follows an invariant timetable. Histogenesis of large principal neurons occurs first, followed by genesis of local circuit neurons. Well-defined germinal zones can be demarcated, giving origin to different types of neurons in a regular timetable. The pattern of histogenesis of the cerebellar cortical neurons is complicated by the fact that cells originate from two separate germinal zones. A zone in the roof of the fourth ventricle gives origin to the Purkinje and Golgi II cells as well as some glial cells, all of which migrate outward toward the pia mater to form the mantle layer of the cerebellar plate. Somewhat later, another germinal zone, called the external granule layer, is formed immediately beneath the pia covering the cerebellar plate, and this gives origin to granule cells, stellate and basket cells, and some glial cells, all of which migrate deeper into the cerebral cortex.

Migration of young neurons out of the ventricular germinal zone to form the cerebellar plate mantle layer occurs before day 6 of incubation in the chick embryo

(Saetersdal, 1956, 1959; Forströnen, 1963; Hanaway, 1967), from days 11 to 13 of gestation in the mouse fetus (Miale and Sidman, 1961), before day 17 of gestation in the fetus of the albino rat (Addison, 1911), and from days 60 to 80 of gestation in the human fetus (Ellis, 1920; Raaf and Kernohan, 1944; Woodard, 1960; Rakic and Sidman, 1969, 1970). In the mouse and rat fetus, by day 17, the cerebellar plate is composed of an inner, ventricular germinal layer, a middle mantle or intermediate layer, and an outer marginal layer. The mantle layer of the cerebellar plate is composed of two strata. The deeper stratum of larger immature neurons differentiates to form the large neurons of the roof nuclei. The young neurons of the more superficial stratum of the mantle differentiate into Purkinje cells.

The Purkinje cells in the chick embryo are generated between days 3 and 6 of incubation, and DNA synthesis ceases in the ventricular germinal zone of the chick on day 12 of embryonic development (Hanaway, 1967). Using [^{3}H]thymidine autoradiography, Miale and Sidman (1961) showed that the Purkinje cells of the mouse cerebellum originate—as postmitotic cells no longer able to incorporate tritiated thymidine—on embryonic days 11, 12, and 13, and migrate out into the superficial part of the mantle from day 17. In pyridine–silver preparations of the 14-day embryonic mouse brain, axons, probably climbing fibers from the inferior olive and possibly also monoaminergic fibers from the locus coeruleus, raphe nuclei, and substantia nigra (Seiger and Olson, 1973; Lauder and Bloom, 1974, 1975), may be seen to have grown into the cerebellum in the path of migrating Purkinje cells (Sidman, 1968).

The other cerebellar cells that are derived from the ventricular germinal zone are the Golgi II neurons, the small neurons of the roof nuclei, and probably some glial cells. The precursors of the Golgi II neurons complete their final DNA synthesis and mitosis on embryonic days 12–15 in the albino mouse and migrate directly from the ventricular germinal zone to the molecular layer of the cerebellar cortex (Miale and Sidman, 1961). In the mouse, cells originating in the ventricular germinal zone after embryonic day 13 differentiate into small neurons of the roof nuclei (Miale and Sidman, 1961; Taber Pierce, 1967*b*). Mitotic activity in the ventricular germinal zone decreases between days 13 and 15 and ceases by day 17 of gestation in the mouse fetus (Miale and Sidman, 1961). Development of cells derived from the external granular layer (the granule cells, basket and stellate cells, and probably some glial cells) will be discussed following the next section on the development of Purkinje cells.

3.4.2. Purkinje Cell Ontogenesis

In all vertebrates the Purkinje cells are derived from the ventricular germinal zone and migrate out into the superficial layers of the mantle of the cerebellar plate; they are initially small and are arranged in irregular rows up to 12 cells thick that become thinned out to a single row during the subsequent growth of the cerebellum. Purkinje cells originate on E14–E17 in the rat fetus, on E11–E14 in the mouse fetus, on E3–E6 in the chick embryo: in all cases the production of Purkinje cells commences and ceases before that of any other type of cell in the cerebellar cortex. The Purkinje cells apparently remain quiescent for several days after their generation and migration. They grow very slowly until the proliferation of external granule cells occurs. The Purkinje cells begin to differentiate rapidly after the granule cells migrate past them from the external granule layer to the internal granule layer. These events occur 4–20 days after birth in the albino mouse and albino rat, and from fetal month 4 to postnatal month 11 in humans. The Purkinje cells form a single row at about 4 days postnatally in the rat (Addison, 1911; Altman and Winfree, 1977) and 10 days postnatally in the mouse (Miale and Sidman, 1961). Their nuclei continue to increase in size until postnatal day 10 in the mouse and postnatal day 14 in the rat, but in spite of earlier reports to the contrary, the Purkinje cells do not become polyploid.

There have been numerous reports of tetraploidy in Purkinje cells: the Purkinje cells are apparently diploid at birth but ostensibly attain a tetraploid DNA content some weeks later (Sandritter *et al.,* 1967; Lapham, 1968; Nováková *et al.,* 1968; Herman and Lapham, 1968; Lentz and Lapham, 1969, 1970). In all these reports the DNA was measured by cytophotometry of thick paraffin or frozen sections stained by the Feulgen technique. However, the reported increases of cellular DNA content are incorrect and are probably artifacts of the cytophotometric method. Mann and Yates (1973*a*) and S. Fujita (1974), who controlled for nonspecific loss of light in their cytophotometric measurements, reported diploid DNA values in Purkinje cell nuclei and in the cerebellum of adult humans. When measured biochemically, the DNA content of Purkinje cell nuclei isolated from 8 to 10-week-old mice was found to be in the normal diploid range (J. Cohen *et al.,* 1973). Consistent with these reports is the finding that developing Purkinje cells show no labeling with tritiated thymidine administered during the period of apparent increase in ploidy as measured by the Feulgen technique (Mareš *et al.,* 1974). Cumulative exposure to tritiated thymidine for 18 days *in vitro* did not result in labeling of Purkinje cells in the cerebellum of the newborn rat (Manuelidis and Manuelidis, 1974). These findings throw doubt not only on previous reports of tetraploid Purkinje cells but also on other reports of polyploidy in neurons (see Section 2.2). The technique of Feulgen cytophotometry is not in question if it is used with proper precautions (S. Fujita *et al.,* 1971, 1972, 1974; Mann and Yates, 1973*a;* S. Fujita, 1974). In fact, polyploid glial cells discovered in the Purkinje cell layer by Lapham and Johnstone (1963) have been confirmed in the human cerebellum by Mann and Yates (1973*b*). They found that polyploidy is not age dependent, and reported a strict numerical ratio between these glia and Purkinje cells: for each Purkinje cell they found 1 octaploid, 50 tetraploid, and 250 diploid glial cells.

The axon of the Purkinje cell can be seen at the time of birth, and the axonal collaterals that spread transversely from one Purkinje cell to the cell bodies of neighboring Purkinje cells develop shortly after birth in the rat. The growth of the dendrites of the Purkinje cells is shown by the increase in width of the molecular layer of the cerebellar cortex (Fig. 3.11). From postnatal days 4 to 10 in the mouse and the first 21 postnatal days in the rat, the Purkinje cells undergo the changes beautifully illustrated by Ramón y Cajal (1909–1911). The growth of the Purkinje cell dendrites and the increase in their branching have been described in detail in the rat by Addison (1911) and Altman (1972*b*). In the newborn rat the Purkinje cells have an apical dendritic process, which may or may not have a few branches. The first outgrowths from the apical pole of the Purkinje cells become resorbed. Growth of the Purkinje cell dendrites is delayed until after birth and occurs over a prolonged period during which the external granular layer gives origin to granule cells. The tips of the Purkinje cell dendrites reach only as far as the inner layer of external granule cells, and as the external granular layer becomes depleted, so do the Purkinje cell dendrites branch and extend closer to the pial surface. In the rat the tips of the dendrites reach the pia at 20–25 days after birth, at the time of disappearance of the external granular layer. According to Addison (1911), the number of terminal branches of Purkinje cell dendrites continues to increase up to 110 days after birth in the rat.

Growth of the Purkinje cell dendrites in the cat has been described by Purpura *et al.* (1964). At birth, the Purkinje cells of the cat have a short, unbranched dendrite. Branching of the dendrites occurs especially between 8 and 12 days after birth, and this happens simultaneously with the inward migration of the granule cells. By postnatal day 40 in the cat, the Purkinje cell dendrites have developed dendritic spines, and the dendrites are fully developed by 60 days after birth.

The differentiation of Purkinje cells in man follows the same sequence as in other mammals, but the human Purkinje cells differentiate and grow more slowly (Zecevic and Rakic, 1976). During the fourth fetal month (12–16 weeks), the Purkinje cells are distributed in several rows, and have smooth somas and dendrites which are short and unbranched. During the period from 16 to 28 weeks of gestation, the Purkinje cells become aligned as a monocellular layer, spines develop on somata, and further branching of dendrites occurs. The first synapses develop on the somatic spines and on the dendritic shafts at about 16 weeks and continue to form thereafter. The somatic spines disappear, the dendrites branch, and spines start appearing on the secondary and tertiary branches between the 24th and 28th fetal weeks and continue to form until the dendrites have completed their growth and assumed the adult form at the end of the first postnatal year.

The relationship between the migration of granule cells, the growth of Purkinje cell dendrites and the synapses between the axons of the granule cells (the parallel fibers), and the dendritic spines of Purkinje cells has been discussed by Ramón y Cajal (1929*a,* Chapter 12). He proposed the "tentative hypothesis" that the growth of the Purkinje cell dendrites is stimulated by the appearance of the parallel fibers and the migration of the granule cells. This is rather similar to Sidman's (1968) notion that an interaction may occur between the Purkinje cells and the granule cells that migrate past them, resulting in the formation of specific connections between them. Although these proposals are still in the realm of speculation, there is evidence that the development of Purkinje cell dendrites is stimulated in some unknown way by the migration of granule cells and the development of parallel fibers. That the matter is not quite so simple as the hypothesis would suggest is shown by the fact that in the human fetus the growth of Purkinje cell dendrites commences before the first migration of granule cells, thus demonstrating an aspect of the Purkinje cell's autonomy (Rakic and Sidman, 1970). The Purkinje cell dendrites do not develop normally but remain stunted if the external granule cells are destroyed by X-rays (Purpura *et al.,* 1964) or by a virus (Kilham and Margolis, 1964, 1965, 1966*a,b*). This does not show the cause of the dendritic malformation, which may be due to the direct action of the radiation or virus on the dendrites or may be indirectly due to destruction of granule cells. The latter may be required to stimulate the growth and branching of the dendrites of Purkinje cells, either as the granule cells migrate past the Purkinje cells or as their parallel fibers form synapses on the Purkinje cell dendrites.

Development of climbing fibers has been described by Athias (1897*a*), Ramón y Cajal (1909–1911), and O'Leary *et al.* (1971). They grow into the cerebellum from the inferior olive, and perhaps also from other sources. The climbing fibers, with their characteristic varicosities, can be seen in reduced silver or Golgi preparations during the early postnatal period from the time of onset of growth of Purkinje cell dendrites. At first, the climbing fibers have numerous redundant branches, which later disappear. Initially, the climbing fibers form a plexus in the granular layer, contributing to the *lamina dissecans,* a layer that appears transiently between the Purkinje and granular layers in the human cerebellum. This is described below. The terminal branches of the developing climbing fibers contact Purkinje cell bodies, apparently making transient synaptic connections there (Mugnaini, 1969, 1970; Larramendi, 1969; Altman, 1972*b*). As the growth of Purkinje cell dendrites occurs, the climbing fibers extend over the surface of all the dendritic branches. At that stage the climbing fibers largely leave the cell body, clearing the way for the later growth of basket cell processes onto the Purkinje cell body. This development extends from the age of 5 days to 30 days postnatally in the rat.

The mechanism of selective association between climbing fibers and Purkinje cells is unknown. Ramón y Cajal cited this as a prime example in support of his theory of chemotaxis, suggesting that the climbing fibers, "upon arriving from distant centers, smell out, so to speak, the bodies of the Purkinje elements, which they embrace by means of varicose nests, which are the rudiments of the future arborizations" (Ramón y Cajal, 1917).

A layer of cytoplasmic processes lying between the Purkinje cell bodies and the internal granular layer develops transiently in the human cerebellum. This layer, called the *lamina dissecans* by Hayashi (1924), has been studied more recently by Verbitskaya (1969) and by Rakic and Sidman (1970). It has also been shown in the developing cerebellum of the blue whale (Korneliussen, 1967) and is probably found in all primates and other mammals with a long period of gestation. In the human cerebellum the lamina dissecans first appears at 20–21 weeks of gestation as an acellular layer 15–20 μm thick. It persists for about 10 weeks and then disappears. Its presence can thus be used as an indication of fetal age. The lamina dissecans contains axonal terminals of mossy and climbing fibers and transient cytoplasmic outgrowths from developing granule and Purkinje cells (Rakic and Sidman, 1970).

3.4.3. Ontogenesis of Cerebellar Local Circuit Neurons

The granule cells, stellate cells, and basket cells, and probably some of the cerebellar glial cells, are derived from germinal cells that originate from the rhombic lip and migrate over the surface of the cerebellar plate to form a germinal zone, the external granular layer. The granule cells are generated in the external granular layer and migrate through the molecular layer and Purkinje cell layer to form the internal granular layer (Obersteiner, 1883; Ramón y Cajal, 1890*a,b;* Schaper, 1894*a,b,* 1895). The external granular cells migrate over the surface of the cerebellum from the rostral part of the rhombic lip, a germinal zone in the alar plate forming the wall of the fourth ventricle (Schaper, 1894*a,b,* 1895; Ramón y Cajal, 1909–1911; Addison, 1911; Raaf and Kernohan, 1944). The germinal zone giving rise to the external granular layer is the most rostral part of the rhombic lip, the more caudal parts of which give rise to cells that migrate to form the inferior olivary nuclei, cochlear nuclei, and pontine nuclei (Harkmark, 1954; Taber Pierce, 1966, 1967*a,b,* 1973). The cells migrating from the rhombic lip form a continuous sheet extending rostrally over the cerebellar plate and medially into the brain stem, where the mass of migrating cells is termed the *pontobulbar body* in the human fetus (Essick, 1907, 1912).

DNA synthesis and mitosis in the ventricular germinal zone decrease during the 13- to 15-day fetal period in the mouse, while at the same time the number of cells increases in the external granular layer (Miale and Sidman, 1961). In the chick embryo, mitotic activity declines in the ventricular germinal zone after day 8 and ceases on day 12, while the external granular layer appears only on day 6 and increases in thickness between days 8 and 15 of embryonic development (Saetersdal, 1956, 1959). Moreover, the DNA content, and hence the number of cells, of the chick cerebellum increases 400 percent between days 11 and 21 of incubation (Margolis, 1969), as is shown in Fig. 3.20. This increase must be due entirely to proliferation of external granule cells because proliferation in the ventricular germinal zone ceases on day 12 of incubation.

The histogenesis of granule cells in the external granular layer has been described in the chick (Ramón y Cajal, 1890*a;* Saetersdal, 1956, 1959; Forströnen, 1963; Hanaway, 1967; Mugnaini and Forströnen, 1967), the mouse (L. L. Uzman, 1960; Miale and Sidman, 1961; S. Fujita *et al.,* 1966; S. Fujita, 1967; Mareš *et al.,* 1970), the rat (Addison, 1911; Altman and Das, 1966; Altman, 1966*b,* 1972*c*), the dog (Ramón y Cajal, 1929*a;* Phemister and Young, 1968), the cat (Purpura *et al.,* 1964), the monkey (Kornguth *et al.,* 1967, 1968), and the human (Ellis, 1920; Raaf and Kernohan, 1944; J. S. Woodard, 1960; Rakic and Sidman, 1970).

The external granular layer appears first over the posterolateral part of the cerebellum and spreads anteromedially to cover the entire cerebellar plate. In all vertebrates the external granular layer increases in thickness from a single layer of cells to a layer six to eight cells deep as a result of proliferation of external granule cells. Mitotic figures are scattered throughout the external granular layer during the period of its increase in thickness. In this respect the external granular layer does not resemble the ventricular germinal zone in which cells retract toward the ventricle during mitosis. Therefore, it appears unlikely that interkinetic nuclear migration occurs in the external granular cells. The external granular layer persists for a period that varies according to the species, but eventually it becomes reduced in thickness to a single layer of cells and ultimately disappears. The external granular layer disappears at about the time of birth or soon after birth in precocial animals such as the chick or guinea pig, but it persists for some time after birth in altricial animals. For example, the external granular layer disappears only 20–25 days after birth in the albino mouse and rat, at about 60 days after birth in the cat, at about 75 days after birth in the dog, and at about 600 days after birth in humans (Fig. 3.12 and 3.13). During the initial period of increase in thickness of the external granular layer, cumulative labeling with [^{3}H]thymidine results in labeling of 100 percent of the external granular cells (S. Fujita *et al.,* 1966). This shows that all the cells are engaged in DNA synthesis and mitosis. However, in the second half of the period of development of the external granular layer, a zone of cells without mitotic figures has been described, lying between the actively proliferating external granular cells and the molecular layer (Ramón y Cajal, 1909–1911; Addison, 1911). The cells in this zone do not incorporate [^{3}H]thymidine (Fig. 3.14), thus showing that they have ceased mitosis (S. Fujita *et al.,* 1966).

Migration of the granule cells was known to pose a difficult problem; because they arise late in development, they have to migrate along paths apparently blocked by obstacles in the form of cells that have developed earlier, and yet, as Ramón y Cajal showed (Fig. 3.15), they follow a straight radial path. This problem has now been solved with the discovery that the Bergmann glia act as guides for migrating granule cells (Mugnaini and Forströnen, 1967; Rakic, 1971*b*), In Golgi preparations, Ramón y Cajal recognized the changes in shape and position of the granule cells as they migrate from the external granular layer (Fig. 3.15). The cells in the superficial half of the external granular layer, which are in various phases of the generation cycle, were named the "phase embryonale ou indifferent" by Ramón y Cajal (1909–1911). In the deeper part of the external granular layer the cells are bipolar, with two processes oriented parallel to the surface in the direction of the folia similar to the parallel fibers of the mature cortex ("phase de la bipolarité horizontale"). Ramón y Cajal recognized that these were postmitotic granule cells at the beginning of their inward migration. By the use of tritiated thymidine autoradiography, it has been shown that these granule cells have ceased DNA synthesis (Fig. 3.14), since they remain unlabeled after a period of exposure to the [^{3}H]thymidine that results in labeling of all the cells in the superficial zone

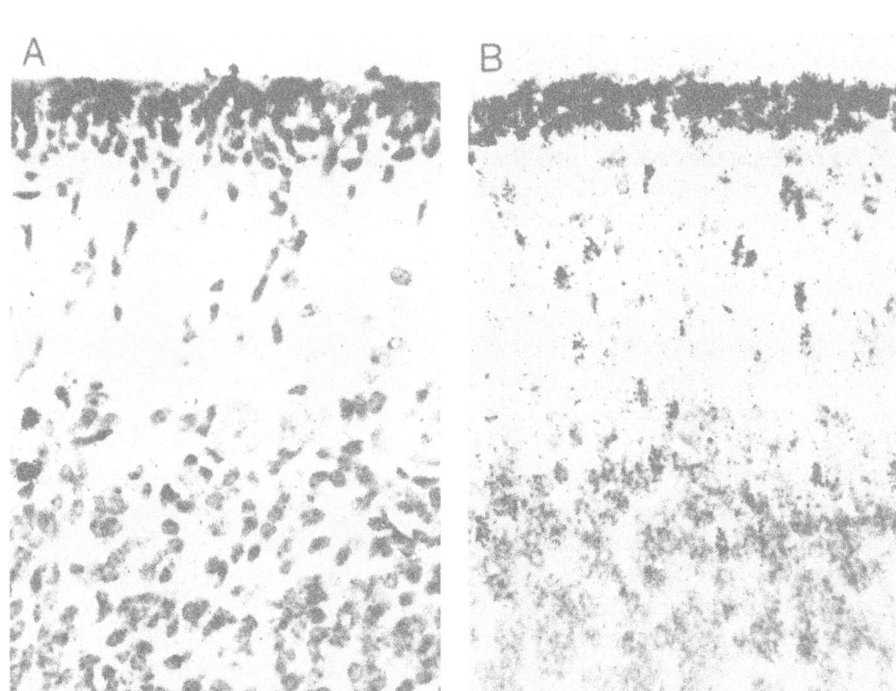

Figure 3.14. Autoradiographs of the cerebellar cortex of the mouse injected with tritiated thymidine at 10 days after birth and killed 10 hr later (A) and 31 hr later (B). In A the cells in the superficial zone of the external granule layer are heavily labeled, and some glial cells in the vicinity of the Purkinje cells are labeled. The cells in the deep part of the external granule layer and the granule cells (with elongated nuclei) migrating down through the molecular layer are not labeled. In (B) the labeled cells have moved from the superficial to the deep half of the external granule layer, and labeled granule cells are in the process of migrating down through the molecular and Purkinje cell layers. EG, External granule layer; M, molecular layer; P, Purkinje cell layer; IG, internal granule layer. From S. Fujita, *J. Cell Biol.* *32*:277–287 (1967).

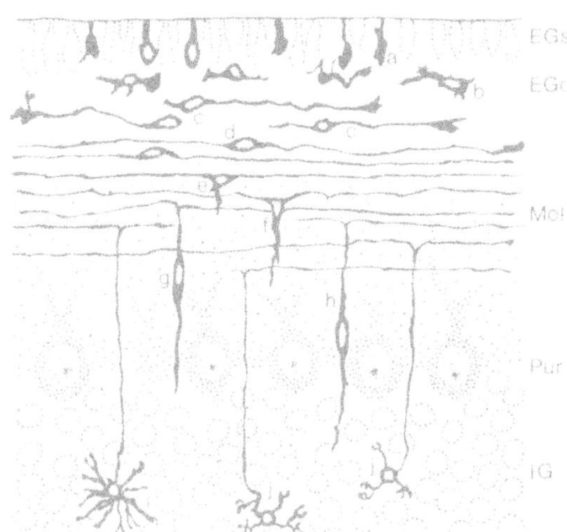

Figure 3.15. Phases in the migration and differentiation of cerebellar granule cells (a–j) from the superficial zone of the external granule layer (EGs) to the deep zone of the external granule layer (EGd), through the molecular layer (Mol) and Purkinje cell layer (Pur) to the internal granule layer (IG) of the mammalian cerebellum. Modified from S. Ramón y Cajal (1909–1911).

of the external granular layer (S. Fujita *et al.,* 1966; S. Fujita, 1967). A third cytoplasmic process grows from the granule cells vertically down into the molecular layer, and the nucleus migrates into this process. The cells assume a T shape ("phase de la bipolarité verticale"), as the nucleus migrates within the vertical cytoplasmic process and through the molecular layer and Purkinje cell layer. When the granule cell reaches its position in the internal granular layer, its migration ends, and some short, clawlike telodendria sprout from the cell body. This was termed the "phase du grain profond ou jeune" by Ramón y Cajal (1909–1911). The telodendria of the granule cells and of the Golgi cells, together with terminals of the mossy fibers, form the cerebellar glomeruli, which are first seen in the inner nuclear layer at 12–14 days after birth in the rat (Addison, 1911). As the granule cells continue to be formed into the third week, and as additional time is taken by their migration and the growth of their dendrites, the formation of glomeruli continues for more than 30 days postnatally (Altman, 1972*c*).

It seems, from the arrangement of the internal granule cells, as if the deepest granule cells are generated first and the internal granular layer is formed in "inside-out" order. The axons of granule cells in the outer layer of the internal granular layer ascend to the surface of the molecular layer, while the granule cells lying progressively deeper send their axons to correspondingly deeper levels of the molecular layer (C. A. Fox *et al.,* 1967; Altman, 1972*b*).

Mugnaini and Forströnen (1967) studied the ultrastructural changes that occur in the cerebellar cortex of the chick embryo at 17–20 days of development and found a continuous series of transitional forms of granule cells between the external and internal granular layers. Electron microscopy has thus confirmed the description of migrating granule cells illustrated by Ramón y Cajal (1890*a,b,* 1909–1911), and has shown that the radially oriented Bergmann glia are used as guides by the granule cells (Fig. 3.15) as they migrate from the external to the internal granular layer (reviewed by Sidman and Rakic, 1973).

Proliferation and migration of cerebellar granule cells have been studied in the newborn mouse by means of [^{3}H]thymidine autoradiography (Miale and Sidman, 1961; Altman, 1966*b;* S. Fujita *et al.,* 1966). S. Fujita *et al.,* (1966) determined the percentage of labeled cells in the internal and external granular layers of the cerebellum of the newborn mouse at different times after a single injection of [^{3}H]thymidine (pulse labeling) and after the cells had been exposed to the labeled nucleotide for longer periods (cumulative labeling). The percentage of cells in the external granular layer which are labeled 2 hours after a single injection of [^{3}H]thymidine increases from 30 percent at birth to 44 percent at day 7 postnatally and then diminishes to zero at 20 days (S. Fujita *et al.*, 1966). Proliferation in the cerebellar ventricular germinal zone ceases after postnatal day 10 in the mouse cerebellum, and labeling after P10 is confined almost entirely to the external granule cells, which makes it relatively easy to follow their migration. Their transit time can be determined from the time of a pulse of [^{3}H]thymidine to the time of first appearance of labeled granule cells in the internal granular layer. Altman (1966*b*) estimated that the maximum transit time of external granule cells over a distance of 200 μm is 3 days; the minimum speed of migration is 1.7–2.5 μm per hour. According to S. Fujita *et al.* (1966), the transit time is 42 hours, and the speed of migration of cerebellar granule cells is approximately 100 μm per day in the mouse (4.2 μm per hour). These rates of migration should be compared with the rate of 5.5 μm per hour of neurons migrating from the ventricular germinal zone to the cortical plate of the rhesus monkey (Rakic, 1974) and the migration rate of 4 μm per hour of neurons in the chick optic tectum (LaVail and Cowan, 1971*b*) and chick isthmo-optic nucleus (P. G. H. Clarke *et al.*, 1976). The similar rates found independently in several different systems and species indicate that the underlying mechanisms of neuronal migration are probably similar in all these cases.

Concerning the origins of cerebellar glial cells, Ramón y Cajal concluded that only neurons are derived from the external granular layer, whereas all cerebellar glia are derived from the periventricular germinal layer. Schaper (1894*a,b,* 1895) proposed that the external granular layer consists of "indifferent cells" that may give rise to glia as well as neurons. From the results of [^{3}H]thymidine autoradiography, S. Fujita *et al.* (1966) concluded that glioblasts originating from the ventricular germinal zone have already dispersed throughout the cerebellum of the mouse at birth before any cells have migrated from the external granular layer. The pulse labeling experiments make it clear that a great deal of cell proliferation occurs in the internal granular layer of the mouse cerebellum from birth to postnatal day 5. Between birth and 5 days, labeling of 5–10 percent of cells in the internal granular layer occurs within 2 hours after a single injection of [^{3}H]thymidine. In that short period, labeled cells could not have migrated into the internal granular layer, and they must therefore be glioblasts, proliferating in the internal granular layer, because cell migration from the external granular layer does not commences until postnatal day 3 in the mouse. S. Fujita *et al.* (1966) concluded that the glioblasts of the internal granular layer originate from the ventricular germinal zone. They suggested that only after the cells of the external granular layer cease producing neurons do they change into glioblasts, which form the oligodendrocytes and astrocytes of the molecular layer. This is supposed to occur several days before the disappearance of the external granular layer, which occurs about postnatal day 20 in the mouse.

Some of the cells produced in the external granular layer migrate only as far as the molecular layer, and there differentiate into basket cells and small stellate cells. According to Altman (1972*a*), the basket and stellate cells are impeded from penetrating deeper than the underlying bed of parallel fibers because their processes are oriented at a right angle to the parallel fibers. In the rat the basket cells originate mainly on postnatal days 6 and 7, while the stellate cells originate mainly on days 8–11 (Altman, 1972*a*).

Some indication of the proliferative activity of the external granular layer may be gained from the observations that the DNA content of the mouse cerebellum increases 580 percent in the first 2 weeks after birth (Howard, 1968) and the DNA content of the chick cerebellum increases 400 percent in the last 10 days of incubation (Margolis, 1969). These increases can be attributed largely to the formation of granule cells and, to a far lesser extent to glial proliferation. With a generation time of 16–20 hours, the external granule cells of the mouse can produce at least 14 generations in the first 14 days after birth, while in fact the total number of cells (DNA content of the cerebellum) increases 6 times. This indicates that many external granule cells cease DNA synthesis and mitosis before day 14.

Early reports of a gradual reduction in the number of cells in the rat cerebellum (Inukai, 1928) and the human cerebellum (Ellis, 1920) from birth to old age have not been confirmed by the more accurate methods of assaying for the total number of cells by measuring the DNA content of the brain. Howard (1973) has shown that the DNA content of the cerebellum of the mouse remains constant from 60 to 470 days of age. As there is no cell production in the cerebellum at that age, the results show that there is also negligible cell death. However, death of up to 3 percent of postmitotic cells occurs in the external granular layer of normal rats up to 21 days after birth (P. D. Lewis, 1975). In support of the concept of stability of the cerebellar cortical cells in the adult is the failure to find any electron microscopic evidence of degenerating cells in the cerebellar cortex of the adult rat, whereas in the same study, degenerating neurons were found in the lateral cerebellar nucleus (Chan-Palay, 1973).

3.4.4. Selective Effects of Harmful Agents on Developing Cerebellar Cortical Neurons

An aspect of the specificity of neuronal types is their selective sensitivity or resistance to infections, cytotoxic agents, and ionizing radiation. Differences in the effect of such agents may thus help to reveal singularities in structure and function or in the developmental programs of the cerebellar neurons. Cells undergoing rapid mitosis and migrating cells are particularly susceptible to damage or destruction by radiation, cytotoxins, or virus infections. The external granule layer of the cerebellum is one of the sites of the most intense proliferative and migratory activity in newborn mammals. Agents acting in the perinatal and early postnatal period are thus likely to interfere with the development of cerebellar granule cells, and the other cerebellar cells may change as a result of loss of granule cells. Such changes have been reported in the mammalian cerebellum as a result of postnatal X-irradiation (Hicks, 1958; Hicks *et al.*, 1961; Hicks and D'Amato, 1966; Altman *et al.*, 1968, 1969; Altman and Anderson, 1972), viruses (Kilham and Margolis, 1964, 1965, 1966*a,b;* Herndon *et al.*, 1971*a,b*), cytotoxic chemicals such as nitrogen mustard, triethylene melamine, and other toxins (Hicks, 1954; Herndon, 1968; Nathanson *et al.*, 1969; Shimada and Langman, 1970; Chanda *et al.*, 1973), the thymidine analogue 5-bromodeoxyuridine (Zamenhof *et al.*, 1971*b*; Webster *et al.*, 1973), and fluorodeoxyuridine, which inhibits DNA synthesis (Maruyama *et al.*, 1968; Shimada and Langman, 1970; Webster *et al.*, 1973). External granular cells that survive the effects of X-rays or fluorodeoxyuridine can proliferate and reconstitute the external granule layer (Altman *et al.*, 1969; Shimada and Langman, 1970; Altman and Anderson, 1972).

After destruction of the cerebellar granule cells, a variety of changes have been seen in the other cells of the cerebellum. Some of the changes, for example, the stunting of Purkinje cell dendrites, may be ascribed to removal of the normal afferents to the dendrites of Purkinje cells. The dendritic spines persist after removal of their afferents, and the deafferented spines remain permanently disconnected as a rule, but in rare cases they have been found making anomalous synapses with mossy fibers (Altman and Anderson, 1972; Llinás *et al.*, 1973). In the cerebellar cortex of ferrets after infection with panleukopenia virus, which destroys the granule cells, Llinás *et al.* (1973) found some evidence indicating that the mossy fibers, deprived of the granule cells which are their normal postsynaptic targets, may form anomalous synapses on stellate, basket, and Golgi cells. This is of interest in relation to mechanisms of development of neuronal connections, but the pathological changes that occur after virus infection should not be extrapolated too freely to normal development, and the term "neuronal plasticity" should not be used in such cases. To apply the term to all reactions of the nervous system in response to injury, regardless of the mechanism of the neuronal reaction, would only corrupt the meaning of the term. The term "neuronal plasticity" is better reserved for adaptive modifications of neurons within the normal physiological range, and is thus a form of homeostasis. In the pathological case, the "specificity" of the mossy fibers themselves or of the cerebellar neurons may have been altered by the virus so that mossy fibers fail to recognize their correct postsynaptic targets. On the other hand, the anomalous connections may be interpreted to support the theory that specificity of connections is not absolute but merely relative: connections may normally be made on the basis of the best fit between pre- and postsynaptic elements, but if the normal best fit cannot be achieved, a second best fit may be a viable alternative. This and other hypotheses of the mechanisms of selective formation of synapses and of neuronal plasticity are discussed in Sections 5.5 and 9.6.

3.4.5. Mutations Affecting the Development of the Cerebellum

Several mutations that affect the cerebellum have been described in the mouse. They represent a small fraction of more than 90 neurological mutations that are known in this species (Sidman *et al.*, 1965). By comparing the normal mice with mutants or by comparing one mutation with another, mechanisms may eventually be found that may be attributed to the action of a single gene.

All known mutations affecting the cerebellum are autosomal recessive mutations. They are not clustered on any chromosome. It is noteworthy that they all have their influence on morphogenesis, not on histogenesis. The various cerebellar neurons originate at the normal times and apparently in normal numbers, but the mutations produce changes in cell migration and differentation. It is likely that mutations that affect histogenesis will have such widespread repercussions as to preclude fetal survival, even in the heterozygous condition. This is entirely in accord with **the concept that almost all mutations affecting development do so at late stages because mutations affecting early stages of development are usually lethal** (Huxley and De Beer, 1934; M. Jacobson, 1974b, 1975a). The salient features of the mutant mice with cerebellar abnormalities are summarized as follows:

Swaying (Sidman, 1968). Mice with the swaying mutation show hypotonia of the limbs and ataxia from birth. Parts of the anterior cerebellar vermis are missing, and the remainder of the vermis is malformed and fused with the colliculi. The cerebellar cortex is broken into islands of cells by aberrant fascicles of nerve fibers. Despite the disruption of the normal morphology, the individual cell types preserve their proper anatomical relationships. This is in marked contrast to the abnormal intercellular relationships found in all the other cerebellar mutants.

Weaver (Sidman *et al.,* 1965; Sidman, 1968). In the homozygous weaver mutant the cerebellum is small due to loss of almost all the granule cells during the first and second weeks after birth. The mice are small, hypotonic, ataxic, and have a severe tremor, but some survive to adulthood. Other parts of the nervous system and other organs are normal. Other abnormalities of the cerebellum include stunting of the dendrites of Purkinje cells, which form several rows. Despite the absence of the parallel fibers that normally synapse on the Purkinje dendritic spines, the latter appear unaffected (A. Hirano and Dembitzer, 1973). There are abnormal connections between mossy fibers and Golgi II cells, and climbing fibers retain their connections with somatic thorns of Purkinje cells (Landis, 1973). The primary defect in weaver was at first thought to be in the granule cells (Sidman, 1968). The granule cells originate at the normal time and apparently in normal quantities, but they die at the inner margin of the external granular layer. Evidence that the defect is not in the granule cells came when Rezai and Yoon (1972) showed that in the heterozygote, which is normal behaviorally, the rate of migration of granule cells is slowed, indicating that the death of granule cells in the homozygote is secondary to failure of migration. The role of Bergmann glia as guides for migrating granule cells first proposed by Mugnaini and Forströnen (1967), and later much amplified by Rakic (1971*b*), indicated that the primary effect of the mutation might be on the Bergmann glia. Rakic and Sidman (1973*a,b,c*) reported that the Bergmann glia are reduced in number and morphologically abnormal. The Bergmann cell abnormalities are first seen after the third postnatal day in homozygotes as well as in heterozygotes. The Bergmann glial cells are enlarged 2–4 times in diameter and have a variety of cytoplasmic abnormalities (Rakic and Sidman, 1973*b,c*; Bignami and Dahl, 1974*b*; Sotelo and Changeux, 1974*b*). These findings indicate that the effect in the Bergmann glia precedes and may be the cause of the death of granule cells. However, it is not known whether the defect in the mutant is a loss of some vital activity of the glial cell or whether it is a failure of the granule cell to respond to the defective glial cell. Indeed, it is not known whether the granule cells normally use the glial cells as a passive guide or whether glial cells play an active role in granule cell migration. In spite of the excellent morphological studies, we still have no indication of the primary gene product that is altered in any of the cerebellar mutants.

Staggerer. The staggerer mutant is clinically similar to weaver, including the ataxia, slight tremor, hypotonia, and a small cerebellum deficient in granule cells, but the pathogenesis is entirely different in the two mutants. Here the defect is first seen in the Purkinje cells, which are small and have stunted dendrites almost devoid of spines (Sidman, 1968, 1972). The granule cells originate on schedule and migrate normally but then die in the second to fifth weeks after birth. Sidman (1974) and Sotelo and Changeux (1974*a*) have suggested that the granule cells die because they are dependent on the formation of connections with their usual postsynaptic elements, the spines of Purkinje cell dendrites, which are absent in staggerer. However, this dependence is not reciprocal, for the Purkinje cell dendritic spines are not dependent on the granule cell inputs. This is demonstrated by the survival of the dendritic spines in the absence of granule cells in weaver as well as after depletion of granule cells by irradiation, virus infection, or cytotoxins (Altman *et al.,* 1969; A. Hirano *et al.,* 1972; Llinás *et al.,* 1973).

Reeler (Falconer, 1951; Hamburgh, 1960, 1963; Meier and Hoag, 1962; Sidman *et al.,* 1965). Reeler mice have ataxia, hypotonia, and a fine tremor. The cerebellum is small and the fissures are greatly reduced. The Purkinje cells are misplaced and misaligned. They have stunted dendrites with few small branchlets and gross disorientation of the dendritic tree. The granule cells are reduced in number, and most lie external to the Purkinje cells. Synaptogenesis appears to occur normally, despite the cellular disarray (Rakic and Sidman, 1972). Similar malformations occur in the hippocampal cortex and cerebral isocortex. Just as the granule cells fail to migrate past the cerebellar Purkinje cells, the granule cells of the fascia dentata fail to migrate to their proper positions (Meier and Hoag, 1962), and the young neurons of the cerebral isocortex fail to migrate outward past the neurons that preceded them (Hamburgh, 1960, 1963; Caviness and Sidman, 1972, 1973; Devor *et al.,* 1975). Electrophysiologically, there do not appear to be abnormal connections in the hippocampus despite cellular malpositioning (Bliss and Chung, 1974). Conservation of normal synaptic associations between malpositioned and disoriented neurons in the cerebral and cerebellar cortex is a good example of the selective growth of axons to their postsynaptic targets in a situation where failure of such selective synaptogenesis might be predicted.

Nervous and Purkinje Cell Degeneration. The two mutants, nervous and Purkinje cell degeneration, are very similar in that death of Purkinje cells is the major abnormality, yet they differ in a number of ways (Sidman and Green, 1970; Landis, 1973; Sidman, 1974). In both mutants the majority of Purkinje cells degenerate in the first 2 months after birth, but they show only moderate ataxia. In Purkinje cell degeneration, cerebellar histogenesis and morphogenesis are normal until cell degeneration begins at about postnatal day 15, reaches a peak at 22–28 days of age, and results in virtually complete loss of Purkinje cells. Later, almost all retinal photoreceptors degenerate, and degeneration of mitral cells of the olfactory bulbs occurs. Nervous mutants show mitochondrial abnormalities in all Purkinje cells at about postnatal day 15, and this is followed by loss of 85–90 percent of the Purkinje cells in the fourth to seventh weeks.

What has been learned from these cerebellar mutants? Perhaps it is best to say what has not been learned: in no case has it been possible to identify the primary gene product that is absent or defective in the mutant. The phenotypic expression is liable to be misleading, as the history of weaver has shown, and we should not be surprised to find that the primary defect is remote from the phenotypic expression of the mutant allele. In defense of the use of mutants that affect the nervous system, it can be said that the only means of mapping the genetic loci that influence development of the nervous system is by finding mutant alleles. In addition, the study of the defective morphogenesis of the brain has led to further understanding of the mechanisms of normal morphogenesis. Thus, while the role of Bermann glia in guiding granule cells was suggested by Mugnaini and Forströnen (1967) from studies of normal material, the concept of guidance of migrating neurons by radial glial cells has obtained greater credence from the studies on the weaver mutant.

The mutants also illustrate the essential autonomy of the Purkinje cells: their phenotype remains recognizable in spite of their gross malpositioning in reeler, and they retain their dendritic spines in spite of the depletion of granule cells in weaver and reeler. In the absence of their normal input these naked dendritic spines rarely accept alternative presynaptic inputs. This and other observations have a bearing on the problem of specificity of synaptic connections. Synapses are formed with surprising normality in mutants in which cells are grossly malpositioned, provided that the cells are present (Rakic, 1975*b*). In weaver mice the mossy fibers target accurately on heterotopic granule cells (Rakic and Sidman, 1973*b*), and the malpositioned Purkinje cells in reeler cerebellum receive all the usual synaptic inputs (Rakic and Sidman, 1972). However, aberrant synaptic connections may be formed by presynaptic cells whose postsynaptic targets are absent. For example, in weaver cerebellum, if the depletion of granule cells is slight, the mossy fibers form synapses correctly on granule cells, although the latter are heterotopic, but if the granule cells are very severely depleted or virtually absent, as they may be after irradiation or in some regions of the homozygous weaver cerebellum, the mossy fibers synapse aberrantly on Golgi II cells. The mutants show the limits of such malconnections, for when the Purkinje cell dendritic spines are devoid of parallel fiber inputs they do not accept anomalous inputs from neighboring axons such as mossy fiber terminals. Nor do the basket and stellate cells, which synapse on the smooth parts of the Purkinje cell dendrites, occupy the synaptic sites on the spines left vacant by the parallel fibers. It is also very significant that, despite malpositioning of the neurons in the reeler cerebral cortex, the appropriate classes of neurons are connected within the cortex, and the interhemispheric connections through the corpus callosum are normal (Caviness, 1976, Caviness and Yorke, 1976). These observations are consistent with the concept that presynaptic terminals will target with great precision and efficiency on matching postsynaptic targets even if the latter are malpositioned (M. Jacobson and Levine, 1975*b*), but if the targets that fit normally are inaccessible the next best fit may sometimes be a viable alternative. One has to proceed cautiously with this line of reasoning in cases where the poisons or radiation might well have disturbed the postsynaptic membrane markers that enable the axon terminals to recognize their appropriate targets. In summary, the mutants may be said to have given considerable evidence of the stability of the mechanism that result in selective synaptic association and to have given some evidence of the formation of functional connections between neurons that do not normally form such connections. The possible rôles of such malconnections in the evolution of the nervous system is discussed in Section 7.12.

3.5. Vascularization of the Mammalian Central Nervous System

Studies of the invasion of the central nervous system by blood vessels have shown that brain capillaries develop from solid cords of endothelial cells which develop a slitlike lumen which increases in caliber slowly over a period of several days (Craigie, 1925; Donahue and Pappas, 1961; Strong, 1961; Otto and Lierse, 1970; Caley and Maxwell, 1970; Bär and Wolff, 1973; Hannah and Nathaniel, 1974). As the mantle layer increases in thickness, it is invaded by new cords of capillary endothelial cells that sprout from more mature capillaries. These strands are separated from the nerve cells by a basement membrane (Bär and Wolff, 1973), and this becomes enveloped by astrocytic processes (Sakia, 1965; Phelps, 1972). The capillaries form a continuous system without fenestrations. The phase of most active capillary sprouting corresponds with the development of dentrites and proliferations of glial cells. It is reasonable to assume that the proliferation of the capillary endothelial cells may be stimulated by the rapid growth of the brain, and it is certain that vascularization develops to satisfy the metabolic requirements of the rapidly growing nervous tissue.

As a general rule, it can be assumed that the density of vascularization of various regions of the nervous system is proportional to the metabolic activity and especially the oxygen consumption of each region (Dunning and Wolff, 1937; Campbell, 1939; Kuhlman and Lowry, 1956; Friede, 1966). However, there are still large gaps in our knowledge of the correlation between vascularization and metabolism of developing nervous tissue. When considering the growth of blood vessels in the developing nervous system, one recognizes how difficult it is to deal separately with such closely interdependent developing systems as the cardiovascular and nervous systems. There has been no definitive study of how much the developing nervous tissue depends on its blood supply, nor is it known to what extent the growth of blood vessels is stimulated by the nervous tissue. Growth of capillaries into the developing central nervous system is maximal at the time during which the nervous system is most vulnerable to malnutrition. However, one can only surmise that vascular insufficiency may play some role in the retardation of brain development resulting from undernutrition (see Section 6.1). In the extreme case of vascular insufficiency, the effects on developing neurons are catastrophic, resulting in infarction of the germinal matrix, the site of the most active cell proliferation. It seems that a collateral blood supply fails to develop in time to save the nervous tissue that is deprived of an adequate blood supply. The effects of less than total failure of blood supply to developing nervous tissue are not well documented, and very little is known about the metabolic requirements of developing nervous tissue and the role of the blood supply in providing these requirements (Friede, 1966, pp. 1–15, review).

3.6. Development of Cortical Folds in the Cerebrum and Cerebellum

Studies of the development of the convolutions may be said to have started with Friedrich Tiedemann (1781–1861), who, in 1816, correctly described the order of development of the main primary, secondary, and tertiary fissures in the human fetus during the final trimester of gestation. The terms *primary, secondary,* and *tertiary* were introduced later by Alexander Ecker in 1869, and an accurate and almost complete description of their development in the human fetus was given by Wilhelm His (1890*a*, 1904). Primary sulci are quite invariant in all members of the species (Connolly, 1950; Bailey and von Bonin, 1951), secondary sulci show more individual variation even in identical twins, and tertiary sulci show great variability. Bailey and von Bonin (1951) list the following primary cerebral sulci: hippocampal, Sylvian, calcarine, parietooccipital, callosomarginal, central, interparietal, superior temporal, olfactory, and rhinal. Secondary sulci include precentral, postcentral, lunate, superior frontal, and orbital.

There is a large literature devoted to the individual and racial variability in the pattern of cerebral convolutions, but in summarizing the literature Bailey and von Bonin (1951) concluded that there is no evidence of racial differences and that the basis of the individual variations, whether genetic or developmental, is not known. This is discussed further in Section 7.12.

The developing primate cerebral cortex is smooth during the period of neuron genesis and migration, and only shallow primary fissures are present at the time when virtually all cortical neurons have been formed. The primary sulci start developing earlier than the secondary sulci, and these fissures and sulci develop between 12 and 26 weeks of gestation. Gyri become well defined between 26 and 28 weeks in the human fetus, and are fairly constant in their positions. The tertiary sulci, which start developing in the eighth and ninth months of gestation and become fully developed only in the first year after birth, are quite variable. Folding does not occur while the neurons are being produced, but only afterwards during the phase of glial cell production, growth of nerve cell processes, and myelination. Development of convolutions is clearly correlated with the maximal rate of increase in the volume of the cortex, but it seems unlikely that the relatively invariant pattern of gyri can be explained simply by differences in rates of growth between the cortex and the underlying tissues.

There are two theories of development of cerebral cortical gyri. The first is that folding occurs because of the greater growth of the flexible cortex relative to the rigid internal structures such as the corpus callosum, thalamus, and basal ganglia (Le Gros Clark, 1945). According to the other theory, cortical folding is due to relative differences in growth within the cortex itself: differences between layers and between regions (Bielschowsky, 1923; D. H. Barron, 1950; Welker and Campos, 1963; Richman *et al.,* 1975).

The only experimental analysis of the problem, by D. H. Barron (1950), shows that the cerebral convolutions develop normally in the sheep fetus after removal of the basal ganglia and corpus callosum or after undercutting of the cortex has separated it from the relatively rigid structures beneath. Barron concluded that the deep brain structures are not involved in cortical folding but that the mechanism of folding is within the cortex. The same conclusion has been reached from a different direction: Richman *et al.* (1975), from a consideration of congenital defects of cortical folding in human fetuses, concluded that gyri develop because of unequal growth of the superficial and deep layers of the cortex. In microgyria the cortex is thrown into an increased number of small folds, whereas the cortex is smooth in lissencephaly. In both malformations the cortex is thinned and the number of layers is reduced (Richman *et al.,* 1973; R. M. Stewart *et al.,* 1975). In the normal cortex the three outer cortical layers grow at a slightly faster rate than the three inner layers. In the lissencephalic cortex the growth of all cortical layers is greatly reduced, and there is no significant difference in growth rate between inner and outer layers, whereas in microgyria the inner cortical layers grow more slowly than normal.

Although the differences in rates of growth of cortical layers can explain why the cortex buckles, it does not indicate why the primary and secondary fissures occur at relatively constant positions. That constancy is likely to result from differences in growth rates between different parts of the cortex. Folding of the cortex occurs during the growth of dendrites of cortical neurons, and it is likely that the geometry of dendritic growth and of the fiber trajectories within the cortex will be found to have a constant relationship to the geometry of the gyri. The shape of each gyrus may give an indication of the functional organization of the underlying cortex in the sense that some cellular elements have a constant geometrical relationship to the axes of the gyrus. Welker and Campos (1963) have cogently reasoned that the invariance of the primary and secondary fissures is due to the differences in the density of thalamocortical projection to functionally distinct regions of the cortex. Gyri receive strong projections from the thalamus, while sulci receive weak thalamic projections. The major gyri tend to receive projections from distinct peripheral body regions, so that the invariant pattern of primary and secondary fissures can be correlated with functional mapping onto the cortex (Fig. 3.16). This concept can be traced back to the phrenological theory of Gall and Spurzheim, whose *Anatomie et Physiologie due Système Nerveux* (1810–1819), especially in Volumes 1 (1810) and 2 (1812), tried to establish a relationship between the intellectual functions and the shape of the cranium and the underlying convolutions. The phrenological theory, while incorrect in the localization of so-called intellectual and moral functions, was based on much correct anatomical observation, especially that of Gall, and its main significance was to have given an impetus to studies of the relationship between structure and function of the cerebral cortex (see E. Clarke and O'Malley, 1968; R. M. Young, 1970). Out of such studies has come the principle that the magnification of cortical representation is proportional to the functional importance of the peripheral sensory or motor fields and that the primary gyri correspond fairly well, although not precisely, with cytoarchitectonic fields and with functional representation in the cortex.

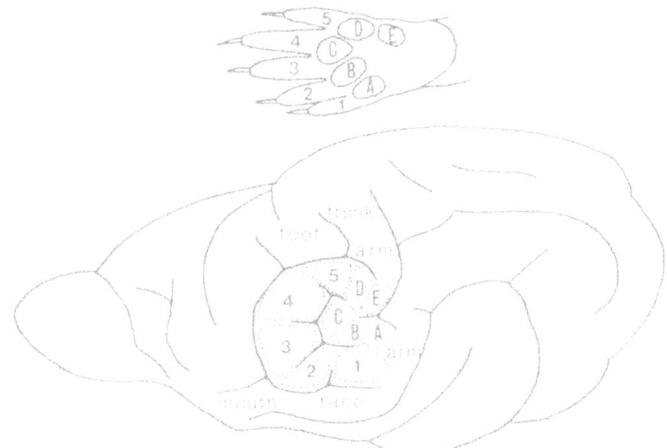

Figure 3.16. Correspondence of gyri with functional sensory representation of one side of the body on the contralateral cerebral cortex (SmI) of the raccoon. The area of cortex representing unit area of skin varies according to the receptor density in each region, which is correlated with the region's functional importance. There is a greatly magnified cortical representation of the plantar skin of the front paw, which is correlated with the raccoon's use of its front paws as a sensory organ. From W. I. Welker and S. Seidenstein, *J. Comp. Neurol. 111:*469–501 (1959).

Folding of the cerebellar cortex must occur as the proliferation in the external granular layer results in tremendous expansion of the cortex over the relatively slowly growing white matter. The main pattern of gyri and sulci is established early in postnatal development. The cerebellar fissures are all identifiable at 2 days of age in the mouse (Mareš and Lodin, 1970), and in the human fetus all the lobules of the cerebellar vermis can be identified as the major fissures develop at about 15 weeks of gestation. Thereafter, the number of folia increases until about 2 months postnatally as shown in Fig. 3.17 (Loeser *et al.,* 1972).

As the cerebellar cortex grows, the fissures deepen and the gyri become more pronounced. The mechanism of gyrification are not known. It is easy to conceive qualitatively of the mechanics of folding of a sheet of tissue as the result of differences in rates of growth within the cerebellar cortex or between the cortex and underlying brain. More rapid growth of the cortex than the underlying brain is considered to be the principal cause of cerebellar folding (Saetersdal, 1956; Haddara and Nooreddin, 1966). The pattern of fissuration may be due to differences in rates of cell proliferation or to growth and cell death at different

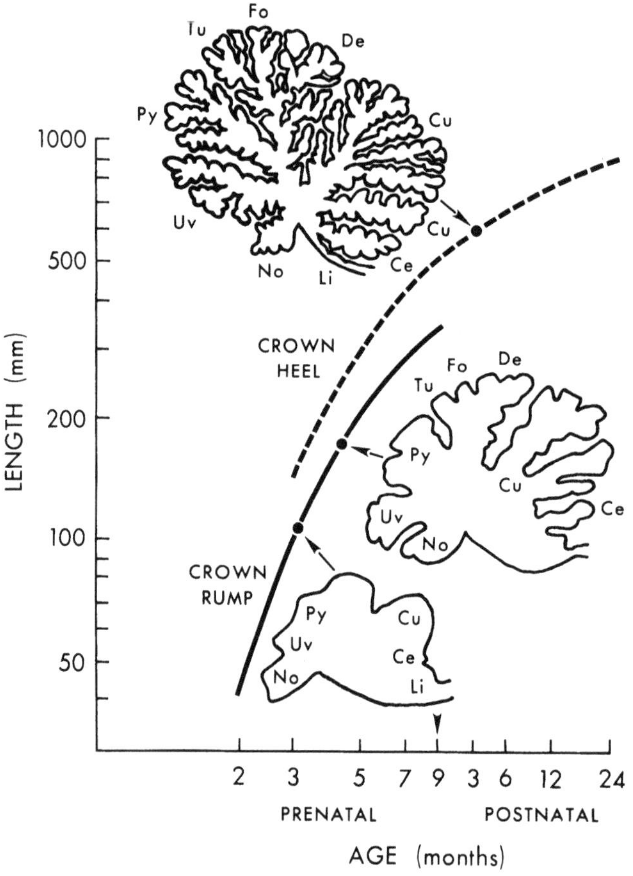

Figure 3.17. Development of folia in human cerebellar vermis in relation to age and length of the fetus and newborn infant. The total number of folia in the cerebellar vermis is about 10 at 15 weeks of gestation, increases to about 50 at 20 weeks, 250 at 40 weeks, and attains the adult number of 300 at about 30 weeks after birth. From J. D. Loeser, R. J. Lemire, and E. C. Alvord, Jr., *Anat. Rec. 173:*109–114 (1972).

depths in the cortex and in different cortical regions. The causes of such regularities of cell proliferation, growth, and death are entirely unknown. In the cerebellar cortex of the mouse the proliferation rate in the external granular layer is slightly greater in the sulci than on the gyri (Mareš and Lodin, 1970), which may be the cause of the cortical thickening in the depth of the sulcus and cortical thinning at the convexity of the gyrus. The pattern of folding of the cerebellar cortex is definitely related to the cellular architectonics: the folia develop in the axis of the parallel fibers, while the Purkinje cell dendrites are in the plane orthogonal to the long axis of the folium. In mutant mice with cerebellar defects that result in reduced growth of the cerebellar cortex, the fissures are also reduced. The secondary cerebellar fissures are almost absent in the reeler mutant mice, in which malpositioning and disorientation of cerebellar cells result in serious disruption of the normal pattern of cortical lamination.

3.7. Histogenesis of Insect Nervous System

Textbooks of invertebrate embryology (Dawydoff, 1928; Pflugfelder, 1958; Kumeé and Dan, 1968) contain little information about the development of the nervous systems of invertebrates. In this regard, a critical friend has described the works on insects by Butt (1941) as the least misinformative and by Hagan (1951) as the least uninformative. From them the following information can be gleaned: the ectodermal cells that give rise to the nervous system in insects are called the *neuroblast mother cells,* which undergo equal division to give rise to two neuroblasts, first so named by Wheeler (1891, 1893). The neuroblasts of insects are aptly named because they are true "blast" cells (Greek *blastos,* a germ or a bud) that divide to give rise to cells named *ganglion mother cells* by Bauer (1904), but which may be called second- or third-generation neuroblasts. The ganglion mother cells divide to form the *ganglion cells,* which are the postmitotic nerve cells (Fig. 3.18).

The first division of the neuroblasts tends to be unequal so that the ganglion mother cells are smaller than the neuroblasts, but later divisions become progressively more equal until, finally, an equal division gives rise to two ganglion mother cells. There are exceptions to this sequence; for example, in the optic lobes of the cockroach and stick insect, the divisions of neuroblasts are equal from the beginning (Malzacher, 1968). Moreover, there is evidence that in some insects the neuroblasts degenerate at the end of the larval stages (Wheeler, 1891; Bauer, 1904; Panov, 1960; Gouin, 1965; Nordlander and Edwards, 1969; Starre-van der Molen, 1974; Bate, 1976). Neurogenesis proceeds in a rostral-to-caudal sequence, and the onset of degeneration of neuroblasts occurs in the same sequence in the locust (Bate, 1976). The same number of neuroblasts gives rise to the large and complex thoracic ganglia as to the small and relatively simple abdominal ganglia of the locust, and selective death of neuroblasts may be a way of controlling the number of neurons in a particular ganglion (Bate, 1976).

As each ganglion mother cell is generated by division of the neuroblast, it displaces those generated earlier, so that a column of cells is formed, with the oldest cells at the head of the column farthest from the neuroblast. Experiments in which insect larvae and pupae have been fixed at progressive intervals after an injection of tritiated thymidine have shown that the age of any neuron can be determined by its distance from the proliferating center, since older cells are

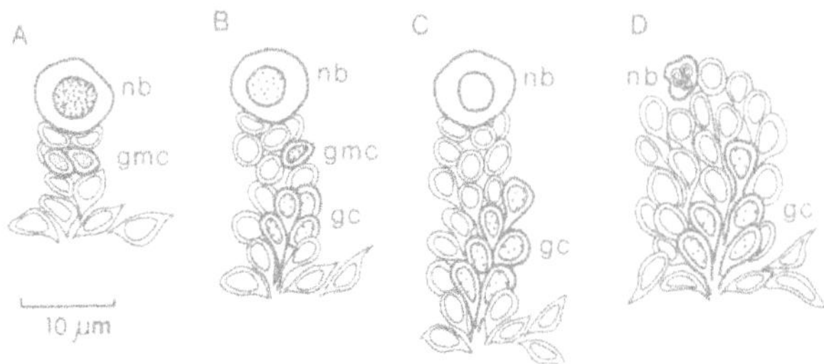

Figure 3.18. Position of labeled cells in a groups of cells descended from one neuroblast (nb) in the brain of the monarch butterfly, fixed at successive intervals after an injection of tritiated thymidine at the beginning of the fourth instar. A: The neuroblast and two ganglion mother cells (gmc) are labeled 2 hr after the injection. B: At the beginning of the fifth instar, the neuroblast is less heavily labeled, another ganglion mather cell is labeled, and the original ganglion cells (gc) are lightly labeled. C: Late in the fifth instar, label is not detectable in the neuroblast, indicating that it has been diluted by cell division. D: Two days after pupation, the neuroblast is degenerating. Note that the density of labeling of ganglion cells does not diminish, indicating that the ganglion cells have not divided. From R. H. Nordlander and J. S. Edwards, Postembryonic brain development in the monarch butterfly, *Danaus plexippus,* L., *Arch. Entwicklungsmech. Organ. 162:*197–217 (1969).

displaced by cells that are generated at later stages (Nordlander and Edwards, 1968*a,* 1969), as is shown in Fig. 3.18. The ganglion mother cells then divide once, with the spindle axis at right angles to the column of cells, each giving rise to two neurons (Bauer, 1904; Baden, 1936; Panov, 1960; Malzacher, 1968; Nordlander and Edwards, 1968*b*).

The maximum number of neuroblasts is rather small, about 110 in the stick insect and 140 in the cockroach (Malzacher, 1968). The number of neuroblasts diminishes during the late larval and pupal stages until they finally disappear in the pupa, either by degeneration or by final division into two mother cells. Mitosis of neuroblasts and mother cells in insects ceases last in the corpora pedunculata. The neurons derived from each neuroblast tend to remain together and form a clonal group, although some neurons become displaced to join groups derived from other neuroblasts. If the morphogenesis of the insect nervous system is similar to that of the imaginal discs, one would predict that clonally related cells would remain together in the nervous system. In the dorsal mesothoracic disc of *Drosophila,* "the spatial relationships among cells developing from the same line is preserved throughout ontogeny, with modifications by differential growth rates" (C. Murphy and Tokunaga, 1970). Factors that determine cell movements in the imaginal disc are regional differences in rates of growth and in mitotic rates. These result in passive displacement of groups of cells and not free migration of individual cells. In general, in neither the vertebrate nor invertebrate nervous system is there any evidence of free migration of individual neurons, but rather the neurons move *en masse* or in groups.

3.8. Lineage of Neurons of Vertebrates and Invertebrates

Cell lineage in the nervous system is a problem that, after a period of neglect, is again receiving the attention that its importance merits. One reason for this curious neglect may be that studies of cell lineage have, until recently, been made almost exclusively on invertebrates, whereas most of the work on neurogenesis has been done on vertebrates. Another reason for the slow progress is that the techniques for studying cell lineage—genetic mosaics, for example,—are not easily applied to the nervous system. To give another instance, *in vitro* cloning of normal nerve cells is not possible, while abnormal cells that can be cloned, such as neuroblastoma cells, may not provide the means to determine how different types of neurons are lineally related. To discover the lineages of the different types of cells in the retina or the cerebellar cortex, to mention only two structures whose development is fairly well characterized, may require genetic analysis of mutations that selectively alter only a single type of cell. Although a large number of mutants affecting the nervous system have been identified (see Section 3.4.5), none has yet been found that lends itself to the analysis of cell lineage. The mutations constitute *forces majeures* that alter normal development of the nervous system so widely as to virtually prohibit analysis of the effect on a single type of cell.

Another method for studying cell lineage depends on being able to follow a marked or identifiable cell line. The most direct approach, to trace a single cell through serial reconstruction of the entire nervous system at different stages of development can be done on simple invertebrates whose nervous system contains hundreds or thousands of cells (Brenner, 1974; J. G. White *et al.,* 1976; Sulsten, 1976). By means of automated methods of tissue reconstruction from serial sections (Ware and Lopresti, 1975, review), it may eventually become possible to study cell lineage in small regions of the vertebrate nervous system.

There is a temptation to use any convenient, even if inadequate technique for studying a difficult problem. Therefore, it is well to emphasize the inadequacy of some techniques that have been used for studying cell lineage in the nervous system. Thus labeling cells with tritiated thymidine ([^{3}H]TdR), the method most often used for analysis of the time of cell origin, has serious limitations for studying cell lineage. In this method, the time of administration of the [^{3}H]TdR to the developing nervous system is systematically varied, and the locations and phenotypes of the labeled cells are later identified in autoradiographs. Cells that were labeled after a brief pulse must have been in the phase of DNA synthesis during their terminal cell cycle, while cells that remained unlabeled after a long period of continuous administration of [^{3}H]TdR must have completed the final round of DNA synthesis before the initiation of labeling. In such studies, cells of a particular type are found to originate over a span of time ranging from hours to days, and cells of different types in the same population generally have overlapping timespans of origin, for example, in the retina (S. Fujita and Horii, 1963; Morris, 1973, 1975), in the cerebellar cortex (see Section 3.1), or in the cerebral cortex (Rakic, 1974, 1975*a*). From such data one can determine the relative temporal order of origin of different types of cells, and these are found to overlap. In a tissue such as the central nervous system, in which several types of cells develop in any one region, the temporal succession of appearance of different kinds of cells cannot show the lineage of the different kinds of cells, and any deductions regarding lineage (e.g., Morris, 1973) are questionable. Attempts to infer lineage solely from morphological similarities (e.g., Hinds and Hinds, 1974) should not be taken seriously, regardless of the merits of other conclusions that may legitimately be drawn from the same observations.

Under favorable circumstances, some limited information about cell lineage can be derived from the thymidine labeling technique. Thus if only one type of cell is labeled by a pulse, or if one cell type alone remains unlabeled after prolonged administration of [^{3}H]thymidine, then it can be safely concluded that the stem cells giving origin to that type of cell do not, at the same time, give origin to another type of cell. For example, because the first cells in the retina to withdraw from DNA synthesis and mitosis later differentiate as retinal ganglion cells, it is safe to infer that the stem cells give origin exclusively to ganglion cells at that stage (M. Jacobson, 1968*b*), but it cannot be determined whether the same stem cells may not also produce other types of cells at later stages of development.

Many questions about cell lineage in the nervous system remain unanswered. For instance, does every type of neuron and glial cell originate from a different type of stem cell or are there stem cells that give rise to more than one type or to all types of nerve cells? Do neurons and glia arise from different stem cells or from a common precursor? If there is a common precursor, does it produce neurons and glia concurrently or sequentially at different stages of development? If a single stem cell can produce more than one type of neuron or glial cell, how is the production of different types of cells regulated? Are the cells in a particular region, regardless of their phenotype, all the descendants of the same stem cell pool or are there different pools for different types of cells in the same region? To what extent is the differentiation of any type of neuron due to its lineage and to what extent do other factors, such as position, control terminal cytodifferentiation?

There are several methods by which lineage has been studied, but the application of these methods to the nervous system is rather limited. Direct observation of marked cells in the early embryo can identify the progenitor cells of a particular part of the nervous system. This approach, which involves vital dye labelling of stem cells in the neural plate, allows the plotting of a fate map. Because of dilution and loss of the label, it is not possible to determine whether the marked cells contribute all their descendents to the tissue in question or whether only some of the cells of that tissue are derived from the marked stem cells while other cells in the same tissue are derived from other, unmarked parts of the neural plate (see Section 1.2). At best, this method permits a map of the presumptive fate of neural plate cells in the sense that, if stem cells are left undisturbed in that position, their progeny will contribute to a particular part of the nervous system. Such fate maps do not show whether, at that stage of development, the stem cells have embarked on a specific program of differentiation or whether this program is reversible.

The information yielded by vital staining can also be obtained from chimeras, in which the animal is a mosaic of genetically different cells. As the mosaic is usually established at very early embryonic stages, before the neural plate stage, and as the pattern of clones in the neural plate is unpredictable, such chimeras are of limited use in studies of cell lineage in the nervous system. There are several causes of such mosaicism. In female mammals only one X chromosome is genetically active; the other is inactivated at early stages of embryonic development, and the inactivated chromosome is transmitted to all the progeny of that cell. This gives rise to a natural mosaicism in females that are heterozygous for X-linked markers. Because of the early stage and uncertain time of X inactivation, this type of mosaic has little or no application to lineage studies in the nervous system.

Construction of composite embryos by sticking together cells derived from two genetically distinct mouse embryos at about the eight-cell stage produces another type of mosaic animal. In such "allophenic mice" (Mintz, 1971; Tettenborn *et al.*, 1971), cells of the adult are derived from one or other of the parents and the distribution of cells will depend on the amount of mingling or of segregation of the two strains of cells at the time at which the presumptive fates of the cells had become established as a map. As J. H. Lewis *et al.* (1972) have pointed out, such experiments "reveal only the relative size of the group of cells giving rise to a tissue, compared with the mosaic patch size, at the time when the presumptive fate of those progenitors first became definite. From this type of investigation the number of progenitors at the time of determination, that is, at the time of the first, decisive step of differentiation, cannot be deduced." The difficulty of deriving the size of the stem cell pool from such experiments greatly reduces the usefulness of this technique. Indeed, the validity of some of the conclusions derived from studies of allophenic mice is questionable, for example, the conclusion that the retinal photoreceptors of the mouse are a clone originating from a group of ten initiator cells near the center of the retina (Mintz and Sanyal, 1970). Because the cells from the two parents are able to mingle before the time of primary neural induction, the pattern of the mosaic in the neural plate is unpredictable and will tend to be fine grained, with the result that cells from both parents will contribute to all parts of the nervous system. This method does not have the certainty and precision provided by xenoplastic transplantation of genetically marked neural crest or neural plate cells, for example, transplantation between quail and chick embryos (see Section 1.4), that has been successfully used to map the prospective fates of parts of the neural crest (Le Douarin, 1973). Xenoplastic transplantation between anuran and urodele amphibian embryos has a long history (summarized in Harrison, 1935), including studies of the fates of parts of the neural plate transplanted between the frog *Bombinator pachypus* and the newt *Triton alpestris* (Roth, 1950). The frog cells have smaller and less chromatic nuclei than the newt cells. In all cases, there is a sharp line of division between the central nervous tissues derived from the transplant and those of the host, with no intermingling of cells at the margins of the graft. The large size of the grafts precludes any conclusions about cell lineage, but, in principle, xenoplastic transplantation of a few stem cells should provide a means of determining cell lineage, and the technical difficulties of such an experiment could be compensated by the advantages of precise localization and timing of the transplant.

In *Drosophila* two types of genetic mosaics have been used to study cell lineage: gynandromorphs and X-ray-induced somatic crossing-over mosaics. Gynandromorphs are produced through loss of an X chromosome at an early cleavage division, with the result that the animal is a mosaic of XO and XX cells. the XO tissues in the gynandromorphs can be identified by means of a genetic marker. X-ray-induced somatic recombination can be initiated at later stages of development than gynandromorphy. The affected cell transmits its abnormality to its offspring, which form a clone. Because clonally related cells stay together during development of insects, the clones form large, compact groups of cells in the later stages of development or in the adult animal (Fig. 3.19). In general, two tissues that share a stem cell pool should be correlated in mosaic composition provided that they did not diverge in development before the onset of mosaicism. Gynandromorphs have been used for determining the part of the nervous system that is affected in behavioral mutants of *Drosophila* (Hotta and Benzer, 1970, 1972, 1973; Ikeda and Kaplan, 1970*a,b;* D. T. Suzuki *et al.,* 1971; Griglatti *et al.,* 1972). In these studies the mosaics consisted of tissues which were heterozygous for a recessive behavior mutation located on the X chromosome and tissues which were hemizygous for the mutation. By testing many such mosaics, it could be determined which region of the animal had to be hemizygous in order to produce the mutant behavior.

There have been several investigations of the genetic determinants of behavior in insects using genetic mosaics. P. W. Whiting (1932) made gynandromorphs (sex mosaics) of the parasitic wasp *Habrobracon,* in which the males and females have different behavior, and showed that the head controls sexual behavior in that species. Using genetic mosaics of *Drosophila,* it has been observed that specific behavioral or functional effects are associated with a mutant gene expressed in a specific tissue. Thus Ikeda and Kaplan (1970*b*) have shown that the hyperkinetic mutation, which causes shaking of the leg when the fly is etherized, is linked to the individual legs, while Hotta and Benzer (1970) have found that various abnormalities of visual behavior are due to defects within the compound eye. However, these studies were limited by the fact that the mosaicism was not directly visible in neurons. The nervous localization had to be indirectly determined from the

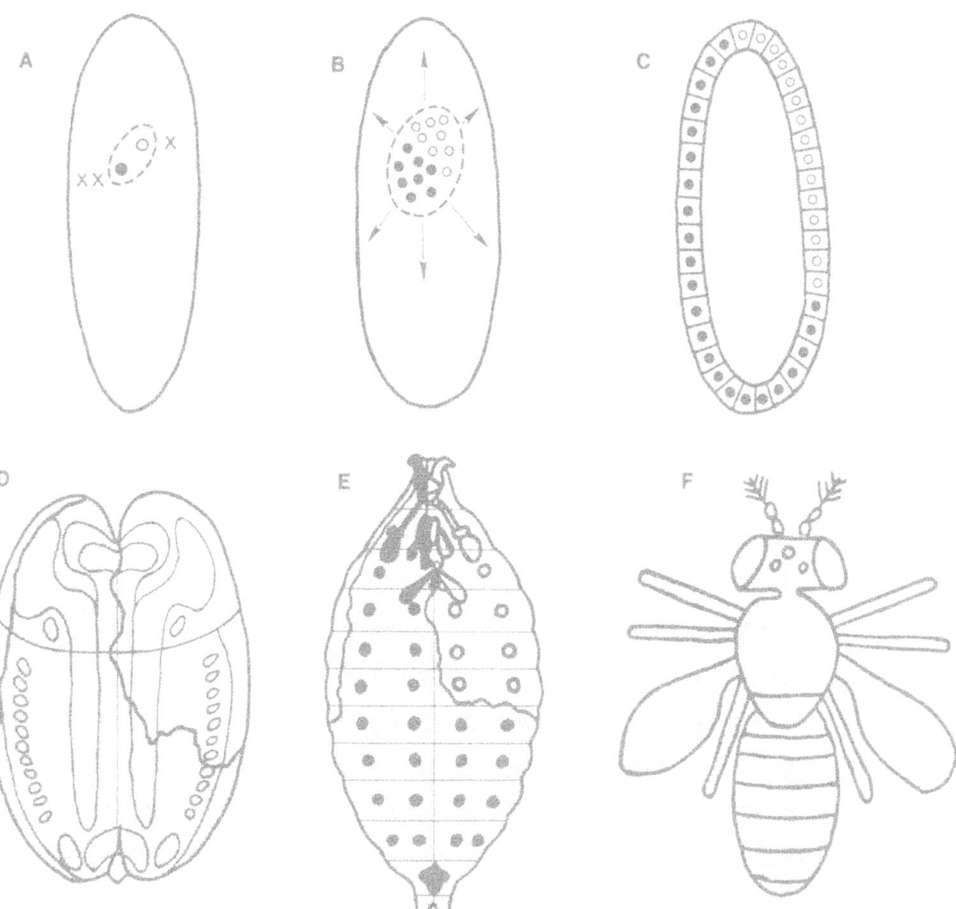

Figure 3.19. Formation of a gynandromorph. A: Starting with a female (XX) egg, one of the X chromosomes is lost during the first nuclear division. This produces one nucleus that contains only a single X, and develops into male tissues. The orientation of the first mitotic spindle is (in *Drosophila*) random so that these nuclei produce, as they divide, descendant nuclei that are variously oriented in different embryos. B: The nuclei divide in a syncytium without cell walls. After about a dozen divisions, the nuclei migrate to the surface of the egg, and (C) cell membranes are laid down to form a blastoderm, the female muclei forming some areas, male nuclei forming others. D: The blastoderm is sketched as if cut along the dorsal side and folded open like a book, showing a fate map of the regions destined to become the various larval organs. In the example shown, the shaded portion will develop into female parts, the unshaded into male parts, eventually hatching as a composite larva. E: A mature larva split dorsally and opened flat, indicating the various imaginal discs which are destined to develop into adult surface structures after metamorphosis. The adult (F) is a composite formed from some female and some male discs. From Y. Hotta and S. Benzer, *Proc. Natl. Acad. Sci. U.S.A. 67:*1156–1163 (1970).

cuticular distribution of the mosaicism and by the construction of morphogenetic fate maps. Hotta and Benzer (1972) mapped the foci in the blastoderm from which the nervous structures arise that produce the mutant behavior: for example, the foci for the ether-induced leg shaking caused by the Hyperkinetic[1] mutation were mapped to the thoracic ganglia. In fact, Ikeda and Kaplan (1970*a,b*) have shown, by electrophysiological recording, that the thoracic ganglion motoneurons are defective in the Hyperkinetic[1] mutants. Combining the genetic mosaics with enzyme markers, Kankel and Hall (1976) have been able to derive fate maps for the nervous system by looking directly at the tissue distribution of the X-linked enzyme activities. Their most significant finding is that only three to ten blastoderm cells give rise to each major ganglion. Because a large population of neurons is derived from each stem cell in the blastoderm, they conclude that gynandromorphs with small clones in the nervous system cannot be obtained. The main limitation of mosaics generated very early in development is that they cannot give the fine resolution required for lineage studies of individual neuronal phenotypes. Indeed, a fate map of the *Drosophila* brain has been achieved by direct embryological observations (Poulson, 1950) that equals and exceeds the resolution of fate maps so far derived from studies of genetic mosaics. The direct method of tracing lineages is possible because of the consistency with which neurons with particular functions and connections can be mapped to specific locations in the ganglia of some insects and because of the regular order in which the neurons originate from identifiable individual neuroblasts.

An important advance in understanding the relationship of cell differentiation to cell lineage and to cell position has come from studies by García-Bellído *et al.* (1973) of the development of the mesothoracic disc in *Drosophila*. X-ray-induced somatic crossing over is used to mark cells whose progeny form clones that are found to be confined to wing compartments. Each compartment has precisely defined borders and is made up exclusively of the surviving descendants of a small group of primordial cells; thus it is termed a *polyclone*. Genetic mosaics of homeotic mutants have shown that each compartment is controlled by a few genes called *selector genes*. An entire compartment is altered in the homeotic mutant, which suggests that the compartment is the unit for genetic control of development of morphological patterns. By irradiating embryos at different stages of development, the progeny of marked cells can be followed in relation to compartment boundaries. Such experiments show that different structures, such as bristles and veins, within a compartment are not determined by a lineage mechanism but apparently by their position with respect to the compartment borders (García-Bellído, 1975). Such experiments have not yet been extended to the nervous system, but they offer the possibility of determining whether individual neuronal phenotypes are determined on the basis of lineage or position or both, and also provide a possible means of understanding the genetic control of cell differentiation in the nervous system.

3.9. Control of the Number and Size of Nerve Cells

The number of neurons that reach maturity is the result of a balance between cell proliferation and cell death during neurogenesis. The limits to these parameters may be set by the genetic constitution, but the final size of the brain and the number of neurons and glial cells in the nervous system must be affected by many factors. These include hormones, growth factors, and nutrients within the developing system, as as well as such external factors as temperature and nutrition. It is often necessary to make accurate counts of neurons and glia in order to determine precisely how and when such factors may affect development of the nervous system. It is also important to obtain an accurate measure of the constancy and variability of the total number of neurons or the numbers in particular parts of the nervous system. In most animals, the total number of neurons is attained in the embryo or fetus, and postembryonic or postnatal increase in cells is largely or entirely due to addition of glial cells. Addition of neurons during a short period after birth is essentially limited to a few restricted regions of the brain in mammals (see Section 3.1). These cases of restricted neurogenesis after birth are in sharp contrast to the cases of addition of neurons as well as glia to all parts of the nervous system throughout life in submammalian vertebrates and in some invertebrates. The addition of neurons throughout life poses the problem of how the newborn cells are integrated into the preexisting circuitry, and how the increase in neuron population affects behavior. All the species in which continuous addition of cells occurs have complete repertoires of behavior in the young adult, and any changes that occur as the animal grows must be very subtle.

There is a wealth of data on the constancy of numbers of neurons, but there are no explanations of how such constancy is controlled or achieved, or of why the number of neurons is constant. Apart from the concept that complex functions require a large number of neurons, we have no definite understanding of the relationship between a particular function of the nervous system and the number of neurons required to perform that function. Collecting data to show that a particular animal or part of its nervous system contains a constant number of neurons is far easier than reaching an understanding of the causes or of the functional significance of such constancy of cell content.

In many invertebrates, the nervous system contains thousands or, at the most, tens of thousands of neurons. Counting the number of neurons by simple histological methods and mapping their locations and interconnections are within the realm of possibility in these invertebrates. The insect nervous system has a neuron count of about the same order of magnitude as that of the submammalian vertebrates, that is, between 10^6 and 10^7. The number is greater again by up to 2 orders of magnitude in mammals, and shows a regular phylogenetic increase until it culminates in man with an estimated 10^{10} neurons.

Ogawa (1939) has counted and measured all the nerve cells and nerve fibers at various stages of development of an annelid worm and has found that the total number of nerve cells in the brain increases from 6000 to 10,000 from hatching to sexual maturity. Wiersma (1957) counted the neurons of the crayfish and found that the brain contains 70,000–80,000 neurons, while the total for the whole nervous system is about 95,000. This does not mean that the nervous system is simple in all invertebrates. The octopus has a brain of exceptional complexity, containing about 10^7 neurons in animals of 600–700 g body weight (J. Z. Young, 1963; Giuditta *et al.,* 1971); this is about the same as the number of neurons in the brains of some fish and amphibians—for example, 1.7×10^7 in the frog *Rana esculenta* (Kemali and Braitenberg, 1969). The numbers of cells in the octopus brain, neurons as well as glia, continue to increase with age allometrically with increase in body weight, reaching a total of 4×10^8 cells in octopus of 4.5 kg body weight (Packard and Albergoni, 1970; Giuditta *et al.,* 1971). The highest nervous centers of the octopus and some insects are more complex than many parts of the vertebrate brain (Ramón y Cajal and Sánchez, 1915; J. Z. Young, 1964). Reference to the work of Ramón y Cajal and Sánchez (1915) on the visual centers of insects is a chastening experience for anyone with a tendency to think of the invertebrate nervous system as simple. Ramón y Cajal was quite explicit in this regard when he wrote:

> The complexity of the insect retina is something stupendous, disconcerting, and without precedent in other animals. . . . Compared with the retina of these apparently humble representatives of life (hymenoptera, lepidoptera, and neuroptera), the retina of the bird or the higher mammal appears as something coarse, rude, and deplorably elementary. The comparison of a rude wall clock with an exquisite and diminutive hunting-case watch fails to give an adequate idea of the contrast, for the "hunting-case eye" of the higher insect does not merely consist of more delicate wheels, but contains besides various highly complicated organs which are not represented in the vertebrates.*

Nevertheless, the simpler invertebrates have some advantages for studies of the factors that control the number of cells in the nervous system. In many invertebrates the total number of neurons is quite constant, their positions are relatively invariant, and there is little variability in their connectivity patterns (Bullock and Horridge, 1965; M. J. Cohen and Jacklet, 1967; J. G. White *et al.*, 1976; Sulston, 1976). Even in arthropods, where the number and positions of neurons are remarkably constant, there are individual variations, particularly in the branching patterns of nerves, as Bullock and Horridge (1965) have emphasized. These are of great interest, particularly if the variations are determined genetically rather than as a result of developmental accidents. Variability of the position of the neuron soma not associated with the variability of the synaptic connections of the displaced neurons occurs in a snail (Benjamin, 1976). Such conservation of essentially normal connectivity in spite of gross malposition of nerve cell bodies has also been found in genetically determined developmental derangements of the mammalian nervous system (see Sections 3.10 and 7.12).

The final number of neurons in insects is reached in the pupal stage, and no further production of neurons occurs later in development. During postembryonic nervous development in insects, only glia increase in number, although neurons as well as glia increase in size (Power, 1952; Panov, 1962; Gymer and Edwards, 1967; H. Korr, 1968; Malzacher, 1968). Neurons present in the larva may not be functionally connected, or the activity of neuronal circuits present in the larva or in the early instars may be suppressed by descending inhibition from the brain (Bentley and Hoy, 1970). The small size of many neurons in insects is an advantage when studying them by electron microscope, but is a disadvantage for electrophysiological investigations.

The size and complexity of the vertebrate brain make it impossible to count the total number of neurons directly in histological sections, although direct counts have been made of neurons in small parts of the brain. For example, the total number of neurons in the ventral cochlear nucleus of man is 48,010 (S.D. 4550), corrected for counting errors (Konigsmark and Murphy, 1970).

An alternative to histological methods of determining the total number of neurons plus glial cells is to measure the amount of DNA in the whole nervous

*A similar view was expressed by von Baer: "I believe that in fact the bee is more highly organized than the fish, although according to another type" (*Entwicklungsgeschichte*, 1828, 1, 208). There is also an echo here of the Cartesian idea of the organism as a clockwork mechanism or living machine. In the extreme form that this idea reached in La Mettrie's *L'homme Machine* (first published in 1748), man is regarded merely as a machine with more wheels and springs than lower organisms. See de Solla Price (1964).

system or parts of it (Santen and Agranoff, 1963; Winick and Noble, 1965; Oja, 1966; E. Howard, 1968; Nováková *et al.*, 1968; Stasný *et al.*, 1968; Margolis, 1969). The number of cells is obtained by dividing the total quantity of DNA in the nervous system by the quantity of DNA in a single euploid cell. The latter is a constant quantity for each species. For example, the DNA content of a single euploid brain cell is 6.4×10^{-12} g in the rat, 7.1×10^{-12} g in the cat, 6.5×10^{-12} g in the dog, and 7.1×10^{-12} g in man (Heller and Elliott, 1954; Santen and Agranoff, 1963). The DNA content of a euploid cell of the chicken is 25×10^{-13} g, and from the total DNA content of the brain Margolis (1969) has calculated that the total number of cells in the chick brain at hatching is about 5×10^{8}. In the chick at hatching, the cerebellum, cerebrum, and optic lobes each contain about 16×10^{7} cells, and the number of cells in these parts of the brain changes in a systematic way during the postnatal period (Fig. 3.20).

The mean cell weight can be computed from the brain weight divided by the total brain DNA, with a correction for the weight of the extracellular fluid. The ratio of brain weight to DNA gives a rough-and-ready estimate of mean cell weight, but a measure of the variability of neuronal size and territory can be obtained only by much more tedious histological methods (Haddara, 1956; Sholl, 1956*a*, Mannen, 1966; Ware and Lopresti, 1975). The mean weight of the brain and the number of neurons are greater in male than in female mammals (Pearl, 1905; Blinkov and Glezer, 1968; Jerison, 1963; Calaresu and Henry, 1971).

The variability of cell size and number in the nervous system of vertebrates is not known because of serious limitations in the accuracy of methods of counting and measuring neurons and glia (Shariff, 1953; Nurnberger and Gordon, 1957; Haug, 1960, 1967*b;* Brizzee *et al.*, 1964). For example, the ratio of glia to neurons

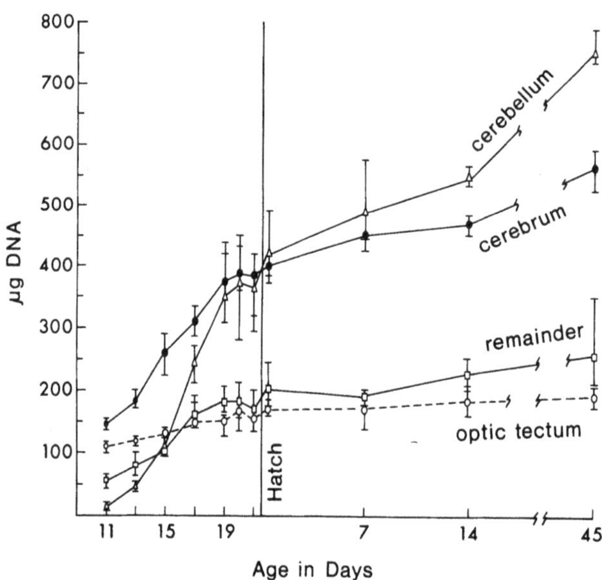

Figure 3.20. DNA content of parts of the brain of the chick at different ages before and after hatching. Each value, reported as micrograms of DNA per brain region (optic tectum, cerebrum, cerebellum, and remainder of the brain), is the average of at least six determinations. The vertical bars show the range of values obtained. From F. L. Margolis, *J. Neurochem. 16:*447–456 (1969), copyright Pergamon Press.

has to be determined by direct counts of cells in histological sections. Different glia-to-neuron ratios ranging from 10:1 to 1:1 have been obtained by different investigators using different counting methods and different methods of correcting for counting errors (Brizzee *et al.*, 1964). Counts of the total number of neurons in the cerebral cortex of man very widely and give an indication of the limitations of the methods that have been employed: The results have varied from 2.6×10^9 (Pakkenberg, 1967), to 5.5×10^9 (Berger, 1921), to 6.9×10^9 (Shariff, 1953), to 9.3×10^9 (H. Thompson, 1899), to 14×10^9 (von Economo and Koskinas, 1925). It is clear that more reliable cell counts, particularly in the mammalian brain, will have to be made before the real variability in the number of neurons and glia can be determined. Better methods of counting neurons (Konigsmark, 1970) are essential for determining the individual and intraspecies variations in the number of brain cells. Such variations between individuals at the same age of the same species may result from genetic, nutritional, hormonal, or other functional differences (Zamenhof, 1941, 1942, 1976; Kuhlenkampf, 1952; Altman and Das, 1964; Zamenhof *et al.*, 1964, 1966, 1968; E. Howard, 1965, 1968; E. Howard and Granoff, 1968; M. C. Diamond *et al.*, 1966). A large genetic variability in the number of neurons in the hippocampal formation of different strains of mice has been demonstrated by Wimer *et al.* (1976). The significance of such variability is discussed in Section 7.12.

Even the body temperature of the pregnant female has a marked influence on the number of cells that survive to birth in the fetus. Increasing the body temperature of the pregnant female guinea pig by 3–4°C on the 18th–25th days of gestation, for 1 hour, results in a 10 percent reduction in fetal brain weight. Two heat stresses, each of 1 hour, produce a 13 percent decrease in brain weight, and a deficit of 26 percent in fetal brain weight follows eight periods of maternal heat stress, each lasting an hour (M. J. Edwards, 1969). The deficit in brain weight is due in large part to a reduction in the number of brain cells (M. J. Edwards *et al.*, 1971), but whether the affected cells are neurons or glia is not known. The effect of hyperthermia is to damage and destroy ventricular germinal cells of the telencephalon, and probably elsewhere in the brain, with resulting decrease in mitotic activity (M. J. Edwards *et al.*, 1974; Wanner *et al.*, 1976). The possible effects of hyperthermia on the human fetus should be kept in mind in cases of fever during pregnancy, although a connection between pyrexia during pregnancy and fetal brain damage or mental retardation in man has not yet been established. An increase in number of neurons has been reported following hyperthermia and a decrease following hypothermia for a short period during incubation of the chick embryo (Zamenhof, 1976). In the chick, too, the period of neuron proliferation is especially sensitive to changes in temperature. Thus raising the temperature from 37.5°C to 40.5°C on days 5–7 of incubation results in a 22 percent increase of the cerebellar cells that originate during those days (Purkinje cells, Golgi II cells, and neurons of the cerebellar roof nuclei). Embryos incubated at 35.3°C on days 5–7 have a 14.6 percent reduction in those neurons at hatching when compared with controls incubated at 37.5°C (Zamenhof, 1976).

The factors that control the number of glial cells are not understood. The concept that more highly evolved brains have a higher ratio of glial cells to neurons goes back to the nineteenth century and found its principal exponent in von Economo (1926). Friede (1954) found that the mean number of glial cells per neuron (glia-to-neuron ratio) in all cellular layers of the mammalian cerebral cortex was 1.7 in man, 1.2 in the horse, and 0.4 in the rabbit and mouse. These findings apparently support the concept of a phylogenetic increase in the glia-to-neuron ratio. However, in contradiction to this view, Hawkins and Olszewski (1957) have shown that the mean glia-to-neuron ratio is 4.5 in the whale, and they conclude that the increase in the number of glial cells per nerve cell is not correlated with phylogenetic status but with the size of the brain. The increase in glia-to-neuron ratio in larger animals appears to be due to the fact that the size of the neurons is correlated with the size of the animal, so that large neurons may require more glia to support them, nourish them, or interact with them in ways that are not yet understood (Hawkins and Olszewski, 1957; Friede and van Houten, 1962; Friede, 1963). Methods of mechanically disaggregating the brain and separating neurons and glia have been devised (Raine *et al.,* 1971; Sinha and Rose, 1971; Capps-Covey and McIlwain, 1975). These promise to clarify the factors that affect the number of cells in the brain and that alter the glia-to-neuron ratio.

The size and number of neurons are partly determined by the size of the animal. In the invertebrates as well as the vertebrates the size of the neurons is generally greater in larger species (Hanström, 1926; Goosen, 1949; Möller, 1950; Schulz, 1951; Nolte, 1953; Neder, 1959). The large neurons, such as the cerebral cortical pyramidal cells, have longer dendrites with more branches in large mammals than in small mammals (Shariff, 1953; Bok, 1959). However, among mammals, the body weight is more significantly related to the number of neurons than to neuron size: a 4-ton elephant is a million times larger than a 4-gram shrew and the brain of the elephant is more than 10,000 times heavier than that of the shrew, yet the differences in the sizes of their neurons are only slight.

There is a good linear relation between the gestation time and the cube root of the brain weight at birth in all the mammalian orders: over a range of 16–655 days, the gestation time varies as the 0.334 power of the neonatal brain weight (Sacher and Staffeldt, 1974). In general, the rate of growth of the fetal brain varies little between mammalian species. The brain is the slowest-growing organ in the mammalian fetus, and it therefore sets important limits on the duration of gestation. To compensate for the longer gestation time, smaller litter size, and hence the slower reproductive rate in large-brained species, the life span is directly proportional to the brain weight (Sacher, 1959).

The brain-to-body weight ratio decreases progressively during postnatal development in mammals (Pearl, 1905; Dubois, 1923; Donaldson, 1925; von Bonin, 1937; Brummelkamp, 1939; Hersh, 1941; Count, 1947). In man the brain is about 18 percent of the body weight at 3 months gestation, 16 percent at 4 months, 14 percent at 5 months and about 12 percent at birth. Thereafter, the brain weight diminishes to 10 percent of the body weight at 1 year of age and to about 2.5 percent at age 20. In the adult human, the brain consumes about 20 percent of the total oxygen consumption of the entire body (McIlwain, 1959). Epstein (1973) has suggested that the main limitation in the size of the human brain at birth is not the size of the maternal birth canal but the inability of the newborn to provide oxygen and glucose for a brain larger than 12 percent of the body weight. This problem does not arise in other mammals because their brain-to-body weight ratio is always less than that in man. For example, at birth the brain-to-body weight ratio is 12 percent in man, 8 percent in the chimpanzee, and only 5 percent in the cat. This difference between man and other mammals persists throughout development (Fig. 3.21).

According to Count (1947), "a fetus of given body size always has a heavier brain than some extant relative of equal body size who is presumably less highly evolved." Statements such as this oversimplify the problem of the evolutionary tendency to increase brain-to-body weight ratio. There are three factors that have to be taken into account. The first, the limitation of size of the mammalian brain by the capacity of the body to supply it with energy, has already been mentioned. In poikilothermic animals, the limit may be set by the oxygen supply available to the embryo in the egg. In mammals, the placenta also sets a limit to brain size. The nutritional requirements of the fetus increase as the cube of its linear dimensions. This sets a limit to the number of fetuses in large animals and limits the growth of the brain in multiple pregnancies. We can say that the Lilliputians in *Gulliver's Travels* could not have had the intellectual abilities they display in Swift's story: they are described as being scaled down to one-twelfth the size of a normal man, but with otherwise normal proportions. In fact, their body size could not have supported a brain larger than that of a dog, and their intellects would have had to be reduced accordingly. Similar misconceptions abound in the literature concerning giants and dwarfs. It occurs, more subtly, in the following proposition by Hans Reichenbach (1951, p. 132): "Suppose that during the night all physical objects, including our bodies became ten times as large. On awakening this morning we should be in no condition to test this assumption, since our measuring rods and other instruments would have undergone congruent changes." This statement ignores the fact that unless the fundamental laws of physics were also changed, a tenfold increase in linear dimensions of the body would have to be attended by

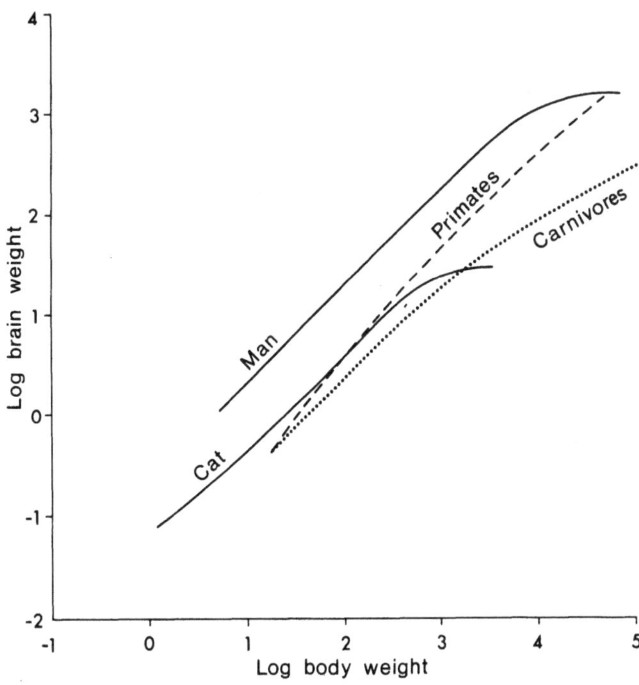

Figure 3.21. Relationship between log brain weight and log body weight during ontogeny in man and the domestic cat (solid lines) and in a phylogenetic series of primates and carnivores (broken line). From E. W. Count, *Ann. N.Y. Acad. Sci. 46*:993–1122 (1947), copyright The New York Academy of Sciences, reprinted by permission.

such great changes in the relative sizes of the parts that the change in form would be noticed immediately. This is because increase in linear dimensions of the body results in increase of the body mass by the cube, but the cross-sectional area of the weight-bearing bones increases only as the square of the linear dimensions. In order to bear the additional weight of the soft tissues, the weight of the skeleton has to increase proportionately more than the increase in body weight. As a result, the ratio of brain weight to body weight is less in large than in small animals (Goosen, 1949; Rensch, 1958). This brings us to the second factor that is often not taken into account in considering the significance of brain-to-body weight ratio, namely, the fact that soft tissues have a much greater innervation than bone. Brain-to-body weight ratios should be calculated on the basis of soft tissue weight when comparing animals with very different skeletal mass (see, for example, Fig. 1 in Jerison, 1970, showing the relation of brain-to-body size in living and extinct animals). The problem of changes in physiological functions that are correlated with changes in body size has been well discussed by Adolph (1949), S. J. Gould (1966), Stahl (1970), Schmidt-Nielsen (1970), and Pilbeam and Gould (1974).

The third factor to take into account in considering the significance of brain size in relation to body size and to the evolution of the brain is the relative number of Type I and Type II neurons. Type I neurons form the main efferent and afferent pathways, and their axons form the peripheral nerves, whereas Type II neurons are local circuit neurons that form the central integrating circuits. I have suggested that the number of Type I neurons is correlated with the total body mass, whereas the number of Type II neurons can be more closely correlated with behavioral complexity than with the size of the animal (M. Jacobson, 1975*a*). Thus the body size might be expected to be closely correlated with the number of nerve fibers passing through the foramen magnum, and, in fact, Radinsky (1967) has shown that there is a coefficient of correlation of 0.976 between body weight and foramen magnum area in representatives of five orders of extant mammals. The increased number of Type I neurons, such as spinal motoneurons and spinal sensory ganglion cells, in large animals is reflected in a linear relationship between the number of axons in peripheral nerves and the body weight (Schnepp and Schnepp, 1971; Schnepp *et al.,* 1971). It is reasonable to expect the number of Type I neurons to be closely related to body weight regardless of phylogenetic position, but the increase in the ratio of brain-to-body weight that occurs during phylogeny is probably due to an increase in Type II neurons. As an example, the ratio of granule cells (Type II) to Purkinje cells (Type I) in the cerebellar cortex is 1500:1 in man, 950:1 in the rhesus monkey, 600:1 in the cat, 140:1 in the mouse, and 100:1 in the frog (Blinkov and Glezer, 1968). The stellate cells of the mammalian cerebral cortex increase from 31 percent of the total number of cortical neurons in the rabbit, to 35 percent in the cat, and to 45 percent in the monkey (Mitra, 1955). These figures indicate a progressive evolutionary increase in the ratio of Type II to Type I neurons. For several additional reasons dealt with elsewhere (M. Jacobson, 1974*b,* 1975*a*), the distinction between Type I and Type II neurons will have to be made in the future when considering evolution of the brain and in making comparisons between brains of different species.

The size of neurons may also be related to the life span and phylogenetic status of the animal. D'Arcy Thompson (1942) pointed out that "such cells as continue to divide through life tend to uniformity of size in all mammals; those which do not do so, and in particular the ganglion cells, continue to grow, and their size becomes, therefore, a function of the duration of life." It should be pointed out that the largest neurons are to be found in invertebrates and that the largest neurons in the vertebrate nervous system are the first to be formed during development. Giant neurons are found only in the lower vertebrate orders—for example, Muller cells and other giant neurons in lampreys (H. P. Whiting, 1957; Rovainen, 1967*a,b*) and Rohon-Beard cells and Mauthner cells in fish and amphibians (Stefanelli, 1951; A. F. Hughes, 1957; Otsuka, 1962, 1964; Moulton *et al.,* 1968; Kimmel and Eaton, 1976). The size of the brain increases during postnatal life, owing primarily to an increase in cell size and myelination and only slightly to an increase in the number of cells. It has yet to be established that there is an increase in neuronal size as a result of learning and experience in mammals, although it is clear that neurons increase in size during normal maturation (Donaldson and Nagasaka, 1918; Kuhlenbeck, 1954; Brizzee and Jacobs, 1959; Schadé, 1959; Schadé and Groeningen, 1961; M. W. Fox *et al.,* 1966; Ford and Cohan, 1968; Blinkov and Glezer, 1968).

The problem of neuron loss with aging is highly controversial—reports of stability of cell number are balanced by other reports of decline of the number of neurons. There is no doubt that the weight of the brain frequently declines sharply during senescence, but the question then is whether there is an inevitable physiological loss of neurons or whether the loss is due to a variety of pathological states—trauma, vascular insufficiency, nutritional deficiencies, toxins, or infective agents. Even in the latter cases, the loss of neurons varies in different parts of the nervous system so that counts made in one region may not correlate with counts made in another region. Even in one region, the different types of neurons may behave differently during aging or in response to infections, poisons, or insufficiency of oxygen or nutrients. Until fairly recently, it was believed that the number of neurons inevitably declines with age and that brain weight declines linearly after middle age in man (reviewed by Wright and Spink, 1959). That view has been challenged in more recent studies (Konigsmark and Murphy, 1970, 1972; E. Howard, 1973), and even in the earlier literature there are reports of failure to find neuron loss. Those reports deal mainly with the number of large, class I neurons. For example, no change in the number of axons in the sciatic nerve is found in rats up to 850 days of age (Birren and Wall, 1956), nor is there a reduction in number of fibers in the ventral spinal roots of cats up to 50 weeks of age (Moyer and Kaliszewski, 1958). Large neurons, too, of the cat's spinal cord are undiminished until 50 weeks of age, and are reduced in number only by 15 percent at 110 weeks (Wright and Spink, 1959). These reports of neuronal stability are supported by the observations that no reduction is found in the total number of neurons in the ventral cochlear nucleus counted in 23 human brains from birth to 90 years of age (Konigsmark and Murphy, 1972). Other brain stem nuclei have also been found to have a cell population that is not diminished in old age: the motor nucleus of the facial nerve (Van Buskirk, 1945), the dentate nucleus (Höpker, 1951), and the main nucleus of the inferior olive (Monagle and Brody, 1974).

By contrast, the cerebral cortex and cerebellar cortex seem to be more susceptible to loss of cells as a result of aging. Loss of neurons in the human cerebral cortex was reported by Brody (1955), and in the rat by Brizzee *et al.* (1968). Loss of Purkinje cells in the cerebellar cortex was reported by Ellis (1919, 1920), Harms (1927), and Inukai (1928). The problems of individual variations and counting errors as well as the causes of death have to be taken into consideration in assessing the meanings of these findings. In healthy laboratory animals there does not appear to be a decline in brain weight or brain DNA content with advanced age (E. Howard, 1973). The constancy of brain DNA content from maturity to very old age in the rat does not support the view that brain cell loss is inevitable. However, loss of neurons in restricted regions or replacement of neurons by glial cells cannot be detected by measuring total brain DNA content.

Increase in functional activity of the nervous system has been shown to produce an increased proliferation of glia, which have the capacity to divide, even in adult mammals (Hommes and Leblond, 1967), but there is no evidence of increased neuronal proliferation due to functional activity. For example, increased motor activity produces an increased proliferation of glia in the ventral horn of the spinal cord of mice (Kuhlenkampf, 1952). The result of enriching the environment and increasing the sensorimotor activity of young rats is an increase in thickness and weight of the cerebral cortex of about 6 percent, particularly in the visual and somatosensory areas of the cortex. This is mainly due to increase in glia in the cerebral cortex (M. C. Diamond *et al.*, 1964, 1966) and in the white matter of the cerebrum and corpus callosum (Altman and Das, 1964).

The size of the neurons is also related to their ploidy. However, reports that many large neurons, such as cerebellar Purkinje cells and hippocampal pyramidal neurons, continue DNA synthesis without cell division and attain a tetraploid quantity of DNA are now thought to be false (Mann and Yates, 1973*a,b*). The large neurons are capable of maintaining themselves with a diploid DNA content. In experimentally produced polyploid salamanders and newts, all the cells (including neurons and glia) are greatly enlarged, but the organs (including the brain) are normal in size and shape. Although the cells are increased in volume, there is a compensatory decrease in their numbers, as shown by Fig. 3.22 (Fankhauser, 1941, 1945*a,b;* Gurdon, 1959; Bradom, 1960). Bradom (1962) has shown that haploid salamanders also have brains of normal dimensions, since the cells, although small, are increased in number (Fig. 3.22). Tetraploid mice at 14½ and

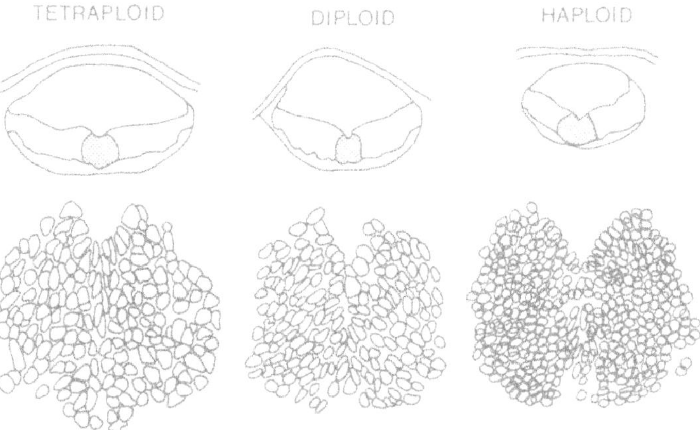

Figure 3.22. Projection drawings of transverse sections through the medulla of tetraploid, diploid, and haploid hybrid newts. The nuclei in the shaded areas of the medulla are shown below in tetraploid, diploid, and haploid newts, to indicate the differences in size of the cells. From W. F. Bradom, *J. Exp. Zool. 143:*323–345 (1960) and *Biol. Bull. 123:*253–263 (1962).

16½ days gestation are found to have about one-quarter as many cells as diploids of the same age, but in the polyploids the nervous system contains many abnormalities (Snow, 1975). The total size of an animal may be set by the limits to protein synthesis, which in turn may be limited by the amount of ribosomal RNA. In fact, the number of ribosomal RNA cistrons per cell has been shown to be twice as great in tetraploid as in diploid fish (Schmidtke *et al.*, 1975).

It is of considerable interest that the maze-learning ability of polyploid salamanders with a reduced number of very large brain cells is considerably worse than the learning ability of diploid salamanders (Fankhauser *et al.*, 1955). In this connection, Vernon and Butsch (1957) concluded that "polyploidy, whether triploid or tetraploid, brings about a decrease in maze-learning ability. It is not possible, however, to state whether such an effect is the result of the increase in cell size, the reduction in the number of cells, or the reduction in the number of neuronal connections that probably results from the reduced number of cells." Unfortunately, the learning ability of haploid salamanders, which have an increased number of neurons, has not been investigated. The relationship between brain size, number of neurons, and learning ability could also be studied very profitably in ants, in which the highest nervous centers, the corpora pedunculata, are very small in the males, larger in the females, and largest in the workers (Pandazis, 1930; Goll, 1967). "The behavior of the three groups corresponds to their brain structure: the males may truly be called stupid, the females are far superior, and the highest faculties are those of the workers" (Goetsch, 1957).

Growth of the nervous system, measured by changes in weight and size, has thus been found to correlate with the size of the species and with its ontogenetic stage and phylogenetic status. The differences in dimensions of the nervous system during development may be termed *ontogenetic relative growth,* whereas the difference in adult dimensions between related species may be termed *phylogenetic differential growth.* The same power function, $y = bx^k$, the allometric or relative growth function (J. S. Huxley, 1932), describes the relationships between homologous parts of a series of adult animals belonging to different species and the increase in size of any part of the brain during development (Hersh, 1941; Grenell and Scammon, 1943; Noback and Moss, 1956).

Written in straight-line logarithmic form, the allometric equation becomes

$$\log y = \log b + k \log x$$

where b and k are constants and x and y represent variable parameters such as body weight, brain weight, the weight or the dimensions of different parts of the nervous system, or of the same part at different times during ontogeny, or in different animals that are closely related phylogenetically. If x and y conform to the relative growth equation and the constants do not change during ontogeny, a straight line with slope k is obtained on a double logarithmic plot, and log b is the y intercept. Often, where the constants change during ontogeny, sigmoid relative growth curves are obtained.

Depending on the values of b and k, the ontogenetic and phylogenetic relationship may be parallel, divergent, or convergent, or a combination of these three. An example of parallel allometry is given by Brummelkamp (1939), who showed that the brain weight to body weight relation in various groups of vertebrates (including fish, amphibians, and mammals) conforms to the allometric equation for each group, with $k = 5/9$ for all groups; however, the value of b for each group differs by some integral power of 2. Jerison (1969) has plotted the brain and body weights for 198 vertebrate species (data from Crile and Quiring, 1940) showing that the data conform to the allometric equation with an exponent of ⅔, close to the value obtained by Brummelkamp. Extending Brummelkamp's findings, Jerison has found that the value of the constant b is 10 times greater in the higher vertebrates (birds, mammals) than in the lower (fish, reptiles), and is clearly related to phylogenetic status of the group. The brain-to-body weight ratio is about twice as large in monkeys as in any other mammals, twice as large in the great apes as in monkeys, and twice as large in man as in the great apes.

Unfortunately, the relative growth curve does not differentiate between growth due to increase in cell size and growth due to increase in cell number and gives no hint of the ratios of neurons to glia or of Type I to Type II neurons. The allometric equation does not tell us anything about the mechanisms that control the growth of the nervous system and that determine its final size and shape. These limitations are generally acknowledged by morphologists. For example, E. S. Russell (1916, p. 312) states: "Pure morphology is essentially a science of comparison which seeks to disentangle the unity hidden beneath the diversity of organic form. It is not immediately concerned with the cause of organic diversity." There may be advantages, for purposes of comparative morphology, in the use of dimensionless numbers (see Stahl, 1962, 1970) and of nonmetric topological analysis (Kuhlenbeck, 1967; Thom, 1974). However, the most important advances in the past have come not from the application of this kind of "pure" morphology but rather from the morphologists who make strong inductions regarding the functional significance of their morphological data.

4

Differentiation, Growth, and Maturation of Neurons

4.1. Introduction

The control of cell differentiation in eukaryotes is exerted at many levels: DNA replication, transcription, and translation, activation of enzymes, and control of membrane permeability by hormones or other intercellular transmitters. Transcriptional control is particularly important in eukaryotes because of the presence of the cytoplasm, which can store and sequestrate factors that control gene expression, and because of the presence in eukaryote chromatin of some proteins that inhibit transcription and others that activate it. As Britten and Davidson (1969, 1971) have recognized, the histones produce a nonspecific, general repression of transcription, whereas differential gene action consists largely of counteracting this repression by means of activators that are specific with respect to their time of action and with respect to the gene loci that they activate. These activators may be hormone–protein complexes and cytoplasmic factors that enter the nucleus and become bound to acidic, nonhistone proteins in the chromosomes (Davidson and Britten, 1973).

The capacity of cytoplasmic factors to control gene expression in the oocyte (Gurdon and Woodland, 1968; Gurdon, 1974) has also been shown to apply to the nucleus of the differentiated cell. Thus the nucleus recommences DNA replication and transcription when transplanted into an enucleated amphibian egg (T. J. King and Briggs, 1956; Gurdon, 1970; Laskey and Gurdon, 1970). Cytoplasmic control of gene activity in developing neurons has not been demonstrated directly. That such controls exist is suggested by the vast body of evidence that differentiation of nerve cells is strongly influenced by cellular interactions and must, therefore, be mediated by the cell membrane and cytoplasm (see Chapter 7).

We have to distinguish between the process of differentiation of neuronal phenotypes from an undifferentiated stem cell and the process of stabilization and continued expression of the differentiated state. We can assay for the former by biochemical, cytochemical, and immunochemical methods of detecting neuronal phenotypes at early stages of differentiation, while the terminal processes of differentiation are usually recognized by the appearance of structures as seen with the microscope.

The identification of distinct neuronal and glial phenotypes has, until recently, required overt cytodifferentiation, and thus the cells could be recognized unambiguously only when they were approaching the final stages of differentiation. This often involved the subjective impressions of the observer, and was especially subject to error in cases where cells have similar appearances during their preterminal stages of differentiation, when transitional forms might arise, or when cell differentiation might be somewhat atypical, as in tissue culture.

Ideally, objective criteria of cell differentiation should obviate many of these difficulties. Several such objective criteria are now available, for example, the use of labeled antibodies to cell-specific proteins, or biochemical or histochemical assays for specific cell products or the enzymes that synthesize such products. There are several proteins that are found only in nerve tissue. One of these, 14-3-2 protein, is specific to neurons of mammals and birds but is probably absent in fish and reptiles (B. W. Moore and Perez, 1968; B. W. Moore, 1972). 14-3-2 protein is probably concentrated at the presynaptic terminals, and its concentration during development of the nervous system increases during the period of synaptogenesis (Grasso and Pirazzi, 1975). Another brain-specific protein, S100, is found in glial cells in all species that have been examined. During development, the concentration of S100 protein provides an index of gliogenesis. The localization of S100 is predominantly in the nucleus (Michetti *et al.*, 1974). Rapid increase of S100 protein in mouse brain between 15 and 21 days after birth is due mainly to increased synthesis (Stewart and Urban, 1972; Stewart, 1975), and correlates well with gliogenesis in the mouse brain. In chick spinal cord, S100 protein increases rapidly after the 10th day of incubation at the time of maximum gliogenesis (Cicero and Provine, 1972).

The use of RNA–DNA hybridization techniques can detect which RNA species are transcribed from repeated sequences and which from unique DNA sequences (R. L. Davidson, 1973, review). Recent reports have shown that brain DNA contains several times as many unique DNA sequences as are found in liver, kidney, or spleen: Hahn and Laird (1971), Grouse *et al.* (1972), I. R. Brown and Church (1972), and Soga and Takahashi (1975, 1976). The last authors also showed, by separating glial cells and neurons, that while neurons and glia contain about the same number of repeated DNA sequences, neurons have more unique DNA sequences than glia.

Another way of studying the differentiative capabilities, in the sense of the genetic information that the cell may express but that is partially repressed, is by somatic cell hybridization (H. Harris *et al.*, 1966) using Sendai virus to fuse neurons with nonneural cells of various types. The heterokaryons divide and can be cultured for many generations. C.-O. Jacobson (1969) seeded mouse brain cells on top of a monolayer of cultured cells such as monkey kidney cells in the presence of Sendai virus and obtained heterokaryons that expressed neuronal phenotypes. The effects of somatic cell hybridization on gene expression permit some inferences to be made about mechanisms of gene control of differentiation (R. L. Davidson, 1973 review). If differentiated phenotypes are extinguished in the hybrids that were previously expressed in one of the parent cell lines, it can be inferred that the genes for those phenotypes are under negative control. Alternatively, genes that code for phenotypes present in only one parent cell line that continue to be expressed in the hybrids may be under positive control.

In hybrids of neuroblastoma cells and various types of fibroblasts, it has been shown that the majority of neuronal phenotypes continue to be expressed (McMorris *et al.*, 1974; McMorris and Ruddle, 1974). These phenotypes, which may thus be under positive control, include neuronal morphology, action potential generation, acetylcholine sensitivity, and neuron-specific 14-3-2 protein. By contrast, the enzyme steroid sulfatase, present in neuroblastoma cells, was extinguished in neuroblastoma–fibroblast hybrids in which the fibroblast cell line did not contain steroid sulfatase, indicating that this protein may be under negative control. Choline acetyltransferase was expressed in one hybrid derived from parents neither of which had choline acetyltransferase activity.

It is not known if there is a definite stage of development at which the neuron becomes committed to a specific developmental program, nor is it known whether the neuron, once committed to one program, is able to change to another pathway of differentiation. The evidence is against such a change: it shows that after the neuron has become postmitotic its phenotype is remarkably stable even under extreme conditions. For example, neurons retain their main phenotypic characteristics after they have been separated into single cells and maintained in culture, or after they have been disaggregated and reaggregated *in vitro*.

The evidence suggests that transcription is necessary during the early but not the later stages of neuron differentiation: a dose of actinomycin D, sufficient to result in more than 90 percent reduction of uridine incorporation into RNA does not prevent outgrowth of the axon after the latter has been started, but does inhibit further neuron differentiation if applied before axonal outgrowth (Partlow and Larrabee, 1971; Burnham and Varon, 1974).

4.2. Ultrastructural Signs of Neuronal Differentiation

The latency between the time of origin and the time at which the various types of neurons attain their full differentiation varies. Some types, such as Purkinje cells and Mauthner's neurons, originate early but have a delayed and prolonged differentiation, while others, such as the cerebellar granule cells, arise late in ontogeny but differentiate rapidly. Many attempts have been made to correlate the maturity of young neurons, usually called "neuroblasts," with their ultrastructure (Duncan, 1957; Lyser, 1964, 1968*a,b;* Tennyson, 1965; S. Fujita, 1966; Wechsler, 1966*b,* 1967; Meller and Haupt, 1967; Sechrist and Lavelle, 1966; Sechrist, 1969; Fisher and M. Jacobson, 1970). It should be clear that there are only very general morphological criteria which may help to determine the age of the neuron, and it is here that pure morphology requires the support of other information such as the functional type of neuron, its time of origin, and the onset of its functional activities culminating in its integration into functional neuronal circuits. There is little to be said in favor of using a blanket term such as "neuroblast" to refer to any type of neuron which is postmitotic but not fully differentiated, without paying regard to its functional relationships. There is no unanimity about the definition of a "neuroblast," and there are differences of opinion about the stage at which the "neuroblast" should be called a neuron. Because various authors have used different criteria for identifying "neuroblasts," it is difficult to compare their results or their conclusions regarding the cytodifferentiation of the precursors of the neuron. Moreover, their criteria for identifying a cell as a neuroepithelial germinal cell, neuroblast, or neuron are much more often implied than defined. In this discussion the postmitotic cell that develops without further division into a neuron will simply be called an immature or young neuron, and the word "neuroblast" will be reserved for the cell that gives rise to neurons in the invertebrates (see Section 3.7).

The appearance of membrane-bound ribosomes or rough endoplasmic reticulum in the cytoplasm of the young neuron is usually taken as one of the criteria for identifying a neuron, or is used to distinguish the young neuron from the neuroepithelial germinal cell, which has very sparse rough endoplasmic reticulum. Most observers have concluded that an obvious increase in the amount of rough endoplasmic reticulum as well as smooth cytoplasmic membranes is the first sign of differentiation of the neuron (Bellairs, 1959; Tennyson and Pappas, 1962; Tennyson, 1965; Eschner and Glees, 1963; S. Fujita, 1966). Our observations have not lent support to such a simple view, for we have found that germinal cells and early neurons are structurally indistinguishable in the retina of *Xenopus* (Fisher and M. Jacobson, 1970). Although the amount of rough endoplasmic reticulum gradually increases during maturation of the neuron concomitantly with an increase in the Golgi complex and in the neurotubules, the time at which these changes are first observed and the rate of increase vary greatly in different types of neurons. Figure 4.1 illustrates these changes as they occur in the spinal dorsal root ganglia of the rabbit (Tennyson, 1965). There are reasons for believing that these changes occur early and rapidly in the type of neuron that forms an axon early in development. This occurs, for example, in motor neurons in the spinal cord of the chick embryo, in which axonal growth commences while the young neuron is still migrating out of the germinal zone. By contrast, in the immature retinal ganglion cells and in other immature neurons that have long period of growth before the outgrowth of the axon commences, the cytoplasm is filled with free ribosomes and polysomes, and the rough endoplasmic reticulum, Golgi complex, and neurotubules are sparse until axonal growth occurs. At that stage there is a great increase in the amount of endoplasmic reticulum, and the Golgi apparatus also becomes larger (Fisher and M. Jacobson, 1970). The ergastoplasmic cysternae that form the Nissl bodies and that are characteristic of the mature neuron are formed only after the growth of the axon has commenced, even before the axon has made terminal connections. While the dendrites are growing, which continues long after the axon has formed terminal connections, there are also abundant free ribosomes and membrane-bound ribosomes in the cytoplasm of the neuron. In neurons in which growth of the volume of dendrites is large in proportion to the increase in volume of the axon, a high proportion of the ribosomes are free, for example, in cerebellar Purkinje cells.

The development of the Nissl substance, which consists of cisternae of rough endoplasmic reticulum (Palay and Palade, 1955), must be considered together with the nucleoli in which the ribosomes are formed (Birnstiel *et al.*,

1963; Perry, 1966). Most mature neurons have a single nucleolus, although some have one or more small nucleoli in addition to the large one. By contrast, multiple nucleoli are the rule in developing neurons. The maximal number of nucleoli per cell is determined by the number of chromosomal nuclear organizers, but most cells contain fewer nucleoli than permitted by the nucleolar organizers, and the factors controlling nucleolar number are not understood.

The early neuron contains very little Nissl substance in the cytoplasm and very little RNA in the nucleolus, but the nucleolar DNA is concentrated as a dense Feulgen-positive body located centrally in the nucleolus. During the development of the neuron, the nucleolar RNA increases and the nucleolar DNA becomes

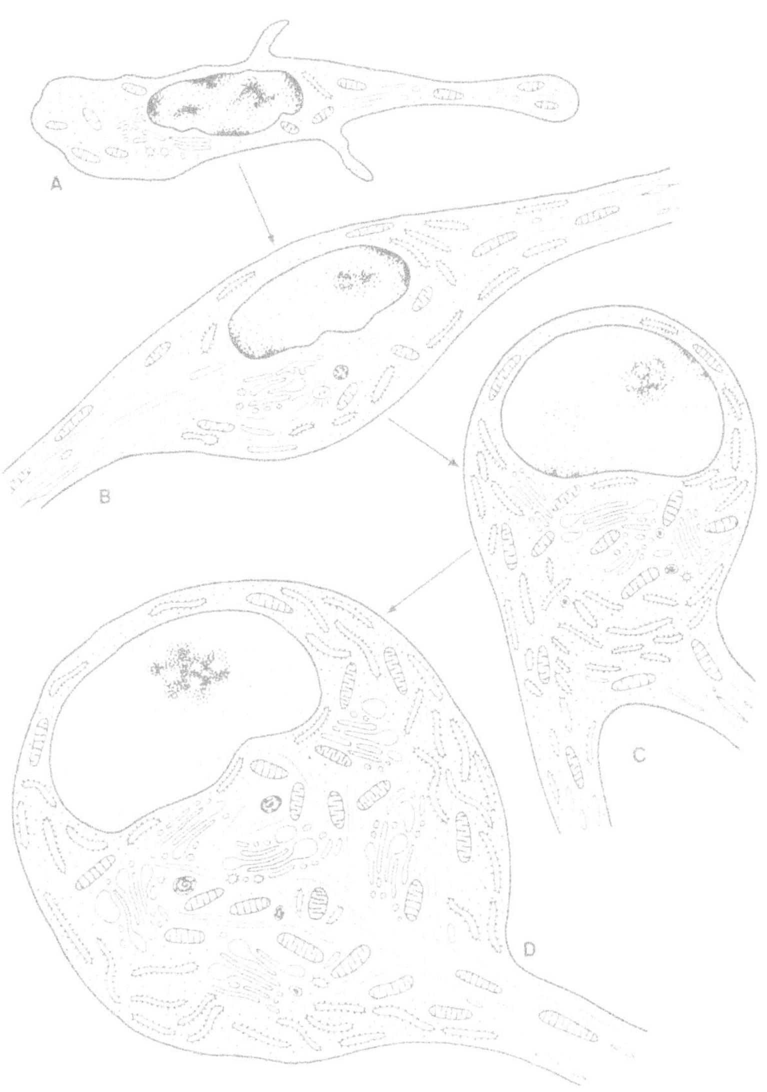

Figure 4.1. Differentiation of the dorsal root ganglion neurons of the rabbit embryo. A to D show progressive stages during development. From V. M. Tennyson, *J. Comp. Neurol. 124:*267–318 (1965).

dispersed around the periphery of the nucleolus but probably remains constant in quantity (Fig. 4.2). Lavelle (1956) showed that in developing neurons, as well as in various types of mature neurons in the guinea pig, the amount of nucleolar RNA is directly proportional to the amount of cytoplasmic RNA in the Nissl substance. The amounts of RNA and DNA were not measured quantitatively, but were estimated from the intensity of staining with thionine or with the Feulgen technique. Lavelle (1956) concluded that "the first sign of nucleolar development is always closely accompanied by the first noticeable increase in cytoplasmic basophilia of Nissl substance. The two processes, therefore, are precisely correlated from the start, as well as in their successive developmental stages. The final degree of development of the nucleolar apparatus is related directly to the characteristic amount of Nissl substance finally attained by a particular type of cell" (Lavelle, 1956).

Nissl substance first appears in the cytoplasm as small granules which stain with thionin and which form a cap on one side of the nucleus close to the nuclear membrane. The Nissl substance later becomes distributed throughout the cytoplasm, and its granules become larger and rougher. However, the degree of development of the nucleolus and the distribution and amount of Nissl granules vary in different types of neurons in the mature nervous system (Lavelle, 1956). Very sparse and fine Nissl granules and nucleoli with little RNA and with compact DNA are found in internal granule cells of the cerebellum, internal and external granule cells of the olfactory bulb, and retinal bipolar cells. Golgi type II neurons in the molecular layers of the cerebral cortex and cerebellar cortex have sparse Nissl substance and nucleolar RNA. The nucleolar RNA and cytoplasmic RNA of these types of neurons seem to have the characteristics usually associated with

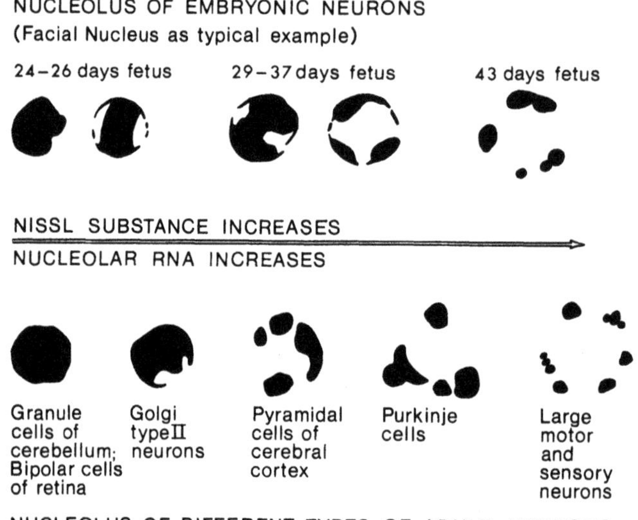

Figure 4.2. Appearance of the nucleolus of embryonic and adult neurons stained for DNA by the Feulgen technique. Top: Embryonic neurons of the facial nucleus of the guinea pig fetus. Bottom: Various types of neurons in the adult guinea pig. Increase in the Nissl substance in the cytoplasm is correlated with dispersion of the nucleolar DNA and with increase in the nucleolar RNA that occupies the unstained space in the center of the nucleolus. From A. Lavelle, *J. Comp. Neurol. 104:*175–206 (1956).

immature neurons (Fig. 4.2.). These types of neurons have relatively more free polyribosomes than membrane-bound ribosomes. This probably indicates that their protein synthesis is geared to growth rather than to secretion and that a larger proportion of the proteins are going into the dendrites than into the axon. The dendrites of these types of neurons continue to grow and probably to form new connections for a long time after their axons have made their connections and have ceased to grow significantly in length (Morest, 1969*a,b*). Cerebellar Purkinje cells (Herndon, 1963) and the large pyramidal cells of layer V of the cerebral cortex (Lavelle, 1951; Pappas and Purpura, 1961; Niklowitz and Bak, 1965) have a moderate amount of Nissl substance, and the DNA forms a beadlike ring around the periphery of their nucleoli. Complete dispersion of the nucleolar DNA is found in cells with great amounts of Nissl substance, such as the large sensory neurons in the spinal ganglia (Tennyson, 1965), large spinal motor neurons (Rapoport and Stempak, 1968), and large neurons in the motor nucleus of the facial or trigeminal nerve (Lavelle, 1956, Fig. 1). In these neurons the Nissl substance extends into the proximal parts of the dendrites but is absent from the axon hillock.

The number of mitochondria increases severalfold in rat brain from birth to maturity as estimated by mitochondrial counts or by measurements of mitochondrial proteins or enzymes (V. R. Potter *et al.,* 1945; Dahl and Samson, 1959; Samson *et al.,* 1960; Pysh, 1970). In immature neurons the mitochondria have a more lucent matrix and fewer and less regularly arranged cristae than in most mitochondria found in mature neurons (Pysh, 1970).

Microtubules and filaments are important organelles whose presence and localization in the immature neuron may be regarded as a sign of the stage of maturity of the cell. Sechrist (1969) considered that the appearance of microtubules and filaments is the first sign of differentiation of the neuron. However, microtubules have been observed in germinal cells in association with terminal bars, centrioles and the mitotic spindle (L. Herman and Kauffman, 1966; Wechsler, 1967; Lyser, 1968*a,b*), and are better correlated with the functional activities of the cell than with its age. Because microtubules and microfilaments are concerned with cellular movement, they are seen in early immature neurons that are migrating. In other types of immature neurons that are not actively motile, the microtubules and filaments develop only at a much later stage of development, when the outgrowth of the axon occurs. The neurofibrils, which can be seen with the light microscope in so-called neuroblasts, neurons, and astrocytes after silver impregnation, are probably artifacts caused by clumps of neurofilaments and neurotubules (E. G. Gray and Guillery, 1961, 1966; Guillery, 1965; Sechrist and Lavelle, 1966). Neurotubules and neurofilaments are homologous with cytoplasmic microtubules and microfilaments, which are seen with the electron microscope in most plant and animal cells (Porter, 1966).

Neurofilaments have a diameter of about 100 Å, are straight and unbranched, and tend to run for considerable distances from the cell body into the dendrite or axon (Wuerker and Palay, 1969). They are characteristic organelles in axons and extend into the growth cone, but are sparse in dendrites and in the cytoplasm of the cell body. They are virtually absent in the finest dendritic branches and in the smallest caliber axons. The giant axons of invertebrates are very rich in neurofilaments. At high magnification, the neurofilaments have a circular cross section formed of three to six globular subunits, each about 30 Å in diameter, with a light core about 35 Å in diameter (Wuerker and Palay, 1969).

They often occur with a regular spacing about 400 A apart. Fine cross-bridges, radiating like spokes from the neurofilaments, appear to link adjacent neurofilaments. The protein of filaments has been characterized in squid giant axons from which uncontaminated axoplasm can be squeezed out (Huneeus and Davison, 1970). It is an acidic protein of molecular weight about 70,000, with a composition different from that of neurofilament protein of mammalian brain, which has a molecular weight of about 56,000. Neurofilament protein has a different amino acid composition from either tubulin or actin (Davison and Winslow, 1974).

Microfilaments are fibrous organelles 40–60 Å in diameter which are found in many different types of cells, including the growth cones of axons and dendrites and in glial cells. They may form a network or may be arranged in parallel to form bundles. A network of microfilaments is found in some invertebrate axons that lack neurofilaments (Metuzals, 1969; H. L. Fernandez *et al.,* 1971; P. R. Burton and Fernandez, 1973; Moran and Rowley, 1974). The observation that molecules of heavy meromyosin from skeletal muscle attach as characteristic oblique sidearms to microfilaments indicates that those filaments behave like actin (Tilney and Mooseker, 1971; Schroeder, 1972; Ludueña and Wessells, 1973). Biochemically, the microfilaments have been characterized as a protein similar to muscle actin (Fine and Bray, 1971). It has been proposed that contractile microfilaments are the motive force for cell movements, including the movement of the tip of the growing axons (Tennyson, 1970; K. M. Yamada *et al.,* 1971). According to Ludueña and Wessells (1973), the network of microfilaments in the growth cone is responsible for elongation of microspikes at the axon tip, whereas bundles of parallel microfilaments not found in axons are responsible for the contractile phase of locomotion, in glial cells, for example.

Neurotubules are long, tubular intracellular organelles 230–250 Å in diameter, 130–150 Å inside diameter, and probably extending in length from the perikaryon to the axonal or dendritic endings, that is, up to a meter or more in length. Evidence that each neurotubule extends continuously without branching from cell body to axon tip is that the number of neurotubules in the cell body equals the sum of neurotubules in all the axonal branches (Weiss and Mayr, 1971). There is a linear relationship between the total number of neurotubules and the cross-sectional area of the axon, indicating that there is a constant ratio of polymerized tubule material to axoplasm in sciatic nerve of adult rats and mice (Friede and Samorajski, 1970), and this relationship also holds for optic nerve axons of different calibers at different stages of development (Lyser, 1971).

Microtubules are fibrous polymers largely or entirely composed of subunits of a protein called tubulin, of molecular weight approximately 110,000–120.000. This is a dimer composed of two different protomers, α- and β-tubulin, each 55,000–60,000 molecular weight and about 40 Å diameter, but the protomers differ from one another in amino acid composition (Ludueña and Woodward, 1975). The dimer is thus 4 × 90 Å, and is wound into a helix with 13 tubulin subunits per turn (L. G. Tilney *et al.,* 1973). Each protomer is tightly bound to guanosine 5-triphosphate (GTP). The "clear zone" which is always seen around neurotubules indicates that there is another component surrounding the neurotubule (Behnke, 1975). Microtubules of the same structure are found in all eukaryotic cells, including neurons and neuroglia. The tubulins from different sources are sufficiently alike for tubulin subunits from different types of cells and different species to polymerize to form hybrid microtubules (Binder *et al.,* 1975). Amino acid sequence studies of tubulin indicate that tubulins evolved from a single ancestral protein some time before the divergence of the echinoderm and chordate lines of descent and that tubulins have conserved their primary structure during evolution (Ludueña and Woodward, 1975). The protein subunits of neurotubules have a different amino acid composition from those of neurofilaments (Davison and Winslow, 1974), which rules out any possibility of their interconversion, as was once proposed (A. Peters and Vaughn, 1967).

Microtubules may be classified as labile or stable: labile microtubules, which include neurotubules, cytoplasmic microtubules, and microtubules of the mitotic spindle, are easily disrupted by colchicine, vinblastine, podophyllotoxin, low temperature, or high pressure (3000 psi), and therefore cannot be isolated intact from cells unless stabilized by D_2O or other agents. Stable microtubules, which are found in centrioles, cilia, and flagella, are not depolymerized by drugs or other agents which destroy labile microtubules.

Microtubules associated with the cilia and centriole are present in all young neurons and many mature neurons and glia. Neuronal cilia and centrioles can be seen very easily by light microscopy in sections impregnated with silver by the Nauta method (H. A. Dahl, 1963). Centrioles can also be shown by light microscopy in neurons stained by other histological methods (Lenhossék, 1895; Hatai, 1901; del Rio-Hortega, 1916). A centriole in which microtubules terminate has been found in immature retinal ganglion cells of the chick embryo (Gonatas and Robbins, 1965), in young neurons of the spinal cord of the chick and rabbit embryo (Lyser, 1964, 1968*a,b;* Tennyson, 1965), in neuroepithelial cells of the chick embryo (S. Fujita, 1966; Lyser, 1968*b*), and in immature cerebellar Purkinje cells (Kornguth *et al.,* 1967; del Cerro and Snider, 1969).

A cilium associated with a pair of centrioles is found in mature neurons—for example, in the lateral geniculate neurons of the macaque (U. Karlsson, 1966*a,b*) and the granular neurons of the fascia dentata of the rat hippocampus (H. A. Dahl, 1963), the granule cells and Purkinje cells of the rat cerebellum (del Cerro and Snider, 1967, 1969), as well as on neurosecretory cells (Palay, 1961; B. G. Barnes, 1961), ependymal cells (Palay, 1958*a;* Tennyson and Pappas, 1962), astrocytes (H. A. Dahl, 1963), and Schwann cells (Grillo and Palay, 1963). The cilium of the ependymal cell has a 9+2 array of microtubules, which is characteristic of motile cilia. However, neuronal and glial cilia have a 9+0 array of microtubules in the proximal part and an 8+1 array distally (H. A. Dahl, 1963), and are probably not motile.

The labile cytoplasmic microtubules, including neurotubules, are in dynamic equilibrium with a cytoplasmic pool of soluble tubulin subunits. Guanosine triphosphate, high Mg^{2+} and low Ca^{2+} are some requirements for the assembly process. It is not known what controls the position and orientation of microtubules in the cell, but it is obvious that there must be such controls because the tubules are located in specific positions and orientations in different parts of the nerve cell. Finally, the function of neurotubules is not as fully known as is widely supposed. They may provide cytoskeletal support and they may play a direct function in transport of materials in the cell. Most studies of the function of microtubules make use of their inactivation by drugs—tubulin binds specifically with colchicine, the vinca alkaloids vincristine and vinblastine, and podophyllotoxin. Tubulin has specific binding sites for these drugs as well as different binding sites for guanine nucleotides and for other tubulin molecules.

Tubulin in axons is transported with the slow flow to the nerve endings, where it constitutes about 28 percent of the soluble protein in axonal terminals (Feit *et al.*, 1971). This correlates with the observation that tubulin is added only at the distal end of the microtubules (Borisy *et al.*, 1974; Olmsted *et al.*, 1974; Dentler *et al.*, 1974); presumably tubulin has to be transported to the growing end of nerve fibers in order to be added to the neurotubules as they elongate. There are indications that the physical properties of brain tubulin may change during embryonic development in the chick, as shown by reduction in the half-time of decay of colchicine binding to tubulin (Bamburg *et al.*, 1973). There is some evidence that nerve fibers are most sensitive to colchicine during their initial outgrowth in tissue culture and that their sensitivity to colchicine diminishes with increasing maturity (Daniels, 1975).

Interaction of drugs with microtubule proteins has been used to block the action of microtubules and so to infer their functions in the cell (L. Wilson *et al.*, 1974, review). Colchicine binds with high affinity to tubulin. Podophyllotoxin, another plant alkaloid, binds to the same site on the tubulin as colchicine. Vinblastine and vincristine bind to a different site. These alkaloids produce their effects by preventing assembly of the tubulin into microtubules, the tubulin assembling instead into nontubular crystalline arrays. The alkaloids do not appear to bind to assembled microtubules, but produce dissociation of microtubules secondary to depletion of the soluble pool of tubulin that is in equilibrium with the microtubules. Lumicolchicines, derivatives obtained by ultraviolet irradiation of colchicine, do not inhibit mitosis and do not block axonal flow, but they do inhibit nucleoside transport across the cell membrane, which is also one of the side effects of colchicine.

Biochemical dissection of the mechanism of axonal flow, using the antimitotic drugs, is restricted by the limits of specificity of action of the drugs (see Sections 2.3 and 4.8). These agents have other effects in addition to their action on microtubules. Colchicine inhibits transport across the cell membrane (Mizel and Wilson, 1972). Colchicine and vinblastine inhibit the release of norepinephrine from sympathetic nerve endings (Thoa *et al.*, 1972). Vinblastine has been found to precipitate a number of proteins in addition to tubulin (L. Wilson *et al.*, 1970). There is thus an element of doubt in all the experiments in which the role of microtubules in the functions of the cell—in axonal flow, for example—has been inferred from the inhibition by colchicine. Misgivings are also raised by the observation that fast axonal flow is blocked by doses of colchicine which do not appear to alter the structure of axonal neurotubules as seen with the electron microscope (Sjöstrand *et al.*, 1970; Hansson and Sjöstrand, 1971; J. L. Karlsson *et al.*, 1971; Norström *et al.*, 1971; Byers, 1974), and by the observation that intact neurotubules persist in crayfish axons after axoplasmic flow has been stopped with vinblastine (H. L. Fernandez *et al.*, 1971).

From these examples it may be seen that the ultrastructure of the developing neuron gives an indication of its functional activities, and a critical assessment of the ultrastructure can give an indication of the maturity of the neuron. The combined appearance of many structures in the young neuron may be of greater help than any single criterion in determining its maturity, but there are no hard-and-fast rules. The usefulness and reliability of these criteria are limited by the hazard of selecting data from a small part of the cell, which is unavoidable when thin sections and high magnifications are used. Random variations in the distribution of various subcellular structures make quantitative and statistical evaluation of changes in the number of subcellular structures extremely hazardous as well as arduous. Pease (1964) has expressed this as follows: "An electron microscopist who is concerned with tissue work simply cannot accept most problems that are primarily statistical. He cannot possibly process enough samples. He can only effectively deal with problems which yield simple qualitative answers. Processes that involve development and change are his anathema."

4.3. Origin and Growth of the Axon

The historical development of knowledge of the outgrowth of the nerve fiber from the young neuron has often been summarized. S. Ramón y Cajal (1908, 1933) reviewed the development of the rival theories and gave a masterful critique of their eristic distinctions. He gives us an insight into the polemical fervor of the disputants, which is in contrast with R. G. Harrison's (1935) more dispassionate survey and with the blandness of recent reviews (Detwiler, 1936; A. F. Hughes, 1968*a*).

At the end of the nineteenth century there was still considerable conflict of ideas about the development of the nerve fiber. There were three main theories of its development. According to the cell-chain theory, originated by Theodor Schwann (1810–1882), the axon is formed by fusion of the cells that form the neurilemmal sheath, namely the Schwann cells. This theory was disproved by R. G. Harrison (1904, 1906, 1924*a*) when he showed that removal of the neural crest, from which the Schwann cells originate, results in the development of normal nerve fibers in the absence of Schwann cells. He also showed that removal of the neural tube, which contains the developing neurons, prevents the formation of nerves, although the Schwann cells are left intact.

The plasmodesm or syncytial theory originated with Viktor Hensen (1835–1924) and was supported by Hans Held (1866–1942). According to this theory, the nerve fiber differentiates from preestablished filaments that connect all the cells of the nervous system into a "neurosyncytium." This theory was founded on various misinterpretations of histology as well as the presence of histological artifacts, and eventually gave way to more accurate histological observations, particularly those of Wilhelm His (1831–1904) and Santiago Ramón y Cajal (1852–1934). The outgrowth of the nerve fiber had first been clearly described in 1887 from histological sections by Wilhelm His: "The fibres which grow out from the nerve cells advance by growing into existing interstitial spaces between other tissue elements. In the spinal cord and in the brain, the medullary stroma already formed, provides pathways for expansion and its structure undoubtedly determines the course of the process of extension. . . ." In the same year, Forel gave additional histological evidence that nerve fibers originate only from nerve cells, depend for their vitality on continuity with the nerve cell, and terminate by contact, not by continuity, with another nerve cell. However, opposition to the neuron theory continued despite these and other demonstrations, and it was not until Ramón y Cajal had presented overwhelming evidence in its favor and Harrison had demonstrated the growth of living nerve fibers that the neuron theory was widely accepted. An inquiry into the origins of the neuron theory shows, in the words of Arthur Lovejoy (1936), "how far, even in the minds of acute and professedly unprejudiced men of science, the emotion of conviction may lag behind the presentation of proof," but it also shows that in the minds of the original proponents of a theory, conviction must always precede the presentation of proof.

In Ramón y Cajal the genius of the artist and scientist were combined to a unique degree. He was able to synthesize his experience of many histological preparations in his drawings, showing relationships between neurons that were seldom if ever seen in a single view through the microscope. In describing and justifying this method, he wrote: "a histological drawing is never an impersonal copy of everything present in the preparation. If that were true our figures would be far too complicated and almost incomprehensible. By virture of an incontestable right, the scientific artist, for the purpose of clarity and simplicity, omits many useless details. . . . In order to decrease the number of figures artists are sometimes forced to combine objects which are scattered in two or three successive sections" (Ramón y Cajal, 1929*a*). In addition, he often grasped the functional significance of the living structure he observed in dead, fixed specimens, and was not averse to making bold inferences. His vivid description of activity of the growth cone (see Section 4.4), which he saw only as a fixed and stained structure, is typical of the strong inductive vein in his mode of thought. Ramón y Cajal's method was akin to that of one school of Chinese artists discussed by March (1935): "natural forms were studied with reference to their typical and permanent, rather than their accidental and transient phenomena; with reference to their functions as well as to their appearances; and certain general principles were deduced. . . . The habits of growth, the effects of seasonal change, the genetic and functional relations of parts were observed. . . ." He had the ability, above all others, to create a kinematic reconstruction of the degenerating, regenerating, and developing neurons that he observed in fixed histological sections. By the turn of the century he had arrived at the modern conception of the dynamics of neuronal growth, and had recognized that the axon was an ameboid outgrowth of the young neuron.

The outgrowth theory was finally proved by Ross G. Harrison (1870–1959) using the technique of tissue culture, which he invented (for Harrison's contributions to experimental embryology, see Oppenheimer, 1966). Harrison (1907*a,b,* 1910) excised pieces of neural tube from early tailbud frog larvae, at a stage before any nerve fibers are present, and explanted the tissue into a drop of frog lymph suspended from a coverslip over a depression slide. Nerve fibers were seen growing out of the explant, in many cases from single isolated cells, for distances up to 1.15 mm, at rates ranging from 15.6 to 56 μm per hour (Fig. 4.3).

Harrison (1910) also gave the first description of the outgrowth of nerve fibers from young neurons *in vivo.* He observed the growth of the axons from the Rohon-Beard cells, which are the primary sensory cells and which can be seen in the dorsal part of the neural tube just beneath the epidermis in living frog embryos. Harrison observed that as the axon grows out of the Rohon-Beard cell into the subepidermal tissue, it slowly increases in length and gives rise to many branches. The tip of the initial outgrowth, as well as the end of each branch, consists of an enlargement from which ameboid terminal filaments are constantly emitted and retracted. These were the first observations of the activities of the

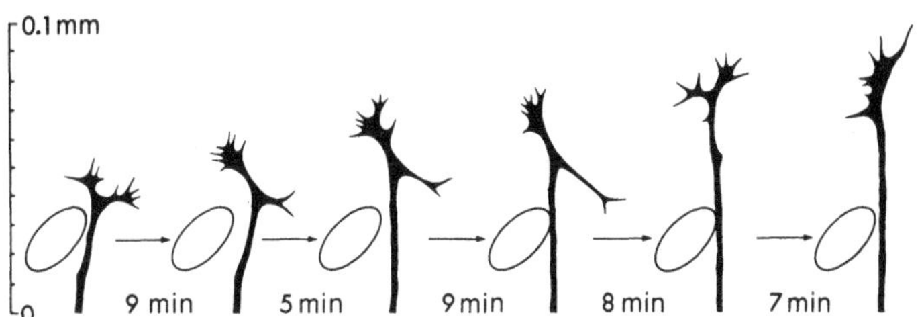

Figure 4.3. Six successive views of the end of a growing nerve fiber, showing its change of shape and rate of growth. The sketches were made with the aid of a camera lucida at the time intervals indicated. The red blood corpuscle, shown in outline, marks a fixed point. The average rate of elongation of the nerve was about 1 μm/min. The total length of the nerve fiber was 800 μm. The observations were made on a preparation of frog embryo ectoderm, isolated in lymph, 4 days after isolation. From R. G. Harrison, *J. Exp. Zool. 9:*787–846 (1910).

growth cone during normal development in a living animal. They fully confirmed Ramón y Cajal's descriptions of growth cones in fixed specimens, and they provided a standard by which to assess whether growth cones in tissue culture were normal or artifactual. The growth of the axons of Rohon-Beard cells occurs in the same way as the growth of axons in tissue culture. The fact that Harrison's description of the growth of living nerve fibers agreed completely with Ramón y Cajal's description of the growth of nerve fibers in histological preparations of the developing nervous system at one stroke established the validity of Ramón y Cajal's observations, which were far more detailed and diverse than any that could be obtained *in vitro* at that time. Harrison's experiments had, in his words, taken the mode of formation of the axon "out of the realm of inference and placed it upon the secure foundation of direct observation." His experiment had completely confirmed the accuracy of Ramón y Cajal's observations and the validity of the outgrowth theory.

Harrison coined the term "exploratory fibers" for the nerve fiber that precedes the rest in the development of a fiber pathway. Ramón y Cajal gives many vivid descriptions of these pathfinders. For instance, during the outgrowth of the dorsal spinal root from the spinal sensory ganglia, he says, "a bundle of precocious bipolar cells strikes with its cones, like battering-rams, on the posterior basal membrane and opens a narrow breach in it. Other sensory fibers, differentiating later, make use of this opening, and assault the interior of the spinal cord along its dorsal portion."

4.4. The Axonal Growth Cone

Ramón y Cajal discovered the growth cone, recognized its functions, and illustrated its various appearances during the 1890s. In his *Recollections of My Life* (1917), he writes: "I had the good fortune to behold for the first time that fantastic ending of the growing axon. In my sections of the three-days chick embryo, this ending appeared as a concentration of protoplasm of conical form, endowed with ameboid movements. It could be compared with a living battering ram, soft and flexible, which advances, pushing aside mechanically the obstacles which it finds in its way, until it reaches the area of its peripheral distribution. This curious terminal club, I christened the growth cone."

The appearance of the growth cone is similar in the Rohon-Beard cells of living frog larvae (Harrison, 1910), the outgrowing axons in the tail fin of the intact, living frog tadpole (Speidel, 1933, 1941), and the axons growing in tissue culture of neurons from amphibians (Harrison, 1907*a,b,* 1910, 1912, 1914), chick embryos (W. H. Lewis and Lewis, 1912; A. F. Hughes, 1953; Nakai, 1956, 1960; D. Bray, 1970; K. M. Yamada *et al.,* 1970, 1971; Wessells *et al.,* 1971*a,b*), and human fetuses (Nakai and Kawasaki, 1959). The tip of the axon is slightly swollen and may have an undulating membrane, or it may give rise to filopodia. The filopodia are motile extensions of the growth cone, with a length of up to 10–20 μm and a diameter of about 0.3 μm. There may be from 1 to 30 filopodia on a single growth cone. The filopodia extend and retract rapidly at a rate of about 6–10 μm per minute, and they are in constant motion. They tend to adhere to other cells or foreign bodies that they touch. The mechanism of extension at the growth cone is quite similar to that observed during the extension phase of movement of many types of cells, but the contraction phase that serves to pull the cell bodily forward is absent in the growth cone, in which the principal cause of extension is insertion of new material into the growth cone. However, other similarities between the advancing tip of the growth cone and the advancing tip of a moving fibroblast are striking. They include forward extension of a ruffling or undulating membrane, extension of filopodia or microspikes, contact with and adhesion to the substratum (Nakai, 1960, 1965), addition of new surface membrane near the advancing tip of the cell, and a movement of surface components of the cell membrane from the advancing tip toward the cell body (D. Bray, 1970; Koda and Partlow, 1976), as shown in Fig. 4.4.

All or most of the interactions of the neuron with its environment take place at the growth cone. Only the growth cone moves—the remainder of the nerve cell is stationary. Thus, as the axon or dendrite elongates, the cell body and proximal segments of the axon or dendrite are, in most cases, attached and stationary. There are exceptions in which the cell body itself migrates, as in the case of the cerebellar granule cells. However, the addition of new material during the elongation of the axon, and probably also of dendrites, occurs at the growth cone, which is solely responsible for the choice of direction, for selecting a pathway, and, finally, for selecting a suitable target at which to stop elongating.

Many studies of growth cones with the electron microscope have confirmed the observations obtained with the light microscope and have added the facts that the growth cones of axons are similar to those of dendrites, containing the usual cytoplasmic organelles, including mitochondria, ribosomes (especially in dendritic growth cones), microtubules, 100 Å neurofilaments and 50 Å microfilaments, and many vesicles and cisternae of smooth endoplasmic reticulum (del Cerro and Snider, 1968; Tennyson, 1970; K. M. Yamada *et al.,* 1971; D. Bray and Bunge, 1973; Skoff and Hamburger, 1974; del Cerro, 1974; G. Q. Fox *et al.,* 1976). Growth cones of glial cells have essentially similar appearances to those of neurons (del Cerro, 1974).

Two observations on growth cones merit further attention. The first is that growth cones can take up proteins (ferritin, molecular weight 500,000, and peroxidase, molecular weight 40,000) from the extracellular space, apparently by pinocytosis (Birks *et al.*, 1972; M. B. Bunge, 1973*a;* del Cerro, 1974). This capacity for pinocytosis persists at the presynaptic and postsynaptic membranes in the adult neuron (U. Smith, 1971). Some of the particles taken into the growing neuron are rapidly transported toward the cell body, and the movement of larger particles inside living nerve fibers in tissue culture can be seen with the light microscope (Burdwood, 1965; Berlinrood *et al.*, 1972).

The second noteworthy observation is that the growth cone contains a network of microfilaments 40–60 Å in diameter, which are the main components of the ruffling membrane, filopodia, and microspikes (K. M. Yamada *et al.*, 1970, 1971; Wessells *et al.*, 1971*a,b;* M. B. Bunge, 1973*b*). There are several lines of evidence that implicate these microfilaments in the mechanism of movement of the growth cone and its filopodia. Ludueña and Wessells (1973) have made the distinction between the microfilaments in the form of a network or lattice, which is present in the growth cone, and a different configuration of microfilaments, in

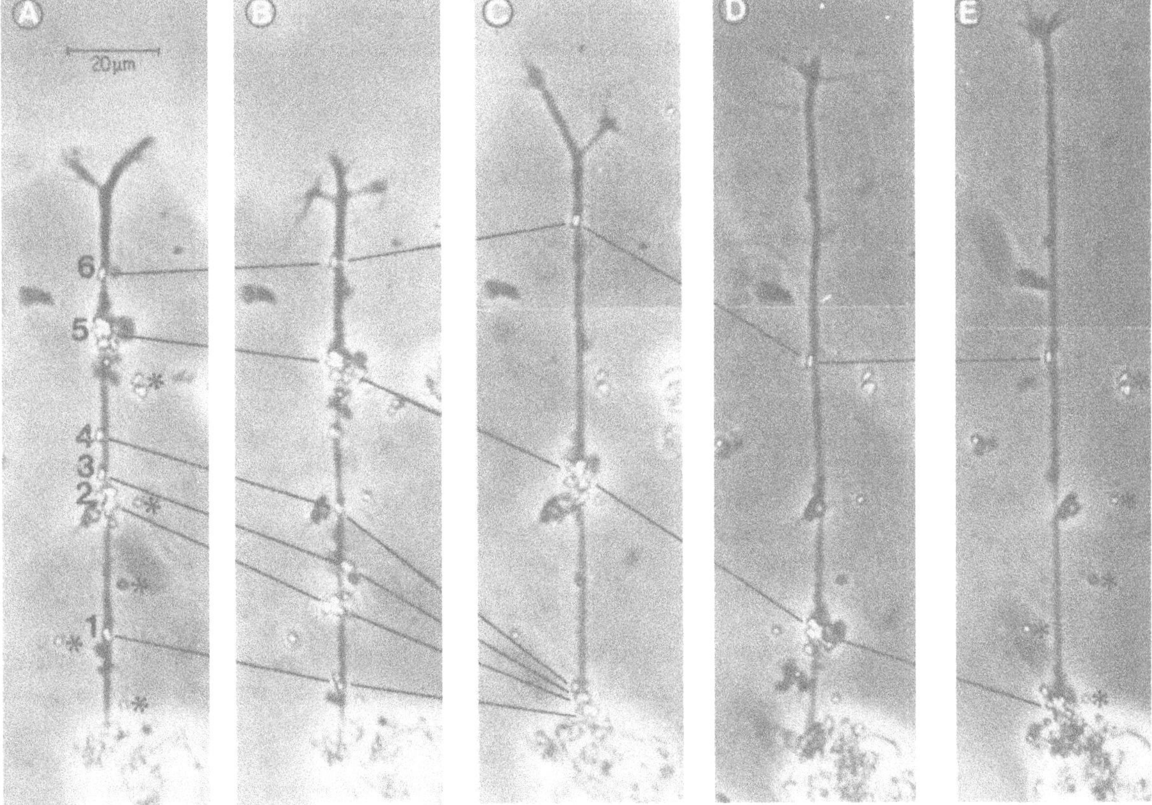

Figure 4.4. Retrograde movement of polystyrene beads attached to growing sympathetic neurites. Movement of six separate clusters of beads is indicated by the solid lines. This series of photographs (A–E) corresponds to 0, 30, 60, 90, and 120 min, respectively, after application of the marker beads. Those beads indicated by asterisks (*) in photographs A and E were attached to the surface and remained motionless during the observation period. Sympathetic ganglia were excised from 12-day chick embryos, enzymatically dissociated, plated on collagen, and incubated for 18 hr. Polystyrene beads (1.1 μm) were attached to the neurons as previously described by Koda and Partlow (1976), and photographs were taken every 10 min. By courtesy of Dr. L. M. Partlow.

bundles, which is found in migrating glial cells but not in the axon growth cone. They propose that the microfilament lattice is involved in the extension phase, while the microfilament bundles, called sheath filaments, function in the contractile phase of cell locomotion. These filaments look like actin filaments. The sheath filaments of glial cells, but not the lattice filaments of axons, react with myosin in the right way: when the cells are made permeable by treatment with glycerol and then treated with heavy meromyosin, the latter attach to the filaments in a characteristic arrowhead pattern (Ludueña and Wessells, 1973). Another bit of evidence that the microfilaments are involved in movements of the growth cone is that addition of cytochalasin B to cultures of actively extending axons results in immediate inhibition of the growth cone and stops elongation of the axon (Wessells *et al.*, 1971*b*).

Further evidence that some of the microfilaments in neurons and glia are composed of actin, in the absence of evidence of the composition of purified microfilaments, came initially from evidence showing that actin as well as myosin is present in mammalian brain (Puszkin *et al.*, 1968, 1972; Fine and Bray, 1971; Berl *et al.*, 1973). Recently, fluorescent antibodies to actin filaments have been used to demonstrate the presence of a network of actin filaments in fibroblasts which correlates with the distribution of microfilaments in the cell (Weber and Groeschel-Stewart, 1974).

4.5. Elongation and Branching of the Axon

That microtubules play a role in supporting the elongation of the axon is shown by experiments in which conditions that inhibit axon outgrowth or cause retraction of the axon also produce a reduction of axonal microtubules and, conversely, conditions that enhance axon elongation also increase the assembly and stability of microtubules. Several agents stimulate growth of nerve fibers and also increase the assembly of microtubules. Nerve fiber outgrowth is stimulated by 10–20 percent D_2O in the culture medium of sympathetic ganglia (M. R. Murray and Benitez, 1968). Increased outgrowth of nerve fibers, associated with increased assembly of microtubules, occurs when chick ganglia or neuroblastoma cells in culture are treated with cyclic AMP or dibutyryl cyclic AMP (Prasad and Hsie, 1971; Furmanski *et al.*, 1971; Roisen *et al.*, 1972*a,b*). Nerve growth factor (NGF) stimulates outgrowth of axons, and this is associated with increased microtubule density.

Reversible inhibition of outgrowth and elongation of nerve fibers in cultures of chick dorsal root ganglia is produced by colchicine in low concentrations (2.4×10^{-8} M to 1.2×10^{-7} M) and retraction of axons occurs within 30 minutes at high colchicine concentration (1.2×10^{-7} M to 2.4×10^{-6} M) (K. M. Yamada *et al.*, 1970; M. P. Daniels, 1972). Recovery from colchicine occurs in about 12 hours after cessation of treatment. Colcemid has the same effect as colchicine, but recovery occurs within hours. Treatment with high concentrations of colchicine, resulting in retraction of the nerve fiber, also results in a reduction in the number of microtubules per unit cross-sectional area (Chang, 1972; M. P. Daniels, 1975). This effect of colchicine can be reversed by addition of NGF or dibutyryl cyclic AMP. Apparently cyclic AMP enhances axon elongation by stimulating the assembly of microtubules from the available pool of tubulin (Roisen *et al.*, 1972*b*, 1975).

However, neither cAMP nor NGF can reverse the inhibitory effect of cytochalasin B on axon elongation.

Several other factors may correlate with initiation of outgrowth of axons from young neurons. In some if not all neurons, axonal outgrowth occurs only after the cessation of DNA synthesis. This has been shown in retinal ganglion cells of frogs (M. Jacobson, 1968*b;* Fisher and Jacobson, 1970) and the chick embryo (A. J. Kahn, 1973, 1974), and in Mauthner's neuron (Vargas-Lizardi and Lyser, 1974), and obviously occurs in such cells as the cerebellar cortical granule cells in which DNA synthesis ceases in the external granule layer before the young neurons migrate deeper into the cortex, spinning out their axons behind them (see Section 3.7). Whether this is a general correlation is not clear, and in any case it is not clear what significance to attribute to the relationship between the postmitotic status of a neuron and the onset of its cytodifferentiation.

Several chemical agents have been shown to induce or increase the outgrowth of neurites (the term used when it is not easy to determine whether the outgrowth is an axon or a dendrite) from neurons in tissue culture. The chief of these is **nerve growth factor** (NGF), which is dealt with separately in Section 6.7. Several lines of evidence indicate that NGF stimulates assembly of neurotubules. Because neurotubules appear to be required for the normal outgrowth of the axon, to provide mechanical support for the axon, and possibly to play a role in axoplasmic flow, axonal outgrowth should be potentiated by any factors that stimulate the synthesis of tubulin and enhance the conditions for assembly of microtubules. Cyclic AMP added to the culture medium stimulates outgrowth of axons from sympathetic ganglion cells as well as from neuroblastoma cells *in vitro,* but the mechanism of action of cyclic AMP appears to be different from that of NGF (Hier *et al.,* 1972; Monard *et al.,* 1973).

Attention has been drawn to the fact that the proliferation of glial cells occurs at the same time as outgrowth of axons in the sympathetic and spinal sensory ganglia (M. Jacobson, 1970*b,* p. 214). Nageotte (1907) was the first to report that in transplanted sensory ganglia the satellite cells appear to exert a strong attraction on the regenerating axonal sprouts. This is what Ramón y Cajal meant when he referred to "the nutritive and tutorial functions of the glial cells." In the past few years various lines of evidence have indicated that glial cells may produce a factor which stimulates outgrowth of axons from neurons of spinal sensory ganglia. The action of glial cells mimics the action of NGF, suggesting that the glial cells may produce NGF (Burnham *et al.,* 1972). However, it seems that glial cells may provide the outgrowing axon with more than NGF because dissociated neurons from sympathetic ganglia fail to survive in culture in the absence of glia, despite the presence of NGF, but survive if glial cells are added to the culture in the absence of added NGF (Burnham *et al.,* 1972; Varon *et al.,* 1974*a,b;* Ebendal and C.-O. Jacobson, 1975). A protein similar to 2.5 S NGF has been isolated from glioma cells (Longo and Penhoet, 1974) which stimulates neurite outgrowth from neuroblastoma cells.

The rate of growth of axons and their appearance are similar *in vivo* and *in vitro,* but there may be considerable variations depending on the species and the conditions, especially the temperature. Amphibian axons grow at the rate of 15.6-56 μm per hour in tissue culture at room temperature (R. G. Harrison, 1910), which is similar to the growth rate of about 40 μm per hour of axons in the tail fin of tadpoles (Speidel, 1941). Temperature dependence is shown by the increase in rate of regeneration of axons from 25 μm per hour at 9°C to 92 μm per hour at 26°C in the frog (Lubińska and Olekiewicz, 1950).

In cultures of chick neurons at 37°C, the rate of axonal growth ranges from 7 to 51 μm per hour (A. F. Hughes, 1953; Nakai, 1956). Similar variability has been observed in the elongation of regenerating mammalian axons, which is usually in the range of 83–124 μm per hour but may reach a maximum of 170 μm per hour (Ramón y Cajal, 1928, p. 23) or a minimum of 5–10 μm per hour. The slowest rates have been observed in the distal parts of the limbs (Sunderland, 1947). This is probably due to the central to peripheral temperature gradient and not to slowing of the growth rate as the axon elongates. Evidence for the latter conclusion is that the rate of axonal growth in tissue culture or in the tail fin does not diminish with distance from the cell body.

The question of where elongation occurs in the developing axon was thoroughly discussed by Ramón y Cajal in his inimitable manner in *Degeneration and Regeneration of the Nervous System* (1928, p. 362 *et seq.*). He concluded that "longitudinal growth of nerve fibres is especially localized in their free ends, where the cone of growth is situated," and "the cone of growth possesses two important functions: to lengthen the conductor (longitudinal growth), and to create new nerve paths." However, "the increase of calibre of the axon is a function of the entire fibre." Prophetic notes sound throughout Ramón y Cajal's works. For example, in the previously cited work (p. 370), he states: "The act of axonic growth and emission of branches imply complex processes of organization of the membrane, the neuroplasma, and the neurofibrillar network.—The neuroplasma must be conceived, not as an inert liquid, but as a complex protoplasmic organ, full of special invisible units."

That the axon does not elongate like a growing hair from its proximal region or at all points along its length was evident from Harrison's (1910) observations of the relationship of the growth cone to fixed external markers, and also was evident from observations by Speidel (1942) on the elongation of axons in the tail fin of the frog tadpole, showing that axonal extension occurs only at the growth cone. D. Bray (1970, 1973*a*) has shown that carmine and glass particles of irregular size, approximately 1–5 μm diameter, are picked up by the growth cone and moved a short distance backward, where they remain attached to the axon at a fixed distance from the cell body despite the increase in length of the axon. Koda and Partlow (1976) showed that polystyrene beads 1.1 μm diameter or erythrocytes coated with concanavalin A become attached to cultured sympathetic nerve fibers and move on the axon surface toward the cell body at rates ranging from 11 to 84 μm per hour (mean 49 ± 6 μm per hour), as shown in Fig. 4.4. This is in the same order as the rate of elongation of nerve fibers under the same conditions. However, the rate of retrograde movement of particles attached to the outside of the axon is 1 or 2 orders of magnitude slower than movement of particles inside the axon. Particles inside the axon generally move at rates of 1–5 μm per second, but some particles have been seen moving at more than 20 μm per second (Burdwood, 1965). The movement of particles inside the axon is not closely coupled to movement of particles attached to the external surface of the axonal plasma membrane.

Growing nerves can be seen easily through the transparent epidermis of the tail fin of frog tadpoles. R. G. Harrison (1904, 1924*a,b*) observed the migration of Schwann cells along these nerves, but it remained for Speidel to describe their growth, the movements of their endings, and their myelination (Speidel, 1932,

1933, 1935*a,b,* 1941, 1942, 1964). Because the growth cones at the tips of the cutaneous nerve fibers behave like those in tissue culture, we may extrapolate from the culture system to the living tissue with more confidence than is usually possible. The axons are at first unmyelinated, but Schwann cells migrate out along the axons and some fibers become myelinated (see Section 4.14). Branching of the axon actually occurs at its end, although collateral branches may occur along its length. During myelination, branches that are not at a node of Ranvier are eliminated.

Speidel observed that retraction of a growing axon may occur spontaneously or may be induced by mechanical obstruction, injury, or noxious chemicals such as alcohol. During retraction of the axon the axoplasm can be seen flowing proximally, and the axon terminal is transformed into a lanceolate retraction club. The rate of retraction is usually the same as that of extension, about 40 μm per hour. Speidel (1941, Fig. 3) noticed that "sometimes a vigorous production of transient knob-like excrescences accompanies the retraction" as if fluid had been squeezed out by the contraction. These look like the syneretic blebs that form on the retracting pseudopod of the ameboid cell *Difflugia* (Wohlman and Allen, 1968, Fig. 3).

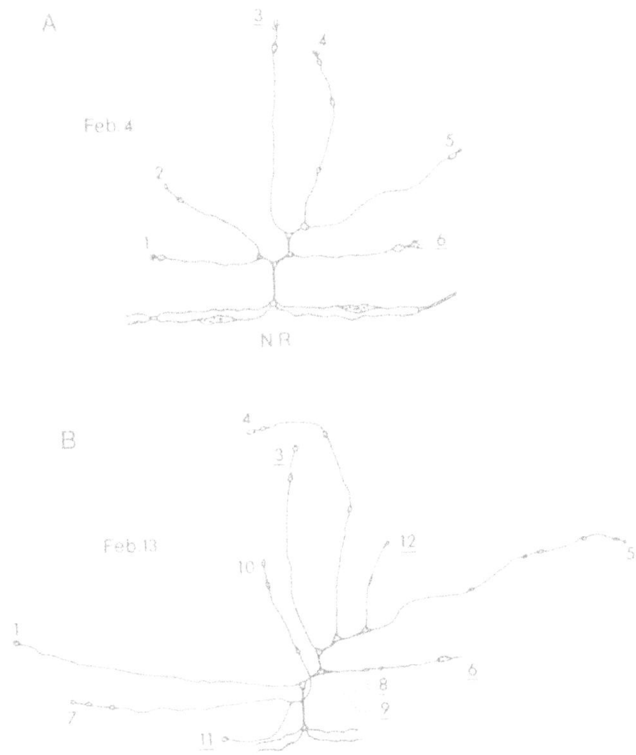

Figure 4.5. A young axonal terminal arborization seen through the transparent skin of the tail fin of the living frog tadpole, showing its growth from February 4 (A) to February 13 (B). The endings are numbered to show the changes of their positions and lengths during the period of observation. An underlined number signifies that the tip of the branch was deeply located away from the skin. Growth cones were present on endings 1, 3, 4, and 6 on February 13. Endings 2, 8, and 9 were eliminated. Six new endings (7–12) developed during the period of observation. From C. C. Speidel, *J. Comp. Neurol. 76:*57–69 (1942).

During normal growth of cutaneous axons of the tadpole, Speidel observed extension, retraction, branching, and elimination of branches by autotomy, all occurring continuously (Figs. 4.5 and 4.6). One can clearly see in Speidel's figures that the lengths of the proximal segments between branching points remain constant as the axon extends distally, thus showing that extension occurs at or close to the growth cones. This has recently been confirmed by D. Bray (1970, 1973*b*), as shown in Fig. 4.7. Speidel observed that most cutaneous nerve fibers grow superficially into the skin but some aberrant fibers grow in the opposite direction. "Aberrant deep sprouts of this type which are of no service as cutaneous endings undergo readjustment along one of the following lines: they may advance further through the tissues and then extend superficially to establish cutaneous connections; they may retract variable distances and then change their direction of growth to reach the skin; they may suffer a variable amount of degeneration or autotomy with subsequent growth to a superficial position; or finally they may be completely eliminated by either full retraction or autotomy" (Speidel, 1941). The morphology of living axonal terminals with growth cones and filopodia is well preserved in histological preparations. The developing terminal arborizations in

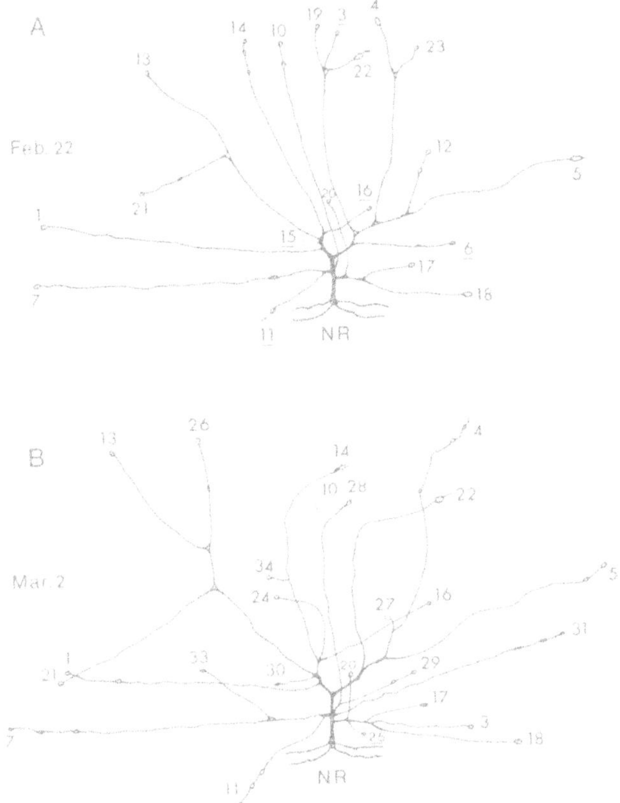

Figure 4.6. The terminal axonal arborization illustrated in Fig. 4.5 observed in the tail fin of the living frog tadpole from February 22 (C) to March (D). Eleven new endings had appeared by February 22, and 11 more new endings had sprouted by March 2. Some endings were eliminated, others retracted, others extended, and some showed no changes during the period of observation. Note that these figures show that elongation occurs at the growth cones, because the lengths of the proximal segments of the branches remained constant. From C. C. Speidel, *J. Comp. Neurol. 76*:57–69 (1942).

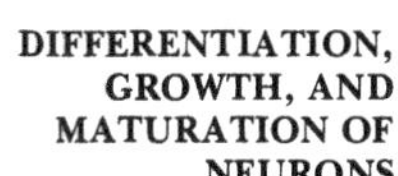

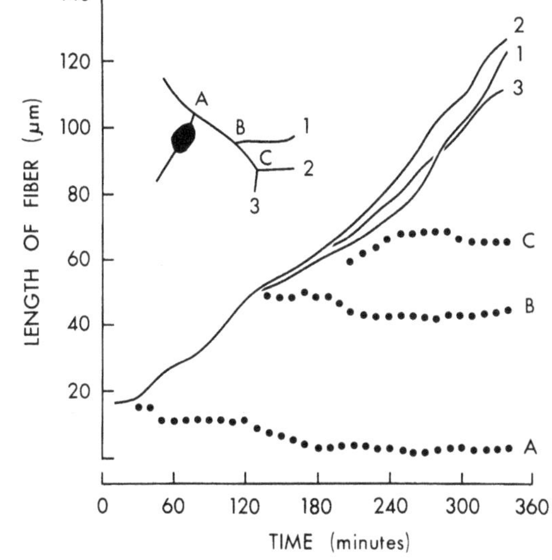

Figure 4.7. Lengths of outgrowing axonal branches of a single sympathetic neuron in tissue culture. Measurements made from time-lapse movie of the cell shown as it appeared at 300 min after the start of the measurements. Lengths were measured from the cell body to growth cones and branch points. From D. Bray, *J. Cell Biol.* *56:*702–712 (1973).

the central nervous system, as illustrated in fixed preparations by Ramón y Cajal (1929*a*) and Morest (1968), show axons and dendrites terminating in growth cones, filopodia, retraction bulbs, resting end bulbs, and signs of degeneration or autotomy which closely represent these structures in living nerves.

The branching pattern of axons must be optimized to give the least resistance to movement of materials in the axon. Therefore, we would expect the optimal form of the axonal tree to be determined to some extent by the principle of least work. Least work is attained for blood flow in arteries (C. D. Murray, 1926*a,b*) if small branches diverge at right angles from large ones, if bifurcation into two branches of equal diameter occurs with an angle of about 75° between them, and if, for angles in the range of 75–90°, the diameters of the two branches have a ratio ranging from 1 to 0.05. C. D. Murray (1926*a,b*) also showed that the cross-sectional area of branches must exceed the cross-sectional area of the parent trunk. In fact, the cross-sectional area of motor nerve fibers to the sternomastoid muscle of the rat increases by a factor of 11 from center to periphery (Zenker and Hohberg, 1973). Such an increase in total cross-sectional area of the axonal tree would be predicted on the basis that narrower branches offer more resistance to axonal flow and, therefore, increased total area of the branches is required to maintain the flow of the same volume of material. Such considerations apply, if at all, only to slow flow, which constitutes more than 80 percent of the mass of material transported in the axon. The rate of fast flow is apparently independent of axonal diameter (Ochs, 1972*a,b*). However, while the cross-sectional area of the axonal tree increases by an order of magnitude, the sum total number of microtubules remains constant. Recent observations of the elongation and branching of nerve fibers in tissue culture (D. Bray, 1970, 1973*b*) have confirmed that the final form of the axonal tree is determined by the frequency of branching, which is a random event in the culture system. Thinner branches subtend a smaller angle than the thick branches as predicted by the principle of least work.

Whether fasciculation of nerve fibers occurs or whether the fibers remain separate depends on the substratum. Nakai (1960) observed that when a filopodium of a growth cone makes contact with another nerve fiber, more filopodia are formed, which shorten while maintaining contact, thus bringing the fibers closer together. Whether a lasting contact is made depends on whether the adhesion between the two axons or retractive force of the filopodia is greater than adhesion between the axons and substrate. By varying the solidity of the substrate, Nakai (1960) showed that axons remain in contact with each other and form fascicles on semiliquid medium, but grow independently of each other on a solid medium. He calculated that the retractive force of a filopodium must be at least 3×10^{-10} dyne. Nakai (1960) and Dunn (1971) showed that nerve fibers growing in tissue culture will remain separate if growing on a solid substratum, but in a liquid medium they attach to each other and form fascicles. The pattern of outgrowth thus depends to a considerable extent on the substratum or medium. Paul Weiss (1934) showed that nerve fibers in culture orient themselves along lines of tension in the plasma clot in which they are growing. He proposed that fibers grow radially from an explant because the explant causes radially oriented stresses in the clot ("one-center effect"), and fibers form a bridge between two explants cultured about 1 mm apart because of the orientation of fibrin micelles between the explants ("two-center effect"). Dunn (1971) has confirmed that the substratum is under stress as Weiss had deduced, but nevertheless that the growing nerve fibers show the "two-center effect" only under conditions that permit fasciculation. In a solid clot the fibers do not fasciculate, but fibers coming into contact mutually inhibit one another's elongation, with the result that their directions of growth are parallel or divergent (Fig. 4.8). The contact reaction of the elongating axons is remarkably similar to the mutual contact inhibition of movement seen in fibroblasts moving on

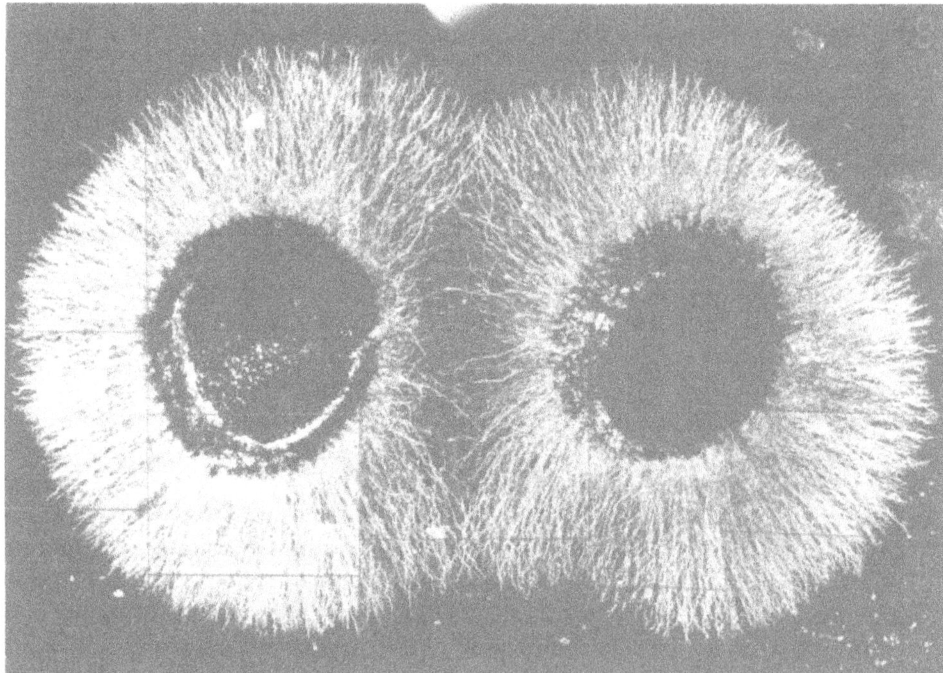

Figure 4.8. Mutual contact inhibition of axon elongation shown by axons deviating from their radial direction of growth after making contact in the zone between two chick embryo dorsal root ganglia explanted in tissue culture. From G. A. Dunn, *J. Comp. Neurol. 143*:491–508 (1971).

glass (Abercrombic and Heaysman, 1954). These observations of nerve fiber interactions in culture suggest that the tendency of axons to fasciculate or to grow separately may depend on the fluidity of the medium in which they are elongating. Axons in the early embryo tend to fasciculate, indicating that they are in a liquid medium, but when the nerve endings arrive at a solid substratum to which they can adhere, they separate into individual fibers and are guided by their contact with the substratum (Weiss, 1934, 1939, p. 527, 1941*a;* Nakai, 1965; Letourneau, 1975*a,b;* Ebendal, 1976*a,b,c*). When there is a high density of axons growing in a solid medium, their direction of elongation is dominated by mutual contact inhibition, but as the density falls and the probability of interaxonal contact diminishes, contact guidance by the substratum becomes increasingly more potent in determining the direction of elongation of the axons (Ebendal, 1976*a*).

It is now 80 years since Harrison's first report on the growth of axons in tissue culture provided the essential information that bridged the observations made of fixed and stained axons with those of nerves growing and regenerating *in vivo.* Meanwhile, tissue culture has continued to offer, even if not to fulfill, the initial promise that it would enable us to discover the mechanisms by means of which axons grow out, select pathways, and find the appropriate postsynaptic targets.

4.6. The Direction of Initial Outgrowth of the Axon

The single major feature that distinguishes nerve cell differentiation and growth from that of all other types of cells is outgrowth of the axon from the nerve cell body in a specific direction, along a specific pathway, to form synaptic connections with specific targets. The proper functioning of the nervous system absolutely depends on the outgrowth of axons to make connections with the correct postsynaptic targets within the central nervous system as well as between the central neurons and peripheral receptor and effector organs. The invariance of the direction of initial outgrowth of the axon, its trajectory, and its targeting on postsynaptic sites are the *sine qua non* of axonal development.

Harrison (1910) considered that the development of the *peripheral nervous system* can be explained in general, if not in detail, by (1) predetermination of the initial direction of outgrowth of the axon from the young neuron, (2) the motive force of nerve growth, and (3) the guidance to nerve fiber growth afforded by solid support. Nevertheless, he recognized that "the specific arrangement of fibers within the central nervous system affords a morphogenetic problem of much greater difficulty." In concurring here with Harrison, I have to add that neither in the peripheral nor in the central nervous system have the mechanisms of axonal growth and pathway selection been revealed by the observations that have been made since Harrison's time. Where the problem has been considered in the central nervous system—for example, in the selection of pathways by optic nerve fibers growing from the retina to the visual centers of the brain—no real understanding of the basic mechanisms has emerged. These observations are considered further in Section 9.10. To Harrison and others at that time, the vertebrate limb seemed sufficiently simple to offer a solution to the problem of development of peripheral nerve patterns. However, this system has been neglected during the past 20 years, probably because the basic mechanisms had not been revealed after decades of effort by very able investigators. An appraisal of their work, however, shows that the limb still offers unique advantages in studying the growth of axons to their targets and that it is still reasonable to assume that the mechanisms of axonal pathway selection and interaction of growing axons with cells along their pathways and at their target zones are likely to be the same in the central nervous system as in the peripheral nervous system. The earliest observations made by Braus (1905) on the innervation of amphibian limbs were interpreted in terms of Hensen's theory (see Section 4.3), namely that the nerve centers and their peripheral organs are connected from the beginning by means of protoplasmic bridges from which the nerve fibers differentiated as a result of use. That theory was disproven by Harrison's (1907*a*) observation that the nerve fibers grow into the limb as outgrowths of the nerve cells in the spinal cord and spinal ganglia. He made the important observation, since repeatedly confirmed (Hamburger, 1928; A. C. Taylor, 1943, 1944; A. F. Hughes, 1968*b*, review; Lamb, 1974, 1976), that the nerve fibers grow into the vicinity of the limb before the limb bud is distinguishable, that the limb bud is innervated from the beginning, and that the basic pattern of innervation of the limb is established before any of the bones, muscles, or digits have differentiated. Harrison also confirmed the observation of Braus, since repeatedly confirmed (Detwiler, 1920*a;* Piatt, 1941), that "a normal limb bud, when transplanted to practically any region of the body of a normal tadpole, will acquire a system of peripheral nerves, which do not differ appreciably from the normal in their arrangement, and which are connected with the nerves of the region into which the limb is implanted, although in the normal individual the latter nerves may have no relation whatever to the limbs." This normal pattern is recovered even when a well-differentiated limb is grafted heterotopically (Weiss, 1937*b*). As Harrison conceded, "This fact, though in other respects of cardinal importance, affords no solution of our problem. . . ." but it does show that any intrinsic tendencies of the axons themselves are dominated by factors in the tissues through which the nerves grow. A normal pattern of innervation develops in an amphibian forelimb that has developed in total absence of innervation when such an "aneurogenic" limb at midlarval stages of development is grafted in place of a normally innervated forelimb at the same stage (Piatt, 1942). However, when an "aneurogenic" forelimb at midlarval stages is grafted in place of a normal hindlimb at the same stage, a chaotic pattern of innervation develops (Piatt, 1958). While definitive conclusions cannot be drawn from these experiments, they show that the original normal innervation creates conditions in the limb that favor reinnervation by heterotopic nerves. I shall not indulge in conjectures about mechanisms because the facts have a tendency to be easily obscured by a growth of speculation.

The reader will be aware that nerves regenerating into a transplanted limb are confronted with a completely different situation than that faced by nerves growing into a normal limb bud. The regenerating nerves have to wend their way from hip to toes through a complex multiple-choice maze. The order with which they connect with target organs in not known. Assays of function after reinnervation of a grafted limb give a crude measure of the normality of reconnection because it is well known that apparently normal movement of amphibian limbs, as observed with the naked eye, can be subserved by a small fraction of the normal innervation, even if a fraction of those are incorrectly connected (see Section 9.3 for further discussion). By contrast, during normal development, the limb bud is innervated from the beginning, and as structures in the limb mature in a proximodistal order they appear to become innervated in the same order (Romanes, 1941, 1946; A. C. Taylor, 1943; Roncali, 1970). However, Landmesser and Morris (1975) found that in the chick embryo most limb muscles and embryonic muscle masses become innervated at the same time, with no clearly defined proximodistal sequence of innervation. Moreover, saturation of the peripheral structures with nerves is achieved initially by a surplus of motor as well as sensory neurons, followed by death of the redundant neurons that fail to find vacant synaptic sites in the limb. There is no evidence that the motoneurons that die have formed incorrect connections, but, on the contrary, there is evidence that the initial connections between motoneurons and muscle are highly selective in the chick embryo before the time of motoneuron death (Landmesser and Morris, 1975). The way is which motoneurons match with muscles in the limb is dealt with in Sections 8.2 and 9.4

Sprouting of axons in the young neuron is not random. The initial outgrowth of the axon normally occurs in the direction it must take to reach its correct destination. For example, all young ganglion cells of the retina of vertebrates send their axons radially inward toward the optic stalk. This cannot be due entirely to mechanical forces within the retina, which would predispose an equal number of optic axons to grow radially outward. This occurs rarely, but optic axons that initially take an aberrant course usually double back to grow in the right direction (Ramón y Cajal, 1910, 1929*a*).

In each region of the central nervous system, the axons grow out in a characteristic and consistent direction, with only slight variations of their direction and course of growth (Szentágothai and Székely, 1956*a;* Lyser, 1966). It is not known to what extent the polarization of the neuron is inherent or the extent to which it is the result of polarizing influences in the cellular environment. There is a formal resemblance between axonal outgrowth from the young neuron and the sprouting of spores and pollen grains, between axonal growth and the growth of tentacles of suctorian protozoa, and between axonal sprouting and the outgrowth of the rhizoid from the egg of *Fucus,* a brown alga. The polarity of *Fucus* eggs can be determined by the differential action of external conditions. Application of a gradient of temperature, auxin, pH, light, or electrical potential will result in the outgrowth of the rhizoid according to the direction of the gradient (E. J. Lund, 1923, 1947; Whitaker, 1940*a,b,* 1941; Jaffe, 1955, 1968; Nakazawa, 1959; Peng and Jaffe, 1976). However, the outgrowth of the rhizoid occurs even when the egg is irregularly rotated in sea water (Whitaker, 1940*b*), showing that action of external gradients is not essential for outgrowth of the rhizoid. In this as in many other cases, including that of the outgrowth of nerve fibers, the developmental processes are genetically programmed and autonomous at first, but later become subject to the contingencies of external forces.

It is not known what predetermines the direction of outgrowth of the axon from the young neuron. This must involve a polarization of the distribution of molecules within the cell. One indication of the polarization of the neuron is the unequal distribution of cytoplasmic organelles. For example, the Golgi apparatus and cisternae of rough endoplasmic reticulum are small and scanty as seen with the electron microscope in the young neuron before outgrowth of the axon, but they become very prominent in the region of initial axonal growth. This was discovered by Ramón y Cajal (1919), who noted that "the location of the (Golgi) apparatus always constitutes the nidus from which emerge both the primordial axonal outgrowth as well as the first dendrons." The outgrowth of the axon depends on a supply of the appropriate materials distributed to the part of the neuron at which the initial axonal outgrowth occurs.

As a rule, the axon emerges from the pole of the neuron nearest the external surface of the neural tube. Mall (1893) first suggested that where this rule does not hold, the young neuron has rotated from its original axis; some observations are consistent with his suggestion. For example, there is some evidence that the pyramidal neurons of the cerebral cortex undergo complete inversion during their development (Stensaas, 1967*b*) so that the axon usually emerges from the basal region of the cell body and grows away from the external surface of the cortex. A small percentage of cortical pyramidal neurons fail to rotate completely (Fig. 4.9), and such neurons may be found in any degree of disorientation. Regardless of the orientation of the neuron, the axon often emerges from the basal pole of the neuron and the main dendrite from its apex, indicating that the initial outgrowth of the axon and dendrite is determined by factors within the neuron and not in the surrounding tissue. The direction of outgrowth of the apical dendrite continues to conform to the axis of the neuron, even when the neuron is inverted (Van der Loos, 1965; Stensaas, 1967*b;* A. Globus and Scheibel, 1967*c*). The axon arises occasionally from an anomalous position on the cell body or a dendrite and grows in its usual direction; or, after having grown a short distance in the direction that had been predetermined in the neuron, it makes a hairpin bend to grow toward its correct destination (Fig. 4.10). Ramón y Cajal (1929*a,* p. 90) described inverted young neurons in the medulla of the chick embryo which have a hairpin bend on the axon but which run in the correct direction regardless of the direction of its initial outgrowth. These observations indicate that the initial direction of outgrowth of the axon is predetermined in the neuron but that the direction of further elongation is determined by factors in the tissue through which the axon grows.

Experiments to elucidate the factors that determine the polarity of Mauthner's neuron have given results that are in harmony with those described above. Rostrocaudal inversion of the presumptive Mauthner's cell in the amphibian gastrula or neurula results in the development of an inverted Mauthner's neuron (Stefanelli, 1950, 1951; C. -O. Jacobson, 1964; Hibbard, 1965*a*). In the majority of cases, the axon grows out for a short distance rostrad and then bends back, decussates normally, and grows down the spinal cord in the usual manner (Fig.

Figure 4.9. Photomicrographs of inverted pyramidal cells in the rabbit cerebral cortex. A: Two pyramidal cells in the cortex of a 5-day-old rabbit. Cell 1 is properly oriented; cell 2 is inverted. In cell 2 the axon origin (ax-o) is at the usual site, the pyramid base. After growing initially toward the pia, the axon makes a hairpin curve (ax-c) to grow in the correct direction. The orientation of the apical dendritic shaft (ad) conforms with the orientation of the cell body. B: Two inverted pyramidal cells in the deeper half of the occipital cortex of an adult rabbit. The axon (ax) in cell 1 originates from the region between the cell body and apical dendrite (ad); the axon in cell 2 originates from the base of the apical dendrite. In both cells the axon runs in the correct direction, but the apical dendritic shaft is incorrectly oriented. C: Pyramidal cell from adult rabbit cerebral cortex showing the axon (ax) growing initially in the wrong direction and then curving to grow in the correct direction. The apical dendritic shaft (ad) is incorrectly oriented. From H. Van der Loos, *Bull. Johns Hopkins Hosp. 117:*228–250 (1965).

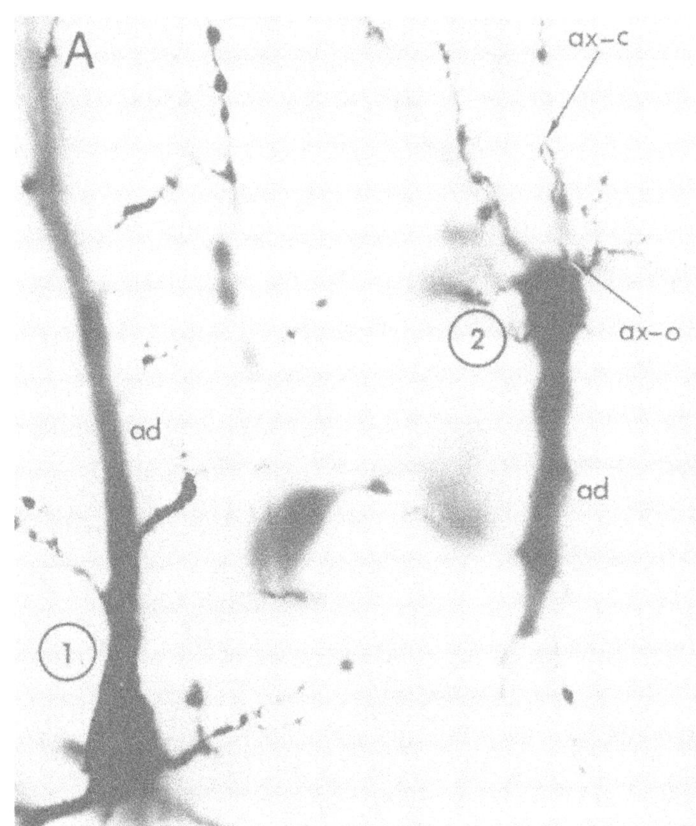
A
ax–c
2
ax–o
ad
ad
1

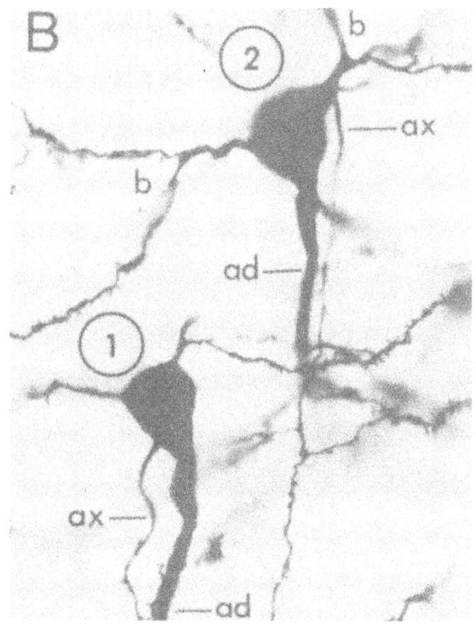
B
2
b
ax
b
ad
1
ax
ad

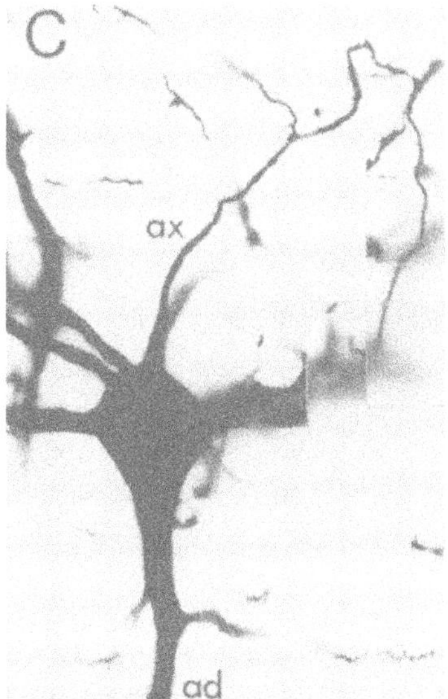
C
ax
ad

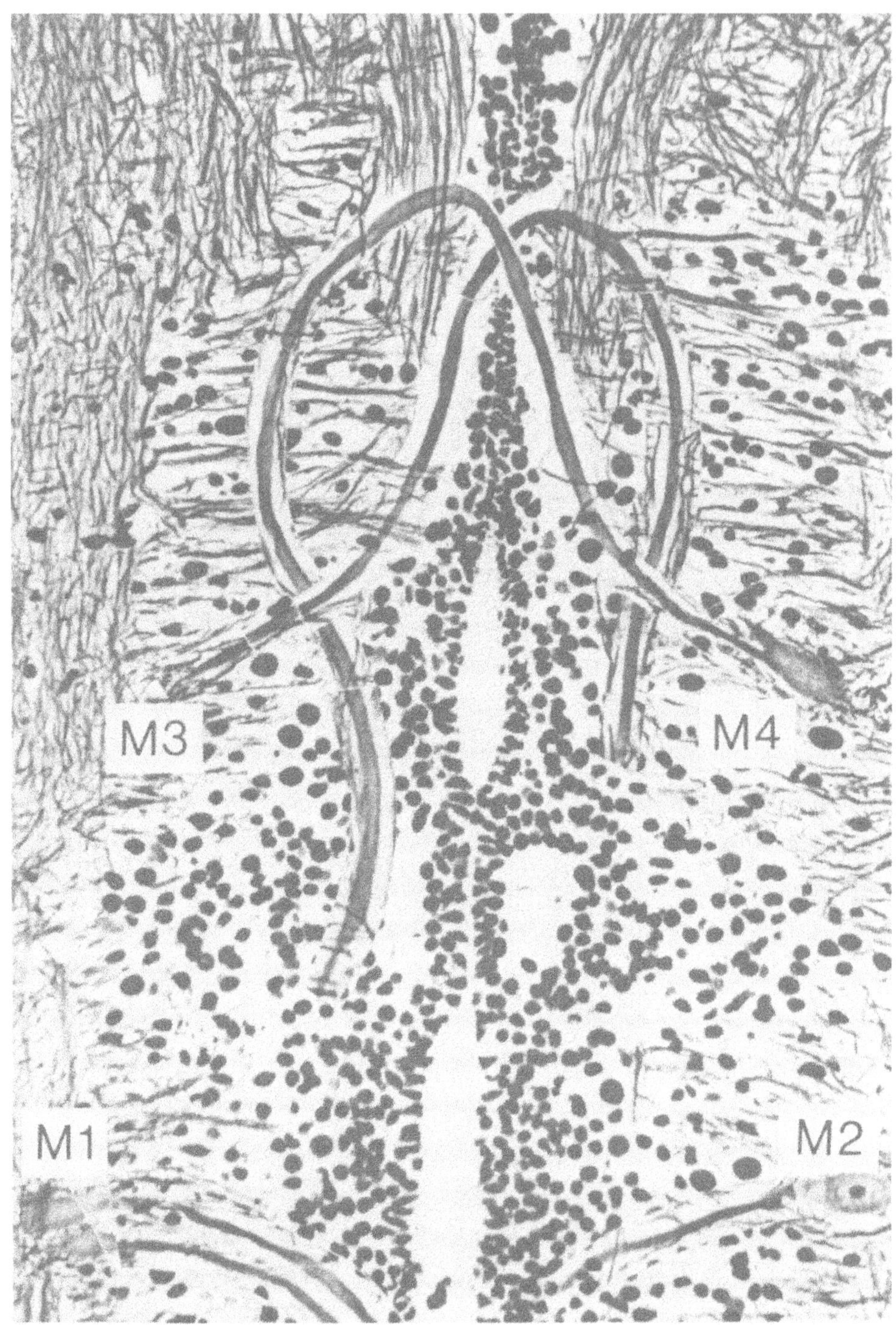

Figure 4.10. Mauthner's neurons in the salamander *Pleurodeles waltii*. M1 and M2 are the normal Mauthner's neurons of the host (duplicated on the left side). M3 and M4 are Mauthner's neurons in a segment of medulla grafted with anteroposterior axis reversed. The axons of the grafted Mauthner's neurons decussate, curve back, and grow in the correct direction. Composite photograph. 190×. From E. Hibbard, *Exp. Neurol. 13*:289–301 (1965), copyright Academic Press, Inc.

4.10). "The dendrites, on the other hand, do not attain their normal destinations, but branch out in the new abnormal location" (Stefanelli, 1950).

From these observations one can draw the following conclusions about the factors that determine the polarity of the neuron:

1. The neuron's polarity is intrinsically determined so that the axon and dendrites sprout in a predetermined manner, irrespective of the orientation of the neuron.
2. After the axon has grown a short distance in the wrong direction, it may reorient itself with respect to its substratum, showing that extrinsic factors override the intrinsic propensity of the axon to continue growing in the direction of its initial outgrowth.
3. The dendrites do not reorient but conform to the orientation of the cell body. In such cases, in the absence of normal axodendritic connections, the dendrites remain stunted and the dendritic tree becomes malformed. The evidence for the latter statements may be found in Section 5.6.

4.7. The Motive Force of Axonal Growth

In sprouting of an axon (and this applies also to sprouting of dendrites), there is an enormous increase in surface area of the neuron and a parallel increase in its surface free energy. During outgrowth of its protoplasmic processes, the neuron changes from a more probable to a less probable configuration, or from a configuration of stable equilibrium to one of unstable equilibrium. A stimulating introduction to the biophysical analysis of cell form in relation to surface energy was provided by D'Arcy Thompson (1942) in Chapter IV of *On Growth and Form,* but little that is new has been added, except by Steinberg and his students, about surface free energy during cell aggregation. The formation of cell contacts during reaggregation is such as to result in the minimum free energy of the aggregate (Steinberg, 1963, 1964, 1970). On the contrary, the surface free energy of the nervous system increases greatly as the nerve cell processes grow out, branch, make synaptic connections, and form an increasingly intricate pattern of neuronal circuits. The nervous system is the most improbable of all aggregates of cells.

The problem of axonal growth may be reduced in part to the problem of selective synthesis and mobilization of the molecules that compose the axon. Unfortunately, nothing is now known about this at the molecular level. We may assume that axonal growth is preceded by differential gene activation, followed by a specific temporal order of synthesis. The molecules necessary for axonal growth must then be distributed into the region of the cell where the initial outgrowth of the axon occurs. Growth of the axon involves not merely synthesis of the proper materials but also differential distribution of the products of synthesis. Synthesis is scalar, having only magnitude and not direction in space. Cytodifferentiation and growth, which involve differential distribution of molecules, are vectorial, since they have both magnitude and direction in space. This may result from bulk flow or from some kind of active transport. In the latter case, the enzymes play the role of Maxwell's demon, converting random movements of molecules into movement in one direction. A vectorial distribution of substrates and products results from the anisotropic arrangement of enzymes in cellular organelles and membranes.

As the axon elongates and as it increases in diameter, the new materials necessary for growth and maintenance are synthesized in the cell body and then transported into the axon. However, the axon may have a limited capacity to synthesize protein, although electron microscopy has shown the absence of ribosomes and granular endoplasmic reticulum in the axoplasm (Palay *et al.*, 1968). RNA has been found in some axons (E. Koenig, 1965; Miani *et al.*, 1966; A. Edström, 1966; J. J. Bray and Austin, 1968; J. A. Peterson *et al.*, 1968; A. Edström *et al.*, 1969; A. Edström and Sjöstrand, 1969). Tritiated uridine has been shown to be incorporated into RNA in the axon, myelin sheath, and Schwann cells of peripheral nerves of the newt (Singer and Green, 1968). Isolated axons in tissue culture have been found to incorporate [^{3}H]leucine into protein (E. Koenig, 1967). Incorporation of [^{14}C]lysine into protein occurs in isolated segments of the sciatic nerve of the rat (Appeltauer *et al.*, 1965). Isolated segments of the axon of Mauthner's neuron of the goldfish can incorporate labeled amino acids into proteins (A. Edström, 1966, 1967).

The type and functions of RNA in the axon are still in question. It is not yet finally established whether the axonal RNA is soluble or is associated with particles, particularly with the mitochondria. Ribonucleic acid has been demonstrated in Mauthner's axon (J.-E. Edström *et al.*, 1962; A. Edström *et al.*, 1969), the axon of the crustacean stretch receptor neuron (Grampp and J.-E. Edström, 1963), cat hypoglossal axons (E. Koenig, 1965), vagus and hypoglossal nerves of the rabbit (Miani *et al.*, 1966), peripheral nerve fibers of the newt (Singer and Green, 1968), and isolated synaptosomes (Balázs and Cocks, 1967; Austin and Morgan, 1967). In Mauthner's neuron the axonal RNA content is 4 times that of the perikaryon (J.-E. Edström *et al.*, 1962). A. Edström (1964*a,b*) found soluble RNA and ribosomal RNA in axons of Mauthner's neurons of goldfish. In the Mauthner axon isolated from the cell body, but *in situ* in the spinal cord, synthesis occurred of RNA sedimenting at 4 S and at 18–30 S, but only 4 S RNA was synthesized in the isolated Mauthner axon stripped of all other cells (A. Edström *et al.*, 1969). Actinomycin D inhibited protein synthesis (A. Edström, 1967) and RNA synthesis (A. Edström *et al.*, 1969) in isolated axons of Mauthner's neuron, showing that axonal RNA synthesis is DNA dependent.

It seems most probable that RNA and protein synthesis in the axon occurs in the mitochondria, which are present in large numbers in the axon and which contain DNA and RNA (Granick and Gibor, 1967; Wagner, 1969; Nass, 1969). Barondes (1966) has demonstrated protein synthesis in mitochondria of nerve endings in the brain of the mouse. Hamberger *et al.* (1970*a*) has shown that mitochondria isolated from neurons are extremely active in protein synthesis, and that neuronal mitochondria are more active in this regard than glial mitochondria. No ribosomes are found in the outgrowing axon even though the cytoplasm of the young neuron has a high density of ribosomes—singly, in clusters, or attached to cytoplasmic membranes. Ribosomes either break down in the axoplasm or cannot enter the axon from the cell body. This cannot be due to their size, because mitochondria and granules of various types that are larger than ribosomes are found in the axon and are known to move in the axon from the cell body to the presynaptic terminals as well as in the opposite direction (Zelená, 1968; Zelená *et al.*, 1968; P. Banks *et al.*, 1969; Geffen, 1969).

Other possible methods of increasing the volume of the axon are pinocytosis of materials into the axon tip from the extracellular fluid (Holtzman, 1971, review) and transfer of materials to the axon from the Schwann cells or glial cells. There is evidence of transfer of the amino acid histidine from Schwann cells to the axoplasm of peripheral nerves in the newt (M. Singer and Salpeter, 1966). Although a considerable time has elapsed since W. H. Lewis (1931) first used the term *pinocytosis* for ingestion of extracellular fluid by macrophages, the study of protein uptake by cells from the extracellular fluid was curiously neglected until quite recently (Ryser, 1968). There are three kinds of evidence for pinocytosis by nerve endings. First, pinocytosis has been observed in neurons in tissue culture (A. F. Hughes, 1953; Nakai, 1956; Klatzko and Miquel, 1960; Burdwood, 1965), but one might contend that the conditions in the culture could have been unphysiological. Second, indentations of the surface membranes of nerve terminals have been seen by electron microscopy, and these are considered to be evidence of pinocytosis (K. H. Andres, 1964; K. H. Andres and Von Düring, 1966; Waxman and Pappas, 1969; Holtzman and Peterson, 1969). Similar "pinocytotic stomata" have been seen in electron micrographs of freeze-etched nerve terminals, which shows that they are not artifacts produced by fixation (Moor *et al.*, 1969; Akert *et al.*, 1972). The objection to this evidence is that it has not been possible to tell whether the indentation of the surface membrane indicates that substances are being pinocytosed or whether they are being released, as they are known to be released at synapses. Additional evidence for pinocytosis is that uptake of electron-opaque tracers from the extracellular space into axons can be seen with the electron microscope. Examples of the uptake of materials from the extracellular space into the axon are the reincorporation of synaptic transmitters by the presynaptic membrane (Devine and Simpson, 1968) and the uptake of exogenous peroxidase into vesicles in the neuron (Holtzman and Peterson, 1969; Zacks and Saito, 1969). Uptake of ferritin into axonal terminals has been demonstrated at the motor end plate (Birks, 1966) and into sympathetic postganglionic axons *in vitro* (Birks *et al.*, 1972). Uptake of ferritin into spinal ganglion cells of the toad has been observed after intraperitoneal injection of the protein (Rosenbluth and Wissig, 1964), and has also been observed in central nervous system neurons after injection into the cerebrospinal fluid (Brightman, 1965). Waxman and Pappas (1969) found that saccharated iron ioxide, injected into cat lateral geniculate body, appeared in membrane-bound vesicles in presynaptic terminals, which suggested that the marker had been taken up by pinocytosis from the synaptic cleft. These observations suggest that the neuron may take up material from the extracellular space by means of pinocytosis and that transfer of materials between glial cells and neurons, or between neurons, may occur in that way.

Apart from small quantities of materials that may enter the axon from outside, the structural proteins required for axonal growth and maintenance, as well as the enzymes required for synthesis of synaptic transmitters, are synthesized in the cell body of the neuron and then transported into the axon. This is discussed in greater detail in the next section.

The perikaryon is the only site of synthesis of proteins required for elongation and growth of the axon and of the proteins of the presynaptic structures. The synaptic and axonal membrane proteins are synthesized on the polyribosomes of the Nissl substance. Some of these polypeptides enter the cisternae of the Golgi apparatus, where they are attached to carbohydrates such as glucosamine, galactose, or fucose, and the resulting glycoproteins are transported into the cisternae of the smooth endoplasmic reticulum (SER). The SER extends as a continuous system of cisternae and tubules from the perikaryon into the growing axon and serves as a conduit for fast transport (40–400 mm per day) of materials to the axonal membrane and to the presynaptic terminals. Not all polypeptides enter the SER. The bulk of newly synthesized protein is composed of subunits of the neurotubules and neurofilaments, and these are transported slowly (1–5 mm per day) in the axoplasm surrounding the SER. The neurotubules and neurofilaments can be demonstrated with the electron microscope from the very beginning of outgrowth of the axon (Lyser, 1964, 1968*a;* Sechrist and Lavelle, 1966). Their subunits are transported to the growth cone of the outgrowing axon, where the subunits are added to the distal ends of the neurotubules. The neurotubules and neurofilaments have been implicated in the mechanism of axonal flow, and they may also provide mechanical support for the axon. The neurofilament protein is also synthesized in the perikaryon and transported with the slow axonal flow to the growth cone, where the microfilaments are essential for the ameboid movements of the growth cone and its filopodia.

4.8. Transport of Materials in the Axon

The concept of the nerve fiber as a hollow tube for conducting vital materials to and from the central nervous system has endured for several centuries. Indeed, despite the flimsiest of evidence to support the concept, it was the prevailing doctrine during the seventeenth and eighteenth centuries (E. Clarke, 1968). The concept was not entirely without experimental evidence to support it. Thus Alexander Monro *primus* (1732) inferred that animal spirits were blocked from entering the diaphragm when a ligature was tightened around the phrenic nerve, and he noted that a few contractions of the diaphragm could be elicited by squeezing the nerve distal to the ligature. This is another example to show that concepts have an existence which is almost independent of the validity of the evidence that goes to support them. Monro's experiment, in principle, was capable of demonstrating axonal flow, and it was only the advantages of modern instruments, particularly the microscope, and not a significant advance in experimental design, that allowed the first modern demonstration of proximodistal flow of axoplasm by Weiss and Hiscoe in 1948. They showed that the swelling and distortion of axons that arise proximal to a ligature tied on a peripheral nerve moved distally at a rate of about 1 mm per day after the ligature was removed. Much of the subsequent work on this problem can be said to be an extended footnote to this classical experiment.

The following treatment of this subject concentrates on aspects that seem especially relevant to developmental neurobiology. The results of the hundreds of research papers on axoplasmic flow that have appeared in the past decade have been summarized in many reviews of the subject (Lubińska, 1964; Lasek, 1970; Ochs, 1972*a,b;* Jeffrey and Austin, 1973; Grafstein, 1975; Heslop, 1975).

Flow of materials within the neuron has a fourfold significance in relation to development of the nervous system. First, flow from the cell body to the axonal and dendritic endings is a way of providing materials for growth and for renewal of components which have a shorter life span than that of the neuron as a whole.

Second, it provides materials for the formation, maintenance, and functions of the synapses. Third, flow of materials to the cell body from the axon terminal may allow recirculation of axonal components and may enable signals to be transmitted from the extracellular environment at the tips of the axon and even from the axon's postsynaptic targets. Finally, axonal flow of labeled material provides a relatively nondestructive means of tracing nervous pathways during development (Cowan *et al.*, 1972).

The velocity of the flow of materials in the axon, in mammals, appears to occur either in the range 1–10 mm per day (40–400 μm per hour), which has been called **slow flow,** or in the range 100–1000 mm per day (4–40 mm per hour), known as **fast flow.** Reported rates of fast axonal flow are not comparable because of different species, different conditions, and different experimental techniques. Several rates of axonal flow have been reported in the same nerve, e.g., the optic nerve (J. O. Karlsson and Sjöstrand, 1971*a*), and these may reflect the heterogeneity of the axons of different diameter and lengths that compose the optic nerve as well as the heterogeneity of the materials that are transported. The rate of fast axoplasmic transport, in a variety of species, has been found to be rather constant at 17 ± 2 mm per hour in mammals, in sensory as well as motor nerves, and in the central nervous system. Apparently the velocity seems to be little affected by, or unrelated to, the diameter of the axon. Bulk flow of any kind would be related to the diameter of the axon. If there is bulk flow, as Weiss (1963) conceives the slow flow to be, the axoplasm would be expected to behave like a viscoelastic, non-Newtonian liquid such as a suspension of fine particles or an emulsion in which the viscosity depends on the shear stress. One might also predict that the dimensions of the axons and the angles of branching would be such as to minimize the work required to propel the axoplasm. This subject is treated well by D'Arcy Thompson (1942, p. 948). The rheology of axoplasmic flow has been investigated by Biondi *et al.* (1972), who found that minute quantities of axoplasm drawn up into a microcapillary tube by a high vacuum behaved as a pseudoplastic fluid with a viscosity 10^6 times that of water. However, channels of fluid with lower viscosity may be present in the axon, and there is now convincing evidence that the endoplasmic reticulum forms a continuous system of channels for fast flow from the cell body to the axonal and dendritic terminals (Droz *et al.*, 1975).

Thirty years after the "discovery" of axonal flow by Weiss and Hiscoe (1948), its mechanism is still the subject of hypotheses which have yet to be verified experimentally. Certain possibilities have been eliminated while others have been made more or less probable. Four main mechanisms that have been proposed are hydrostatic pressure, diffusion, axonal peristalsis, and the action of neurotubules.

Hydrostatic pressure, generated in the cell body, might be responsible for the initial outgrowth of the axon, as in the contraction–hydraulic theory of ameboid movement in which the propulsive force is delivered by contraction of a network of contractile protein filaments at the rear, driving fluid components of the cytoplasm into the pseudopod (Jahn and Bovee, 1969). This is what Ramón y Cajal might have had in mind when he proposed that *vìs a tergo* (force from behind) propelled materials into the growing axon. A similar model was suggested by J. Z. Young (1944, 1945). However, this model is not consistent with the following empirical data: bidirectional movement of granules and mitochondria in the axon (Lubińska, 1964; Burdwood, 1965; Zelená, 1968), and transport of materials in the distal part of the axon separated from the cell body by a ligature (A. Dahlström, 1967*a,b;* P. Banks *et al.*, 1969).

Diffusion of materials down a concentration gradient created by synthesis in the cell body and utilization or release of materials at the axon terminals have been ruled out by experiments which show that there is no concentration gradient of proteins in the axon and that transport of proteins in the axon continues normally after total inhibition of protein synthesis in the cell body (R. P. Peterson *et al.*, 1967). Moreover, transport of catecholamine granules, with a diameter of 500 Å, at a velocity of 200 mm per day (A. Dahlström and Häggendal, 1966, 1967) or of mitochondria (Scharf and Blume, 1964; Weiss and Pillai, 1965; Zelená, 1968; Khan and Ochs, 1974) could not possibly be the result of diffusion.

Axonal peristalsis has been seen in neurons cultured *in vitro* (Pomerat, 1961; Weiss *et al.*, 1962; Burdwood, 1965; Weiss, 1972). Weiss (1963, 1964, 1972) has suggested that a periaxonal wave of contraction might produce a pressure wave in the axoplasm, which might result in propulsion of materials within the axon. Axonal peristalsis might be intrinsic to the axon or transmitted from glial or Schwann cells, which have been seen pulsating in tissue culture (D. A. Russel and Bland, 1933; Lumsden and Pomerat, 1951; Ernyei and Young, 1966). Although theoretical calculations show that slow axonal flow could be produced by the observed peristaltic waves (Biondi *et al.*, 1972), it is hard to see how peristalsis could result in orthograde and in retrograde flow unless there were valves in the channels. Materials moving at different velocities could, in principle, be propelled by axonal peristalsis if the materials flowed in different channels—the fast flow in the endoplasmic reticulum compartment and the slow flow in the axoplasm as a whole. At present, the evidence does not show whether the observed axonal waves are directly related to axonal flow and, if so, whether they are the effect of axonal flow rather than its cause.

The mechanisms that have to be considered seriously are, first, peristaltic pumping, possibly involving the axolemma and subadjacent axoplasm, propelling material in the axoplasm as well as in special channels, and, second, a transport mechanism involving interactions between actin and myosin, in which the neurotubules play a part. In either case, the channels for rapidly flowing materials seem to be in the tubules of smooth endoplasmic reticulum. The role of neurofilaments in axonal flow is uncertain—they are said to be unnecessary for axonal flow on the evidence that neurofilaments are sparse or absent in mammalian axons less than 1 μm in diameter and are absent from axons of some arthropods such as the cockroach and crayfish.

Neurotubules have been implicated because they are universally present in axons and dendrites, because they are found in various cells in relationship to materials moving in the cytoplasm, and because such movements, including axoplasmic flow, are inhibited by colchicine and related drugs that bind to microtubules (Wuerker and Kirkpatrick, 1972; L. Wilson *et al.*, 1974, reviews). Local injection of colchicine into the sciatic nerve of the rat inhibits the rapid transport of amine storage granules in the adrenergic nerve fibers (Dahlström, 1968). Injection of colchicine into the hypoglossal or vagus nerves completely blocks both slow and fast transport of protein (Sjöstrand *et al.*, 1970). Colchicine has also been found to inhibit slow transport of protein in the crayfish nerve cord (H. L. Fernandez *et al.*, 1970) and fast transport of neurosecretory material in the supraoptic neurons of the rat (Norström *et al.*, 1971). Apparently the concentration of colchicine is important: fast flow is more sensitive than slow flow, but both are inhibited by colchicine. The concentration of colchicine that is required to totally inhibit fast axonal flow is large enough to have numerous other toxic effects. These include inhibition of nucleoside transport (Mizel and Wilson, 1972) as well as a variety of abnormalities seen with the electron microscope in glial cells as well as in neurons: infolding of the nuclear membrane and alterations of the appearance of the endoplasmic reticulum, Golgi apparatus, and mitochondria (J. O. Karlsson *et al.,* 1971; Hansson and Sjöstrand, 1971). The fact that lumicolchicine, which has some of the toxic effects of colchicine but does not bind to tubulin, does not block axonal flow (M. T. Price, 1974) is evidence in support of the role of neurotubules in axonal flow. However, there are other findings that do not support that hypothesis. Thus local anesthetics block axonal flow when applied as a cuff around the nerve but have no apparent effect on neurotubules (Bisby, 1975). Moreover, colchicine applied to the vagus nerve of the rabbit allows rapid transport at the normal rate despite substantial loss of neurotubules, and total loss of neurotubules in some cases (Byers, 1974). Labeled proteins continued to accumulate in cisternae of smooth endoplasmic reticulum in such nerves that had been treated with colchicine.

Thus the evidence implicating neurotubules in axonal flow is merely circumstantial, not direct. Moreover, if the neurotubules play a role in axoplasmic flow, do they provide the motive force (Schmitt, 1968) or do they merely act as passive cytoskeletal supports for the flow of axoplasm? There is, at present, no evidence to show whether slow and fast axonal flow both share the same mechanism or whether they use different mechanisms.

One widely accepted model of the role of neurotubules in axonal flow invokes changes in the conformation of molecular bridges between the neurotubules and a protein that packages the material that is transported. This change of conformation of the cross-bridges gives the materials a thrust in the direction of flow, either toward or away from the cell body.* This mechanism, rather like the action of cross-bridges between the thick and thin filaments in skeletal muscle, is supported by no more than circumstantial evidence, such as the reports that bridges linking neurotubules and vesicles are occasionally seen in electron micrographs and have been convincingly illustrated in lamprey axons (D. S. Smith, 1970). Also consistent with a variety of models is evidence showing that fast axonal flow requires a local source of energy, mediated by ATP, derived from oxidative metabolism (Ochs, 1971*a,b,* 1972*a,b*).

While the neurotubules were considered the structures most likely to be involved in the motile force of axoplasmic flow, little attention was paid to other structures that might serve as channels for flow. It has been suggested that the smooth endoplasmic reticulum might extend from the cell body continuously in the axon to the presynaptic terminals, and thus serve as a channel for flow of materials (Palay, 1958*b;* A. Peters *et al.,* 1970). Recently, evidence has accumulated showing that materials transported rapidly in the axon, either to or from the cell body, are localized within tubules and cisternae of the smooth endoplasmic

*Compare Descartes' description of the flow of humors in relation to fibrils: "As fast as any particle is detached at the extremity of each fibril, another is attached at its root" (*La Description du Corps Humain,* first published 1664). Modern theories of cellular movement echo the micromechanical models of the eighteenth-century theorists such as Boorhaave, Haller, and Bonnet and their antecedents going back to antiquity. In his *Contemplation de la Nature* (first published 1764), Bonnet described the organism as "a marvellous assemblage of an almost infinite number of tubes differently figured, calibrated and twisted."

reticulum. Herpes simplex virus, transported from the nerve endings to the perikaryon, is localized within endoplasmic reticulum (ER), and its localization can be made without ambiguity (Kristensson *et al.,* 1974). Likewise, horseradish peroxidase, ferritin, or thorium dioxide is taken up by pinocytosis into vesicles which form multivesicular bodies that apparently coalesce to form cisternae in the preterminal part of the axon (Holtzman, 1971; Birks *et al.,* 1972). Horseradish peroxidase is always surrounded by smooth endoplasmic reticulum and is localized within tubules and cisternae of ER as it flows in the axon (Sotelo and Riche, 1974). Catecholamine granules, transported from the cell body in the fast phase of axonal flow, are also confined within the smooth ER (Taxi and Sotelo, 1973). Finally, Droz *et al.* (1975) have confirmed that the smooth ER forms a continuous system of channels from the perikaryon to the axonal terminals. Tubules of smooth ER, 60–120 nm in diameter, apparently provide channels for fast flow in both directions in the axon. These ER tubules come into close apposition with the plasma membrane of the axon, indicating that an exchange of materials may occur at such points of contact. In the preterminal region the smooth ER forms a network of fine tubules, 20–30 nm in diameter, from which synaptic vesicles appear to bud. Radioactive labeled proteins, conveyed by fast axonal flow from the cell body, are difficult to localize unambiguously to the smooth ER because such localization is almost at the limits of resolution of electron microscopic autoradiography. However, by compressing the axon to impede axonal flow temporarily, Droz *et al.* (1975) have shown by means of high-resolution autoradiography that radioactive labeled proteins, conveyed by fast axonal flow, are localized to regions containing accumulations of smooth ER.

The evidence, taken as a whole, shows that the smooth ER probably provides channels for rapid transport of a diversity of materials from the axonal terminals to the cell body, as well as from the sites of their synthesis in the cell body to the axon and presynaptic terminals. Bidirectional transport implies some sort of valve. The same propulsive mechanism could, in principle, suffice to propel all materials, the differences in velocities arising from other variables such as molecular or particle size. The mechanism of flow of material inside the ER channels is unlikely to involve neurotubules directly, although they may be implicated indirectly, for example, by involvement of the axoplasm surrounding the endoplasmic reticulum.

The total quantity of material transported by slow flow has been estimated to be about 5 times the quantity transported by fast flow in chicken sciatic nerve (J. J. Bray and Austin, 1969; Sjöstrand and Karlsson, 1969).

The fate of the transported material is uncertain, but it might be supposed that some material may be utilized for renewal of axonal structures, some may be metabolized, some may be recirculated by retrograde axonal flow, while other material may be released at the terminals (Droz, 1973). There are growing indications that proteins or peptides released from nerve terminals may be taken up by postsynaptic cells (Korr *et al.,* 1967; Alvarez and Püschel, 1972; Grafstein and Laureno, 1973; Droz *et al.,* 1973), or transferred directly from pre- to postsynaptic cell via gap junctions. By showing label in the postsynaptic cell after inhibition of protein synthesis, Droz *et al.* (1973) have excluded the possibility, left open in other studies, that the label in the postsynaptic cell was derived from radioactive breakdown products of protein in the presynaptic terminals.

Local synthesis in synaptic terminals can occur from amino acids taken up from the extracellular fluid or transported along the nerves (Concalon and

Beidler, 1975). Axonal transport of soluble precursors and transfer to postsynaptic neurons have been demonstrated (Schubert and Kreutzberg, 1974).

It can be said, without any injustice, that all the claims to have demonstrated flow of RNA in optic nerves have failed to demonstrate that the RNA is transported intraaxonally (J. J. Bray and Austin, 1968; J. A. Peterson *et al.*, 1968; Casola *et al.*, 1969; Bondy, 1972; Bondy and Madsen, 1973; Bondy and Marchisio, 1973; Jarlstedt and Karlsson, 1973). Most of the RNA in nerves is outside the axon, in glial or Schwann cells (Autilio-Gambetti *et al.*, 1973). The only species of RNA present in axoplasm is 4 S, whereas 4 S, 19 S, and 28 S RNA is found in the neuronal and glial cell bodies (A. Edström *et al.*, 1969). A well-controlled study (Autilio-Gambetti *et al.*, 1973) failed to find evidence of RNA transport in rabbit optic nerve, and concluded that the RNA that accumulated in the nerve after intraocular injection of [^{3}H]uridine was due to diffusion of the uridine in and around the axon followed by incorporation into RNA in adjacent glial cells. Therefore, conclusions about the role of messenger RNA transported from the nucleus to the axonal endings are purely speculative.

Subcellular localization of various materials that flow in axons has been studied, either by autoradiography, using light and electron microscopy (Figs. 4.11 and 4.12), or by fractionation of homogenates of brain or nerve after the

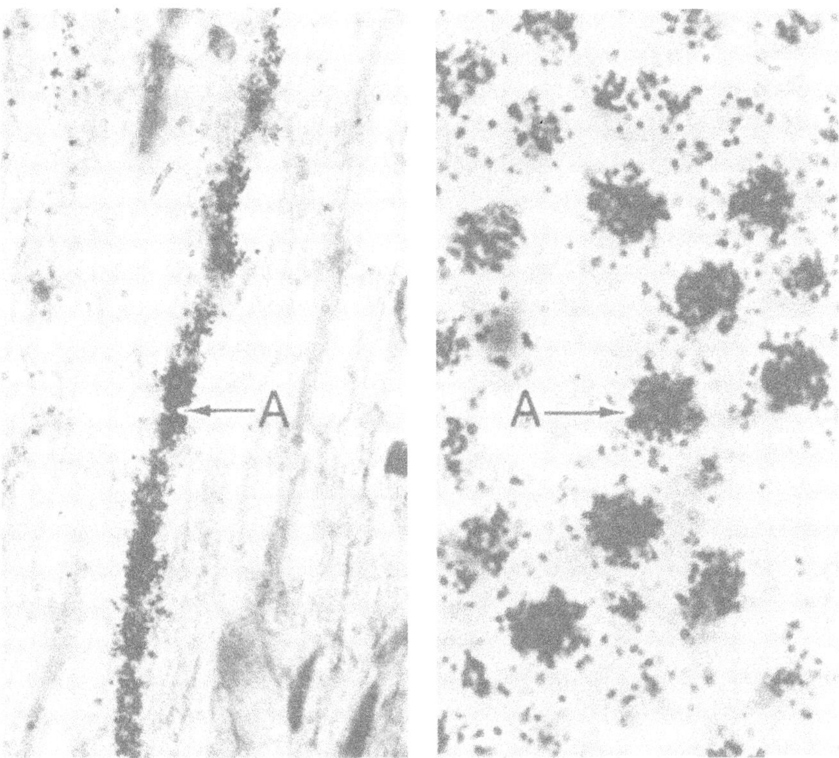

Figure 4.11. Autoradiographs of spinal roots showing labeling of axons (A) following an injection of tritiated leucine. Left: Dorsal root of a cat, 12 hr after injection, 2 mm from site of injection into dorsal root ganglion. 800×. Right: Ventral root of a rat, 4 days after injection into spinal cord, 4 mm from cord. 2100×. From R. J. Lasek, *Brain Res.* *7*:360–377 (1968), and R. J. Lasek, *Exp. Neurol.* *21*:41–51 (1968), copyright Academic Press, Inc.

administration of radioactive materials that are incorporated into identifiable components of the nerve cell. Electron microscopic autoradiographs made after injection of radioactive amino acids have shown that the **fast-moving proteins** in the axon on the way to the nerve endings are located in the plasma membrane, smooth endoplasmic reticulum, and amine storage granules. The mitochondria as a whole move with the slow flow, but components of mitochondrial membranes are conveyed with the fast flow. Glycoproteins are transported exclusively with the fast flow, and virtually all glycoproteins move directly to the nerve endings (J.-O. Karlsson and Sjöstrand, 1971*a,b,c;* G. Bennett *et al.,* 1973; Droz *et al.,* 1973). By contrast, the bulk of the fast-moving protein is deposited in the axon *en route* (Concalon and Beidler, 1975). In the nerve endings, the fast-moving proteins and glycoproteins are located principally in synaptic vesicles and the presynaptic plasma membrane (Fig. 4.13).

The **slow-flowing proteins** have been localized, in electron microscopic autoradiographs, to bundles of neurofilaments, neurotubules, mitochondria, and plasma membrane. In contrast to the fast-flowing materials, which largely arrive at the nerve endings, most of the slowly flowing protein is deposited along the entire length of the axon, and probably less than 5 percent enters the nerve endings (Droz *et al.,* 1973).

In homogenates of brain and nerves, the fast-flowing proteins and glycoproteins are associated with "particulate" fractions thought to contain plasma mem-

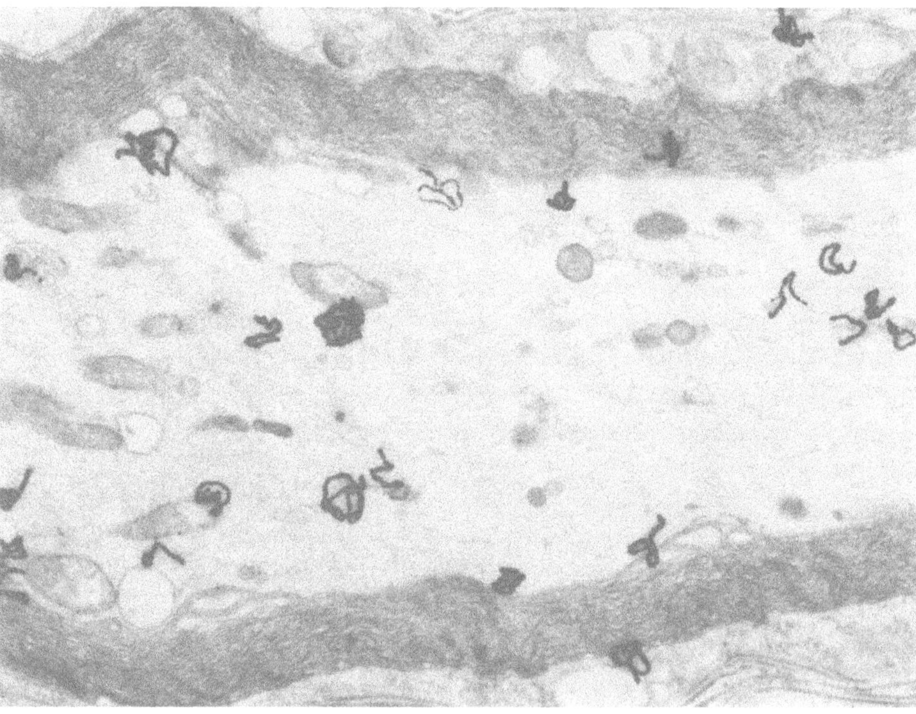

Figure 4.12. High-resolution autoradiograph of a postganglionic axon excised 3 mm from the ciliary ganglion of a chicken injected with tritiated leucine 24 hr before. The silver grains are associated with neurofilaments, mitochondria, and multivesicular bodies in the axoplasm. By courtesy of Dr. B. Droz.

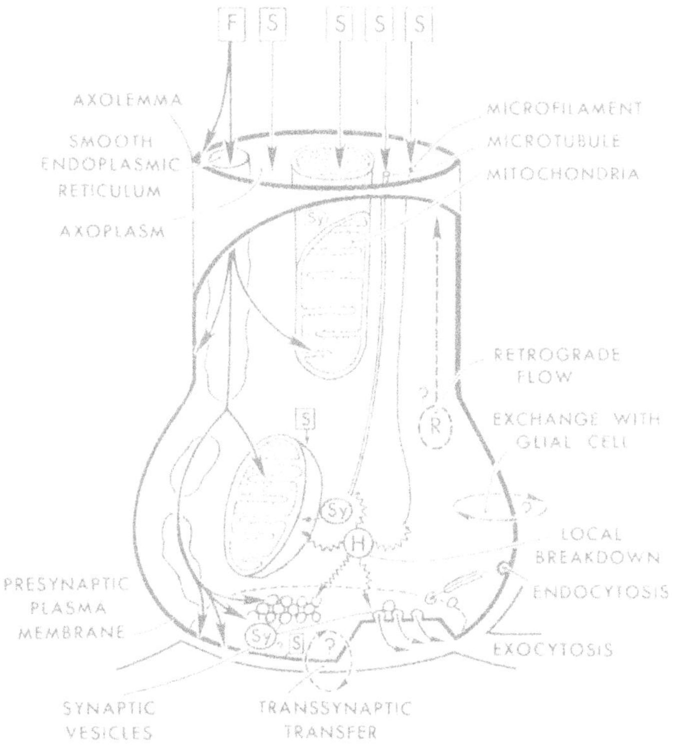

Figure 4.13. Dynamic condition of synaptic proteins in an axon terminal. F, Fast phase of the axonal flow; S, slow phase of the axonal flow; Sy, sites of local protein synthesis or of local incorporation of labeled amino acids; H, hydrolytic enzymes such as proteinases and peptide hydrolases; R, retrograde flow. From B. Droz, *Brain Res. 62:*383–394 (1973).

branes, synaptic vesicles, and other particles, whereas the slow-flowing proteins are found in the "soluble" fraction (which does not indicate that they are soluble *in vivo*) consisting of nonparticulate components of axoplasm and microtubule and microfilament proteins (Cuénod and Schönbach, 1971; J.-O. Karlsson and Sjöstrand, 1971*a,b,c;* DiGiamberardino *et al.,* 1973). The neurotubule and neurofilament proteins compose more than 75 percent of the slow component of axonal flow in mammals (P. N. Hoffman and Lasek, 1975).

In studies that set a standard of excellence in this field, Droz *et al.* (1973), G. Bennett *et al.* (1973), and DiGiamberardino *et al.* (1973) characterized the axonal flow of protein and glycoprotein from the preganglionic cell bodies in the third nerve nucleus to the giant calyciform terminals in the ciliary ganglion. They found that fast-flowing proteins, moving at a rate of about 288 mm per day, are mainly used for renewal of various membranes (synaptic vesicles, mitochondria, endoplasmic reticulum, and plasma membrane, particularly the presynaptic membrane). These proteins turn over in about 17 hours. They observed a wave of slowly flowing protein moving down the axon at a rate of 1.5–10 mm per day, most of which is deposited in the axoplasm along the entire length of the axon, and less than 5 percent arriving at the nerve endings. These proteins are deposited in regions of axoplasm devoid of synaptic vesicles and mitochondria.

The life span of materials in the neuron has been studied by determining the rate of disappearance of material pulse-labeled with radioactive precursors. These kinetic studies, using high-resolution autoradiography and cell fractionation techniques, have shown that various components of the neuron are continually replaced, and that the proteins and glycoproteins of the nerve endings turn over at various rates and are replaced by material that flows from the cell body. The subject of renewal of synaptic proteins has been reviewed by Droz (1973). Not surprisingly, in view of the heterogeneity of materials that flow in nerve fibers, their turnover times range from hours to months. Proteins conveyed by slow flow turn over slowly, with half-lives of about 3 weeks in the axon and 10–18 days in the presynaptic region (J.-O. Karlsson and Sjöstrand, 1971*a;* Droz *et al.,* 1973; H. L. Koenig *et al.,* 1973; Droz, 1973). Rapidly transported proteins turn over at varying rates in nerve endings: one fraction turns over in less than 1 day (Cuénod and Schönbach, 1971; J.-O. Karlsson and Sjöstrand, 1971*c*), another fraction containing fucosyl glycoproteins turns over in about 10 days (Marko and Cuénod, 1973; G. Bennett *et al.,* 1973), while another component appears to have a turnover time of several months (Elam and Agranoff, 1971).

Whether there are **changes in the rate of axonal flow during development** is quite controversial. We have to ask the question whether the reported changes in rate of flow are due to maturation and aging or whether they are due to differences in temperature (particularly as a result of cooling of embryos and newborn animals), changes in dimensions of the nerves (rate of change in length and in diameter may be independent variables), or other variables that are usually uncontrolled or not even considered. The addition of new axons to the developing nerve and the elongation of axons that occur during the experimental period have to be taken into account when studying slow axonal flow in growing nerves.

Many reports of changes in rate of slow flow do not take all these factors into consideration. For example, in one of the more carefully controlled studies of changes in rate of fast axonal flow during maturation, Hendrickson and Cowan (1971) reported an increase in rate of fast flow of protein in optic nerve fibers of the rabbit. They determined the earliest time of appearance of labeled protein in the superior colliculus after injection of [^{3}H]leucine into one eye. In 6-day-old rabbits, they found a rate of flow of 120 mm per day, increasing to 150 mm per day by the end of the third week postnatally, and attaining the adult level of about 200 mm per day at the end of the fourth week. This is almost twice the value obtained by essentially the same method by J.-O. Karlsson and Sjöstrand (1968) in adult rabbits. The rate of slow flow, reported by Hendrickson and Cowan (1971), diminished from 5 mm per day at the end of the first week to 2 mm per day in rabbits greater than 4 weeks of age. Increase in the rate of fast flow of protein was also found in the chick embryo, where no fast flow of protein could be detected at 7 days of incubation (Marchisio and Sjöstrand, 1972), and the rate almost doubled between 10 and 18 days of incubation (Marchisio *et al.,* 1973). On the other hand, Ochs (1973), in a careful study, found that the rate of fast flow in sciatic nerve remained remarkably uniform in cats 2 weeks of age (389 ± 29 mm per day) and 6 weeks of age (426 ± 26 mm per day) compared with adult cats (430 ± 27 mm per day) and adult dogs (439 ± 34 mm per day). Ochs (1972*a,b*) reported similar rates, about 410 mm per day, for fast flow in peripheral motor and sensory nerves as well as in central tracts of a variety of mammalian species.

In experiments on chick embryos and newborn mammals, the rate of fast axoplasmic flow is likely to be reduced significantly by cooling the animals even slightly. Fast axonal flow has a Q_{10} of 2–2.6 (Ochs and Smith, 1971, 1975), which means that a change of temperature of only 0.5°C will change the rate of fast flow by 15 mm per day. This seems to be the main or only reason for the slower rates of rapid axonal flow found in cold-blooded as compared with warm-blooded animals. Neither the species, type of nerve, nor caliber of the axons appears to affect the rate of fast axonal flow, if allowance is made for temperature differences. In the light of the evidence now available, the changes in rate of fast flow that have been reported during development may well be due to lowering of the body temperature of embryos or newborn animals during the experiment. The reported changes in rate of slow flow also need to be corrected for changes in the number and dimensions of the axons during development. In brief, inadequate controls of the varying parameters of the developing nerve make it impossible to draw reliable conclusions about changes of rate from the published reports on flow rates in developing nerves.

Flow of protein in dendrites* is a controversial and unresolved problem. It is difficult to obtain good evidence of transport of materials in dendrites. The presence of microtubules might tempt one to infer that dendritic flow occurs, but then the presence of ribosomes in dendrites makes local synthesis of proteins in dendrites equally probable, and flow might be difficult to detect against a background of local synthesis. In one study, dendritic transport of protein at a rapid velocity was inferred from the observations that a proximodistal gradient of dendritic labeling was found after a brief survival following application of radioactive amino acids to the nerve cell body (Schubert *et al.,* 1971). A gradient, rather than a peaked distribution of protein, is more consistent with diffusion of amino acid, which is incorporated locally into protein, than with the somatofugal flow of protein.

4.9. Retrograde Axonal Flow

Many different substances of diverse chemical composition are taken up at axonal endings and transported back to the nerve cell body. Although most such substances are foreign, it is very likely that axons serve as a route for retrograde transfer of physiologically significant materials. Probably the first report of retrograde movement of materials in nerve fibers was made by Matsumoto (1920), who observed the movement of material stained with neutral red in sympathetic nerve fibers in tissue culture. Since then, there have been several reports of particles moving visibly in both directions in living nerve fibers (Burdwood, 1965; Pomerat, 1961; Berlinrood *et al.,* 1972; Forman *et al.,* 1971; P. D. Cooper and Smith, 1974) and of materials dammed up at both sides of a constriction on a nerve Lubińska,

*The spinal ganglion sensory nerve fibers are axons structurally and in their mode of development, and to refer to them as dendrites is misleading and serves no useful purpose. For example, the ratio of neurofilaments to neurotubules is much greater in axons, both motor and sensory, than in dendrites (Wuerker and Palay, 1969).

1964, review; Partlow *et al.,* 1972). In fact, retrograde movement of poliomyelitis virus in nerves had been shown as early as 1940 by Bodian and Howe. They demonstrated that movement of poliomyelitis virus was blocked by freezing and then thawing a short segment of the nerve, which disrupted the axons without affecting the periaxonal space, indicating that the virus moved within the axons rather than between them (Bodian and Howe, 1941*a,b*).

Certain viruses are specific for nerve and/or glial cells. Poliomyelitis and rabies viruses are selective for neurons. Herpes simplex virus (Types 1 and 2) infects both neurons and glia. The virus can enter peripheral axons and travel in the axon at a rate of 30 mm per day to the cell body, where it may remain latent but can be reactivated by damaging the peripheral nerve (Walz *et al.,* 1974). The virus is localized within cisternae of the smooth endoplasmic reticulum (Kristensson *et al.,* 1974), and there is evidence that other neurotropic viruses use the smooth ER as channels for their transmission within the neuron.

Tetanus toxin is taken up by nerve fibers, apparently nonselectively because it accumulates in motor, sensory, as well as sympathetic nerves, and is transported retrogradely to the cell body at a rate of about 7.5 mm per hour. (Stoeckel *et al.,* 1975). Prior administration of neuraminidase abolishes the uptake of tetanus toxin, indicating that the toxin binds to gangliosides of the axonal membrane.

Radioactive material injected into the tongue muscles appears in the nerve cell bodies of the hypoglossal nucleus (W. E. Watson, 1968). This was confirmed by Kristensson and Olsson (1971, 1973), who showed that Evans blue-labeled albumin and horseradish peroxidase (HRP) appear in the hypoglossal neurons or spinal cord motoneurons after those protein tracers are injected into tongue muscles or gastrocnemius muscle, respectively. The rate of transport of these exogenous proteins was calculated as 120 mm per day.

Horseradish peroxidase has been used to show that retrograde axonal flow occurs in peripheral nerves as well as in axons in the central nervous system. Retrograde flow of HRP has thus become a useful neuroanatomical technique for tracing pathways (Kristensson, 1975, and LaVail, 1975, reviews).

Little is known about the mechanism of transport of HRP, which is a protein of molecular weight 44,000. It is apparently taken up by pinocytosis into a variety of cell types, including glia and neurons (Sellinger and Petiet, 1973), where its reaction product can be identified by light or electron microscopy (R. C. Graham and Karnovsky, 1966). In the axon, HRP is taken up at the nerve terminal (Holtzman *et al.,* 1971), accumulates in vesicles and multivesicular bodies, and is transported within cisternae of smooth endoplasmic reticulum in the axon (Sotelo and Riche, 1974). Electrical stimulation of motor nerves has been found to increase the uptake of HRP into the motor nerve terminals at the neuromuscular junction (Holtzman *et al.,* 1971; Heuser and Reese, 1973; Heuser *et al.,* 1974). HRP flows toward the cell body and flows in much smaller quantities in the opposite direction (LaVail and LaVail, 1974). Colchicine and vinblastine block the transport of HRP, which has been taken as evidence that its transport may be mediated by neurotubules. However, the evidence that HRP is transported inside channels of smooth endoplasmic reticulum makes it unlikely that neurotubules are directly involved in its transport. Like the other techniques for tracing nerve pathways, the use of HRP is liable to errors of omission and of commission (Guillery, 1970), so that conflicting reports are not surprising. Thus there are some reports that retrograde flow of HRP diminishes or is lost with maturation in peripheral nerves of rats and mice (Kristensson and Olsson, 1971; Kristensson *et al.*, 1971; LaVail and LaVail, 1972) and in the avian isthmo-optic system (LaVail *et al.*, 1973), but Bunt *et al.* (1974) found retrograde flow of HRP as readily in adult as in immature rat optic nerves.

Retrograde transport of normally occurring materials in the axon has been studied by tying one or two ligatures on peripheral nerves and measuring the accumulation of material distal to the ligature. In this way, retrograde transport of acetylcholinesterase has been found at a rate of about 134 mm per day in dog peroneal nerve (Lubińska and Niemierko, 1971) and 70–120 mm per day in rabbit vagus nerve (Sjöstrand and Frizell, 1975). Retrograde transport of choline acetyltransferase in the rabbit hypoglossal nerve was found at a rate of 50–60 mm per day (Sjöstrand and Frizell, 1975).

Nerve growth factor (NGF) is taken up at the nerve ending and is transported back to the cell body in adrenergic sympathetic neurons and spinal sensory neurons, but not in spinal motor neurons (Hendry *et al.*, 1974*a,b;* Paravicini *et al.*, 1975; Stoeckel and Thoenen, 1975; Stoeckel *et al.*, 1975). This transport is blocked by colchicine. The rate of retrograde transport of NGF in sensory neurons is about 13 mm per hour, while in adrenergic sympathetic neurons it is about 2.5 mm per hour. This selectivity of uptake of NGF apparently is due to the presence of receptors for NGF on the spinal sensory and adrenergic sympathetic neurons but not on motoneurons. The function of the NGF in the sensory neurons of adult mammals is not known—uptake of NGF by sensory neurons in adults persists, although the major response of these neurons to NGF occurs during a short period of their development during the phase of axonal outgrowth. In adrenergic neurons the NGF has the function, throughout life, of inducing the synthesis of tyrosine hydroxylase and dopamine-β-hydroxylase, which catalyze the rate-limiting steps in the synthesis of norepinephrine (Thoenen *et al.*, 1972; Stoeckel and Thoenen, 1975). This is the only case known at present of the uptake and retrograde transport of a substance with known physiological functions. However, the concept of uptake and retrograde axonal transport of materials with a trophic action on the neuron or carrying a signal to the perikaryon from the innervated structures has been well established by indirect evidence obtained over a period of several decades (see Sections 7.4 and 7.5), and it is very probable that such substances will be identified in the near future.

4.10. Guidance of Axonal Growth

There is a great deal of anatomical and physiological evidence of specific connectivity within the central nervous system. Nerve fibers grow relatively long distances, bypassing many other neurons on the way, to connect with a specific group of cells. In some cases, the connection is made with a specific neuron or even with a specific part: axon, soma, or dendrite. Peripheral nerves grow to make contact with specific muscles or with specific sense organs.

Some nerves in the adult run a long and tortuous course from origin to termination. This might lead one to suspect that, in the embryo, potent forces must have guided the nerves to their destination. However, the first peripheral nerve fibers have to grow very short distances in a straight line to reach their terminals. For example, the first motor nerves grow almost directly from the spinal cord into the myotomes, which move away from the cord only later. In the limb bud of the chick embryo, the motor axons have to grow less than 1 mm to reach the limb muscles, and develop rapidly, so that the fresh nerve fibers penetrate the limb bud on the fourth day of incubation and the gross pattern of limb innervation has developed by 6½ days (Fouvet, 1973). Such peripheral nerves as the facial or the recurrent laryngeal branch of the vagus are obvious examples in which the course of the nerve has been distorted by the growth of other structures. In the case of the facial nerve, in addition to deformation of the pathway of the peripheral nerve, the nerve cell bodies become displaced after they have formed connections with the periphery.

The final course of peripheral nerves, as well as central tracts, is the result of stretching and passive displacement of the nerves due to growth and movement of the tissues through which they run. This has been called "passive stretching" by R. G. Harrison (1935) and "towing" by Weiss (1941*a*). An extreme case of passive stretching is that of the lateral line nerve, which innervates the lateral line sensory placode while it is in the head and is then towed as the placode migrates into the tail (R. G. Harrison, 1903).

The problem of selective connectivity is discussed at greater length in Chapter 9. At this point, we are trying to account for the mechanisms of axonal guidance which might be at work in determining that axons grow along the appropriate pathway and arrive at the correct destination. The latter phase of axonal growth might be a matter of random search: after the axon has arrived close to its destination, it might at first branch profusely in all directions, but later all unnecessary branches might be eliminated after one or more branches have made the correct terminal contacts and formed connections. Before this process can be effective, however, the axon has to grow to within striking distance of its target. Short-range forces acting over a distance of several hundred micrometers might then guide the axon tip to its target. It is not known how this occurs, and several theories have developed to account for the oriented growth of axons and dendrites.

The main factors that may affect the direction of growth of nerve fiber are electric fields, chemical difference in the medium, and the physical nature of the substrate. It seems likely that all of these factors, as well as others, may play some part. Unfortunately, the proponents of special theories of nerve growth have each emphasized one factor to the exclusion of all others. Their theories may thus be named electrical, or mechanical, or chemical. Here I concur with Mencius (Mêng Tzu, 7 A.26): "What I dislike in these 'unique positions' is that they make a travesty of the Way. They make one point and overlook a hundred others."

4.11. Electrical Theories of Nerve Tropism

There is little evidence that electrical potential differences or electric current flow may be concerned with the orientation and direction of growth of axons and dendrites. S. Ingvar (1920) reported that nerve cells in tissue culture grew along the lines of force of a very weak d-c current ($2–4 \times 10^{-6}$ amp) between two wick electrodes. Ariëns Kappers (1921) regarded this as good evidence that supported his theory of "neurobiotaxis." However, neither Karssen and Sager (1934) nor

D. Ingvar (1947) was able to confirm the effect of a d-c current on the growth of nerve cells *in vitro.* Peterfi and Williams (1933), using direct currents of 2–55 × 10^{-5} amp on nerve cells *in vitro,* observed a movement of the cytoplasm toward the anode. Similar results were obtained by Marsh and Beams (1964*a,b*) and Sisken and Smith (1975). Weiss (1934) suggested that the primary cause of the oriented growth is mechanical guidance of the nerve processes by oriented micelles which form in the culture medium between the electrodes. Electric currents may have multiple effects on the culture, producing electrophoretic movement of ions and molecules as well as orienting dipoles along the lines of force of the electric field.

The fact that nerve fibers are often seen crossing at right angles, or making U-turns, or sending branches in opposite directions is inconsistent with any theory of galvanotropism unless it is assumed that fibers have differential or timed growth responses to electricity.

It is not at present possible to determine whether the intensity and direction of current flow in the developing nervous system are sufficient to orient the growth of nerve fibers. There are insufficient data about the size of the potential differences in the embryonic nervous system, the disposition of current sources and sinks, and the electrical characteristics of the tissues, all of which will play a part in determining the pattern of current flow in a volume conductor such as the brain. Theories of galvanotropism are thus based mainly on speculation and on indirect evidence from phenomena that may have no relevance to galvanotropism. This criticism applies to the theories of "stimulogenous fibrillation" (Bok, 1915) and "neurobiotaxis" (Ariëns Kappers, 1917, 1921, 1932) as well as to Burr's (1932, 1947) "electrodynamic theory of development." These theories are vaguely formulated, but their gist is that the development of some parts of the nervous system depends on electrical stimulation by other parts. It is not made clear how this could occur. In theory, electrophoresis of substances that stimulate or inhibit nerve growth may control the development of the nervous system in a manner analogous to the differential localization of auxin by electric fields, which has been postulated to control plant morphogenesis (W. G. Clark, 1937*a,b,* 1938; Went, 1937; Burr, 1947).

The assumption that the development of one part of the nervous system depends on stimulation by another part may seem to be self-evident and simple. However, the available evidence shows that the combined effects of many influences must be taken into account; therefore, what seems to be the effect of one neuron on another at a distance may really be the result of a complicated combination of many influences. While the effect of electricity on the presumptive neurons is very uncertain, there is evidence that several other factors such as interactions between cells in contact, as well as chemicals and hormones, influence the proliferation of neuroepithelial cells and maturation of neurons. These will be considered elsewhere. Here it is appropriate to draw attention to some of the evidence that some parts of the nervous system may develop autonomously and independently of action potentials originating from sense organs or other parts of the nervous system.

Sensory stimulation and reflex activity are not essential for the development of the nervous system in amphibian embryos, which develop normally while totally anesthetized, and which start normal movements and have normal behavior after they are removed from the anesthetic. This shows that many reflex circuits can develop while normal impulse traffic has been greatly reduced in the developing nervous system (S. A. Matthews and Detwiler 1926; Carmichael, 1926).

4.12. Mechanical Factors Affecting Axonal Growth

The locomotion and growth of epithelial cells, young neurons, and nerve fibers in tissue culture occur only when they are in contact with a surface such as fibrin fibers in a fluid medium, or are at the interface between the solid substratum and liquid medium, or are at the liquid–air interface (Loeb, 1902; Harrison, 1910, 1912; W. H. Lewis and Lewis, 1912). This phenomenon was called *stereotropism* by Loeb (1902) and Harrison (1911, 1912), *contact sensibility* by Dustin (1910), and *tactile adhesion* by Ramón y Cajal (1910, 1928). Wilhelm His was the first to recognize the importance of mechanical factors in embryonic development. This and many other important contributions of Wilhelm His to developmental neurobiology are reviewed by Picken (1956). His clearly understood and described cases of axonal guidance by the tissue substratum and his 1894 review of the mechanical basis of animal morphogenesis contain numerous aperçus of the concepts and mechanism of nerve growth later propagated by Ross Harrison and by Paul Weiss.

Loeb and Fleisher (1917) pointed out that tension in the substratum can orient fibrils along which cells prefer to grow. This was verified experimentally by Weiss (1929, 1934, 1941*a*), who showed that when nerve fibers grow in a plasma clot that has been stretched, the direction of the outgrowing axons follows the pattern of tension in the substratum. Weiss (1941*a*) called this phenomenon *contact guidance.* The tension need not be exerted from outside. Proliferating tissue itself produces tensions in the substratum, resulting in oriented migration of young neurons and other cells and in oriented growth of nerve processes. This is vividly illustrated by the experiment in which two pieces of nerve tissue explanted some distance apart on a plasma clot became connected by outgrowing axons oriented in almost parallel fascicles joining the explants (Weiss, 1934). However, this could have been the result of changes in pH, oxygen tension, or other chemical alterations in the substratum; or it could have been due to the release of growth-promoting substances by the explanted tissue; or it could have been due to the release of enzymes by the explants, which changed the physicochemical nature of the substratum between them; or it could have been due to an electric field between the two pieces of tissue; or, as Weiss concluded, it may have been caused by mechanical stresses in the substratum. This experiment may serve to illustrate the difficulty of separating electrical, mechanical, and chemical factors in the growth of cells in tissue culture. Exactly the same difficulties arise in connection with the observation that nerve fibers tend to grow preferentially along other nerve fibers and so form fascicles and nerve trunks (see page 136).

Mechanical guidance seems to be important in the development of peripheral nerves and central tracts. However, some other factors must control the selective growth and direction of nerve fibers to their proper destinations. Mechanical factors alone cannot account for the way in which nerve fibers continue separately toward their destinations after close contact with other nerve fibers with which they intermingle or which cross their path. This should be kept in mind when considering any theory of nerve growth, such as that proposed by Weiss (1941*a*, 1955), in which mechanical factors are regarded as predominant and electrical and chemical factors are considered to be of secondary importance.

Mechanical guidance by contact with the substratum gives the cell two equal and opposite choices of direction, but it cannot alone determine the direction of cell movement or growth. To accomplish that, some kind of selectivity is required, such as selective adhesion or repulsion of the nerve by the substratum or stimulation or inhibition of growth of the nerve by physical or chemical differences in the substratum. Moreover, it is hardly worth arguing whether the guidance of nerve fibers is mainly chemical or mechanical, for at short range they boil down to the same thing: the physicochemical interaction between the nerve fiber and its environment. This interaction necessarily involves contact between molecules in the nerve, particularly at its surface, and molecules in the surroundings.

The evidence that nerve fibers in tissue culture are oriented by the interfaces and by the disposition of micelles or fibrous molecules in the substratum has led to the conclusion that the same mechanical factors are important in guiding neurites *in vivo.* This conclusion cannot be accepted without many reservations because of the differences between the physicochemical conditions *in vivo* and in tissue culture.

In nervous tissue prepared for light microscopy, the neurons and glial cells are shrunken and distorted so that there appear to be large intercellular spaces between the cells. This makes it seem that growing neurites encounter factors in the "intercellular material" which are similar to those in the tissue culture medium. This is one reason why the behavior of axons growing in tissue culture has often been equated with axon growth *in vivo.*

The cells of the central nervous system at all stages of development appear to be separated by narrow intercellular clefts. After glutaraldehyde fixation and the usual methods of preparing tissues for electron microscopy, the intercellular clefts are about 200 Å wide in the mature brain and the extracellular volume of the brain is less than 5 percent (Horstmann and Meves, 1959). Extracellular clefts as seen with the electron microscope in the developing nervous system may be larger than in the adult (U. Karlsson, 1967; Caley and Maxwell, 1968*a,* 1970; del Cerro *et al.,* 1968). The extracellular clefts, often exceeding 1000 Å in width, are seen in the cerebellum of the rat at birth, but by the 17th postnatal day only a few clefts greater than 200 Å are found (del Cerro *et al.,* 1968). On the other hand, the extracellular clefts in the cerebellum of the chick embryo are found to be 100–400 Å wide (Mugnaini and Forströnen, 1967). Wechsler (1966*a,b,c*) found no change in the 200 Å intercellular clefts of the chick spinal cord during development. However, larger intercellular clefts have invariably been seen after preparing nervous tissue for electron microscopy by freeze substitution, which is a technique consisting of rapid freezing of the tissue followed by substitution with osmium tetroxide in acetone (Van Harreveld *et al.,* 1965, 1966; Malhotra and Van Harreveld, 1966; Bondareff, 1966, 1967*a,b;* Bondareff and Pysh, 1968; Van Harreveld and Khattab, 1969; Pysh, 1969). Therefore, it is possible that the clefts are reduced to 200 Å by swelling of the cells during fixation with aldehydes. When examined with the electron microscope after preparation of the tissue by freeze substitution, the extracellular space appears to occupy 40 percent of the volume of the cerebral cortex of the rat at birth. The extracellular space decreases to 32 percent at 14 days of age and to 26 percent at 21 days, which approaches the adult value of 22 percent as determined by freeze-substitution electron microscopy and by other methods of measuring the volume of extracellular space in the nervous system (Vernadakis and Woodbury, 1965; Bondareff and Pysh, 1968).

The conditions that the axon encounters in the developing nervous system are very different from those in tissue culture. Instead of having a wide expanse of culture medium in which to grow, the axon has to penetrate the intercellular clefts. It does not grow on the surface of the culture medium but between two surfaces which form a complex three-dimensional maze. If the axon were merely guided by contact with the cell wall, it would grow at random in the maze of intercellular clefts, but in fact it appears to pick its way through the clefts, moving toward a specific target. The contents of the intercellular clefts are not known (Bondareff, 1966, 1967*a,b;* Van Harreveld, 1972), but they offer a free passage for diffusion of ions and small molecules (Kuffler and Nicholls, 1966*a,b*). The chemical specificity of the intercellular matrix may provide the growth cone with specific cues to guide it or may supply growth factors or might provide physical conditions that either stimulate or inhibit axonal elongation. Mechanical guidance by macromolecules on the cell surface or in basement membranes, as well as collagen fibers oriented in the intercellular material, may guide the growing axon through the maze of intercellular clefts. The axon may respond differentially to various molecular species on the cell surface (Martínez-Palomo, 1970), particularly to those molecules that project into the intercellular cleft.

4.13. Chemotropism

Under the rubric of *chemotropism* we lump together many phenomena that seem to show that nerve fibers grow up a concentration gradient toward the source of some diffusible substance—that is, they exhibit positive chemotaxis. There is little evidence that nerve fibers might exhibit negative chemotaxis. Chemotaxis involves action at a distance and should therefore be distinguished from chemoaffinity, which involves contact or short-range chemical attraction between cells.

Numerous observations on the regeneration of peripheral nerves indicate that the nerve fibers from the proximal stump of the nerve show a preference for entering the peripheral stump (Ramón y Cajal, 1928). Forssman (1898, 1900) coined the term *neurotropism* to describe the attractive influence of the distal stump. Ramón y Cajal (1910, 1928) thought that the regenerating nerve fibers might be attracted by chemicals released from the degenerating nerve or from Schwann cells.

Many attempts to determine whether the "alluring substances" postulated by Ramón y Cajal (1928, p. 278) are released from degenerating nerve have given negative results, and it is only in the past few years that convincing evidence has been obtained of stimulation of nerve fiber outgrowth by target tissues acting at a distance of up to 1 mm *in vitro.* Nerve fibers in tissue culture are not deflected by a piece of degenerating peripheral nerve (Weiss, 1934). This experiment is obviously merely a preliminary to many more refined investigations of the effects of various tissues, tissue extracts, and chemicals on the growth of axons in tissue culture which are now being attempted.

Negative results were obtained by Weiss and Taylor (1944), who performed experiments to determine the effect of the peripheral nerve stump on the outgrowth of nerve fibers from the proximal stump. After transecting the sciatic or tibial nerve of the white rat, they used a Y-shaped arterial cuff to join the cut ends. The nerve fibers were given a choice between growing into a branch containing the distal nerve stump or into a branch containing a blood clot or tendon. Abundant regeneration occurred into both branches, irrespective of whether the "neurotropic lure" was present or not, or whether the branch was open or closed (Fig. 4.14). These experiments show that neurotropism does not occur in peripheral nerves during regeneration, but they should not be overinterpreted to rule out neurotropism during the initial outgrowth of the developing nerve.

There are many phenomena of selective nerve growth and connection in which it is not possible, at present, to sort out the relative importance of chemotaxis, chemoaffinity, or mechanical guidance. For example, there are several instances where nerves that have been deflected surgically into the wrong pathway follow an aberrant route to their correct destinations. This occurs after transplantation of the abdominal cerci to the thorax of the cricket *Acheta domesticus* (J. S. Edwards and Sahota, 1967). The sensory neurons of insects have their cell bodies in the cuticle, and their axons regenerate back to the central nervous system. Microelectrode recording has shown that the sensory nerves from the transplanted cerci grow back selectively to the giant axons with which they normally connect. Another example to illustrate the complexity and multiplicity of factors that have to be taken into account when considering outgrowth, pathway selection, and target selection by embryonic axons is the following relatively "simple" case. In the eye of the *Daphnia* a bundle of eight optic nerve fibers grows from each ommatidium into the optic lamina. One of the fibers precedes the others into the lamina. The growth cone of this leading or pioneer fiber makes surface contact with undifferentiated neuroblasts, which extend processes to form a wrapping around the pioneer nerve fiber (Macagno *et al.*, 1973; Lopresti *et al.*, 1973). Gap junctions form for a short time between the growing pioneer fiber and the neuroblast that wraps around it (Lopresti *et al.*, 1974). These gap junctions may mediate a cellular interaction, or information exchange, between the nerve fiber

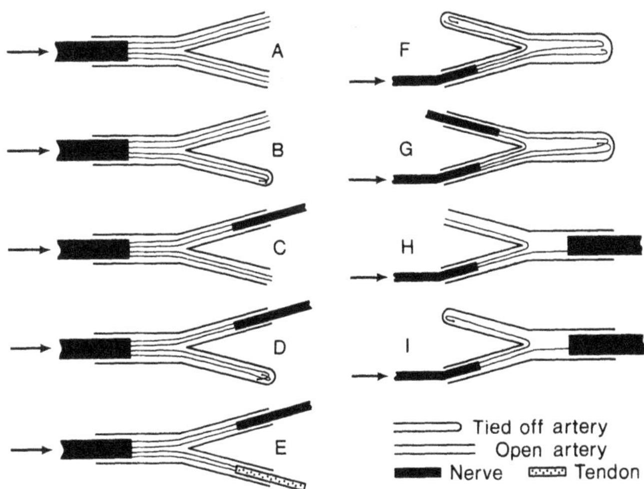

Figure 4.14. Regeneration of nerve fibers in the rat from the proximal cut end of the sciatic nerve or its tibial branch (arrow) into a Y-shaped arterial cuff with one arm containing degenerating nerve and the other arm tied off, left open, or containing tendon. The entire cuff was filled with blood clot. Nerve fibers regenerated nonselectively into both arms of the arterial cuff. From P. Weiss and A. C. Taylor, *J. Exp. Zool.* *95*:233–257 (1944).

and neuroblast, which occurs hours before the appearance of synapses. The five neurons that form a cartridge differentiate in the order in which they make contact with the pioneer fiber, which appears to show that the contact with the presynaptic nerve ending triggers differentiation in the postsynaptic neurons.

As in all other examples to be given below, there is evidence here of specific interaction between the presynaptic and postsynaptic neurons. However, there is no evidence that chemicals released from the postsynaptic neurons will attract the presynaptic terminals from a distance. In some cases the axons may grow directly to their targets, while in other cases the approach to the target may be more indirect. Only careful observations of the intermediate states can reveal the mode of approach to the postsynaptic cells. The correct connections might have been formed by widespread branching of the presynaptic axons, resulting in many random and transient contacts. The correct contacts might be made on the basis of chance and permanent connections formed as a result of chemoaffinity. Speidel has seen this process during development of the innervation of the tadpole's tail fin: The ingrowing axons branch profusely before some terminals make connections with skin or muscles and the unwanted branches are subsequently eliminated by autotomy or withdrawal (Speidel, 1935*a,b,* 1941, review). Preterminal branching of axons also occurs in the skin and in muscles after partial denervation, reinnervation occurring as a result of collateral sprouting (Edds, 1953, review).

A similar explanation might be given for the specific regrowth of sensory nerves from the heteromorph antennule which occasionally develops in place of an amputated compound eye in the adult lobster. The sensory nerves from the heteromorph antennule form synapses on the same neurons as the afferents from the normal antennule (Maynard, 1965; Maynard and Cohen, 1965). Preformed channels in the optic stalk in which the axons grow would be expected to guide them mechanically back to the optic ganglion. However, the selective growth of axons from the antennule toward their correct central neurons in the cerebral ganglion cannot be explained on the basis of mechanical guidance alone.

There are several examples in fish and amphibians of the growth of optic nerve fibers along aberrant pathways to make selective connections with neurons at specific positions in the optic tectum of the midbrain. In the goldfish, optic nerve fibers have been surgically deflected into an abnormal route to the tectum, and have been seen histologically to have grown back to their correct terminal loci, bypassing all other tectal neurons on the way (Arora and Sperry, 1962; Attardi and Sperry, 1963).

Optic nerve fibers may also grow back to the tectum after surgical union of the peripheral stump of the oculomotor nerve (Hibbard, 1967). This occurs very rarely; in most cases, the optic nerve fails to grow back to the tectum. There is no reason to suspect that the rare cases of recovery were due to chemotaxis. The tortuous course of the regenerated optic fibers and the infrequency with which they reached their destination suggest that correct connections are the result of chance encounters between regenerating fibers and tectal cells with which they have some specific affinity. These experiments would have been compelling evidence of chemotaxis if it had been found that the axons grew toward their correct places in the tectum from the start, as if "direction bound." However, it was not known whether the latter was the case or whether the initial outgrowth of axons occurred randomly in all directions, followed by the survival of only those that had made the correct connection.

The inference usually drawn from the experiments described in the previous paragraphs is that chemicals released from the target cells attract certain nerves so that the nerves are guided directly toward specific targets. This conclusion is debatable because "alluring chemicals" have not been demonstrated in any of the experiments reported and because evidence relating to the behavior of the nerves during the period of growth is lacking. Neither is there evidence that the same end result could not have been an outcome of trial and error. One is therefore inclined to be skeptical of the conclusion that the nerve fibers are guided to their destinations by chemotaxis. This conclusion has been reached by a risky process of backward reasoning from the final results to their presumed causes, without any observations of intermediate states.

The possibility of chemotaxis of nerve fibers is strengthened by the fact that some other kinds of cells have been shown to move up a concentration gradient toward the source of some diffusible substance. Chemotaxis of bacteria (see Adler, 1966; Adler and Tso, 1974) and of leukocytes toward bacterial products (McCutcheon, 1946; H. Harris, 1954; Grimes and Barnes, 1973; S. H. Zigmond, 1974) was well known at the end of the nineteenth century, and these examples are cited by Ramón y Cajal (1909–1911, Vol. 1, p. 658) in support of his theory of neurotropism. Other examples of chemotaxis are provided by the ameboid forms of the cellular slime molds which move up a concentration gradient of cyclic AMP (Bonner, 1947; 1959; Konijn *et al.*, 1968; M. H. Cohen and Robertson, 1971; Gerisch *et al.*, 1975), by the chemotaxis of spermatozoa to female gonophores in some hydroids (Miller, 1966; Miller and Brokaw, 1970), and by the attraction of the miracidia of *Schistosoma* by amino acids released from snails (MacInnis *et al.*, 1974). Evidence is growing that "powerful alluring substances," to use Ramón y Cajal's words, are involved in selective growth and connectivity of some types of nerve fibers. However, it seems likely that not all types of nerve fibers show chemotaxis but that selective nerve growth depends on contact between the axon terminal and cells along its path of growth. Cell contact phenomena, such as selective cellular affinities or selective inhibition or stimulation of cell growth or mobility, play an important part in the choice of a pathway by the growing nerve fiber (Nakai, 1960; Ebendal, 1976*a,b;* Letourneau, 1975*a,b*). Unfortunately, a discussion of the physicochemical basis of cellular affinities is impossible within the confines of this book, but there are several reviews (Curtis, 1962; Steinberg, 1963, 1964; Humphreys, 1967; Revel and Ito, 1967) and a monograph by Curtis (1967) which deal with various aspects of this important topic. The role of intercellular recognition in the morphogenesis of the nervous system is considered in Section 9.2.

Whatever skepticism one may entertain on the matter of chemotropism of nerve fibers tends to be softened, but not abolished, by reading Ramón y Cajal's persuasive arguments based on his very extensive observations given in his 1910 paper. His paper on the neurotropic action of epithelia (1919) is most persuasive, but as the matter cannot be resolved by mere observation of histological preparations, even by the master histologist, a justifiable skepticism persists. However, doubts are almost completely allayed by the reports of stimulation of axon outgrowth toward various tissues, over a distance of 0.5–1 mm in tissue culture (Chamley *et al.*, 1973; Ebendal, 1976*a,b;* Ebendal and C.-O. Jacobson, 1976). In such experiments, sympathetic ganglia or other nervous tissue from chick embryos is confronted by one or more target tissues separated by about 1 mm from one another in the same culture medium, and the outgrowth to different target tissues is observed. Ebendal and C.-O. Jacobson (1976) found that fibers grow out of spinal, trigeminal, sympathetic, and Remak's (colon) ganglia preferentially toward the following tissues, listed in diminishing order of their stimulatory effect: heart, kidney, colon, liver, skin, skeletal muscle, spinal cord. That the colon has the strongest stimulating effect on Remak's ganglion may indicate a specific chemotaxis. These results indicate that a substance or substances, emanating from the target tissues, stimulate growth of axons toward the targets.

The distance of 1 mm is the maximum over which a concentration gradient can be set up within a few hours in developing tissues (Crick, 1970, 1971; Munro and Crick 1971). Coughlin (1975) has shown that growth of parasympathetic nerve fibers is specifically stimulated by their normal target organ, the submandibular gland. The submandibular ganglion of the fetal mouse shows little axonal outgrowth when grown alone *in vitro,* but vigorous outgrowth occurs toward a piece of submandibular gland epithelium when the ganglion and epithelium are separated by up to 0.5 mm. This stimulation occurs through a filter with 0.1 μm pores. The stimulation of axonal growth is not potentiated by NGF and is not inhibited by NGF antiserum. Considerable but not absolute specificity is shown: stimulation of axonal outgrowth is greatest toward the normal target organ, the submaxillary gland, but less outgrowth occurs toward the preputial gland and no outgrowth is seen toward a variety of other embryonic mouse tissues. Neither in this nor in any of the other demonstrations of stimulation of axonal outgrowth has the chemotropic agent been identified. However, the history of discovery of the nerve growth factor (see Section 6.8) should remind us that such agents may be present in such low concentrations in normal embryonic tissues that it may be virtually impossible to extract them without some prior information about their chemical nature, and that the neurotropic agents may be found in high concentration in totally unexpected places. More than 50 years ago, the inventor of tissue culture wrote:

> If it could be shown in tissue culture that there is an attraction between growing nerve fibers taken from a certain part of the nervous system and a particular kind of peripheral cell, and between another type of central neuroblast and a different peripheral cell, then we should have direct evidence for the existence of those more subtile factors which seem to be necessary to account for the definitive establishment of particular nervous connections. The few experiments which I have directed to this end have given negative results, which is not surprising when the crudities of the method are borne in mind, but since it is possible to introduce many refinements into these methods, an ultimate solution of the problem in this way does not seem to be beyond hope of attainment. (Harrison, 1910)

That ultimate solution now seems to be well within the realm of possibility.

4.14. Myelination: Interactions between Neurons and Glial Cells

One of the most tantalizing aspects of the development of the myelin sheath is that we know that vital interactions must be occurring between the myelinating cells and the neurons whose axons they ensheath, and yet, in spite of careful observations of the changes in morphology during myelination and of the changes in the composition of the myelin sheath, the basic intercellular interactions which initiate and sustain myelination remain unknown. It might be thought that the interaction between Schwann cells and peripheral nerve axons or between oligodendrocytes and optic nerve axons should be ideal systems for such studies: the nerves are separated from other structures, their components are well known, and the interaction in question can be simply defined as a stereotyped response of the oligodendrocyte or Schwann cell to a particular type of axon. In spite of these advantages, and in spite of a rapid accumulation of observations on the changing morphology and composition of the myelin sheath during development, the basic cellular mechanisms remain to be discovered. This is emphasized here because the rapid accumulation of data has tended to obscure the paucity of understanding of the basic cellular mechanisms involved in myelination. Even the initial condition for myelination, namely the proliferation of oligodendrocytes and Schwann cells, is little understood, and the mechanisms of control of the onset and cessation of their proliferation are virtually unknown. Other large gaps in our understanding of myelination will be apparent in the following section.

Schwann cells, which are solely responsible for myelination of peripheral nerves, are derived from the neural crest and migrate into the peripheral nerves. The mechanism of their migration is poorly understood (Weston, 1963). The evidence that Schwann cells originate solely from the neural crest is that excision of the latter results in total absence of Schwann cells (Harrison, 1924*a;* Detwiler and Kehoe, 1939; Hilber, 1943).

After removal of the neural crest the peripheral nerves develop normally in the complete absence of Schwann cells. Nerve regeneration in the absence of Schwann cells also occurs in the unmyelinated nerve fibers of the cornea (Zander and Weddell, 1951). Although peripheral axons can grow out and form functional connections in the absence of Schwann cells, evidence that the Schwann cells play an important role in maintaining axons will be given below. However, myelination is not essential for the development and functioning of axons. Impulse conduction in axons commences, during development, before the formation of myelin sheaths (Ulett *et al.,* 1944; del Castillo and Vizoso, 1953; Carpenter and Bergland, 1957). Although myelination greatly increases the conduction velocity of the nervous impulse, normal impulse traffic occurs in unmyelinated axons.

Schwann cells migrate out proximodistally along the growing nerve fibers. This was first observed by R. G. Harrison (1904) in living nerve fibers visible through the skin of the tadpole's tail. Later, Speidel used the same preparation, and summarized the results of more than 30 years of research on the development of nerve fibers observed *in vivo* (Speidel, 1964). A short summary is given here of his main findings relevant to Schwann cell activities. Schwann cells migrate at a rate of 40–90 μm per 24 hours in the tail fin at about 20°C. They attach to an unmyelinated portion of the axon and never to a region that is myelinated. Myelination occurs in a proximodistal direction, although sometimes a gap is left between two myelinated internodes, which becomes filled in later. Myelination starts near the nucleus of the Schwann cell and spreads from there in both directions. The myelin close to the nodes is most unstable, and breaks down under unfavorable conditions, leaving the remainder of the internode intact, closer to the Schwann cell nucleus.

The activities of Schwann cells can also be studied conveniently after cutting a nerve or after explanting a piece of peripheral nerve to tissue culture (summarized by Causey, 1960). After nerve section there is a delay of several days before

Schwann cells begin migrating out of the cut ends of both stumps (Ramón y Cajal, 1928; J. Z. Young, 1942; Guth, 1956*b*). They migrate at a rate of about 0.3 mm per day in mammalian peripheral nerves (Rexed, 1944). Eventually, the cells bridge the gap and, with the plasma clot and fibroblasts, they provide mechanical support and guidance for the axons growing out of the proximal nerve stump. Rexed (1944) has found that if an already degenerated nerve is cut again, there is no delay before migration of Schwann cells; thus their migration appears to be inhibited by the presence of normal nerve or accelerated by products of nerve degeneration.

In tissue culture, practically no migration of Schwann cells occurs when the axons are intact, but the Schwann cells migrate away from the nerve when the axons degenerate (Abercrombie and Johnson, 1942, 1946; Abercrombie *et al.*, 1949). In tissue culture, some inhibition of movement of Schwann cells occurs when they come into contact with a regenerating axon. However, the Schwann cells still move about on the surface of the axon *in vitro,* as Speidel has observed in the living tissue. Full inhibition of movement of Schwann cells occurs only after they have formed a myelin sheath around an axon.

There is a remarkable similarity between the behavior of Schwann cells *in vivo* and *in vitro.* According to Lubińska (1961), the rate of migration of Schwann cells in tissue culture of mammalian nerves at 37°C is 30 ± 3.3 μm per hour, which is the same as the rate Rexed (1944) observed *in vivo.* A reduction in temperature diminishes the rate of migration to a few micrometers per hour at 20°C, which is the same as the rate reported by Speidel in the tail fin of the tadpole. In tissue culture, the Schwann cells constantly change their shape. Their movement is intermittent. Schwann cells, like glial cells, pulsate in tissue culture (Russel and Bland, 1933; Lumsden and Pomerat, 1951; Ernyei and Young, 1966; Lumsden, 1968). Migration of Schwann cells ceases during mitosis in tissue culture and *in vivo.* Mitosis is completed at 37°C, *in vitro,* in about 1½ hours from the time of rounding up to the time of separation of the daughter cells (Lubińska, 1961).

Schwann cells continue dividing after migrating into dorsal roots and peripheral nerves. Most of the Schwann cells are formed by mitosis in the peripheral nerves rather than by migration of postmitotic cells from the neural crest (A. Peters and Muir, 1959; Asbury, 1967). The axis of the mitotic spindle in Schwann cells is always parallel to the long axis of the nerve (J. R. Martin and Webster, 1973). Control of the proliferation and number of Schwann cells may be regulated by an interaction with the axon, since proliferation of Schwann cells continues as long as the axon grows in length and ceases after axonal growth in length has terminated. Precisely the correct number of Schwann cells are formed to enclose the axons, but if a peripheral nerve is repeatedly crushed the Schwann cells continue dividing with a resulting overproduction of Schwann cells (P. K. Thomas, 1970). Schwann cells that have begun to form myelin no longer divide (A. Peters and Muir, 1959; Asbury, 1967). The mitotic activity of Schwann cells declines almost to zero in adults, but they retain their ability to divide as they start proliferating in response to degeneration of the axon. The mitotic activity in Schwann cells reaches a maximum at 15–20 days after transection of a peripheral nerve in mammals, and the proliferation ceases after the axons have completed their regeneration (Abercrombie and Johnson, 1946; Abercrombie and Santler, 1957).

Mobility and mitotic activity are characteristic of Schwann cells in the embryo and in certain pathological conditions in the adult. Inhibition of migration and proliferation of Schwann cells is probably due to the axon. It is not due to the presence of myelin, because Schwann cells associated with unmyelinated axons are also sedentary and nonproliferative. However, in demyelinating diseases, the Schwann cells migrate and proliferate when the myelin breaks down, even though the axon appears to be intact. According to Lubińska (1961), the Schwann cells may migrate and proliferate in a region of the nerve that has been demyelinated, but will remain sedentary in normal regions of the axon. Lubińska (1958, 1961) has described replacement of a Schwann cell at a single intercalated internode after death of one Schwann cell, either spontaneously or after injury. The mechanisms underlying the control of migration and proliferation of Schwann cells are unknown.

Schwann cells appear to have some kind of territorial right to a particular length of axon. It appears that the initial length of all internodal segments in myelinated axons is the same. In newly regenerated axons the length of all internodal segments is about 300 μm (Hiscoe, 1947; Vizoso and Young, 1948). The number of internodal segments does not change, but as the nerve elongates during growth of the animal, the nerves are passively stretched and the internodal segments become lengthened (Vizoso, 1950). After regeneration of peripheral nerves in adult rabbit, myelination of axons occurs without subsequent stretching, and all the internodes are 300 μm long (Hiscoe, 1947; Vizoso and Young, 1948). However, stretching of nerves due to growth of the animal cannot be the only cause of elongation of the internodes because all nerve fibers are stretched equally, yet the internodes of large-caliber axons increase more than those of small-caliber axons. During development the length of the internodal segment and the diameter of the axon increase proportionately so that in adult mammals there is a linear relationship between the two, as Fig. 4.15 shows (Vizoso and Young, 1948; P. K. Thomas, 1955; Gurtrecht and Dyck, 1970). Unmyelinated nerve fibers do not

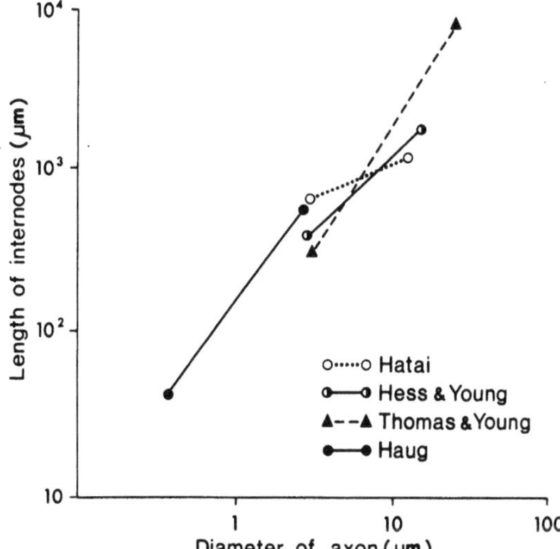

Figure 4.15. Diameter of . myelinated axons and the length of their internodes shown on a double logarithmic plot. The measurements were made on adult animals and the data were abstracted from the following sources: Hatai (1910), frog peripheral nerve; Hess and Young (1949), rabbit spinal cord; Thomas and Young (1949), fish peripheral nerve; Haug (1967*a*), cat cerebral cortex.

show a proportionality between their diameters and the internuclear distances of their Schwann cells (Peyronnard *et al.,* 1975).

The increase in diameter and internodal length of growing axons has interesting functional implications. The velocity of conduction of the nerve impulse is directly proportional to the diameter of nerve fiber: for myelinated nerve fibers this ratio between conduction velocity and fiber diameter is 6.1 (Hursh, 1939; G. Schnepp *et al.,* 1971). Rushton (1951) concluded that, for axons less than 1 μm diameter, conduction is faster without myelin, but Waxman and Bennett (1972) have shown that even for axons of 0.2 μm, which is about the smallest diameter at which axons in the central nervous system are myelinated, the conduction velocity is faster with than without myelin. For an excellent review of increases in conduction velocities during development, see Hildebrand and Skoglund (1971). Because the propagation of the action potential in myelinated axons is saltatory, from node to node (A. F. Huxley and Stämpfli, 1949), the conduction velocity increases with maturation of the axon (Sanders and Whitteridge, 1946; Ridge, 1967). As a result, the time taken for the action potential to traverse the peripheral nerve fiber tends to remain constant as the animal grows. Presumably, the increase in conduction velocity in myelinated axons in the central nervous system also compensates for lengthening of the axons. The conduction time in axons tends to remain constant during growth of the nervous system in spite of the great increases in distances that the nerve impulses must traverse (see Scherrer *et al.,* 1968).

Whether the Schwann cell does or does not form a myelin sheath is determined by the type of axon with which it associates. All the evidence shows that the axon, in some unknown way, stimulates the Schwann cells to form myelin. This capacity of the axon depends on its continuity with the perikaryon, for the Schwann cells disassociate from the axon if it is disconnected from the perikaryon (Ramón y Cajal, 1928, and many later authors). This may indicate that the Schwann cell requires a substance that is made in the neuron cell body and transported down the axon (Speidel, 1964). The experiments in which myelinated and unmyelinated nerves are cross-united show that Schwann cells are able to associate as easily with axons that become myelinated as with those that remain unmyelinated. The myelination of regenerated axons depends on the type of neuron and not on the type of Schwann cell: only myelinated nerves become remyelinated, regardless of the nature of the peripheral nerve stump into which they grow (Langley, 1898; Langley and Anderson, 1904*a,b;* Simpson and Young, 1945; Weinberg and Spencer, 1975; Aguayo *et al.,* 1976*a,b*). These conclusions have recently been confirmed by the joining of a proximal stump of a myelinated nerve to the distal end of an unmyelinated nerve, in which the Schwann cells in either the proximal or distal stump had been prelabeled with [^{3}H]thymidine (Weinberg and Spencer, 1976). The labeled Schwann cells do not migrate from the proximal to the distal stump, and axons regenerating into the distal stump are myelinated by the Schwann cells of the unmyelinated nerve.

The formation of a myelin sheath is also determined by the diameter of the axon (Duncan, 1934*a,b*). In mammalian peripheral nerves, axons smaller than about 1 μm are unmyelinated, and in myelinated nerves the number of lamellae of myelin is proportional to the diameter of the axon (Sanders, 1948; M. A. Matthews, 1968; Friede and Samorajski, 1968; Friede, 1972, 1973*a,b*). In the central nervous system axons of diameter 0.2 μm may be myelinated, although it is uncommon to find myelinated axons less than 0.4 μm (M. A. Matthews, 1968; Waxman and Pappas, 1971; Franson and Hildebrand, 1975). This is another example of the difference between central and peripheral myelination which will be enlarged upon in the following section. These observations indicate either that small axons do not stimulate the Schwann cells to myelinate them or that Schwann cells are incapable of forming a myelin sheath around small axons. It is not known whether Schwann cells can ensheath artificial fibers. Ernyei and Young (1966) have reported the formation of myelin sheath by Schwann cells around fibers of glass, nylon, rayon, and tungsten, 5–30 μm in diameter, in cultures of sympathetic and dorsal root ganglia of mice. However, Field *et al.* (1968*b*) failed to confirm this. It is important to distinguish between simple ensheathment of the fiber and the formation of lamellae of compact myelin. Tissue culture provides an excellent means of studying the development of myelin, as myelination proceeds normally in pieces of the central nervous system cultured *in vitro* (E. R. Peterson and Murray, 1955; Hild, 1957, 1966; Bornstein and Murray, 1958; Wolf, 1964; Field *et al.,* 1968*a;* Crain, 1976). Tissue culture studies have also shown that axons can stimulate the proliferation of Schwann cells in culture (P. M. Wood and Bunge, 1975).

Dramatic demonstration of the influence of the Schwann cell on the caliber of its associated segment of the axon has been given by Aguayo *et al.* (1976*c*). They grafted a segment of sciatic nerve reciprocally between a normal mouse and a trembler mouse. The trembler is a dominant mutant in which a defect of Schwann cells causes widespread deficiency of myelination and reduction of axon caliber. Transfer of normal Schwann cells to a segment of sciatic nerve of the trembler mouse results in normal myelination of that segment and in an increase of the caliber of the trembler axons in the myelinated segment. Conversely, the segment of normal sciatic nerve populated by trembler Schwann cells has a deficit of myelination and a local reduction of axonal caliber. This shows that axon caliber is controlled to a considerable degree by the local influence of the Schwann cell. The mechanism of this influence is not known. It may be due to a local change in the axon resulting in local increase in neurofilaments or neurotubules. It may be due to transfer of macromolecules from the Schwann cell to the axon, as has been reported in the squid giant axon (Lasek *et al.,* 1974). It may be due to transfer of amino acids and other precursors from the Schwann cells to the axon, and local synthesis of axonal components (Singer and Salpeter, 1966; Singer, 1968, review; Krishnan and Singer, 1973). In this connection, it may be significant that ribosomes are more frequently found in myelinated than in unmyelinated axons (Zelená, 1972*a,b*). However, more than 90 percent of RNA in the axon is apparently transfer RNA, and local protein synthesis in the axon is considered insignificant.

One of the most promising experimental strategies for studying interactions between Schwann cells and axons has been to graft a segment of one type of nerve into a gap in another type. The Schwann cells originate locally in such peripheral nerve grafts and do not enter the graft with the regenerating axons from the proximal stump or migrate into the graft from the distal nerve stump. Such experiments have proved that the neuropathy in trembler mice is due to a primary disorder of Schwann cells and is not due to a disorder of the axons, as is shown in Fig. 4.16 (Aguayo *et al.,* 1977). Similar experiments, in which segments are grafted

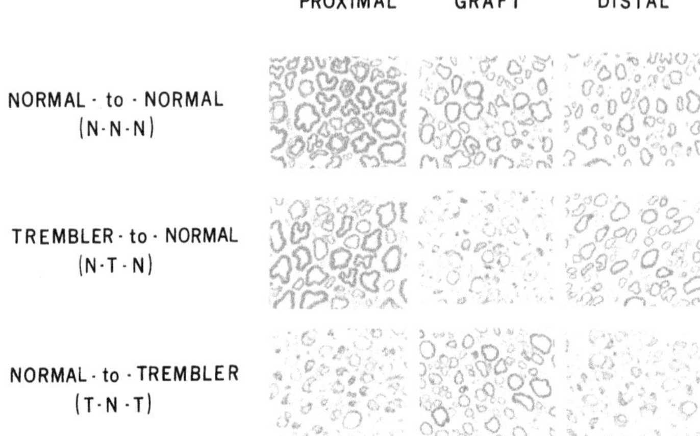

Figure 4.16. Grafting of Schwann cells between segments of the sciatic nerve of normal and trembler mice. Two months after grafting, cross sections were made of sciatic nerves 3 mm proximal to the graft, in the middle of the graft, and 3 mm distal to the graft. Phase micrographs show myelinated and unmyelinated axons: normal-to-normal graft (top row), trembler-to-normal graft (middle row), and normal-to-trembler graft (bottom row). Normal grafted Schwann cells myelinate trembler host axons growing through the graft, but trembler grafted Schwann cells fail to myelinate normal axons. From A. J. Aguayo, M. Attiwell, J. Trecarten, S. Perkins, and G. M. Bray, *Nature 265:*73–75 (1977).

between myelinated and unmyelinated nerves, have shown that myelin production is determined by the axon with which the Schwann cell interacts. Thus Schwann cells from unmyelinated cervical sympathetic nerves will produce myelin when in contact with regenerating axons of sural nerve (Aguayo *et al.,* 1976*a,b*).

4.15. Structure of the Myelin Sheath

X-ray diffraction studies (Caspar and Kirschner, 1971; Blaurock, 1976) have shown that the myelin membrane consists of a lipid bilayer sandwiched between monolayers of protein. The lipid molecules have their hydrocarbon portions oriented radially into the membrane and their polar groups exposed to a protein–aqueous phase which has a different composition on the internal and external surfaces of the membrane. The width of one unit membrane is about 80 Å, consisting of the bimolecular layer of lipid (about 50 Å) and two protein layers (about 15 Å each). The repeating unit of myelin consists of two fused membranes, and this results in a 156 Å periodicity in mammalian central myelin and a 180 Å periodicity in mammalian peripheral nerve myelin (reduced to about 120 Å in electron microscopic preparations due to shrinkage). Electron micrographs of fixed and stained myelin show a periodicity consisting of two electron-dense bands, the major dense line and the intraperiod line separated by a lucent zone. The electron-dense lines are due to proteins, while the lucent regions are due to lipids. The major dense line is formed by apposition of the two inner lamellae of the plasma membrane of the Schwann cell in peripheral nerve, or oligodendrocyte in the central nervous system, with the cytoplasm squeezed out. The intraperiod line is formed by apposition of the two outer lamellae of plasma membrane, with the extracellular space obliterated. A potential extracellular space remains, because the extracellular marker, lanthanum, may penetrate between the myelin lamellae. Hypotonic solutions increase the extracellular space, causing separation of the myelin lamellae at the external surfaces.

The major constituents of myelin are phospholipids, glycolipids, sterols, and proteins (Norton, 1976, review). In mammals, the phospholipids, chiefly phosphatidyl ethanolamine and lecithin, constitute 26–44 percent of dry weight; glycolipids, including sphingomyelin, cerebroside, and ganglioside, constitute 12–22 percent of dry weight; sterols, mainly cholesterol, range from 11 to 22 percent of dry weight in different mammals. Three kinds of proteins that are specific for myelin have been identified. They constitute about 20 percent of the dry weight of myelin.

There are differences between the lipid and protein compositions of central and peripheral myelin, as is to be expected, because they are formed by different types of cells, the Schwann cells in peripheral nerves and the oligodendrocytes in the central nervous system. The myelin period is about 10 percent less in central than in peripheral myelin of the same animal. The lipid compositions differ: peripheral myelin has double the sphingomyelin content of central myelin; the ratio of cerebroside to sphingomyelin is about 1 in peripheral myelin but about 2 in central myelin.

The proteins also differ in central and peripheral myelin. The major protein of central myelin, composing 54 percent of the total protein, is a proteolipid protein named Folch-Lees after its discoverers. It is moderately basic, with a molecular weight of about 34,000. The major protein of peripheral nerve myelin is the so-called Wolfgram protein, which is a neutral proteolipid protein. Very basic proteins constitute 20–30 percent of the protein in both central and peripheral myelin. The basic protein has a molecular weight of about 18,000. The basic protein is antigenic when it enters the blood and gives rise to experimental allergic encephalomyelitis.

The composition of myelin changes during development (Norton and Poduslo, 1973). In the rat, the myelin galactolipids increase by about 50 percent and lecithin decreases by a similar amount from birth to about 2 months of age. At the same time, the polysialogangliosides decrease and the monosialoganglioside, G_{M1}, increases to become the main ganglioside of adult myelin. Myelin protein and proteolipid protein increase during maturation.

4.16. Development of the Myelin Sheath

The early literature dealing with the origin of the myelin sheath has been reviewed by Ramón y Cajal (1928), H. Lehmann (1959), and R. P. Bunge (1968). The history of this subject provides yet another example of a problem being hotly disputed by eminent neurohistologists for almost a century before it was finally resolved in a few years by the use of a new technique. The application of electron microscopy put an end to the debate and confusion that existed before 1953 by showing that the myelin sheath is a tongue of the Schwann cell wrapped around the axon like a scroll around a rod (Geren and Raskind, 1953; Geren, 1954; Robertson, 1955; A. Peters and Muir, 1959; A. Peters, 1960, 1964*a,b*). Geren

(1954) was able to show all stages in the ensheathment and myelination of axons in the sciatic nerve of the chick. The initial stage consists of enfolding of the axon by the Schwann cell, leaving a channel (the mesaxon) open to the extracellular space (Gasser, 1958). Then a tongue of cytoplasm extends from the Schwann cell as a spiral around the axon, ensheathing the latter in many turns of Schwann cell cytoplasm and membranes. Finally, compaction of the Schwann cell membranes occurs as the cytoplasm is squeezed out of the internodal portion and remains only as an inner collar close to the axon, as perinodal loops of cytoplasm near the nodes of Ranvier, as an outer collar containing the nucleus of the Schwann cell, and as the bridges of cytoplasm forming the Schmidt-Lantermann clefts (Figs. 4.17 and 4.18). Initially, the Schwann cells surround bundles of many axons, but as the Schwann cells proliferate they each associate with fewer axons. If the axons remain unmyelinated, they are merely enfolded by cytoplasmic processes of Schwann cells, but axons destined to be myelinated establish a one-to-one relationship with Schwann cells which stop dividing and start wrapping around the axon, which results in myelination (A. Peters and Muir, 1959; A. Peters and Vaughn, 1967; H. Webster, 1971; H. Webster *et al.,* 1973). Myelin continues to be formed while peripheral nerves elongate and increase in caliber during growth of the body, and a single peripheral nerve axon may finally have up to 100 layers of myelin. The growth of the myelin sheath thus necessarily requires very considerable expansion and slippage of myelin lamellae over each other (H. Webster, 1971; Friede, 1973*a,b*). The expansion in the central nervous system is less than that required in peripheral nerves, but must, nevertheless, also occur as the axons increase in length and in caliber.

The role of glia in myelination of axons in the central nervous system also remained an area of uncertainty and disputation until recently. Several investigators had produced circumstantial evidence that interfascicular oligodendrocytes are involved in myelination: The rapid increase in oligodendrocytes in central

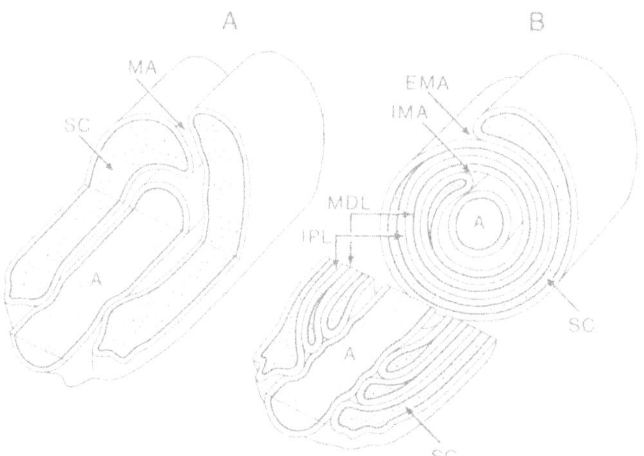

Figure 4.17. Myelination of axons in peripheral nerves by Schwann cells. Left: The axon enclosed by the Schwann cell, before the development of myelin. Right: The cytoplasmic process of the Schwann cells wrapped around the axon and the formation of lamellae of compact myelin. A, Axon; EMA, external mesaxon; IMA, internal mesaxon; IPL, intraperiod line; MDL, major dense line; SC, Schwann cell.

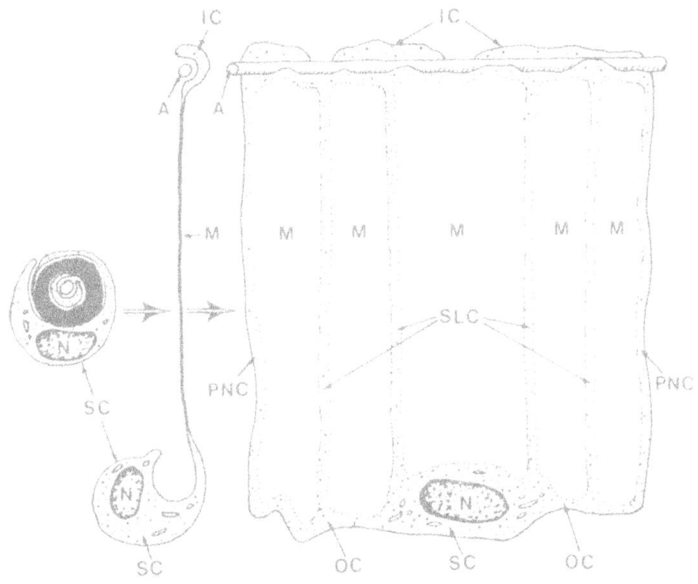

Figure 4.18. "Unrolled" Schwann cell and myelin sheath. A, Axon; M, myelin; IC, inner collar of Schwann cell cytoplasm; N, nucleus of Schwann cell; PNC, perinodal cytoplasm of Schwann cell; OC, outer collar of Schwann cell cytoplasm; SC, Schwann cell; SLC, Schmidt-Lantermann cleft. Modified from H. deF. Webster, *J. Cell Biol. 48:*348–367 (1971).

tracts prior to their myelination and the invariable presence of oligodendrocytes during myelination in the central nervous system were very suggestive observations (del Rio-Hortega, 1924, 1928; Penfield, 1924; Linell and Tom, 1931; Morrison, 1932). As the role of oligodendrocytes in myelination could not be proved, other hypotheses were entertained in which the role of myelin production was assigned to the axons themselves or to the astrocytes (Alpers and Haymaker, 1934; Scharf, 1951; Hild, 1957). Blunt *et al.* (1972) reached the same conclusion. However, electron microscopy showed conclusively that there is continuity between the membrane of the oligodendrocyte and the myelin sheath and that the wrapping of the oligodendrocyte membrane around axons in the central nervous system is essentially the same as the process of myelination in peripheral nerves (Luse, 1956, 1960; Maturana, 1960; A. Peters, 1960, 1964*a,b,* 1966; M. B. Bunge *et al.,* 1962; Kruger and Maxwell, 1966; Knobler and Stempak, 1973; C. Meier, 1976). The structure and development of the central myelin sheath have been thoroughly reviewed by R. P. Bunge (1968).

The structure and composition of central and peripheral myelin sheaths are slightly different, reflecting their formation by different types of cells. In peripheral axons, the Schwann cell cytoplasm consists of a broad tongue forming an outer collar containing the cell nucleus and an inner collar adjacent to the axon, as shown in Fig. 4.17. In central axons the cytoplasm of the oligodendrocyte is connected to the sheath by a process that is prominent early in development but which later becomes very slender and may be as long as 10 μm. Unlike the Schwann cell, a single oligodendrocyte may myelinate more than one axon, and the glial cell body may not be adjacent to its myelin sheath (Fig. 4.19). The main difference at the nodes of Ranvier is the presence of processes of Schwann cell cytoplasm covering the nodes in peripheral axons, whereas the axon is exposed at the nodes of central axons (B. G. Uzman and Villegas, 1960). The point of exit of the cranial nerves and spinal roots is a boundary at which a transition between central and peripheral myelin occurs. We do not know when and how this transition develops, and little attention has been given to this problem. The transition is not hard and fast, because Schwann cells can invade the central nervous system in order to myelinate axons that have been demyelinated, for example, by diptheria toxin, or to myelinate regenerating central axons, for example, after spinal cord compression (McDonald, 1974, review).

Before the onset of myelination there is a period of intense proliferation of interfascicular oligodendrocytes in the central nervous system and of Schwann cells in peripheral nerves. During this period the satellite cells are most sensitive to irradiation. X-irradiation of neonatal rats and mice results in defects in myelination and changes in the composition of myelin (Diller *et al.,* 1964; Schjeide *et al.,* 1968). The intense proliferation of oligodendrocytes in central fiber tracts prior to myelination has been called *myelination gliosis* by Roback and Scherrer (1935). This proliferation ceases at the onset of myelination (Dekaban, 1956; Majno and Karnofsky, 1958; Friede, 1961). Myelination in each region of the brain is always preceded by an increase in vascularization (Craigie, 1925, 1938; J. F. Feeney and Watterson, 1946; R. M. Barlow, 1969). Histochemical studies have shown an increase in the activity of several oxidative enzymes such as cytochrome oxidase, succinic dehydrogenase, NAD-diaphorase, and DPN-diaphorase in Schwann cells and oligodendrocytes during myelination (Friede, 1961, 1966; Yonezawa *et al.,* 1962; Blunt *et al.,* 1967; Schonbach *et al.,* 1968; R. M. Barlow, 1969), as is shown in Fig. 4.20.

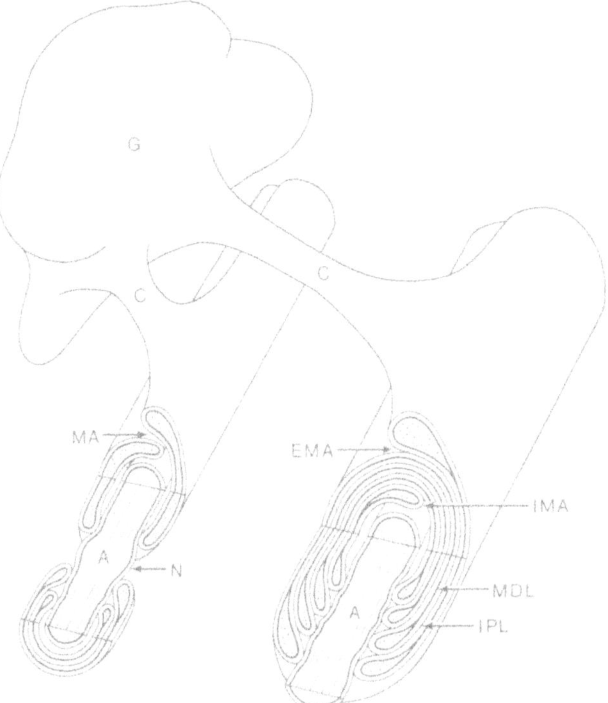

Figure 4.19. Myelination of axons in the central nervous system by an oligodendroglial cell. Myelination is farther advanced on the axon at the right than on the axon at the left. A, Axon; C, cytoplasmic process of oligodendrocyte; EMA, external mesaxon; IMA, internal mesaxon; IPL, intraperiod line; MA, mesaxon; MDL, major dense line; N, node; G, oligodendroglial cell.

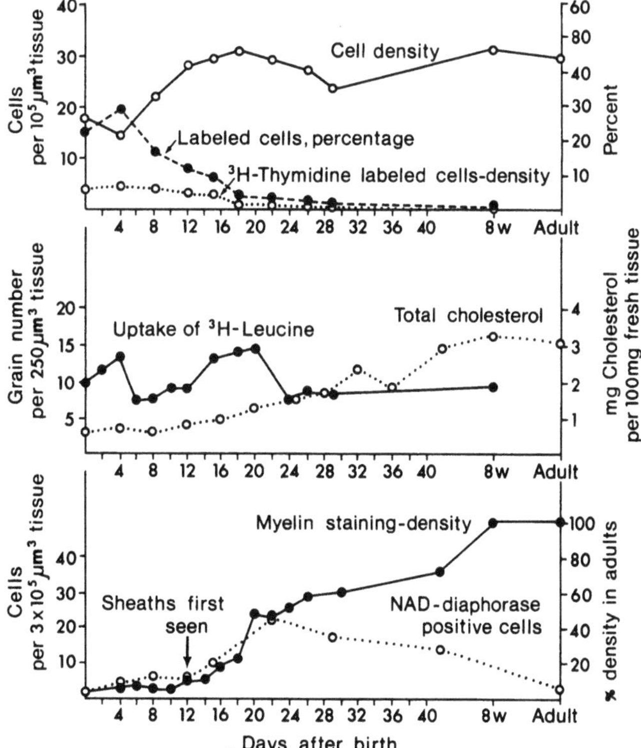

Figure 4.20. Changes in cell density; [^{3}H]thymidine and [^{3}H]leucine incorporation determined by autoradiography; total cholesterol determined biochemically; staining density of myelin and density of cells containing NAD-diaphorase determined histochemically in the corpus callosum of the mouse from birth to maturity. From J. Schonbach, K. U. Hu, and R. L. Friede, *J. Comp. Neurol. 134*:21–38 (1968).

Prior to the formation of myelin lamellae there is a period of greatly increased lipid synthesis in the Schwann cells and interfascicular oligodendrocytes that can be detected histochemically and biochemically. The intense synthetic activities of oligodencrocytes during the period of maximum myelination result in a 1500 percent increase in the total quantity of myelin in the brain of the rat during the period from 15 days to 6 months after birth. During this period the increase in brain weight is largely due to the accumulation of myelin. A biochemical index of the degree of myelination in any part of the nervous system can be obtained from the phospholipid content at any stage of development relative to the phospholipid content of the same region in the adult. Although phospholipids are not restricted to myelin, they are most abundant there, and phospholipids continue to increase while myelin is forming. Therefore, the incorporation of ^{32}P into brain lipids can be used as a rough index of the rate of myelination during development. In the brain of the rat, accumulation of cholesterol and phospholipid increases dramatically 7–10 days after birth, but the increase of cerebroside occurs only during the period when myelin lamellae first appear, that is, from the 10th to the 20th day after birth (Cuzner and Davison, 1968). The accumulation of cerebroside, the most characteristic lipid in myelin, is a useful index of the development of compact myelin.

Once compact myelin has been formed, its lipid constituents appear to be remarkably stable, with very slow turnover; otherwise, there might be very efficient local reutilization of myelin lipids. The evidence for this is that radioactive lipids and other myelin precursors, injected during the period of myelination, persist in the myelin until adult life in chicks, rats, and rabbits (A. N. Davison and Dobbing, 1960*a,b,* 1966; B. G. Uzman and Hedley-Whyte, 1968). Reported turnover times of myelin proteins vary greatly, but it appears that while the proteolipid proteins have a long half-life (about 100 days) another protein component, with high molecular weight, turns over more rapidly, with a half-life of about 40 days (Wood and King, 1971; C. A. Fischer and Morell, 1974).

Because myelination involves a sequence of proliferative and synthetic activities of satellite cells and probably also requires the cooperative activity of the axon, abnormalities of myelin development might result from a variety of disturbances in proliferation and motility of satellite cells or from deficiencies in enzymes or substrates required for the synthesis of myelin. During the time of myelination the central nervous system is especially vulnerable to undernutrition (Dobbing, 1963; Culley and Mertz, 1965; Benton *et al.,* 1966; A. N. Davison and Dobbing, 1966; H. P. Chase *et al.,* 1967; Clos and Legrand, 1969, 1970). Insufficient nutrition during that period results in a delay in myelination and a deficiency in the total quantity of myelin. The effect is on synthesis rather than degradation of myelin. It is also probable, although not fully demonstrated, that undernutrition results in reduced proliferation of oligodendrocytes as well as in a reduction in the quantity of myelin that they synthesize. During the peak period of myelination in the rat, it is established that each oligodendrocyte synthesizes 3 times its own weight of myelin daily (Norton, 1976). It is also evident that the oligodendrocytes require a large supply of the precursors necessary for myelin synthesis. Although malnutrition results in reduced synthesis of myelin, its composition is normal in experimentally undernourished rats and in undernourished humans (J. H. Fox *et al.,* 1972; Krigman and Hogan, 1976). Recovery of myelination is not complete in rats fed *ad libitum* after 20 days postnatal undernutrition (Wiggins *et al.,* 1976). The effects of malnutrition on the developing nervous system are protean and are considered at greater length in Section 6.1.

Defects in the oligodendrocytes are known to occur in mutations that affect myelination in mice. These mutations are known as jimpy, quaking (Sidman *et al.,* 1964), dilute-lethal (Kelton and Rauch, 1962), wabbler-lethal (Dickie *et al.,* 1952), and the *msd* mutant (Meier and MacPike, 1970). The mutants are all deficient in central but not in peripheral myelin. Quaking, dilute-lethal, and wabbler-lethal are autosomal recessives, and jimpy and *msd,* which are very similar, are sex-linked recessive mutants. In dilute-lethal and wabbler-lethal, degeneration of myelin starts at 2 weeks after birth and affects the vestibular, cerebellar, and spinal tracts. Jimpy and *msd* hemizygous males die at about 3 weeks after birth, but quaking mice survive, although they are stunted. In quaking, the defect is a delay and deficiency rather than total absence of myelination. Other defects, such as vacuolation of glial cells and hydrocephalus, also occur in quaking mice (Samorajski *et al.,* 1970). The biochemical lesion is a deficiency in the synthesis of lipids, especially of cerebrosides, which are markedly reduced in the myelin of the jimpy mutants (Nussbaum *et al.,* 1971) and in the quaking mutants (Gregson and Oxberry, 1972). Wolf and Holden (1969) showed that deficient myelination occurs *in vitro* in the jimpy cerebellum, while normal myelination occurs in normal brain cultured on the same coverslip. This shows that the defect is not due to a diffusible agent. The defect seems to be in the oligodendroglia, which do not mature in jimpy mice

(Farkas-Bargeton *et al.,* 1972). By contrast, in quaking mice there is hyperplasia of oligodendrocytes, which may be an attempt to compensate for the deficient myelin production by the oligodendrocytes (Friedrich, 1975). The mutant mice show that central myelination and peripheral myelination are under separate genetic controls.

Abnormal behavior and mental retardation also occur in several metabolic diseases in which deficiencies in the formation of myelin have been reported in humans, as in phenylketonuria (Crome *et al.,* 1962) and inherited disorders of amino acid metabolism (Prensky *et al.,* 1968). In those cases, it is not known whether the myelin deficiency and the behavioral impairment are causally related or merely coincidentally associated. Thyroidectomy of rats at birth results in 30 percent reduction in the dry weight of myelin obtained from the whole brain at 43 days of age, but there is no change in the time course of myelination or the composition of myelin as compared with normal rats (Balázs *et al.,* 1969).

As regards the timing of myelination, there are regional differences and species differences that do not seem to indicate a general principle. The emphasis on myelination as an indication of functional maturation of the brain (Flechsig, 1920; F. Tilney and Casamajor, 1924; Langworthy, 1928*b,* 1930, 1933; F. Tilney, 1933; Windle *et al.,* 1934) was once popular, but should now be regarded as an oversimplification. See Huttenlocher (1970) for correlation of myelination and development of function in the pyramidal tracts. Although it is obvious that the behavioral capacities of newborn animals increase during the period of myelination, there is no reason to regard the former as a direct consequence of the latter. Obviously, myelination cannot be taken as an index of maturity of the unmyelinated fibers, which are merely enfolded by satellite cells without developing a sheath of compact myelin. Impulse traffic starts in axons during development, before they develop myelin sheaths (Ulett *et al.,* 1944; J. del Castillo and Vizoso, 1953; F. G. Carpenter and Bergland, 1957). Langworthy (1928*a*) has shown that precocious motor activities develop in the newborn opossum before myelination commences.

The studies of Flechsig (1920) and others have shown that myelination occurs at specific times in various parts of the nervous system. Flechsig was the first to use this as a means of delineating fiber tracts and was, in this way, able to demonstrate the course of the pyramidal tracts from the cerebral cortex to the anterior horn of the spinal cord. In 1876, Flechsig wrote: "during certain periods of fetal life fibers, which in the adult are of uniform consistency and differ little from one another, can be distinguished from each other in a very striking manner. This is because some of them already have a complete myelin sheath, whereas others still exhibit their naked axis cylinders. Thus we are in a position, especially in the compact white matter, to follow for a considerable distance fibers and fiber bundles that later on, owing to the uniformity of their components, become masked in their course."

In rats, rabbits, and mice, myelination begins only 2 days after birth in the ventral roots and in ventral and lateral tracts of the spinal cord, and then extends in a rostrocaudal direction, with the first myelin appearing in the brain in the internal capsule and posterior commissure at 10 days and starting last in the corpus callosum and association areas of the cerebral cortex at 15–21 days of age (J. B. Watson, 1903; F. Tilney, 1933; S. Jacobson, 1963; A. N. Davison *et al.,* 1966). The sequence of myelination is similar in the opossum (Langworthy, 1928*a*), cat

(F. Tilney and Casamajor, 1924; Langworthy, 1928*b*), sheep (Romanes, 1947; R. M. Barlow, 1969), and man (Flechsig, 1920; Keene and Hewer, 1931, 1933; Langworthy, 1930, 1933; Conel, 1939–1963; Yakovlev and Lecours, 1967), although the time scale differs in different species. Myelination not only starts late, when cellular proliferation and migration in the nervous system have virtually ceased, but also continues until at least 16 weeks of age in the rat and until well into the first decade of life in man. As a first approximation, the sequence of myelination of neurons occurs in the same order as their time of origin and differentiation. Phylogenetically older regions of the nervous system are myelinated before those that have arisen more recently in phylogeny, and in each region the large neurons with long axons are myelinated before small neurons with short axons. However, this orderly sequence becomes obscured with time because the duration of myelination occupies a fairly large fraction of an animal's postnatal life.

5

Elaboration of Dendrites and Synaptic Connections

5.1. Development of Dendrites

The dictum that "Nature geometrizeth, and observeth order in all Things" (Sir Thomas Browne, *Religio Medici,* 1643) cannot be applied more aptly than to the developing nervous system, and it is in the geometry of their dendrites that neurons express their most characteristic features. Yet it is a mere century since those features could first be discerned with the aid of the Golgi technique. Rapid progress could be made only after 1873, when Golgi introduced his techniques for impregnating neurons with metallic salts. Before then, it is true that Deiters, in 1865, had first illustrated the dendrites, which he called protoplasmic processes, in spinal motoneurons, but he could not see the detailed geometry of the dendritic tree. Before the application of the Golgi technique, even the Purkinje cell dendritic tree remained hidden. In 1837, Purkinje illustrated only the perikaryon and proximal part of the dendrites of the cerebellar cells that bear his name, and he did not draw attention to their dendrites. In Koelliker's great three-volume *Mikroskopische Anatomie* (1850–1852), the dendrites are not identified as such. In fact, it was not until 1890 that Wilhelm His introduced the term *dendrite.*

Efforts to understand how dendrites develop have always been cramped by limitations of histological techniques. The Golgi technique of filling the neurons with metallic precipitates was, until the advent of electron microscopy, the only reliable method of studying dendritic morphology. In the century after the invention of the Golgi technique, the study of dendritic growth and form has barely advanced to the stage that the plant and animal taxonomists had surpassed two centuries ago. Attempts at classification of the forms of dendritic trees are based on the concept of the neurophenotype and on the conviction that the form of each neuron, especially the form of its dendritic tree, is a characteristic and invariant feature of a distinct neuronal type. Individual neurons belonging to the same type may exhibit a limited variability, but they are assumed to share certain invariant features that make it possible to assign that cell to its proper type. Such a system of classification of neurons can easily become an artifice, based merely on differences or on similarities of form that are useful as an aid to identification but that have no other functional or developmental significance. The danger of dwelling on externals alone is well shown in the history of taxonomy (Goerke, 1973, pp. 89–105). The danger is greatest when the classification is based on a single technique such as the Golgi method. This has resulted in arbitrary and artificial classifications of dendrites, such as that of Ramón-Moliner (1962, 1968), which are reminiscent of the efforts of the taxonomists before Linnaeus to classify plants into trees, bushes, and herbs.

Investigation of the growth of dendrites would be impossible without the Golgi methods of metallic impregnation of neurons, and a brief summary of the advantages and limitations of these methods may be of assistance in assessing the value of the results obtained with Golgi methods. The **Golgi-Cox method** consists of the precipitation of metallic mercury in the neuron after fixation in a mercury salt. This method impregnates the cell body fully, impregnates the dendrites for most of their length but not into their terminal branches, and shows only the initial portion of the axon. The metal rarely penetrates into the fine dendritic branches or into dendritic spines or filopodia on growing dendrites. About 1–5 percent of the neurons are impregnated by the Golgi-Cox method, apparently at random without any selectivity (Smit and Colon, 1969; Pasternak and Woolsey, 1975). Therefore, the method can be used for obtaining the frequency of different types of neurons and for quantitative studies (Sholl, 1956*a,b*).

The **rapid Golgi method** involves precipitation of silver chromate within the neurons after fixation in a solution of osmium tetroxide and potassium dichromate. The rapid Golgi method generally impregnates the entire neuron, but it is more capricious and results in more unusable sections than the Golgi-Cox method. The reliability and speed of the rapid Golgi method are greatly increased by buffering of the fixing solution (Kemali, 1976). The rapid Golgi method cannot be used for counting the frequency of different types of neurons, but its great advantage is that it impregnates axons and dendrites to their tips. Dendritic spines, growth cones, and filopodia are made visible by this method. The entire axon is often impregnated down to the finest branches so that they can be traced to their synaptic terminals.

In spite of its limitations, the Golgi method has given more information about the growth and form of neurons than any other technique. No alternative to the Golgi method was available until the recently invented technique of filling neurons with fluorescent dyes such as Procion yellow (Stretton and Kravitz, 1968; Milburn and Bentley, 1971) and Procion brown (Christensen, 1973), or with cobalt chloride, which can be precipitated intracellularly as cobalt sulfide (Pitman *et al.*, 1972; Scalia and Fite, 1974). These tracers either can be injected into the neuron through a micropipette or may enter the cell to a more limited extent by diffusion through the cut end of the axon (Iles and Mulloney, 1971; Kater *et al.*, 1973).

The Golgi technique and other methods of filling the entire neuron have brought us within reach of attaining the goal set by Descartes of geometrizing the brain, which has proved too laborious, if possible at all, without their aid. Now that the three-dimensional geometry of the neuron can be derived with the aid of the computer from reconstructions of serial sections (Levinthal and Ware, 1972; D. R. Reddy *et al.*, 1973; Rakic *et al.*, 1974), it may be possible to correlate the form of the neuron with its ontogeny and with its function in ways that were extremely difficult in the past. Computers are useful, but they are neither indispensible nor sufficient, and it has been possible to correlate neuronal geometry with function (e.g., by Pomeranz and Chung, 1970; Kelly and Van Essen, 1974) and with ontogeny, most notably in work done by Ramón y Cajal (1909) without the aid of the computer. Such studies have shown that a keen eye for recognizing patterns in nature and for accurately identifying different types of cells and the knack of interpreting structure in functional terms cannot, at the present time, be supplanted by the computer, but creative interactions with a computer can greatly extend our ability to deal with complex, developing systems.

5.2. Regularities of Dendritic Development

Outgrowth of dendrites always occurs after the outgrowth of the axon. In most cases, as discussed on page 197, it is fairly certain that the axon has formed connections before the differentiation of dendrites commences. Thus, after the neurons have migrated to their final positions, there is a long delay before full differentiation of the dendrites occurs. The young neuron has relatively short and thick dendritic processes, but these develop a complex system of branches which resemble the branching of multiaxiate plants. It is not certain whether branching occurs only at the tips of existing dendrites or whether branches also or only emerge preterminally. Branching results in a great increase in the surface area of the dendrites, which form more than 90 percent of the postsynaptic surface of the neuron (Sholl, 1955; Schadé and Baxter, 1960; Mannen, 1965, 1966; Mungai, 1967). The size, shape, and pattern of dendritic branching seen in neurons impregnated by the Golgi method seem to be characteristic for each type of neuron. There are differences in proportion and structure of different types of neurons, and particularly in the pattern of dendritic branching, on which a system of classification may be based.

Other striking spatial and temporal regularities in the development of dendrites have been observed. There are differences between the developmental chronology of neurons with long axons (Golgi type I, or principal neurons) and those with short axons (Golgi type II neurons) which support the validity of the distinction between them, first made by Golgi (1886). The development of large neurons, in general, occurs earlier than the development of small neurons in any particular region of the nervous system. It is important when making comparisons of different developmental stages to restrict the comparison to corresponding regions of the nervous system. In any region of the brain, the dendrites of neurons with short axons (Golgi type II) differentiate later than dendrites of the principal neurons, which have long axons. For example, in the dorsal nucleus of the lateral geniculate body the principal neurons that send their axons to the visual cortex mature before the Golgi type II neurons, which have short axons that end within the lateral geniculate nucleus. In the lateral geniculate nucleus of the cat the principal neurons have almost completed their development by the end of the second postnatal week when differentiation of dendrites of Golgi type II neurons begins (Morest, 1969*b*).

Maturation of dendrites tends to occur in ventrodorsal or inside-out sequence: dendrites of neurons in the ventral nucleus of the lateral geniculate body mature before those in the dorsal nucleus; the dendrites of the cortex of the brain mature later than the dendrites of the central nuclei projecting to the cortex; and within the cortex the dendrites of deeper layers tend to develop before those in more superficial layers (Schadé *et al.,* 1962; Morest, 1969*b*). Morest found no evidence of a gradient of development of dendrites of a single neuron. Instead, different portions of the dendrite and different dendrites of the same neuron show different degrees of differentiation.

According to Morest (1969*b*), "there is a tendency for the dendrites of neurons in the motor field of the neuropil to begin to differentiate before those in the sensory field at the same anteroposterior level of the brain stem." In general, the motor neurons develop before the sensory neurons in the same region of the nervous system. Within ascending sensory systems (auditory, somatosensory, visual, and olfactory) the neurons mature in ascending order, beginning with those nearest the peripheral receptors and terminating with the neurons at the highest level of the neuraxis.

The shapes of dendritic trees may give an indication of their evolutionary history, but it is in the nature of such hypotheses about the evolution of structures which have left no fossil record that inferences about evolution can be made only tentatively from the evidence of comparative and developmental studies. The well-known figure drawn by Ramón y Cajal (Fig. 5.1) is an early attempt to show a relationship between the development of the dendrites of pyramidal neurons of the mouse and a phylogenetic series of pyramidal cells from the frog, lizard, mouse, and man. The concept of dendritic ontogeny recapitulating its phylogeny has been implicitly accepted since Ramón y Cajal's time (Noback and Purpura, 1961; Poliakov, 1965; Stensaas, 1967*a;* Sanides, 1969). In particular, the notion has gained general acceptance that the forms of dendritic trees have become increasingly elaborate during evolution, and that, for pyramidal cells, there has been a general evolutionary tendency for the basal dendrites to expand more than the apical dendrites.

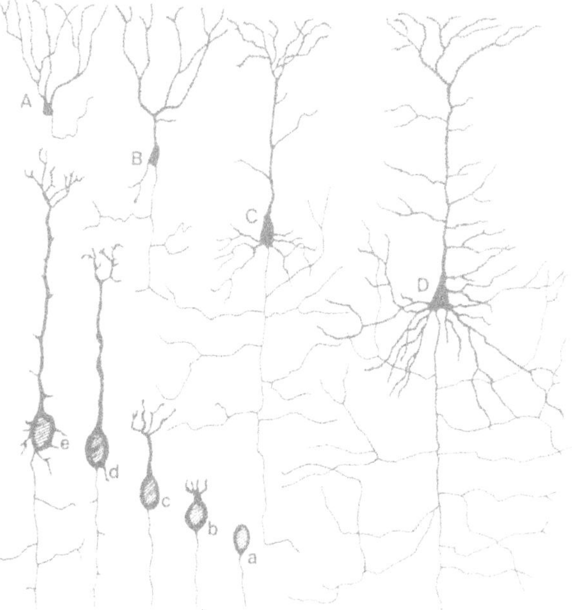

Figure 5.1. Ontogeny of pyramidal neurons, especially their dendrites, recapitulates their phylogeny, according to Ramón y Cajal (1909–1911). A–D: Pyramidal cells of various vertebrates. A, Frog; B, lizard; C, rat; D, man. a–e: Progressive stages in development of a pyramidal neuron.

Ramón y Cajal (1909–1911) observed that the dendrites of spinal motor neurons and cerebellar Purkinje and granule cells undergo great changes during development, some of them regressive. He distinguished an initial phase of outgrowth of an excessive number of dendritic branches, apparently directed at random, followed by a phase of regulation and resorption of the redundant dendrites. He proposed that a selection among the dendritic outgrowth takes place during development, presumably on a functional basis. That is, those dendritic branches that play an essential part in the functions of the dendrites persist, while those that are functionally inappropriate disappear. Ramón y Cajal's description in his autobiography is more picturesque: "I noticed that every ramification, dendritic or axonic, in the course of formation, passes through a chaotic period, so to speak, a period of trials, during which there are sent out at random experimental conductors most of which are destined to disappear. . . . What mysterious forces precede the appearance of the processes, promote their growth and ramification . . . and finally establish those protoplasmic kisses, the intercellular articulations, which seem to constitute the final ecstasy of an epic love story?"

The proper functioning of the dendrites depends on their coming into the proper relationship with axons that are destined to form synapses on them. Ramón y Cajal suggested that the dendrites might grow in response to the presence of axonal terminals and that the survival of dendritic branches would depend on the formation of functional synaptic connections between axons and dendrites. This is referred to in sections 5.7 and 7.11 in connection with growth adjustments of axonal terminals as the "theory of natural selection of neuronal connections." In summary, this theory proposes that the mechanism of selection of connections includes the formation of an excessive number of axonal and dendritic branches, followed by degeneration or resorption of all those branches that fail to make the correct connections.

Many of Ramón y Cajal's conclusions regarding the growth of dendrites have received support from later investigations. The pruning of the shaggy, spinelike branchlets from cerebellar Purkinje cells is described in Section 3.4.2. A similar process occurs in the dendrites of neurons of the brain stem reticular formation of cats: at birth, the dendrites as well as the cell bodies are covered with spines which are almost entirely lost by the third postnatal month (M. E. Scheibel *et al.*, 1973). It is not known what happens to the synapses on the dendritic spines which disappear. It seems very likely that in such cases there are temporary synaptic connections which later disappear or are displaced to other parts of the neuron. This has been shown to occur for the transient climbing fiber connections which are initially made with the spines on the Purkinje cell body but which later move to the dendrites when the spines disappear from the cell body (see Section 3.4.2).

In a study of the development of dendrites in the mammalian brain with the rapid Golgi technique, Morest (1968, 1969*a,b*) showed that dendrites differentiate in conjunction with the specific axonal terminals that are destined to synapse on them, and he suggested that the afferent axonal terminals might stimulate the development of dendrites. For example, the dendrites of the principal neurons of the lateral geniculate nucleus differentiate at the time of arrival of the optic axons in the lateral geniculate nucleus. A terminal growth cone can be seen at the growing tip of the dendrites impregnated by the rapid Golgi method (Fig. 5.2), and preterminal growth buds are seen on the shaft of the dendrites (Morest, 1969*a,b*). Filopodia, similar to those found on axonal growth cones, are seen on the terminal growth cones and on the growth buds on the dendritic shafts (Fig. 5.2). The afferent optic axons in the dorsal nucleus of the lateral geniculate body have growth cones and filopodia that are in "intimate association, possibly actual physical contact" with growth cones and filopodia of the dendrites of Golgi type II neurons (Morest, 1969*b*). The filopodia and growth cones diminish in number as the dendrites mature, but they can still be seen on many mature dendrites. This suggests that some growth adjustments are still occurring, even in mature dendrites, and this possibility has obvious implications for theories of neuronal plasticity and of learning. The dendrites of Golgi type II neurons of the medial geniculate body of the adult cat have growth cones (Morest, 1971). The evidence that Golgi type II neurons continue to grow in an adult mammal supports Ramón y Cajal's speculation that these cells play a role in the higher nervous activities of man (Ramón y Cajal, 1952). Morest cogently argues against the artifactual nature of dendritic growth cones and filopodia. One of the best arguments is that the Golgi technique demonstrates progressive changes in the dendrites with increasing age, which form a developmental sequence culminating in the fully differentiated neuron (Fig. 5.3).

Dendritic growth cones have also been recognized with the electron microscope (del Cerro and Snider, 1969; Kawana *et al.*, 1971; Hinds and Hinds, 1972; Skoff and Hamburger, 1974). They are enlargements of some, but not all, growing tips of the dendrites. They resemble axonal growth cones (see Section 4.4) except that dendritic growth cones lack the undulating membrane seen on some axonal growth cones. Instead, dendritic growth cones possess one to four filopodia. However, the ultrastructure of dendritic and axonal growth cones is similar. They contain a network of 50 Å microfilaments and a variable number of vesicles and cisternae of smooth endoplasmic reticulum. They contain few or no ribosomes, mitochondria, or microtubules. The main identifying features of den-

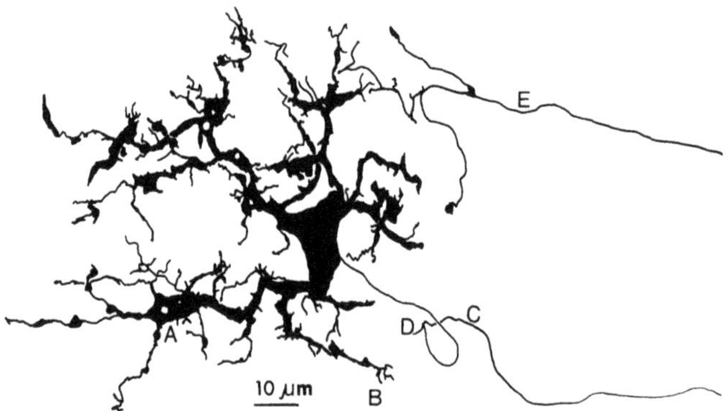

Figure 5.2. Immature stellate neuron from an intermediate layer of the developing cerebral cortex of an opossum fetus (33 mm crown to rump length). A, Dendritic growth cone with lacunae, short filopodia, and larger incipient branches; B, tip of partially differentiated dendritic branch; C, stellate cell axon extending as far as the deepest layer of the cortical plate; D, collateral of the stellate axon; E, afferent axon with growth cones, traced from the underlying presumptive white matter of the intermediate cortical zone. Rapid Golgi technique. A camera lucida drawing from D. K. Morest, The growth of dendrites in the mammalian brain, *Z. Anat. Entwicklungsgesch. 128:*290–317 (1969).

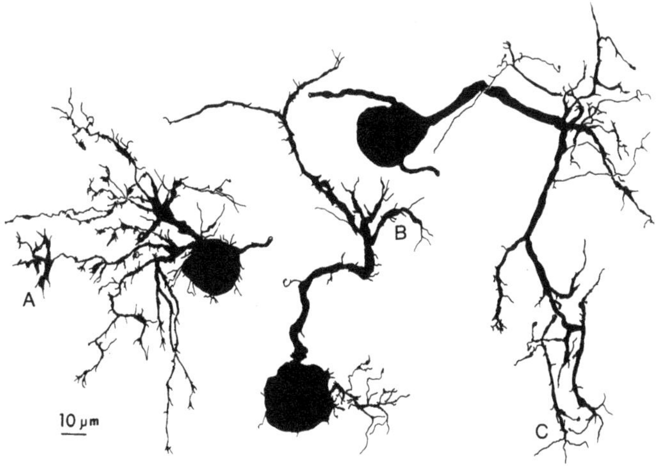

Figure 5.3. Dendritic development of the principal neurons in the medial trapezoid body of young opossums taken from the pouch at different ages. A, From an opposum 42 mm crown to rump; B, 57 mm crown to rump; C, 100 mm crown to rump. A shows growing dendrites with terminal growth cones (near A) and preterminal buds with sprouts. The dendrites and cell body are covered with filopodia. B shows a more mature neuron with a reduction of somatic and dendritic filopodia. The larger dendrite has apparently just begun to form a tuft of branches near B, and the smaller dendrite, with long radiating filopodia, has just begun to form. C shows a neuron with mature dendrites with spicules and spines and well-developed terminal plumes (for example, near C). Rapid Golgi technique. A camera lucida drawing from D. K. Morest, The differentiation of cerebral dendrites: A study of the postmigratory neuroblast in the medial nucleus of the trapezoid body, *Z. Anat. Entwicklungsgesch. 128:*271–289 (1969).

dritic growth cones are their continuity with a dendrite and the presence of microfilaments, one or more filopodia, and axodendritic synapses. It should be noted that all these features are apparently also seen in dendritic retraction bulbs. If, as much evidence shows, dendritic branches are retracted as well as extended, the problem arises of the fate of the synapses that are present on the dendritic growth cones. Skoff and Hamburger (1974), not taking dendritic retraction bulbs into account, made the suggestion that the synapses that are initially formed on the growth cone may later be incorporated into the dendritic shaft. It seems equally probable that during the period of "trial and error" some transient synapses are eventually eliminated. It is in the nature of such evanescent structures to be elusive, and at present there is no good evidence for such temporary connections.

Development of the dendrites occurs at the same time as the development of axodendritic and dendrodendritic synapses, and it will have become clear from the previous discussion that synaptogenesis and dendritic growth are interdependent processes. As a general rule, axodendritic synapses tend to start developing before axosomatic synapses on pyramidal cells of the cerebral neocortex and on cerebellar Purkinje cells, although in the latter case there are transient connections of climbing fibers on somatic spines before dendritic synapses develop (Pappas and Purpura, 1961; Voeller *et al.*, 1963; Purpura *et al.*, 1964; Marty and Scherrer, 1964; Meller *et al.*, 1968*a,b;* Molliver and Van der Loos, 1970). Moreover, axodendritic synapses are formed over an extended period during postnatal growth of dendrites. However, new axodendritic synapses continue to form in the mammalian cerebral cortex and cerebellar cortex. The growth of dendrites and the formation of axodendritic synapses in the cerebral cortex have been correlated with changes in the electroencephalogram and in evoked cortical electrical responses (Ellingson and Wilcott, 1960; Huttenlocher, 1966, 1967; Myslivecek, 1968; G. H. Rose and Lindsley, 1968; Molliver and Van der Loos, 1970). Little is known about the development of dendrodendritic synapses, which are numerous, especially in the mammalian brain, and which are thought to have important functions (Shepherd, 1972; Schmitt *et al.*, 1976). As the following section will show, knowledge of the mechanisms of formation of synaptic connections is at the crux of our understanding of the development of the nervous system as a functioning system. It is not too farfetched to regard the specialized structures and functions of each type of neuron as arrangements mainly designed to support the synapses in their proper spatial and functional relationships.

5.4. Development of Synapses

Development of synapses is indisputably one of the central problems in developmental neurobiology. It is also indisputable that very large gaps in our knowledge of the mechanisms of synaptogenesis remain to be filled in, and that these areas of ignorance impede progress toward understanding how neuronal circuits develop and how they are related to the development of neuronal functions and to the ontogeny of behavior of the organism as a whole.

The mechanisms that control the formation of synapses are largely unknown. Therefore, before discussing the present knowledge in detail, it may be advantageous to consider some general aspects of the development of synapses. Synaptogenesis may be controlled directly by the cell body as well as indirectly by the environment of the developing dendrites and axonal terminals. It is unlikely that the perikaryon exerts a direct control of all the synapses made by its axonal terminals, because many neurons have axonal branches that terminate in a variety of ways. For example, the auditory nerve fibers branch to form several different types of endings in different parts of the cochlear nucleus (Lorenté de Nó, 1933*a;* M. L. Feldman and Harrison, 1969). It seems unlikely that different instructions can be issued by the cell body to different branches of the same axon. The local conditions at the axonal terminals, and especially the nature of the postsynaptic neuron, must play an important part in controlling the formation and differentiation of the synapse.

The development of the synapse almost certainly involves an interaction between the presynaptic and postsynaptic elements. It would not be correct to attribute the primary or determinative role to either component. It is also unlikely that the specificity of synaptic connections depends only on a single factor such as the biochemical compatibility or affinity between presynaptic and postsynaptic elements, as Sperry (1963) has proposed. This is not to deny that specific affinities and disaffinities between presynaptic and postsynaptic elements are necessary for the formation of some or even all synaptic connections, but such affinities may not be sufficient. The two elements must first come into close proximity or even into contact, and the time at which the nexus is made may also have to be specific.

Functional activity may be necessary to ensure full maturation and permanent stability of the synapses. A number of factors, each of which is necessary but not sufficient, may have to act in combination to result in the functional development of the synapse. The preestablished harmony of normal development ensures that all the components are present in the right places at the right times. Thus it is best to observe the processes of synaptogenesis under normal conditions, using probes that perturb normal development as little as possible. However, the disadvantage of inferences made from observations of normal development is that they tend to be weak because they can show only whether events are correlated in time and space, and not whether they are causally related. On the other hand, experimental intervention may result in changes that are not part of normal development. Extreme caution should be exercised in trying to interpret such results in terms of normal developmental processes. Even "gentle" interference may alter normal development, while heroic manipulations of the developing nervous system, such as exposure to chemical toxins, irradiation, virus infection, or surgery, may inhibit normal developmental processes as well as create ones that do not exist under normal conditions.

In addition to physicochemical compatibility of the axonal terminals and the dendritic branches with which they connect, the correct timing of the nexus may be of great importance. If the axon and dendrite fail to make contact at the right time, their subsequent development may be abnormal. Moreover, termination of different types of axons on specific regions of the postsynaptic membrane may occur as a result of the restricted availability of synaptic sites during the time of arrival of axonal terminals at the postsynaptic membrane. As each fresh contingent of axons arrives at the postsynaptic membrane, it may be excluded from the synaptic sites that have been occupied, and may be constrained to occupy synaptic sites that remain vacant on the most recently developed dendritic branches. This is one of the ways in which a topographically organized projection may develop, for example, between the retina and midbrain tectum (M. Jacobson, 1977). This is discussed in Section 9.9.1.

Another example of spatial patterning of synaptogenesis which may be due to the time of arrival of different presynaptic endings is seen in the formation of axodendritic synapses on granule cells of the hippocampal dentate gyrus. D. I. Gottlieb and Cowan (1972) found that the ratio of crossed to uncrossed inputs to the hippocampal granule cells correlates with the time of origin of the granule cells: the earlier their origin, the greater the proportion of uncrossed inputs. Thus at the time the first-formed granule cells are ready to receive synapses on the proximal portions of their dendrites, the only afferents present are those from the same side of the hippocampus, with the fibers from the opposite side not approaching the dentate gyrus until some days later. From such evidence it has been inferred that recognition between the specific afferents and the dentate granule cells is unnecessary; all that seems to be required is that the axons arrive at a time when the granule cell dendrites are ready to receive them.

The obvious truth that both the pre- and postsynaptic components of any synapse must be present at the same time in the same place before they can form a synapse does not necessarily mean that the temporal coincidence is the cause of the formation of the synapse. The observations are equally consistent with a neuronal recognition mechanism, and for that mechanism to be effective it is also necessary for the components to come together and be ready to interact at the right time in development. I have labored this point only because the relationship between cause and effect is often hard to define clearly in the analysis of the development of the nervous system. I am taking the common-sense view that a cause should be a necessary and sufficient condition that invariably accompanies an event—in this case, the formation of a synapse. In most cases, nerve cells come together during development without forming synapses. That the proper components are present at a certain time and place is a necessary but not sufficient condition for the formation of a synapse. It seems as if there must be some degree of mutual affinity between the neurons, or **neuronal recognition,** before the "correct" synaptic associations can develop. Neuronal recognition, therefore, as a mechanism of achieving association between the "correct" neurons, requires that the neurons be prelabeled before they form any association. This introduces the problem of the origin of the labels and their spatial deployment in sets of neurons and their expression during neuronal recognition in the formation of synaptic connections. Neurons, usually at some considerable distance apart initially, grow toward each other to form a synaptic connection; this raises the problem of the mechanisms of targeting of pre- upon postsynaptic elements in the development of neuronal connections and the precision of such neuronal targeting. This theme is taken up more amply in Sections 9.1 and 9.6.

Precise coordination of the development of pre- and postsynaptic elements may be necessary in some cases, but microprecise timing is not required if the growth of dendrites occurs in response to the arrival of the appropriate axonal terminals. One may imagine a situation in which the ingrowing axons stimulate the growth of dendrites on which they are destined to terminate, or stimulate a mutual interaction between axons and dendrites. Situations in which one type of migrating neuron moves through the dendritic field of another type with which it is destined to synapse also invite speculations about possible interactions between the two neurons. For example, the cerebellar granule cells migrate through the dendritic field of the Purkinje cells with which the granule cell axons (the parallel fibers) are destined to synapse (Ramón y Cajal, 1909–1911).

Specificity of connections to a restricted part of the neuron is well established by anatomical and physiological methods. In the pyramidal cells of the cerebral cortex, the excitatory synapses are mainly restricted to specialized postsynaptic structures, the dendritic spines, whereas inhibitory synapses occur on dendritic shafts and on the cell body (Anderson *et al.,* 1963, 1966; Blackstad and Flood, 1963). In these pyramidal neurons the dendrites comprise 96 percent and the cell body only 4 percent of the surface area, whereas the dendritic spines alone account for up 43 percent of the total surface of the neuron (Mungai, 1967). In stellate neurons of the cerebral cortex, the dendrites, which have bulbous dilations but no spines, occupy up to 87 percent of the surface area (Mungai, 1967).

Topographical specificity of presynaptic terminals on the dendrites and cell body seems to be universal. For example, the central three-fifths of the apical shafts of pyramidal cells in the striate cortex receive geniculostriate afferents, and oblique branches of the apical dendrites and the basal dendrites receive intracortical afferents from Golgi type II neurons and axons that cross in the corpus callosum (A. Globus and Scheibel, 1966). Ultrastructural differences between presynaptic terminals on different parts of the neurons in the cat visual cortex have been demonstrated by Colonnier (1968). He found that the dendritic spines of the pyramidal cells in the visual cortex receive only presynaptic terminals containing spheroidal synaptic vesicles, which are presumed to contain excitatory synaptic transmitter (Uchizono, 1965, 1966). Presynaptic terminals containing flattened vesicles, presumed to contain inhibitory synaptic transmitter, are the only type seen on the cell body and are occasionally found on the dendritic shafts but not on the spines (Fig. 5.4). The first synapses to differentiate on motor neurons of monkey spinal cord are axodendritic synapses with spheroidal vesicles (Bodian, 1966*a*,*b*).

Probably the best-documented example of topographic specificity of synaptic connections is provided by the pyramidal cells of CA1 and CA2 of the mammalian hippocampus (Blackstad, 1956; Andersen *et al.*, 1966; D. I. Gottlieb and Cowan, 1973). The distribution of afferent connections is very strikingly segregated on different parts of the hippocampal pyramidal cells. Commissural and septal afferents synapse on the basal dendrites. Intrahippocampal inputs from the basket cells synapse on the cell bodies of the pyramidal cells. These two inputs are probably inhibitory, as indicated by the ellipsoidal or flattened synaptic vesicles. The inputs to the apical dendrites of the pyramidal cells are excitatory as evidenced by their spheroidal synaptic vesicles. On the pyramidal cell apical dendrites, the inputs are also segregated as follows: entorhinal afferents synapse on the tips of the dendrites, commissural and septal afferents are confined to the central parts of the dendrites, while the proximal part of the apical dendrites receive dentate afferents (Fig. 5.5).

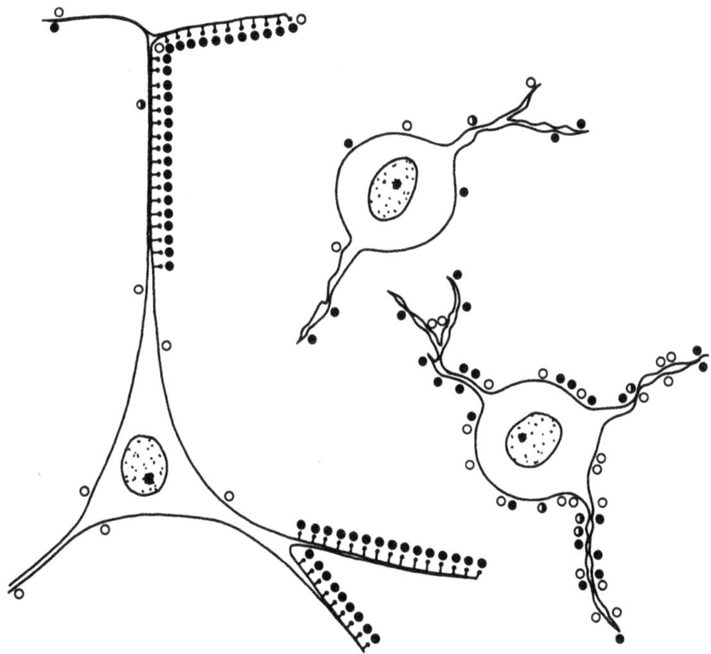

Figure 5.4. Distribution of synaptic types on pyramidal and stellate cell bodies, dendrites, and spines. Closed circles represent asymmetrical contacts with spheroidal vesicles. Open circles represent symmetrical contacts with flattened vesicles. Half-closed circles represent contacts difficult to classify. From M. Colonnier, *Brain Res.* *9:*268–287 (1968).

The onset of synaptogenesis occurs according to a remarkably invariant timetable. In each region of the mammalian nervous system there is usually a difference of less than 1 day between individuals in the appearance of the first synapses on any particular neuron. Synapses appear very suddenly and increase rapidly in numbers thereafter. The stupendous increase in connectivity, which mainly consists of axodendritic synapses, does not occur at random. All the evidence shows that it is highly selective. Most of the evidence indicates that neuronal connections are determined by genetic and developmental processes that operate without any control from the outside world. However, some synapses require functional validation for their normal maturation or even for their survival (see Chapter 9). The development of functional synapses in tissue culture indicates that some synapses can develop in the absence of the neuronal activities that accompany behavior and learning (Crain *et al.*, 1964*a,b;* Crain, 1966; Crain and Peterson, 1967; M. B. Bunge *et al.*, 1967; Model *et al.*, 1971). Tissue culture of neurons may eventually provide a means of discovering the nature of the physicochemical specificities on which the formation of synapses are believed to depend.

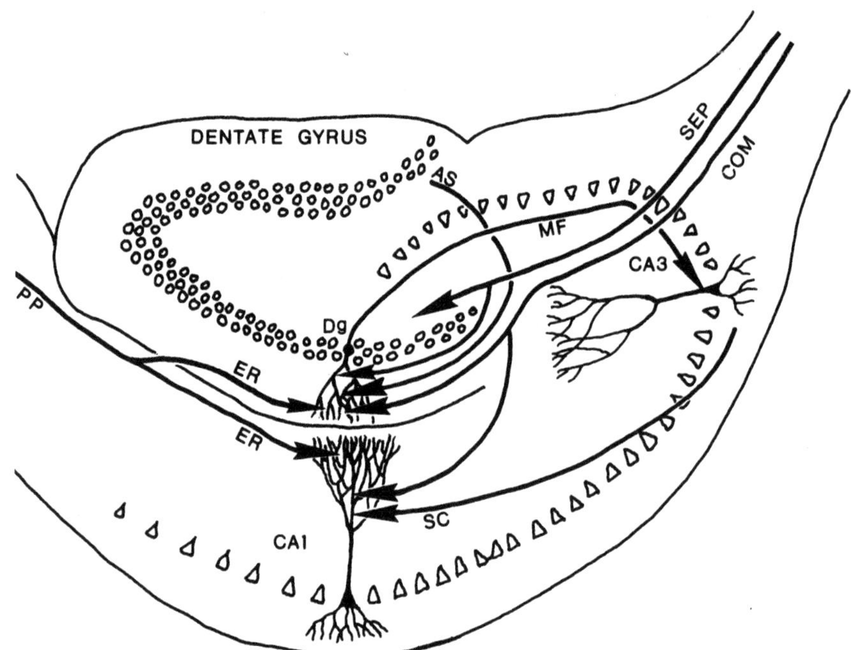

Figure 5.5. Specificity of connections in the hippocampal formation of the rat shown diagrammatically by the location of presynaptic endings (arrowheads) on dendrites at specific levels. The plane of the section is as shown in Fig. 3.8. AS, Association fibers arising from CA3 pyramidal cells, terminating in the midzone of the dentate granule cell dendritic field; COM, commissural fibers from contralateral CA3 pyramidal cells terminating on midzone of dendritic fields of dentate granule cells and CA1 pyramidal cells; Dg, granule cells of dentate gyrus; MF, mossy fibers of granule cells terminating in the inner zone of the dendritic fields of CA3 pyramidal cells; PP, perforant path containing fibers (ER) originating in the entorhinal cortex and terminating in the outer zone of the dendritic field of CA1 pyramidal cells; SC, Schaeffer axon collaterals of CA3 pyramidal cells terminating in the midzone of dendritic field of CA1 pyramidal cells; SEP, septal fibers terminating in the inner zone of the dendritic field of dentate granule cells.

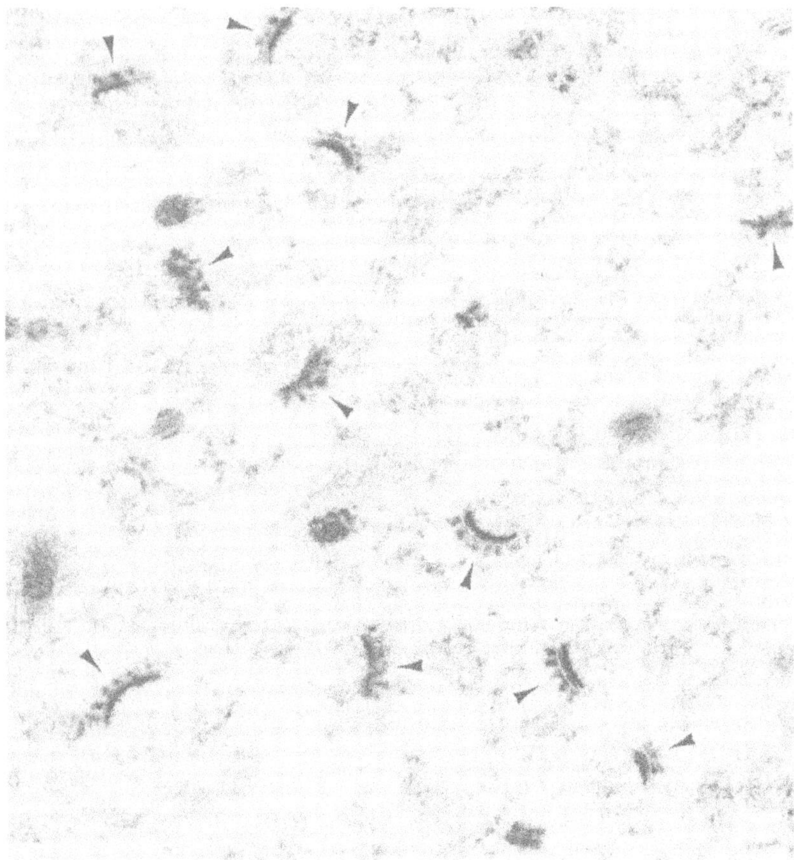

Figure 5.6. Molecular layer of the parietal cerebral cortex of the rat 26 days after birth. Ethanolic phosphotungstic acid stain. Arrows point to synaptic junctions that are much more deeply stained than the background. 24,000×. By courtesy of Dr. F. E. Bloom.

Estimates of the increase in connectivity in the developing cerebral cortex have been obtained from the cell-to-gray coefficient (von Economo, 1926; V. B. Peters and Flexner, 1950; Shariff, 1953; Sholl, 1953). The cell-to-gray coefficient was introduced by von Economo (1926) as an index of connectivity or functional capacity of the cerebral cortex, the rationale being that more neuronal interconnections might be present when the cell bodies are widely spaced. The value of the cell-to-gray coefficient for comparative studies is limited by its variability, owing to slight technical differences in the hands of different investigators (Haug, 1956; Eayrs and Goodhead, 1959). A rough estimate of neuronal connectivity may also be obtained from qualitative estimates of the frequency of synaptic profiles seen with the electron microscope. More accurate counts have been obtained in electron microscopic sections stained with ethanolic phosphotungstic acid, which selectively stains synaptic junctions, as Fig. 5.6 shows (Bloom, 1972; D. G. Jones, 1973, D. G. Jones *et al.*, 1974).

All estimates have shown a very dramatic increase in the connectivity of the mammalian cerebral cortex during the early postnatal period of development.

Eayrs and Goodhead (1959) estimated that a tenfold increase in connectivity occurs between days 12 and 30 after birth in the cerebral cortex of the rat. Aghajanian and Bloom (1967) calculated a sevenfold increase, amounting to 12×10^8 synapses per cubic millimeter, in the molecular layer of rat parietal cortex from the 12th to the 26th day after birth (Fig. 5.7). In the molecular layer of the hippocampal dentate gyrus of the rat, less than 1 percent of the adult number of synapses are present at 4 days after birth, but the number doubles every day until it attains more than 90 percent of the adult value at 30 days after birth (B. Crain *et al.,* 1973). In the olfactory bulb of the mouse, the total number of synapses increases more than 1000 times during the 16-day period from E14, when the first synapses appear, to P10 (Hinds and Hinds, 1976*a*). Even more rapid postnatal increases of the number of synapses have been reported in the cat visual cortex (Cragg, 1972*b*) and the rat cerebellar cortex (Woodward *et al.,* 1971; Cragg, 1972*a*). These observations suggest that synapses must form rapidly, but they do not allow any estimate to be made of the time of formation of a single synapse. They show that there is a net increase of synapses but do not show whether individual synapses persist or are lost.

The problem of turnover of synapses has received very little attention. However, there are several examples of transient synapses in the mammalian central nervous system and they should alert one to the possibility that other types of synapses, which are generally considered permanent, are continually degraded and replaced *in toto.* The transient synapses on the somatic spines of cerebellar Purkinje cells are described in Section 3.4.2. The spinal motoneurons of the newborn kitten have synapses on the initial segment of the axon, but no synapses are found on this region in the adult cat. These synapses are removed and phagocytosed by glial cells during the second week after birth (Ronnevi and Conradi, 1974). Removal of other synapses on the cell body and dendrites of

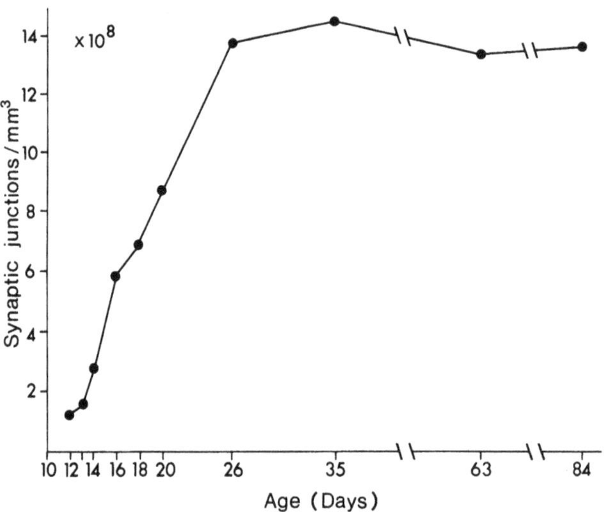

Figure 5.7. Number of synapses per cubic millimeter in the molecular layer of rat parietal cerebral cortex at various ages after birth. Synapses were counted with the electron microscope in thin sections stained with ethanolic phosphotungstic acid. From G. K. Aghajanian and F. E. Bloom, *Brain Res.* *6:*716–727 (1967).

spinal motoneurons also occurs in the kitten during the second postnatal week (Conradi and Ronnevi, 1975). There is also evidence that, after axotomy and anterograde axonal degeneration, the degenerating presynaptic boutons are pinocytosed by the dendrites (Walberg, 1963).

A phenomenon that is hard to understand is the stripping of boutons from the dendrites and cell body of axotomized motoneurons (Blinzinger and Kreutzberg, 1968; Hamberger *et al.*, 1970*b*) and autonomic postganglionic neurons (M. R. Matthews and Nelson, 1975) undergoing chromatolysis (see Section 7.4). This disconnection of boutons occurs as the dendrites of the injured neuron retract (Grant, 1965; Grant and Westman, 1968) so that the density of boutons is only slightly reduced, although their total numbers are reduced to about 50 percent in adult rat hypoglossal neurons (Cull, 1974), or to almost nil in facial neurons of newborn rabbits (Torvik and Söreide, 1972). In the neurons undergoing chromatolysis in the hypoglossal nucleus of the adult rat, the boutons containing spherical vesicles (therefore probably excitatory) are disconnected, whereas boutons containing flattened vesicles (probably inhibitory) are not disconnected (Sumner, 1975). In the adult rat these changes occur during the second to the fifth week after cutting the hypoglossal nerve. They occur more rapidly in the adult rabbit hypoglossal neurons, beginning within 4 days and increasing to a maximum in the second week (Hamberger *et al.*, 1970*b*). The boutons do not retract far, but they are separated from their postsynaptic sites by glial cell processes that grow into the widened synaptic clefts. The boutons reconnect with the postsynaptic membrane after regneration of the injured axon has restored contact with its target cells (Sumner and Watson, 1971). The disconnection and reconnection of boutons as part of the response to axotomy of the postsynaptic neuron are correlated with a block in synaptic transmission to the injured neuron. This has been observed in the ciliary ganglion after section of the ciliary nerves (Pilar and Landmesser, 1972). Depression of synaptic transmission through other sympathetic ganglia after section of the postganglionic nerve (G. L. Brown and Pascoe, 1954; Acheson and Remolina, 1955; C. C. Hunt and Riker, 1966; Pilar and Landmesser, 1972) indicates that disconnection of some presynaptic terminals occurs after section of the postsynaptic nerve. A similar interpretation can be made of the altered presynaptic input to spinal motoneurons undergoing chromatolysis (Eccles *et al.*, 1958*b;* Kuno and Llinás, 1970; Kuno *et al.*, 1974*a,b;* Mendel *et al.*, 1974). Electron microscopic observations of disconnection of boutons from spinal motoneurons after cutting the sciatic nerve in the rat has been made by Kerns and Hinsman (1973*b*). The disconnection and reconnection of boutons occurring during chromatolysis are always accompanied by marked glial cell proliferation in the vicinity of the chromatolytic nerve cell. Because neuroglial proliferation is not seen around normal neurons, it is unlikely that normal synapses undergo periodic disconnection and reconnection as Sotelo and Palay (1971) have suggested. The turnover, if it occurs, must be very slow or it must not provoke a glial cell response. There is, at present, no evidence of loss of synapses in the healthy adult brain.

If there are rules that apply to synaptogenesis, they remain elusive, and it is likely that they will not be revealed by studying synaptogenesis with the electron microscope alone. Biochemical, histochemical, and immunochemical studies of synaptogenesis are required before further progress can be made in identifying the components of developing synapses. Electrophysiological recording from identified synapses during their development is required in order to determine their functional development and to correlate their function with structure as revealed with the electron microscope. All such studies have been severely limited by sampling problems: the heterogeneity of the cell population and the asynchrony of development of cells in the same population. The changes in a single synapse may be very rapid, occurring in hours, while the sequence of events is, at best, inferred from observations made at intervals of days.

The evidence that is at present available deals statistically with large numbers of synapses. It does not give more than a rough approximation to the time taken for development of a single functional synaptic connection, and there are even fewer data which give an indication of the time taken for elimination of a single synapse. This information might be obtained from continuous recording from identified pre- and postsynaptic neurons in low-density tissue culture. Continuous recording during the development of synapses is also possible in amphibian embryos. Blackshaw and Warner (1976*b*) have followed the initial appearance of sensitivity to applied ACh and the onset of functional innervation of muscles in the myotomes of *Xenopus* embryos. Functional ACh receptors develop on the muscle about 0.5–2 hours before flexion movements of the embryo begin. However, miniature endplate potentials, indicating that a functional neuromuscular junction has developed, can be recorded 0.5–2 hours after the appearance of functional ACh receptors in the muscle. This preparation should permit a very precise correlation to be made between development of structure and development of function in the neuromuscular synapse.

Synaptogenesis starts before neurogenesis is completed, and thus newborn neurons migrate to their definitive levels in the cortex, bypassing cortical neurons upon which synapses have already formed or are in the process of formation. However, synaptogenesis may, in some cases, be delayed. The presynaptic endings and the cells on which they will synapse may be juxtaposed for days before they form synaptic connections. For example, in the cerebellum of the mouse, the stellate cells lie closely surrounded by parallel fibers before the latter connect with the stellate cells. This is not due to some inability of the parallel fibers, because they connect with Purkinje cell dendrites while delaying the formation of synapses with stellate cells (Larramendi, 1969). In the olfactory bulb of the mouse there is a delay during which both the presynaptic and postsynaptic elements are close together before the olfactory axons synapse on the mitral cells (Hinds and Hinds, 1976*a*). A similar delay in formation of synapses between optic axons and neurons in the tectum of the chick embryo has been reported (Crossland *et al.*, 1974*a*).

All types of synapses are already present in the mouse olfactory bulb at birth, which is a sign of the precocity of the olfactory system. This should be compared with the delayed, postnatal synaptogenesis in the neocortex (Molliver and Van der Loos, 1970; Cragg, 1975*a,c*). The majority of the synapses in the mouse olfactory bulb are axodendritic, but dendrodendritic synapses are also present at birth (Hinds and Hinds, 1976*a,b*).

The fact that synapses are commonly seen on dendritic as well as on axonal growth cones shows that neither need be completely mature to enable synaptogenesis to commence. There may be cases, however, in which the onset of synaptogenesis is delayed until some essential components of the pre- or postsynaptic membranes are synthesized or take up their positions in the synaptic membranes. It has been suggested that development of the dendrites of some neurons is delayed until the axon has reached its target (Barron, 1943), and that a signal, transmitted from the axon terminals to the cell body, is required for the initiation of dendritic growth. In the sympathetic preganglionic neurons and the spinal ganglion cells, this signal may be nerve growth factor, which is transported to the cell body from the axonal terminals (see Section 6.7.5). There are several other cases in which the axons form synaptic connections before or at the same time as the dendrites make connections. The mitral cells of the mouse olfactory bulb make axonal connections on the same day, E15, as synapses form on its dendrites (Hinds and Hinds, 1976*a*). The axons of association neurons of the rat spinal cord make connections 1 day earlier than synapses form on their dendrites (Vaughn *et al.*, 1974). The fact that dendrites of spinal motor neurons sprout only after the motor axon has grown into the muscles has led to the general acceptance of the notion that dendritic growth is dependent on axonal connections (Ramón y Cajal, 1909–1911, p. 611; Barron, 1943, 1946; Hamburger and Keefe, 1944). This is in accord with the "modulation theory" of Paul Weiss (1936, 1947, 1952), according to which the motoneuron modulates its dendritic connections to match the muscle with which its axon connects. This theory is discussed in Section 9.4, but here it can be noted that the evidence for such central modulation is weak and that, in general, there is growing evidence that the motor axon may associate selectively with an appropriate muscle.

Correlation between structure and function of developing synapses has been made in the chick ciliary ganglion by Landmesser and Pilar (1972). Synaptic transmission begins at embryonic Stage 26½ but few synapses can be seen with the electron microscope at State 33½ when all ganglion cells show synaptic potentials. In the ciliary ganglion there are two classes of cells, choroid and ciliary, with different preganglionic inputs, which can be distinguished functionally and morphologically. Their functional specificity is evinced from the start of synaptogenesis, indicating that the preganglionic axons selectively connect with the proper postganglionic cells. The morphology of the synapses in the ciliary ganglion undergoes marked changes during development. Synaptic connections are initially made by fine terminal branches of presynaptic axons and at those stages (26½–33), synaptic transmission is chemical. These processes appear to retract, and from Stage 36½ are displaced by calyces, so that by Stage 40 all ciliary cells have calyces. At the same time there is an increase in electrical transmission until, at 2 days after hatching, 80 percent of synapses are electrically transmitting. The calyces are temporary structures which disappear by 2 weeks after hatching and break up into a cluster of boutons. This morphological transformation does not impair electrical transmission.

There is no general rule about the order of development of the presynaptic and postsynaptic structures, but in each case the order is apparently invariant. Thus, in the spinal cord of the amphibian embryo, increased density of the presynaptic membrane is seen before the postsynaptic specializations are visible (Hayes and Roberts, 1973, 1974). Synthesis of transmitter in the presynaptic neuron and, presumably, its release at the presynaptic terminals occur independently of development of the postsynaptic specialization during normal development of the chick spinal cord (Zukin *et al.*, 1975) and mouse cerebellum (McLaughlin *et al.*, 1975).

On the other hand, development of the postsynaptic structures is sometimes seen before the arrival of the presynaptic terminals, and development of the postsynaptic membrane specialization is often seen before presynaptic specialization can be seen with the electron microscope. For example, in the olfactory bulb of the mouse, Hinds and Hinds (1976*a,b*) verified in serial sections that postsynaptic specializations develop before presynaptic membrane thickenings are apparent, but the presynaptic endings are, nevertheless, close to the developing postsynaptic structures. The best evidence that postsynaptic structures can develop before presynaptic membrane thickening occurs has been obtained by Rees *et al.* (1976) in the isolated superior cervical ganglion and spinal cord of the rat fetus (Fig. 5.8).

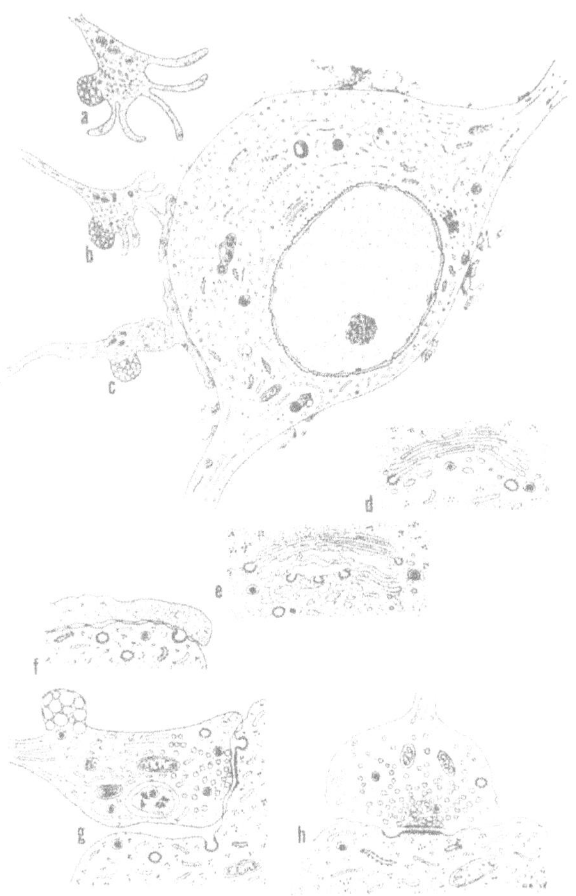

Figure 5.8. An isolated neuronal soma from the superior cervical ganglion as it appears after 2–3 days in culture. Some cellular debris resulting from the mechanical dissociation process clings to the plasmalemma. The nucleus is eccentric, and the cytoplasm is characterized mainly by polysomes, smooth and rough endoplasmic reticulum, Golgi apparatus, mitochondria, multivesicular bodies, and other lysosomal structures. At (a), the soma is approached by a growth cone of a neurite growing out of the spinal cord exhibiting filopodia, a mound area, branched membranous reticulum, and several large lysosomes. At (b), a single filopodium of this growth cone is shown contacting the neuronal surface. Other filopodia are withdrawing. At (c), only the highly flattened, contacting process remains, and its surface membrane has developed many close contacts with the somal plasmalemma. Inset (d) shows the typical Golgi apparatus of a cultured superior cervical ganglion neuron before contact. A few coated vesicles are in continuity with cisternae or present in the adjacent cytoplasm together with an occasional large dense-cored vesicle. Changes occurring in the Golgi complex of a contacted neuron are shown in (e). A greater number of coated vesicles are present, some being continuous with the region of the maturing face of the Golgi complex. These coated vesicles migrate to the neuronal surface in the area of filopodial contact and there fuse with the plasmalemma (as at f), thereby contributing membrane with undercoating (postsynaptic density). This is considered to be the first definitive sign of synaptic specialization. A more advanced stage of synaptogenesis is diagrammed in (g). On the presynaptic side, synaptic vesicles and large dense-cored vesicles appear among the growth cone organelles and cluster at that part of the membrane apposed to the postsynaptic density. In (h), the large amount of membranous reticulum, lysosomes, and mound area typical of the grwoth cone is no longer present. A few mitochondira, some reticulum, occasional large dense-cored vesicles, and numerous synaptic vesicles now characterize the ending. Presynaptic dense material gradually appears, some cleft material is seen, and the cleft widens. Postsynaptic membrane density increases in length as the addition of large coated vesicles continues. From R. P. Rees, M. B. Bunge, and R. P. Bunge, *J. Cell Biol. 68:*240–263 (1976).

They found a series of stages in the formation of synapses after the spinal cord axons arrive in the ganglion. Soon after the initial contact between axonal growth cones and the ganglion cells, the latter show an increase in the size of the Golgi complex and an increase in the number of coated vesicles adjoining the postsynaptic membrane. This is followed by thickening of the postsynaptic membrane, and only later is the specialization of the presynaptic membrane shown by the appearance of presynaptic dense projections and synaptic vesicles. Another indication of the precocity of the postsynaptic membrane is that immature cerebellar Purkinje cells of the rat respond to several putative synaptic transmitters on the first and second days after birth, whereas synapses can first be seen on the third day postnatally (Woodward *et al.,* 1971). That presynaptic stimulation is not required for development of synapses is shown by the fact that synapses develop normal morphology in the cerebellum of the 17-day mouse fetus continuously exposed to xylocaine in culture (Model *et al.,* 1971).

Development of asymmetrical axodendritic synapses seems to go through an intermediate stage in which the pre- and postsynaptic membrane thickenings are equally dense. Hinds and Hinds (1976*b*) found that, early in development of the mouse olfactory bulb, there are more symmetrical axodendritic synapses on growth cones, and later in development the number of asymmetrical synapses increases. This sequence has also been found in the mammalian cerebral neocortex (R. Johnson and Armstrong-James, 1970; Adinolfi, 1972*a,b;* Cragg, 1972*b,c*), in the cerebellar cortex of the chick (Foelix and Oppenheim, 1974), and in the spinal cord of the rat fetus (M. K. May and Biscoe, 1973).

Development of dendritic spines usually occurs after the formation of axodendritic synapses, but the spines can develop and persist in the absence of synapses on them. For example, synapses form first and the spines develop later in the dentate gyrus of the rat (Cotman *et al.,* 1973*a*). The same sequence is seen on the gemmules (which resemble spines) of granule cells in the olfactory bulb of the mouse embryo, but a gemmule without synapses has been seen (Hinds and Hinds, 1976*b*). Conversely, there are other cases where spines are found in the absence of synapses on dendrites of cerebellar Purkinje cells in culture (Seil and Herndon, 1970; Kim, 1975) or after granule cells have been killed, either by a virus infection (Herndon *et al.,* 1971*a,b;* Llinás *et al.,* 1973) or in mutant mice (Rakic and Sidman, 1973*b;* A. Hirano and Dembitzer, 1973).

5.5. Plasticity in the Development of Axons, Dendrites, and Synapses

The term "plasticity" is used to refer to certain types of adjustments of the developing nervous system to changes in the internal or external milieu. For the present purposes, the term is limited mainly to the adjustments that are adaptive, that is, that tend to return the system to its former state or enable the system to function and the organism to survive under the changed conditions. Some derangements of the normal organization, produced by injury, are considered because they may reveal developmental processes that are more difficult to investigate during normal development. This discussion is mainly concerned with structural changes such as the growth of new axonal and dendritic branches and the formation of new synaptic connections. Functional plasticity, such as changes in function of preexisting synapses or changes in behavior without recognizable neuronal changes, are not included here but are referred to briefly in Sections 8.2 and 9.12 and page 214.

The diverse phenomena that go by the name of plasticity are unlikely to be the result of one mechanism, and there are particular cases of anomalous growth resulting in dysfunction when the use of the term is exasperatingly inappropriate. Changes in response to injury that are nonfunctional or malfunctional may have the same relationship to adaptive or constructive plasticity as pathological processes in general have to physiological functions. History shows that in the many cases when the study of deranged function has advanced the knowledge of physiological processes there has been no doubt about which processes were deranged and which were normal. This distinction, which needs to be sharply defined, is frequently blurred in the literature on plasticity in the developing nervous system. The result is that the term is often applied equally to the destructive and maladaptive as well as to constructive and adaptive changes in the nervous system. In such cases, unless the term is used with proper qualifications, it loses much of its heuristic value. **Whenever the term *plasticity* appears in the literature, the reader is called upon to exercise his discernment to the maximum to give a meaning to the term that is appropriate to the context in which it appears.**

5.6. Plasticity and Rigidity of Developing Dendrites

One of the main problems of development of dendrites is to understand the processes that give the dendritic tree its characteristic shape in each type of neuron. Since each cell has the same genotype, how does this become expressed as a variety of phenotypes? How important are factors that are intrinsic to the neuron, including its genetic endowment, and how important are factors that arise progressively during development of the dendrites through interaction between the neuron and its environment? To what extent is the pattern of branching and the distribution of synapses on the dendritic tree a matter of chance and to what extent is it determined by the genome? During normal development we may regard the invariant features of the dendrites of any given type of neuron as indications of the rigid components of development, and the variable features may be regarded as indications of the plastic elements. The role of chance, which may be the basis of such plasticity, is quite limited during normal development. The conditions within the developing organism, which are known to influence the development of the nervous system, are not normally a matter of chance, although they may become contingent on the whim of the experimenter. Similarly, the conditions in the environment that normally affect development of the nervous system are not subject to large random variations but are conditions to which animals are invariably exposed in their natural habitat. By experimentally increasing the range of the conditions it is hoped to reveal the full range of the resulting responses in the developing nervous system. Responses that are qualitatively similar to, although quantitatively greater than, the normal responses of the nervous system to physiological challenges are properly termed plastic changes to distinguish them from pathological changes that obviously result in malfunctions. This is emphasized here because in many experiments the conditions which are imposed on the organism often exceed the range of conditions to which the developing nervous system can respond adaptively, and the plastic responses to such extreme conditions not only are magnified quantitatively but also may be qualitatively different from normal plasticity. For this reason, the experiments in which plasticity is studied in response to changes in sensory stimulation are preferable to those in which the plasticity occurs in response to surgery. The latter sort of experiment can be designed to show which functions and structures are rigid under defined experimental conditions and can show the full range of compensatory and adaptive changes that can be achieved before maladaptive changes occur.

That dendritic growth has a large measure of rigidity or autonomy is shown by the conservation of many features of normal dendritic morphology in neurons that are deprived of their normal axonal inputs and in neurons that are improperly aligned or are malpositioned. In the mammalian cerebral cortex, 15–20 percent of the pyramidal cells in the rabbit, cat, and macaque monkey are improperly oriented, and in some cases are totally inverted. In these neurons the pattern of dendritic arbors conforms with the axis of the cell body and not with the axis radial to the cortical surface, whereas the axon often arises from an unusual position on the cell body or from a dendrite and arches back to run in the usual direction, as is shown in Fig. 4.9 (Van der Loos, 1965; A. Globus and Scheibel, 1967*c*). This indicates that the orientation of the dendrites is intrinsically determined for each class of neurons, but the direction of axonal growth is more under the control of external factors. Such inverted pyramidal cells in the visual cortex of the mouse have a normal distribution of spines on their apical dendritic shafts, but the absolute number of spines is diminished (Valverde and Ruiz-Marcos, 1969). This shows that the distribution of dendritic spines on pyramidal cells may depend on factors that are intrinsic to the neuron and may be relatively independent of external factors such as axonal contacts, or that the appropriate axonal connections with the spines are made regardless of their orientation. The latter alternative is more likely in light of the evidence that normal synaptic connections form on disoriented and misplaced cells in the cerebral cortex of the reeler mutant mouse (see Sections 3.4.5 and 7.11).

Failure of neurons to develop fully in the absence of axons that normally terminate on them is discussed at length in Section 7.2. A few examples taken from several species and different types of neurons should suffice to show the dependence of developing dendrites on transsynaptic stimulation. For example, dendrites of neurons in the acousticovestibular centers of the chick embryo fail to develop fully in the absence of the afferent acoustic nerve fibers (Levi-Montalcini, 1949). Failure of development of dendrites in the optic tectum as the result of removal of an eye during embryonic development has been reported in the frog (Larsell, 1931) and the chick (Filogamo, 1950). The regressive changes that occur in dendrites deprived of afferent connections during development may be illustrated by the effects of destruction of the cerebellar granule cells whose axons (the parallel fibers) normally synapse on the dendritic spines of the Purkinje cells. If the cerebellar granule cells fail to develop because of a genetic abnormality (see Section 3.4.5), or are destroyed by a virus infection, irradiation by X-rays, or cytotoxins (see Section 3.4.4), the Purkinje cell dendrites fail to develop normally. After removal of the granule cells in neonatal mammals, the immature pattern of Purkinje cell dendritic branching persists in the adult, the dendritic spines survive but are reduced in size, and the Purkinje cell dendrites are not oriented toward the outer surface of the cerebellum but are deflected laterally and downward as if an attempt to contact fibers in the deeper layers of the cerebellum (Fig. 5.9). It seems as if the synaptic sites on the Purkinje cell dendrites left vacant by the horizontal fibers may be occupied by synapses from mossy fibers. Such heterologous synapses have been seen with the electron microscope (Altman and Anderson, 1972; Sotelo, 1975). This is supported by the electrophysiological evidence that after virus destruction of granule cells there is abnormal direct excitation of Purkinje cells by mossy fibers (Lliná *et al.,* 1973). In spite of the failure of the Purkinje cell dendrites to develop fully, they remain surprisingly typical and are unmistakable even when they are incorrectly positioned and disoriented in the weaver mouse, as discussed in Section 3.4.5. The effects of such insults to the Purkinje cell provide a measure of its plasticity in the sense of its dependence on the external environment and especially its dependence on normal synaptic inputs, while the residual structural and functional integrity of the Purkinje cells gives a measure of its rigidity or autonomy.

Studies of the effects of sensory stimulation and deprivation on development of dendrites and synapses leave no doubt that long-lasting changes occur as a result of experience. However, the experiments are often poorly controlled so that it is impossible to attribute the changes to any single factor with any certainty.

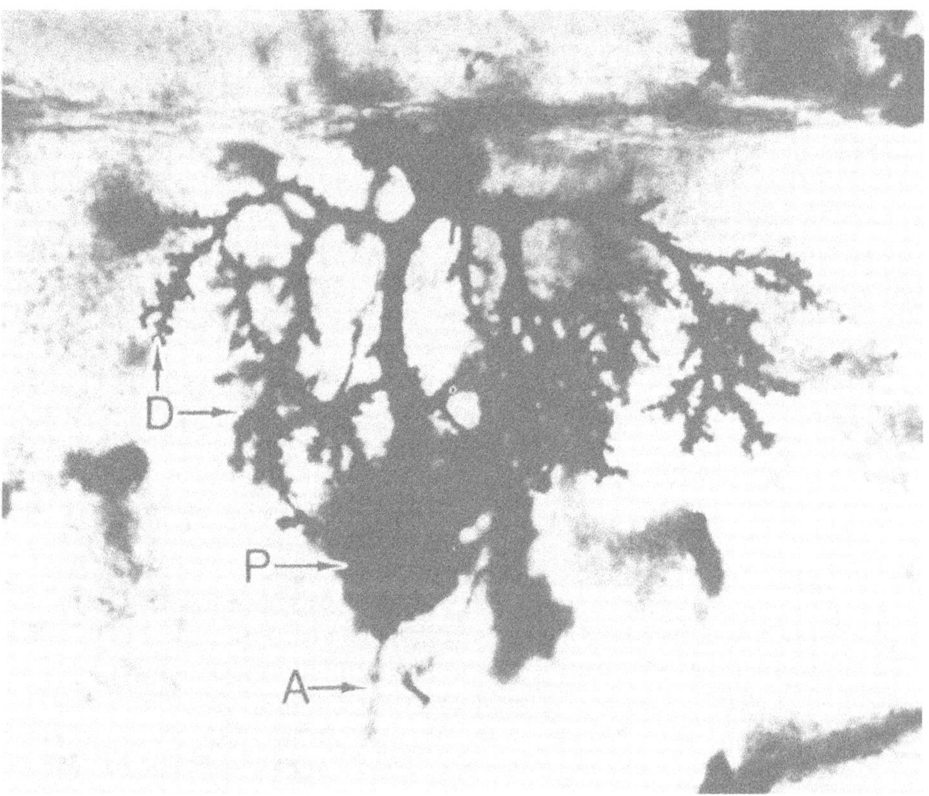

Figure 5.9. Purkinje cell in cat cerebellum at 12 days after birth, after X-irradiation at 1 day of age. Large dendrites are deflected laterally and away from the surface. This abnormal growth is probably related to loss of the external granular layer. A, Axon; D, dendrites; P, Purkinje cell. From R. J. Shofer, G. D. Pappas, and D. P. Purpura, in *Response of the Nervous System to Ionizing Radiation,* T. J. Haley and R. S. Snider (eds.), Little, Brown, Boston, 1964.

Moreover, the results are often given in terms of changes in cell density or cell size without further qualification of the type of cells or their precise location, for example, in the cerebral cortex. Furthermore, in many cases the observations of morphological changes cannot be given a definite functional interpretation because the structures that have altered as a result of sensory deprivation or enrichment have no clearly defined functions. For example, rearing rats in a complex environment that increases their sensory input and motor activity is reported to result in increased complexity of branching of third- and fourth-order bifurcations of the basal dendrites of pyramidal cells, mainly in the occipital cortex, and to a lesser degree in the temporal cortex, but not in the frontal cortex (Volkmar and Greenough, 1972; Greenough and Volkmar, 1973; Greenough *et al.,* 1973). While the functional significance of such changes may eventually be understood, they stand as mere epiphenomena at present. Even further from an explanation in terms of mechanisms are other reports of the effects of enriched experience on the increased weight and thickness of the cerebral cortex and number of cortical glial cells (E. L. Bennett *et al.,* 1964; M. C. Diamond *et al.,* 1964, 1966).

As Darwin (1868) was the first to point out, the size of the brain tends to be considerably reduced in animals as a result of domestication. The effects of an "enriched" environment on brain weight appear to have relevance to the well-known observation that domesticated animals have smaller brains than the same species in the wild. This has been shown by comparing captive and wild birds (Senglaub, 1959), rabbits (Choinowski, 1958), European polecats and ferrets (Schumacher, 1963), cats (Röhrs, 1955), alpacas and llamas (Herre, 1958, 1966; Herre and Thiede, 1965), sheep (Ebinger, 1974), pigs (Herre, 1936; Stephan, 1951; Lunau, 1956; Kruska, 1970*a,b,* 1972; Kruska and Röhrs, 1974), and donkeys (Herre, 1958, 1966). In all these species the brain weight of the domesticated animals is 15–30 percent less than the brain weight of those in the wild. The maximum effect is on the cerebral isocortex, while the allocortex is less severely affected. The most marked effect is on the visual cortex, which may be reduced by 35 percent in domesticated animals compared with those in the wild. This may be related to the smaller size of the eye and retina in domesticated animals (Wigger, 1939). The cerebellum is reduced by about 15 percent and the medulla by about 10 percent in animals in captivity compared with those in the wild. These differences are much greater than those reported between animals exposed to "enriched" and "impoverished" environments in the laboratory. The difference between brain size in domesticated and wild animals is probably a combination of inherited and environmental effects. An environmental effect is indicated by the fact that the brain weight of the first generation of animals born in captivity is 10–20 percent less than the brain weight of the parents raised in the wild (Herre, 1966, review). The effect seems to be produced by factors acting early in life, since animals born in the wild and domesticated later have the same brain size as animals raised in the wild. However, the conditions required to stimulate brain growth in the wild and the critical period during which the environment might stimulate growth of the brain have not been investigated. An inherited effect is shown by the fact that the return of domestic pigs to life in the wild several generations ago has produced no increase in brain size (Kruska and Röhrs, 1974).

The most revealing studies on the effects of sensory input have been on development of the visual system, because the quantity and quality of the visual stimulus can be precisely controlled, because the anatomy of the system is known in sufficient detail to permit accurate localization of any effects, and, above all, because the relationship between structure and function is securely established for many types of identified neurons and synapses in the visual system. The pertinent information about the various types of neurons in the visual pathways of mammals is given in Section 9.12.

Synaptogenesis occurs in the retina of the cat and the rat before birth, although the receptor outer segments become evident only on the fifth day after birth (Cragg, 1975*a*). This shows that synaptogenesis can occur without visual experience. Other studies have shown that all types of retinal cells and synapses develop in rats reared in total darkness for up to 3 years (Burke and Hayhow, 1968). Rats raised with the eyelids sutured closed for 12–18 months develop normal retinal ganglion cell activity (Sherman and Stone, 1973). The only changes that have been found consistently in rats raised from birth in darkness or with the eyes occluded is an *increase* in the number of amacrine cell to bipolar cell synapses in the inner plexiform layer of the retina (Fifková, 1972, 1973; Sosula and Glow, 1970) and an increase in the number of amacrine to ganglion cell synapses in the inner plexiform layer (Sosula and Glow, 1970; Chernenko and West, 1976).

In Section 9.12 further information is provided to show that the effects on the developing visual system are mainly confined to the Y cells and their projections. The Y cells are binocularly activated and respond best to rapidly moving stimuli, and their target cells in the visual cortex show orientation selectivity. Thus binocularity and orientation selectivity are vulnerable to visual deprivation in the neonatal period. The early studies of the effects of visual deprivation did not make the distinction between the plastic and the rigid components (Y cells are plastic while X and W cells are rigid), that is, between those components whose development is sensitive and those that are insensitive to visual stimulation and deprivation. This is well illustrated by the effects of visual experience on the visual cortex. Thus the reports that visual deprivation produces a reduction in the thickness of layers II and IV of the visual cortex (Gyllensten, 1959; Gyllensten *et al.*, 1965), a reduction in the number of synapses in the visual cortex (Cragg, 1967, 1969, 1972*c*, 1975*a,b*), or a reduction in the dendritic spines of pyramidal neurons in layer IV of the striate cortex (Valverde, 1967; A. Globus and Scheibel, 1967*b*; Ruiz-Marcos and Valverde, 1969; Parnavelas *et al.*, 1973) do not provide any clues as to the functional operations performed by the affected neurons. Other reports of changes in the dendrites or axons have the same limitation. For example, Coleman and Riesen (1968) reported that stellate cells in layer IV of the visual cortex of cats reared in darkness have fewer and shorter dendrites than the same cells in normal cats. Valverde (1976) found shorter axons of local circuit neurons in the visual cortex of mice reared in darkness for 19 days.

In the cat's visual system, the majority of synapses develop in the absence of stimulation. Cragg (1975*b*) reported that binocular lid suture in cats from the time of opening the eyes to 45 days of age results in 30 percent reduction of the number of synapses in the visual cortex.

A number of studies show that some dendritic spines develop in the absence of visual stimulation while other spines depend on visual input for their development. Thus the dendritic spines and synapses on them start developing before birth in all mammals, and the number of dendritic spines continues to increase after birth before the eyes open in mice, rats, and cats (Cragg, 1975*a,b*). However, a large increase in the number of dendritic spines occurs at the time of eye opening on postnatal days 10–19, and this increase is almost completely prevented by keeping the mice in the dark, as is shown in Fig. 5.10 (Ruiz-Marcos and Valverde, 1969). In mice reared in the dark, the characteristic spatial distribution of dendritic spines is maintained (exponential increase in numbers of spines with increasing distance from the cell body), but the absolute number of spines is reduced along the whole length of the dendritic shafts (Valverde and Ruiz-Marcos, 1969). The majority of spines are apparently unaffected by visual deprivation. The effect is reversible: returning the dark-reared mice to normal visual stimulation results in a return to nearly normal numbers of spines within a week (Valverde, 1971). The number of spines on pyramidal cells in layers IV and V of the rat's visual cortex can be increased above control levels by raising the rats in constant dim light (Parnavelas *et al.*, 1973).

A very striking effect of monocular visual deprivation in newborn monkeys is seen in the cortical ocular dominance columns: those of the deprived eye are reduced in width while there is a proportional increase in width of the ocular dominance columns of the normal eye (Hubel *et al.*, 1975). This is correlated with severe reduction of cortical neurons driven by the deprived eye (see Section 9.12). The changes in ocular dominance columns can be demonstrated autoradiographically by transneuronal labeling of geniculostriate neurons after injections of [^{3}H]fucose and [^{3}H]proline into one eye. The effect is probably due to enlargement of the dendritic and synaptic fields of the functional eye at the expense of those of the deprived eye.

The effects of visual deprivation on the visual cortex that have been described so far are largely or entirely on pyramidal cells while there is little evidence of any

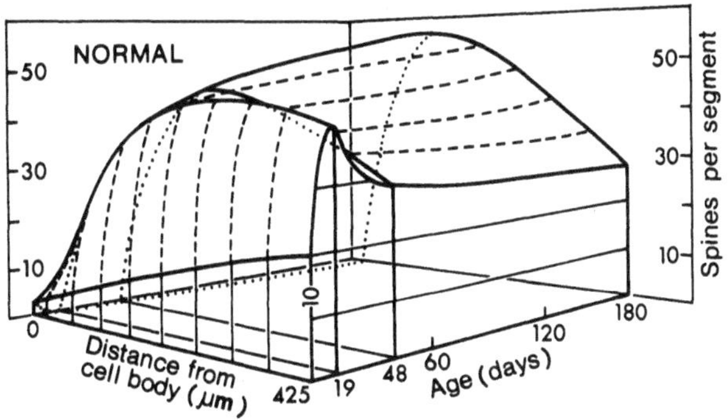

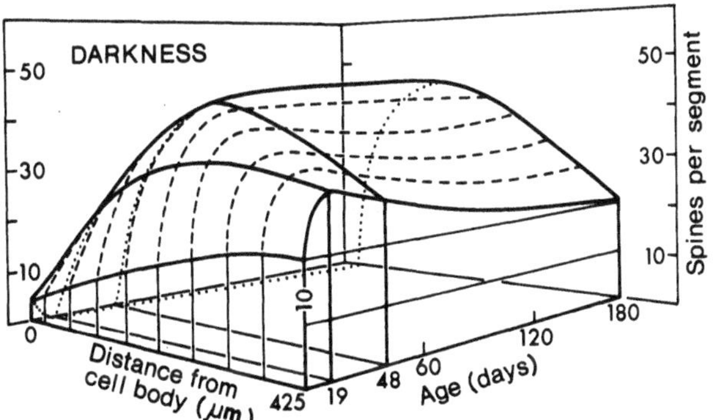

Figure 5.10. Distribution of dendritic spines on the apical dendritic shafts of pyramidal cells in the visual cortex of normal mice at different ages compared with mice raised in the dark. From A. Ruiz-Marcos and F. Valverde, The temporal evolution of the distribution of dendritic spines in the visual cortex of normal and dark raised mice, *Exp. Brain Res.* *8*:284–294 (1969).

changes in stellate cells. This can be correlated with the observation by J. P. Kelly and Van Essen (1974) that pyramidal cells are complex cells while stellate cells are simple cells (see Section 9.12). There is considerable evidence that the pyramidal neurons receive input from Y cells while the stellate neurons receive input from X cells (J. Stone and Dreher, 1973). This evidence is consistent with other evidence that visual deprivation has a selective effect on neurons receiving input from Y cells.

Removal of an eye results in the well-known transneuronal degeneration of lateral geniculate neurons (Minkowski, 1920; M. R. Matthews *et al.*, 1960) and transneuronal changes in the striate cortex. These consist of diminution of dendritic spines at the base of the apical dendrites of pyramidal cells in layer IV of the striate cortex (A. Globus and Scheibel, 1966, 1967*a,b,c,d;* Valverde, 1968; Valverde and Estéban, 1968). Changes in the orientation of dendrites of stellate cells in the visual cortex have been seen after removal of the eye of the mouse at birth (Valverde, 1968). The stellate cells have dendrites that normally radiate in all directions through layers III, IV, and V of the striate cortex. After removal of the eye at birth, layer IV is rendered virtually free of stellate cell dendrites, which radiate mainly into layers II and III. The geniculostriate visual afferent axons are also absent from layer IV; hence Valverde concluded that the dendrites of stellate cells that normally connect in layer IV undergo compensatory growth to connect in layers II and III with recurrent collaterals of superficial pyramidal neurons and in layer V with horizontal collaterals of deep pyramidal cells. The adjustment of synaptic associations in the striate cortex deprived of afferent optic fibers seems to be similar to the occupation by aberrant presynaptic terminals of synaptic sites on dendrites that have been left vacant by the failure of development of the normal contingent of afferent fibers. Many other examples are given below of relocation of nerve endings from their normal synaptic sites to occupy vacant postsynaptic sites. In general, these examples show that degeneration of developing presynaptic terminals may leave synaptic sites vacant and, therefore, "up for grabs." Ingrowing axonal terminals may occupy the vacant postsynaptic sites and form aberrant connections. The formation of these synapses is limited in several ways that are discussed on the following pages.

5.7. Plasticity of Axonal Growth and Terminal Connections

It is a general rule that axons rarely give off collateral branches except near their peripheral field. However, the growing axon sprouts vigorously when it reaches the field which it is destined to innervate. This observation led Ramón y Cajal (1919, 1928) to postulate that axonal sprouting is stimulated by neurotrophic factors produced by the cells in the terminal field. His concept was that the axons that enter a peripheral field compete for the available neurotrophic factors, using them or neutralizing them in the process of collateral sprouting. Thus, according to the hypothesis, the sprouting is self-limiting and results in each terminal field having a characteristic and fairly uniform density of axon branches, with little overlap between the terminal domains of neighboring axons. This hypothesis has been supported and extended by evidence obtained by Aguilar *et al.* (1973) that axon terminals are supplied by means of axonal transport with an antisprouting factor. When axonal transport is blocked by applying colchicine to a nerve in the salamander's leg, adjacent nerves sprout and invade the terminal field of the blocked axon. Neither the hypothetical sprouting factor released by the target tissue nor the antisprouting factor released by the nerve terminal has been identified. Nevertheless, this hypothesis has tremendous heuristic value: it provides an explanation of the differences in the density of innervation of different tissues and in different regions of the central nervous system. These differences are determined by the amount of sprouting factor released by the target cells in proportion to the amount of antisprouting factor released by the afferent nerves. The hypothesis also provides an explanation of the sprouting of neighboring afferents into a surgically deafferented region. This tendency to sprout collaterals from uninjured axons at the margins of a zone of surgically deafferented skin (Weddell *et al.,* 1941; Livingston, 1947; Edds, 1953; Aguilar *et al.,* 1973; J. Diamond *et al.,* 1976) is discussed in Section 8.7 in connection with the development of cutaneous innervation. The same tendency is seen for neighboring, uninjured axons to sprout collaterals after surgical deafferentation of nuclei in the central nervous system. Many examples of this will be given below. Here it should be emphasized that those examples of sprouting in the central nervous system can be more easily understood in relation to the hypothesis that has been outlined above. Collateral sprouting of neighboring axons into a denervated zone is probably due to disinhibition of their tendency to sprout in response to sprouting factors released by the cells that they innervate.

This hypothesis also provides an explanation for the apparent competition between axons for terminal space. This concept was further elaborated by Ramón y Cajal. He first suggested that the stimulus for collateral sprouting is frequently excessive during the initial phase of innervation, and that the number of nerve endings thus tends to exceed the number of synaptic sites that can be occupied by them. This results in a competition between the nerve endings for synaptic sites on their target cells, followed by resorption of the endings that fail to find a site at which to form a synapse. His view of thinking about this is revealed in the following quotation from *Studies on Vertebrate Neurogenesis* (1929):

> There is no question that every strayed axon or dendrite (one which fails to establish a functional connection because it inhabits a foreign cellular territory or because it follows a route which completely prevents it from attaining its proper destination) is progressively resorbed starting from the peripheral or terminal end. . . . We must therefore acknowledge that during neurogenesis there is a kind of competitive struggle among the outgrowths (and perhaps even among the nerve cells) for space and nutrition. . . . However, it is important not to exaggerate, as do certain embryologists, the extent and importance of the cellular competition to the point of likening it to the Darwinian struggle. . . .

In this quotation the explicit reference to Darwin reveals the source of the idea of competition for survival. The reference to "certain embryologists" undoubtedly was meant to refer to Wilhelm Roux, who, in his book *Der Kampf der Theile im Organismus* (1881), had developed the idea of a cellular struggle for survival in the developing organism. Charles Darwin considered this "the most important book on Evolution which has appeared for some time" and noted that its theme is "that there is a struggle going on within every organism between the organic molecules, the cells and the organs. I think that his basis is, that every cell which best performs its functions is, in consequence, at the same time best nourished and best propagates its kind" (F. Darwin, 1888, Vol. 3, p. 244). As

Darwin had recognized, competition is keenest between individuals that are most similar, and will finally result in one type completely displacing another.

This concept of the overproduction of axonal connections can be generalized to include any other components of the developing nervous system that are initially produced in excess and later reduced by death of redundant components. This is considered further in Sections 7.6 and 7.12 in relation to cell death in the developing nervous system. Elimination of redundant neurons may be regarded as a means of error correction or, in the present context, as a mode of developmental plasticity (see Section 7.11).

Collateral sprouting has been most thoroughly studied in the skin, as described in Section 8.7. The development of collateral sprouts from motoneuron terminals as they grow close to muscles is also well documented. During the initial innervation of mammalian skeletal muscle, there is an excess formation of neuromuscular connections, most of which are destined to disappear during early postnatal life, eventually leaving each muscle fiber connected to a single nerve terminal (M. R. Bennett and Pettigrew, 1974; M. C. Brown *et al.,* 1976). This is described in Section 8.2 in relation to development of neuromuscular connections. In that situation, the ratio of nerve terminals to muscle fibers changes as new muscle fibers are formed after birth (Chiakulas and Pauly, 1965). It is conceivable that a similar process may occur in the central nervous system: afferents are present in advance of the stream of migrating neurons and they may make temporary connections with the first neurons to arrive in their field, only to change their connections as more neurons arrive. This may occur in the mammalian cerebral cortex (see Section 3.2). A similar process of transfer of connections in the cerebellar cortex occurs: the climbing fibers form temporary connections with the somatic spines of Purkinje cells before making their permanent synaptic connections on the Purkinje cell dendrites (see Section 3.6).

There is very good evidence that reinnervation of partially denervated muscle occurs as a result of collateral branching of the remaining motor axons. This evidence has been discussed in reviews by Edds (1953) and Coërs and Woolf (1959). In all mammals so far studied, experimental partial denervation of a skeletal muscle is followed, after a few days, by the sprouting of collateral nerve branches by the surviving intramuscular axons. These collaterals arise from the subterminal nodes of Ranvier or from the end plate (Barker and Ip, 1966) (Fig. 5.11). They grow into the neurilemmal sheaths of the severed axons and are mechanically guided directly to the denervated end plates, where they form functional neuromuscular junctions. The branches have only to grow a few hundred micrometers to reach the end plates, and reinnervation is rapid and efficient. The collateral branching starts within a few days of partial denervation, but is most abundant during the third week, and continues for several weeks. As a result of reinnervation, the tension developed by the muscle on stimulating its residual motor nerve almost completely regains the tension developed by stimulating the normal innervation of the muscle on the other side (Van Harreveld, 1945; Weiss and Edds, Jr., 1946). The individual muscle fibers that have been reinnervated become 50–60 percent larger in cross-sectional area than the fibers of the opposite normal muscle (Van Harreveld, 1945). Initially, the collateral branches are of fine caliber, but they rapidly increase in diameter and in the second postoperative month reach diameters within the range of normal nerve fibers

(Edds, 1950*a;* H. Hoffman, 1950). The axons that have become overloaded as a result of forming an excess of terminal branches then increase in diameter after several months (Edds, 1950*b;* Cavanaugh, 1951).

The collateral sprouting of residual axons which occurs after partial denervation of the sartorius muscle is increased by total denervation of the neighboring quadriceps muscle (Van Harreveld, 1947). This indicates that collateral sprouting in the sartorius may be stimulated by a diffusible substance liberated from the denervated quadriceps. However, initial attempts to extract such a substance from denervated muscle and inject it into a partially denervated muscle did not produce clear evidence of increased or accelerated reinnervation (Van Harreveld, 1947). Unambiguous evidence of such an effect was obtained by H. Hoffman (1950) following intramuscular injection of ether extracts of egg yolk, muscle, or peripheral nerve or the white matter of the brain. Any of these substances injected into the anterior tibial muscle of the rat results in new outgrowth of collaterals from motor axons and from 30–50 percent of the motor end plates within 3 or 4 days after the injection. The active substance appears to be in the Schwann or glial cells or in the myelin. Ether extracts of the gray matter of the brain are as inactive as extracts of heart or liver. H. Hoffman (1950) postulated that a lipid is released from degenerating nerve fibers and stimulates sprouting of collaterals from surviving axons and end plates; he called this hypothetical substance *neurocletin* (neuron = a nerve; clesis = a call). The active molecule has not been identified. Mixtures of various fatty acids are inactive. The active extract produces collateral sprouting in the muscle into which it is injected, or, less frequently, in neighboring muscles, but has no effect when injected intraperitoneally or intravenously. Although their attempts to identify the active molecule were unsuccessful, H. Hoffman and Springell (1951) obtained evidence that indicated the molecule to be "a glyceride fatty acid of moderately unsaturated character—probably possessing one double bond."

It should be noted that during development the nerves that invade the muscles and the skin precede the migration of Schwann cells. The Schwann cells cannot therefore play any part in stimulating terminal branching of motor or sensory axons during their initial growth toward the muscle fibers or skin. If there are neurotropic substances attracting the nerves to their proper terminals, as

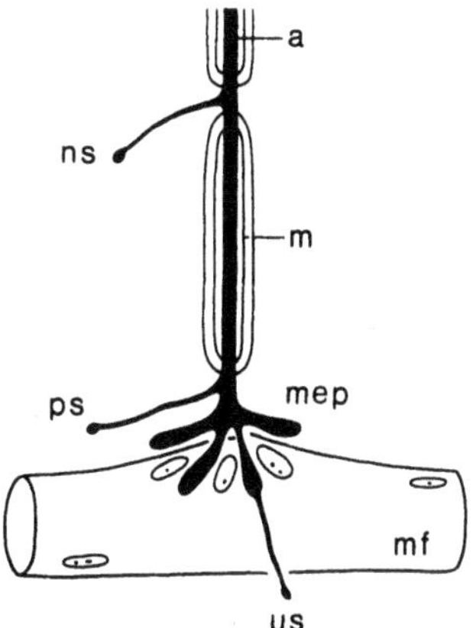

Figure 5.11. The three positions at which axonal sprouts may arise at preterminal and terminal parts of the motor axon. a, Axon; m, myelin sheath; mep, moter end plate; mf, muscle fiber; ns, nodal collateral sprout; ps, preterminal sprout; us, ultraterminal sprout. From D. Barker and M. C. Ip, *Proc. Roy. Soc. (London) Ser. B 163:*538–554 (1966).

Ramón y Cajal postulated, the neurotropic substances cannot be produced by the Schwann cells.

Collateral and ultraterminal sprouts are seen in the axons supplying the skeletal muscle fibers as well as those supplying the intrafusal muscle fibers in healthy muscles of cats and rabbits where the motor supply is intact (Barker and Ip, 1966) (Fig. 5.11). Such sprouts, which end blindly, have previously been regarded as embryonic vestiges that persist after failing to make functional connections (Ramón y Cajal, 1925; Tello, 1922*b*). However, Barker and Ip (1966) suggest that the motor nerve endings in normal muscle may have a limited life span and may be replaced by collateral ultraterminal sprouting. The population of nerve terminals may be in a state of dynamic equilibrium (Weddell and Zander, 1951). It seems to be a property of vertebrate sensory nerve terminals to undergo cycles of degeneration and regeneration, particularly in sites where the sense organelles and nerve terminals are subject to wear and tear, as in the epithelium of the tongue (Beidler, 1963; Beidler and Smallman, 1965).

5.8. Axonal Collateral Sprouting in the Central Nervous System

The development of collateral sprouting from uninjured axons in the vicinity of central nervous system injuries has been copiously documented, but the stimulus for this outgrowth and the mechanism of sprouting and possible functions of the sprouts are not known. In the first modern study of collateral sprouting in the central nervous system, C. N. Liu and Chambers (1958) partially denervated the spinal cord of adult cats by cutting dorsal roots or by section of the corticospinal tract on one side. About 10 months later, after all debris of degeneration had been removed, an adjacent dorsal root was sectioned bilaterally. The animal was killed 4–5 days later, and the axonal degeneration resulting from the section of the final dorsal root was determined. The authors reported an increase in the quantity and extent of degeneration on the side opposite the severed corticospinal tract and on the same side as the chronically sectioned dorsal roots. This shows that sprouting of axons in the spinal cord occurs from the intact dorsal roots. This has been confirmed autoradiographically (M. Murray and Goldberger, 1974) in cats and monkeys. McCouch *et al.* (1958) found that presynaptic dorsal root potentials are increased below a hemisection of the spinal cord compared with the normal side, and they suggest that this arises from sprouting of dorsal roots in the spinal cord.

The most detailed study, using electron microscopy, of collateral sprouting in the central nervous system has been done by Raisman (1969) and Raisman and Field (1973*b*) on the septal nuclei of the adult rat. The two main inputs to this nuclear complex are from the brain stem via the medial forebrain bundle and from the hippocampus via the fornix. Their synaptic endings are sufficiently different to be easily distinguishable in electron micrographs. Removal of the hippocampal afferents results in their replacement by collateral sprouts from septal afferents from the medial forebrain bundle (Fig. 5.12). Other cases of preemption of vacant synaptic sites by axonal sprouts from neighboring afferents show that the conditions under which sprouting occurs are similar in all cases. Such sprouting has been demonstrated with the electron microscope in the ventral cochlear nucleus of the adult rat (Gentschev and Sotelo, 1973) and in the nucleus gracilis of the cat (Rustioni and Sotelo, 1974). In all these cases, the sprouting occurs over a distance of about 250 μm or less. The reinnervation is heterologous (as the ultrastructure of the reinnervating synaptic boutons in each case is different from the original synaptic terminals) and does not lead to functional recovery. There is no evidence, except the presence of normal components of the synapse, that effective transmission occurs at these new synapses.

Extensive collateral sprouting of intact adrenergic neurons occurs after neighboring adrenergic neurons in the central nervous system have been cut (Stenevi *et al.,* 1973; R. Y. Moore *et al.,* 1973, review). These adrenergic neurons also regenerate vigorously. Their axons can innervate tissues that normally receive adrenergic innervation, such as the iris, when these tissues are implanted in the region of cut central adrenergic neurons in the medial forebrain bundle and adjacent nigrostriatal tract of adult rats and rabbits.

The hippocampal formation lends itself particularly well to studies of specific formation of synapses on granule and pyramidal cells and for studies of the plasticity or rigidity of those axodendritic synapses. There is a topographically organized arrangement of inputs to the granule cells of the fascia dentata as shown in Fig. 5.5, and each of the inputs can easily be removed. The dentate gyrus serves as a relay between the entorhinal cortex and the regio inferior of the hippocampus. In the adult rat, lesions of the entorhinal cortex, from which the perforant or temporoammonic pathway originates, denervate the distal half of the granule cells of the fascia dentata. This results in sprouting of the cholinergic endings, which originate in the septum and normally end on the distal segment of the granule cell dendrites. It also results in sprouting of the commissural fibers that normally terminate on the proximal part of the granule cell dendrites. The same phenomenon occurs when other afferents to the granule cell dendrites are removed. In all cases, the deafferented dendrites are reafferented by sprouts from neighboring terminals on the same dendrites (Lynch *et al.,* 1973*a,b,c,* 1974). These sprouts are, therefore, no longer than 250 μm. Somewhat more extensive sprouting has been seen from the entorhinal system of the opposite side, which normally sends a very sparse projection to the contralateral dentate gyrus. These sprouts

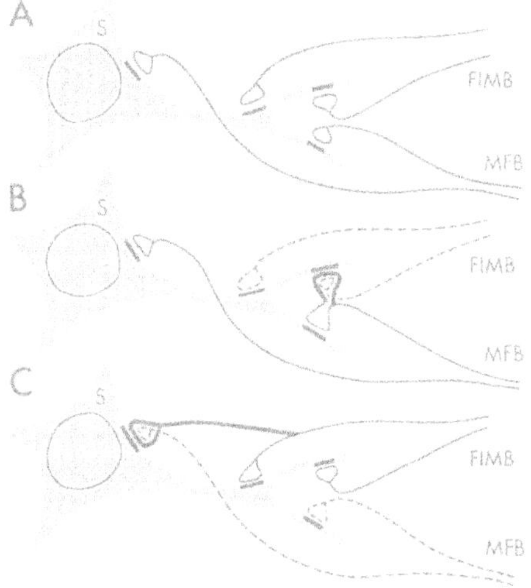

Figure 5.12. A: Rearrangement of synaptic connections in the septal nuclei. In the normal situation, afferents from the medial forebrain bundle (MFB) terminate in boutons on the cell soma (S) and on dendrites, while the fimbrial fibers (FIMB) are restricted in termination to the dendrites. B: Several weeks after a lesion of the fimbria, the medial forebrain bundle fiber terminals extend across from their own sites to occupy the vacated sites, thus forming double synapses. (Degenerated connections are represented by a discontinuous line, presumed plastic changes by a heavy black line.) C: Several weeks after a lesion of the medial forebrain bundle, the fimbrial fibers now give rise to terminals occupying somatic sites, which are presumably those vacated as a result of the former lesion. From G. Raisman, *Brain Res. 14:*25–48 (1969).

may extend as much as 2 or 3 mm across the hippocampal fissure to reinnervate the deafferented granule cell dendrites (Steward *et al.,* 1974). The cells of origin of these reinnervating sprouts from the contralateral cortex are of the same type as those which normally innervate the dentate granule cells from the ipsilateral cortex (Steward *et al.,* 1976).

These experiments show that the precise regional localization of the different inputs to the granule cell dendrites is unlikely to be due to an exclusive biochemical affinity of each type of afferent for a specific dendritic zone. Rather, the topographical segregation of afferents on the dendrites may develop as the result of a temporal order of arrival each type of afferent in relation to outgrowth of the dendritic tree and possibly to a competition between the afferents for the available synaptic sites on the dendrites (D. I. Gottlieb and Cowan, 1972).

The anatomical correlate of the formation of new connections is the almost complete reappearance of dendritic spines 20–80 days after entorhinal lesions (Parnavelas *et al.,* 1974). These experiments also show that the number of spines is a function of the dendrites—deafferentation results in a reduction of spines and therefore the axons are required for their maintenance, but regardless of the type of reinnervating axons the number of dendritic spines returns to a constant density. These observations show that in the cerebral cortical granule and pyramidal cells the dendritic spines are very labile and dependent on synaptic input for their development and survival. For example, removal of the entorhinal afferents, which occupy the distal half of the dendrites of granule cells in the dentate gyrus, results in loss of 30 percent of spines. However, the spines return to normal by 60 days after the lesion (Parnavelas *et al.,* 1974). Valverde (1971) has shown that there is a loss of spines from the apical dendrites of pyramidal cells of mice raised in the dark from birth to 20 days of age. However, when these animals are returned to normal visual experience, there is a partial recovery of the number of apical dendritic spines. Raisman and Field (1973*b*) have reported that the spines in the septal nuclei are reduced by 50 percent 7 days after removal of their hippocampal afferents, but the spine density returns to normal by 30 days postoperative. In the cochlear nucleus of the adult rat, removal of the primary afferents results in reinnervation by sprouting of uninjured afferents in 5–9 days (Gentschev and Sotelo, 1973). Functional connections are formed by sprouts which can first be detected on the dendrites of granule cells in the hippocampal dentate gyrus 10–14 days after a lesion of the entorhinal cortex (Steward *et al.,* 1974). Sprouts from central adrenergic neurons can be detected histochemically 5–7 days postoperative (R. Y. Moore *et al.,* 1971). In all these cases, the recovery is quite rapid, because the distance over which sprouts have to grow is quite small, usually less than 250 μm, and because the degenerating boutons which the sprouts replace are removed rapidly. However, delayed reinnervation has been reported in the nucleus gracilis of the cat: the primary afferents degenerate within a few days but reinnervation, by axons of unknown origin, occurs only after 1–6 months (Rustioni and Sotelo, 1974).

Another type of synaptic reorganization occurs after removal of the primary visual cortex of the rabbit. This operation results, during the following 2 weeks, in death of almost all the neurons in the dorsal nucleus of the lateral geniculate body (LGN). One year postoperative, Ralston and Chow (1973) observed synaptic reorganization in the LGN so that the optic afferents that form axodendritic synapses on the LGN neurons, when deprived of their normal postsynaptic sites, form axoaxonal synapses, probably with surviving interneurons of the nucleus. Such synaptic reorganization can hardly be regarded as a form of physiological compensation or adaptation, as it is certain that no recovery of function occurs.

Anomalous connections in the visual system of the golden hamster develop if lesions are made in the optic tract in the newborn animal but not when similar lesions are made in adults. No reconnections appear to form after lesions of the visual system in adult mammals. By contrast, when the superior colliculus is damaged soon after birth, some optic axons grow into the residual part of the colliculus. Others cross the midline to form functional connections in the opposite, undamaged colliculus. Here the axons from the two eyes segregate in separate regions of the colliculus. These connections result in maladaptive turning of the head away from a visual stimulus. Other optic axons connect anomalously with two regions of the thalamus, the nucleus lateralis posterior and the ventral lateral geniculate nucleus, which normally receive inputs from the superior colliculus but do not normally receive direct retinal projections. In the review of his observations, G. E. Schneider (1973) attributes these anomalous sprouts to the tendency, first noted by Ramón y Cajal (1928), for axons to conserve the total quantity of their terminal arborizations. It should be noted, however, that not all the optic axons have reached the colliculus at the time of the operation, and the anomalous projections might arise not as a result of pruning of their axonal terminals in the colliculus but as a result of misrouting before arrival at the colliculus. Such misrouting of optic axons to the wrong side of the brain has been found after removal of an eye in newborn rats, an effect that is not observed when the eye is removed after the tenth day after birth (R. D. Lund *et al.,* 1973; R. D. Lund and Lund, 1973). As in the initial report of axonal sprouting in the visual system following eye removal in the 3-month-old rat (D. C. Goodman and Horel, 1966), all subsequent reports have confirmed and extended the evidence showing that the anomalous sprouts are more extensive when the eye is removed shortly after birth. The effects are due to a combination of sprouting from the optic tract of the remaining eye in areas that normally receive inputs from both eyes, and also due to misrouting of retinal axons that have not yet completed their growth to the visual centers (D. C. Goodman *et al.,* 1973; Stanfield and Cowan, 1976). Removal of an eye in newborn rabbits results in enlargement of the ipsilateral projection from the other eye to the deafferented tectum (Chow *et al.,* 1973). These new axonal growths are not activated either by visual or any other sensory stimulation or by electrical stimulation of the retina.

The functional effectiveness of collateral sprouting varies from nonfunctional, as in the last example, to grossly malfunctional, as after lesions to the visual pathways of newborn hamsters. These animals are extremely immature at birth and show the most rapid and extensive collateral sprouting that has been observed in the central nervous system of mammals. Yet, despite considerable recovery of function, the ultimate effect is maladaptive behavior. For example, after unilateral removal of the superior colliculus in the newborn hamster, G. E. Schneider (1970, 1973, review) found that optic axons destined for the ablated superior colliculus form functional connections with the remaining superior colliculus. This results in misdirected visual pursuit behavior which is not corrected by experience. A functional deficit also follows partial transsection of the lateral olfactory tract in the newborn hamster: mating behavior in adult life is impaired, apparently as a result of collateral sprouts from residual axons that form aberrant connections

(Devor, 1975). Another sort of malfunction resulting from collateral sprouting is the spasticity and hyperreflexia that occur after lesions of the descending spinal fiber tracts: these tracts do not regenerate and thus their target neurons are reinnervated by sprouting of segmental afferents (Chambers *et al.*, 1973; M. Murray and Goldberger, 1974). The synaptic reorganization that occurs to a limited extent after loss of parallel fibers does not result in any improvement of the cerebellar ataxia (see Section 3.4.4). These observations are consistent in principle, if not in all details, with Ramón y Cajal's pessimistic appraisal of the functional value of the abortive regeneration he observed in the mammalian central nervous system (also see review by Clemente, 1964) as expressed in the frequently cited statement that "In adult centres the nerve paths are something fixed, ended, immutable. Everything may die, nothing may be regenerated" (Ramón y Cajal, 1928).

Recovery or reorganization of function can occur after damage to the mammalian central nervous system without detectable reorganization of structure (Lashley, 1937; Goldman, 1974). This is mentioned here because it may be very difficult to distinguish between structural and purely functional mechanisms by observing behavior or even by neurophysiological techniques. For example, Wall and Egger (1971) reported that some days after destruction of nucleus gracilis of the adult rat, the cells of the ventral posterior lateral nucleus of the thalamus (VPL) that normally respond to stimulation of the hindpaws begin to respond to stimulation of the forepaws. By 3 weeks after the operation, there is an expansion of the responses from the forelimb into areas of VPL that normally respond only to hindlimb stimulation. Initially, this was though to be due to sprouting of afferents from the forelimb onto neurons of VPL whose inputs from the hindlimb had been removed. This conclusion had to be revised when it was found that the deafferentation from the hindlimbs unmasks forelimb afferents that are normally present (Merrill and Wall, 1972). The possibility that injury may disinhibit or unmask latent functions has to be considered in all cases. The possibility has also to be considered that injury can temporarily inhibit certain functions or retard their development. Injury to the developing nervous system may be followed by recovery due to development of entirely new structures rather than to regeneration or collateral sprouting (M. Jacobson, 1974*a;* Goldman, 1974).

Reinnervated synapses are either nonfunctional or dysfunctional if they are nonspecific, that is, heterologous, and in none of the cases of collateral sprouting with the formation of heterologous synaptic connections is there any evidence of recovery of normal or useful functions. This is in sharp contrast to the selectivity of formation of synaptic connections that occurs during development. There is no evidence of random or nonselective formation of connections under normal conditions, but the selectivity can be thwarted or impaired by various surgical operations. Even when nerves are cut and allowed to regenerate into their distal stumps, there is considerable reconnection of axons with their proper targets. For example, selective reinnervation of fast-twitch and slow-graded muscle fibers occurs after nerve regeneration in the toad *Bufo marinus* (Hoh, 1971). Reinnervation of the superior cervical ganglion after cutting the preganglionic fibers results in selective reinnervation of ganglion cells by preganglionic fibers from particular levels of the spinal cord (J. N. Langley, 1895, 1897), and, in the ciliary ganglion, the reinnervating fibers form the correct synaptic connections from the beginning (Landmesser and Pilar, 1970). Even if there is collateral sprouting from neighboring fibers onto denervated ganglion cells, the inappropriate connections are displaced when the appropriate presynaptic fibers regenerate (Guth and Bernstein, 1961). However, several foreign nerves, including peripheral motor nerves and the vagus nerve, can regenerate to form functional heterologous synapses with superior cervical ganglion cells whose own presynaptic fibers have been removed (J. N. Langley, 1898; J. N. Langley and Anderson, 1904*a,b;* Guth, 1956*a,b;* Ceccarelli *et al.,* 1971; McLachlan, 1974; Ostberg *et al.,* 1976; Purves, 1976). The specificity of connections in these cases is relative: a variety of foreign cholinergic nerve fibers can take the place of the native presynaptic fibers. When both foreign vagal and native sympathetic fibers innervate the superior cervical ganglion of the guinea pig simultaneously, about half the ganglion cells receive synapses from both sources after about 1 month, and the proportion of doubly innervated cells remains constant for at least 14 months, showing that the foreign synapses are as stable as the native ones on the same neuron (Purves. 1976).

There is now considerable evidence that foreign innervation persists and remains functionally effective after the normal nerves are allowed to reinnervate their postganglionic cells. This result has been reported in mammalian skeletal muscle (Tonge, 1974*a,b,c;* Frank *et al.,* 1974, 1975), frog fast muscle (Miledi, 1963), and perch gill muscles (Frank and Jansen, 1976). Marotte and Mark (1970*a*) provided behavioral evidence that correct reinnervation suppresses foreign synapses after cross-innervation of goldfish extraocular muscles, but S. A. Scott (1975) showed by electrophysiological recording that both native and foreign nerves remain functionally connected to the cross-innervated muscles. The only instance in which there is unchallenged evidence that suppression of foreign synapses may occur is in skeletal muscles of urodele amphibians when they are innervated both by native and foreign nerves (Mark, 1974*a,b,* 1975, reviews). This is dealt with further in Section 8.2.

The problem of the long-term function of heterologous synapses remains unsolved. The little evidence that is now available shows that some heterologous synapses may persist structurally and functionally although they result in dysfunction, while other heterologous synapses are eliminated or become functionally ineffective. In terms of the hypothesis of functional validation of synaptic connections (M. Jacobson, 1970*a,b,* 1974*b;* Hirsch and Jacobson, 1975), newly formed synapses are labile unless stabilized by function (see also Changeux and Danchin, 1976). Some heterologous synapses may not become stabilized and may therefore degenerate or become functionally ineffective. For example, in the cerebellum of the staggerer mutant mouse, there is a failure of development of Purkinje cell dendritic spines that normally connect with the parallel fibers of the granule cells. The parallel fibers develop and form transient contacts with the dendritic shafts of Purkinje cells, but eventually, as the animal matures, the parallel fibers degenerate and the granule cells die.

To balance these examples of reinnervation in the central nervous system, there are as many cases where sprouting and reinnervation have not been detected following partial deafferentation of central nuclei. For example, in adult cats and kittens, no sprouting of cervical primary afferents onto the spinal nucleus of the trigeminal nerve could be found a year or more after trigeminal denervation (Kerr, 1972, 1975*a,b*). In that instance, sprouting of cervical primary afferent axons was expected because it is known that trigeminal denervation results in deafferentation of the dorsal horn of the spinal cord at the level of C1. Absence of sprouting has also been reported in the dorsal column nuclei after chronic deafferentation (Rustioni and Molenaar, 1975). Sprouting of the auditory nerve into the medial superior olive is not seen after removal of the anteroventral cochlear nucleus (C. N. Liu and Liu, 1971; E. L. White and Nolan, 1974). In the adult cat, after removal of the optic input, the lateral geniculate nucleus is not reinnervated by collateral sprouts (Guillery, 1972*b*), although in kittens a slight amount of translaminar sprouting has been reported (Hickey, 1975). In general, reinnervation of deafferented neurons in the mammalian visual system does not occur in the adult. Finally, there are many cases, reviewed by Stenevi *et al.* (1973), of failure to detect sprouting of central aminergic neurons into deafferented regions such as the superior colliculus, lumbar spinal cord, hypothalamus, and other regions of the central nervous system in which there is a low density of adrenergic innervation. These regions are far removed from a region of high density of adrenergic nerves, and no sprouting can be expected over such distances. There are thus almost as many reports of failure to find sprouting as there are reports of successful sprouting in the mammalian central nervous system, and there seems to be a reason for this difference. In the cases where sprouting is expected but is not found, the axons which are expected to sprout are in close proximity to the denervated zone but they are segregated from the axonal terminals that are removed, whereas in the successful cases the sprouting axons share part of the same postsynaptic zone. The lack of sprouting may be due to a failure of release, transmission, or reception of the signal that must arise from the denervated zone. Obviously, the transmission of the necessary signals will be facilitated if the responding axonal terminals are already connected to the denervated cell, and that is the situation in most cases of sprouting in the central nervous system. In all cases, proximity is a vital factor, and the distances are very short (usually less than 250 μm) over which sprouts have to grow for reafferentation to occur. In most cases, the sprouts arise from axons that belong to the same system as the axons that they replace. For example, rearrangements within the hippocampus, septal nuclei, or spinal cord are confined in each case to a single functional system. This is also true of the visual system: optic tract axons sprout to anomalous positions but remain confined to the visual system. An instance which appears to break this rule that sprouting is confined to the nucelar region to which the axons normally connect has been reported by Kalil and Schneider (1975). They found that when a lesion damages both the superior and inferior colliculus in the newborn hamster, optic axons sprout short distances (less than 250 μm) into the medial geniculate body and form axodendritic synapses on deafferented medial geniculate neurons. In this case, it should be remembered that hamsters are extremely immature at birth. One should think of such results not in terms of adaptive mechanisms designed to bring about recovery of function but rather as a derangement of the developmental program.

The stimulus for collateral sprouting in the central nervous system is still a matter of conjecture. There are three alternative hypotheses: first, that sprouting is stimulated by products of degeneration; second, that sprouting is stimulated by a factor produced by the postsynaptic cells or their associated glial cells; third, that sprouting is due to an inherent tendency of neurons to conserve their protoplasmic volume. One observation makes it unlikely that sprouting is stimulated by products of degeneration, namely that the sprouts can grow into a region that is not denervated. For example, in the newborn hamster, after unilateral removal of the superior colliculus, sprouts of optic nerve fibers grow into the residual, uninjured superior colliculus.

Suggestive of the hypothesis that the postsynaptic cells (and associated glial cells) release a sprouting factor that is neutralized by nerve endings is the observation that reinnervation of vacated synaptic sites is delayed until the original nerve endings have disappeared. This mechanism also has the virtue of parsimony in that it applies to sprouting in the central nervous system as well as to sprouting in the peripheral nervous system. The hypothesis that sprouting is due to an inherent tendency of the neuron to conserve its original protoplasmic volume applies only to cases in which part of the axon is cut away and sprouts emerge from the residual part to compensate for the loss of volume. This hypothesis cannot account for the cases in which sprouting occurs from uninjured neurons in the neighborhood of a denervated region. Neither can that "pruning" hypothesis (G. E. Schneider, 1973) account for sprouting of motoneuron endings after treatment with botulinum toxin (Drachman, 1976, review). On the other hand, the latter observation is consistent with a mechanism in which botulinum toxin prevents the release of antisprouting factors from the nerve ending (Aguilar *et al.*, 1973; J. Diamond *et al.*, 1976), thus allowing uninhibited action of the sprouting factors produced by the postsynaptic cells.

The critical reader will have asked how phenomena such as axonal sprouting, which are the result of experimental disruption of normal development, can be related to the mechanisms of normal development. The genuinely perplexed may not be willing to accept the commonsense answer that the similarities between axonal sprouting after surgery and normal axonal growth during development are sufficient to use the former as a model of the latter. Rather, the critical reader will admit that such extrapolations from disruptive experiments can be made only tentatively and provisionally, subject to constant revision as more information is obtained from studies of *normal development.* Additional information obtained from other disruptive experiments is of little use in checking the relevance of such information to normal development.

Much of this book is devoted to assessing how normal developmental mechanisms can be understood from the evidence obtained from analytical experiments in which the processes of development are greatly perturbed. For example, culture of isolated parts of the nervous system, the use of toxins or of surgery, and even genetic analysis using mutants involve some destructive interference with the normal processes of development. Such experiments are understandable only because the results of different types of experiments are convergent and, finally, because they can be interpreted in relation to normal, relatively undisturbed developmental processes. Thus the patterns of nerve growth seen in tissue culture or the sprouting and regeneration of axons after surgery become intelligible only when they are seen in relation to histological observations of normal axonal growth patterns and to direct observations of the growth of nerve fibers in living organisms. The primacy of the observations of normal development should never be denied: the results of disruption or destructive analytical experiments are intelligible only when they are consistent with observations of normal development, but the reverse does not hold. We should never let it out of our minds that this entire enterprise is aimed at understanding *normal development.*

6

Dependence of the Developing Nervous System on Nutrition and Hormones

6.1. Vulnerability of the Brain to Malnutrition

While in the uterus, the fetus is relatively well protected from changes in the external environment, and the development of its nervous system is largely but not entirely under genetic control. However, the fetal nervous system is vulnerable to trauma, toxins, hyperthermia, infections, radiation, placental insufficiency, and severe maternal malnutrition. These risks increase greatly during and after birth, and the developmental processes that occur in the neonatal period are especially sensitive to external conditions. Some of the conditions which may damage the developing nervous system are considered elsewhere in this book: virus infections (Section 3.4.4), poisons (Sections 2.3 and 3.4.4), radiation (Section 3.4.4), hyperthermia (Section 3.8), and hormonal insufficiency or excess (Sections 6.2 to 6.6). Here, further consideration is given to the **effects of malnutrition** on the developing nervous system in mammals, and particularly in humans.

The vulnerability of the developing nervous system to radiation, poisons, viruses, undernutrition, or hyperthermia is determined by the cellular activities in the developing system that respond to the insult under consideration. Therefore, the effects of the agents or conditions will be different at different times in development, and the vulnerable periods may not be the same for all agents and may differ according to the timetable of developmental events in the nervous system in different species (Dobbing, 1971, 1976).

It is fairly obvious that nutritional deprivation is most likely to have maximum effects on those developmental processes that are most active at the time of the deprivation. Thus malnutrition produces severe deficiencies in the number of neurons if it occurs during the period of neuronal production, maximal effects on glial cell number if it coincides with the period of glial cell proliferation, and maximal effects on myelination if it occurs during the period of myelination.

However, these processes occur in different species at different times in relation to the time of birth, so that the outcome of neonatal malnutrition will be considerably different in the mouse than in man. Therefore, when making extrapolations from experimental animals to humans, one should try to relate the effect of malnutrition to the developmental processes occurring during the time of malnutrition rather than to the time of birth.

At least half the world's population has suffered a period of nutritional deprivation during childhood, and at present about 300 million children throughout the world are malnourished (World Health Organization, Scientific Publication No. 251, 1972). There is no doubt that severe malnutrition in infants and young children during the period of maximal brain growth results in a slowing of the rate of neurological development. If the duration and severity of malnutrition are sufficiently great, the result may be permanent reduction in brain weight, and possibly mental retardation. However, severe malnutrition is infrequent, even in underdeveloped countries, and while such severe clinical malnutrition unquestionably may result in retardation of nervous development, it is more questionable whether marginally undernourished children suffer any permanent damage to the nervous system. Assessment of any direct effects of chronic but not severe malnutrition on the nervous system is almost impossible because of the other disadvantages that poor children suffer. The fact that sociocultural factors play such an important role in intellectual and scholastic development makes it difficult to assess the contribution of malnutrition to the retardation of impoverished children (Cravioto and DeLicardi, 1972; Herzig *et al.,* 1972). "In short, malnutrition and socio-cultural factors are likely to act synergistically to depress both growth and development; however, in the absence of truly experimental studies it is scarcely possible to assign causal significance to specific factors" (Tizard, 1974).

Prenatal nutritional deprivation of the fetus may occur in multiple pregnancy in humans as a result of competition between the fetuses for nutrients. Birth weight of twins is lower than that of singletons, and birth weight is significantly correlated with later intelligence (Churchill *et al.,* 1966). Twins average about 7 IQ points below singletons (Stott, 1960; Vandenburg, 1966; Inouye, 1970). The importance of intrauterine competition for nutrients is shown by the fact that identical twins with the same birth weight have the same IQ, but if their birth weights are unequal the twin with the lower birth weight has the lower IQ in later life (Willerman and Churchill, 1967). The number of variables that enter into human intelligence makes these results difficult to interpret. Thus in a review of the effect of very low birth weight (1500 g or less) on later intelligence, Francis-Williams and Davies (1974) point out that as many of the harmful factors in the treatment of such infants have been eliminated (excessive use of oxygen, hypothermia, prolonged starvation, infections), there has been progressive improvement of the ultimate IQ attained by these children. When babies with low birth weight are cared for under optimal conditions, mental retardation or significant deficits in IQ do not occur (P. A. Davies and Stewart, 1975). In man, it is not known whether twins have a lower brain weight or fewer brain cells than singletons, as would be predicted if animal experimental results, to be described below, can be extrapolated to man. The deficit is unlikely to be due to failure of nerve cell production because production of nerve cells has ceased by 25 weeks of gestation (Dobbing and Sands, 1970), whereas differences in the weight of multiple fetuses compared with a single fetus become apparent only after 26 weeks of gestation (McKeown and Record, 1952). The deficit is more likely to be due to some failure of cell growth and differentiation rather than to a reduction in cell numbers.

Nevertheless, there is good evidence that loss of brain cells can occur after severe malnutrition in human infants. Children who die of severe malnutrition in the first 2 years after birth have greatly reduced quantities of DNA in the cerebrum, cerebellum, and brain stem (Fig. 6.1) compared with well-nourished children of the same age (Winick and Rosso, 1969; Winick *et al.,* 1970). It is not known whether the deficit is in the number of neurons or glial cells.

The effects of maternal undernutrition on fetal brain development have been studied most often in rats, which differ significantly from humans in several important ways: multiple births are the rule in rats, and production of neurons continues throughout gestation. By contrast, production of neurons in humans is virtually completed by about the midpoint of gestation, after which glial cell production continues to the end of gestation and into the second postnatal year. As neurons and glia in the fetal nervous system may not be equally susceptible to the effects of maternal undernutrition, and as the latter may have different secondary effects on the placenta and on the endocrine system in different species, extrapolation from the rat to man should be made with considerable caution.

Myelination is one of the few processes that can be studied best in rats and can be extrapolated to man. Myelination in the central nervous system as well as in peripheral nerves of rats is greatly reduced as a result of neonatal malnutrition (Dobbing, 1963; Culley and Mertz, 1965; Benton *et al.,* 1966; H. P. Chase *et al.,* 1967; Clos and Legrand, 1969, 1970). The ultrastructure of Schwann cells is abnormal and the number of myelin lamellae is reduced in the sciatic nerve of 12-day-old rats underfed from birth (Clos and Legrand, 1970). There is evidence that similar deficits occur in severely malnourished human infants. J. H. Fox *et al.* (1972) found that the total quantity of myelin is reduced in malnourished infants, but the chemical composition of the myelin is not altered (see Section 4.16).

Zamenhof *et al* (1968) pioneered the study of the effects of maternal nutrition on fetal brain development by showing that restriction of protein in the diet of rats for a month before mating and during pregnancy results in 30 percent reduction in body weight and 10 percent reduction in brain DNA of the offspring compared with normal newborn rats. Similar results have been obtained by Winick (1969) and by Zeman and Stanbrough (1969). The authors recognize that their results neither show which types of brain cells are reduced nor show their regional

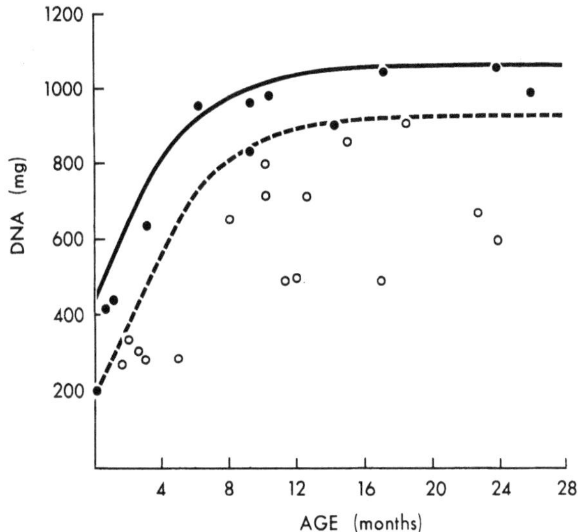

Figure 6.1. DNA content of the cerebrum of normal children (•) and marasmic children (○). From M. Winick, P. Rosso, and J. Waterlow, *Exp. Neurol. 26:*393–400 [1970], copyright Academic Press, Inc.

distribution. These experiments also do not show whether the reduction in DNA (cell number) results from nutritional deficiency directly or indirectly, for example, due to placental insufficiency or hormonal effects.

To determine the time of maximal susceptibility of the fetus to maternal malnutrition and the extent of recovery if normal nutrition is restored, Zamenhof *et al.* (1971*d*) deprived groups of pregnant female rats of protein for 5-day periods at different times during gestation. Abortion occurred in the majority of cases deprived before 10 days of gestation, and in all groups the offspring had significant reductions of body weight, cerebral weight, and cerebral DNA. The effect cannot be due to the protein requirement of the fetuses, which constitutes a very small fraction of the maternal protein requirement, but must be due to other factors such as placental insufficiency and deficiency in maternal gonadotropic hormones, which results in lower levels of estrogen and progesterone. These results also show that even a short, 5-day period of maternal protein deprivation results in irreversible loss of fetal brain cells. That hormonal factors may play a role in this effect is shown by the reversal of the effect of undernutrition by growth hormone (somatotropin) injections (Zamenhof *et al.,* 1971*c*).

The needs of the fetus are diverse and complex, and to a large extent limited by the functional capacities of the placenta. There is considerable evidence that placental growth is affected by maternal malnutrition (Winick, 1967, 1970*a*; Winick *et al.,* 1967; Dayton *et al.,* 1969; Zamenhof *et al.,* 1971*a*), and it is very likely that fetal brain development is affected by impaired placental growth and function (McKeown and Record, 1952; Zamenhof *et al.,* 1971*a*). The complexity of the effects of maternal malnutrition is shown by the phenomenon of transfer of the effects from one generation to the next. It has long been suspected that poor nutrition of the female infant may affect the neurological development of her offspring born much later (Cowley and Griesel, 1963; R. H. Barnes *et al.,* 1966). In rats, Zamenhof *et al.* (1971*e*) obtained evidence that the normally nourished female offspring (F_1) of a mother (F_0) which had been malnourished during pregnancy will produce offspring with significantly reduced brain DNA. The transfer is not genetic, as it occurs only through F_1 females but not through F_1 males. The most likely explanation is that the F_1 females, although well nourished postnatally, had suffered some permanent physical deficiency *in utero* that restricted the development of their (F_2) progeny. The physical defect in the F_1 generation has not been discovered, but the effect might be caused by a deficiency of pituitary hormone releasing factors in the F_1 females. Even in experimental animals the effects of malnutrition may be difficult to separate from those of hormones, even when well-designed control experiments are performed.

Assessment of the effects of malnutrition on nervous development in children is bedeviled by at least two main difficulties. First, the effects of malnutrition cannot be entirely separated from the effects of concomitant insults such as maternal neglect, environmental impoverishment, and lack of stimulation and incentive. Second, the effects of malnutrition on the human brain can rarely be assessed directly by postmortem physical and chemical measurements. Instead, less reliable indices, such as intelligence quotient (IQ) and head circumference, are generally used. These indices are themselves complex variables, and their interpretation is usually difficult and frequently ends in controversy. For example, general intelligence is a complex product of many variable factors, one of them being the size of the brain. As a result, authorities disagree about the relationship between brain size and intelligence—the relationship can be shown in animals (see

Section 3.9) but in man it tends to be overridden by other factors that vary in different sociocultural contexts. In those cases where IQ is found to be reduced in malnourished children, it is often difficult if not impossible to determine whether the reduced IQ is the result of retarded brain development due to malnutrition and associated conditions such as disease, or whether the poor performance is largely or entirely due to social and economic disadvantages. Moreover, a single IQ test has little value, particularly if it is done at an early age; IQ at 1 year of age has no correlation with the IQ at age 17 (B. S. Bloom, 1964). Besides, the IQ is subject to change during childhood: changing the educational level of children can result in increase or reduction of their IQ by as much as 28 points (Skeels, 1966). Obviously, the rate of development of general intelligence is a more revealing index than a single measurement. Circumference of the head is another index that is often used to assess the effects of malnutrition on brain development. However, the circumference of the head is also related to thickness of the skull and scalp and the size of the temporal muscles, so that there is a poor correlation between head size and brain size (Eichhorn and Bayley, 1962). The poor correlation between head size and intelligence is illustrated by the fact that intelligence is normal in a small percentage of microcephalic children (H. P. Martin, 1970). Finally, reduced head circumference in infants and young children may not be irremediable (H. P. Martin, 1970; Stoch and Smythe, 1976).

The difficulties of measuring the effects of malnutrition on human intelligence should not obscure the fact that children can suffer large reductions in IQ from a period of severe malnutrition during the first few years after birth (Waterlow *et al.,* 1960; Stoch and Smythe, 1963, 1967, 1976; G. Graham, 1964; Cravioto, 1966; Cravioto *et al.,* 1966; Coursin, 1967; Scrimshaw and Gordon, 1968; Eichenwald and Fry, 1969; Frisch, 1971; Tizard, 1974). In one such study, Stoch and Smythe (1963, 1967) found that severely undernourished South African children from 1 to 8 years of age were 20 points lower in IQ than well-nourished children of similar parentage. When these children were studied 15 years later, the same severe intellectual deficits were found, showing that the effect is permanent (Stoch and Smythe, 1976). Similar conclusions were reached in another study of the effects of severe undernutrition during infancy on subsequent intellectual functions in Yugoslavian children (Cabak and Najdanvic, 1965; Cabak *et al.,* 1967). In 36 children between the ages of 4 and 24 months who had been hospitalized because of malnutrition but had not suffered from chronic illness thereafter, and who had no significant reduction in body growth, there were marked deficits in IQ. The mean IQ of the malnourished children was 88, in contrast to 101 and 109 for two groups of comparable normal children. Significantly, none of the malnourished children had an IQ above 110 (Fig. 6.2).

These studies of children who have been very severely undernourished show that irreversible brain damage may result, and if malnutrition is so severe that death ensues it can be determined that considerable loss of brain cells had occurred (Fig. 6.1). This type of damage to the nervous system produced by extremely severe nutritional deprivation appears to be similar to the effects of severe hypoxia or hypoglycemia. Severe, chronic nutritional deprivation during infancy and childhood, which in some cases results in impairment of intellectual development, may be analogous to the effects of severe undernutrition in experimental newborn rats which leads to stunting of dendritic growth, reduced synaptogenesis, and deficient myelination. However, these deleterious effects have not been shown to occur in infants and children who suffer from the chronic but

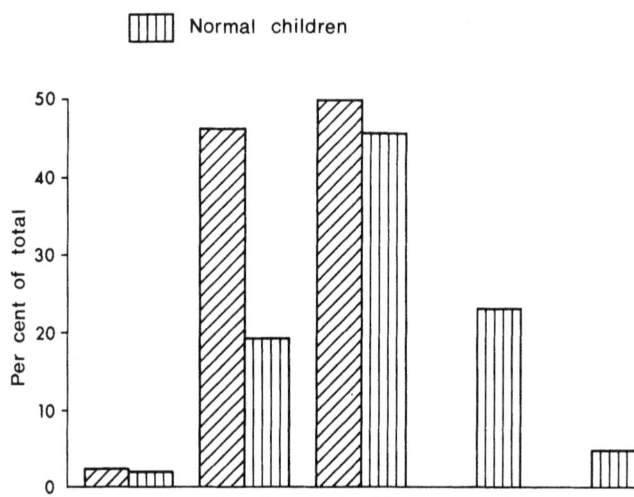

Figure 6.2. Distribution of intelligence quotients of 36 children aged 7–14 years who had been malnourished between the ages of 4 and 24 months compared with the intelligence quotients of normal children of the same ages. Adapted from V. Cabak and R. Najdanvic, *Arch. Dis. Child.* *40*:532–534 (1965).

moderate undernutrition that affects a large percentage of the human species. However, if it were found that such moderate undernutrition damages the developing human brain, it would justify the statement by Brillat-Savarin in his classic of gastronomy, *Physiologie du Goût* (1825): "La destinée des nations dépend de la manière dont elles se nourrissent."

6.2. Role of Hormones in Neural Ontogeny

Two general modes of action of hormones on their target cells have so far been recognized. In the first of these, shown by epinephrine and many peptide hormones, the hormone binds to a specific receptor at the cell surface and then activates the nucleotide cyclase system to stimulate the conversion of a nucleoside triphosphate, such as adenosine triphosphate (ATP), to the corresponding 3′,5′-monophosphate, for example, cyclic adenosine monophosphate (cAMP). The cyclic nucleotide then functions as a "second messenger" which stimulates various intracellular processes. In the second type of action, which occurs with steroid hormones and probably with thyroid hormones, the hormone enters the cell and binds to a cytoplasmic receptor protein which transports the steroid hormone to the cell nucleus where specific RNA synthesis is stimulated.

The effects of hormones on brain development depend primarily on the distribution of target cells, carrying specific receptors, in various parts of the nervous system. Secondarily the role of hormones in neural ontogeny is determined by the availability of the hormones and their accessibility to the target cells.

Thus, in mammals, the influence of maternal hormones on the fetus is restricted by the ability of the hormones to cross the placenta: while steroid hormones, thyroid hormones, and epinephrine do so, peptide hormones do not pass from the maternal to the fetal side of the placenta (Gitlin *et al.*, 1965; Laron *et al.*, 1966). However, maternal hormones can affect placental size and function, and these, in turn, affect brain development (McKeown and Record, 1952; Zamenhof and Van Marthens, 1971; Zamenhof *et al.*, 1971*a,c,f*).

Because hormones exert their effects by binding to specific receptors located selectively on certain target cells, their effects may be localized to particular brain regions and to specific types of cells at restricted times during development. With the exception of the effect of thyroid hormones on myelination (Balázs *et al.*, 1969), which may be a nonspecific effect, and the induction by corticosterone of glycerophosphate dehydrogenase in glial cells (de Vellis, 1973; de Vellis and Kukes, 1973), hormones appear to act primarily on neurons, although glial cells may react to the changes in the neurons. The effects of hormones may be on cell proliferation, cell death, differentiation, growth, and synaptogenesis, and on the synthesis, release, and uptake of synaptic transmitters. It is important to recognize that the effects of hormones on the brain may, and usually do, depend on the dose, stage of development, and type of neuron. These dependencies are shown in the effects of corticosteroids on the rat brain (Vernadakis and Woodbury, 1971) and even more markedly in the effects of thyroxine on the tadpole nervous system. Thyroxine produces stimulation of neuron production in some neuron populations while it retards neuron production in others; it stimulates differentiation of some neurons while it results in death of others (Kollros, 1968*a,b;* Hamburgh, 1968; Decker, 1976).

The effects of thyroid hormone on neuron production during amphibian metamorphosis, especially in the cerebellar cortex (Gona, 1976) and retina (M. Jacobson, 1976*b;* Beach and Jacobson, 1978), are striking cases of the effect of a hormone on production of neurons. As production of neurons has terminated in most parts of the mammalian brain before birth, the effects of hormones on neuron production after birth are restricted mainly to the granule cells of the cerebellar cortex, the dentate gyrus of the hippocampal formation, and the olfactory bulb (see Section 3.1). However, proliferation of granule cells in these regions of the mammalian brain does not appear to be altered by hormones, although the total number of granule cells that ultimately survive may be altered (P. D. Lewis *et al.*, 1976). Glial cell production continues in most regions of the mammalian nervous system after birth, but there is little evidence that, except for the effect during myelination, any hormone acts on glial cell proliferation directly, although glial cells may react to the effects on neurons. With the exception of an effect of thyroid hormones on nerve cell death during amphibian metamorphosis, there is no evidence that hormones directly control or modify cell death in the nervous system, but death of neurons may be secondary to the failure of growth of other neurons with which they connect. Thus death of cerebellar granule cells deprived of their postsynaptic targets has been found as a result of stunting of Purkinje cell dendrites due to deficiency of thyroxine.

The most marked effects of hormones on the nervous system are to stimulate differentiation in the target neurons and particularly to stimulate dendritic growth and synaptogenesis. Growth of dendrites and synaptogenesis appear to have a general dependence on adequate levels of thyroxine, corticosterone, and somatotropin, and deficiency in any of these hormones during the period of dendritic growth results in stunting of dendrites and reduction in the number of dendritic spines and the number of axodendritic synapses. These effects have been reported in the mammalian cerebral and cerebellar cortex, where dendritic growth and synaptogenesis coincide with the period of maximum dependence on thyroxine, sex steroids, and somatotropin (Eayrs, 1955, 1960; Clendinnen and Eayrs, 1961; Balázs *et al.*, 1968; Rebière and Legrand, 1972*a*,*b*).

The fact that either an excess or a deficiency of thyroid hormone or of corticosterone may exert such general effects as reduction of brain DNA content, reduction of growth of dendrites, and reduction of synaptogenesis suggests that these are not the primary effects of the hormones but are produced as secondary effects of metabolic and nutritional disturbances. In such cases, the lecturer may be excused for telling his class: "I wish to correct the statements I made in the last lecture about the effects of hormones on the brain. Whenever I said a 'deficiency' of hormone I meant an 'excess' and whenever I said 'cerebral' cortex I meant 'cerebellar' cortex." Where the effects of the hormone are studied in the intact animal, it is exceedingly difficult to determine the primary effect on the nervous system. There are two methods of avoiding some of these difficulties. First, local implants of the hormone can show effects on brain cells in the vicinity of the implant that are absent elsewhere and thus support a conclusion that identified nerve cells are directly affected by the hormone. The use of tritiated hormones can increase the resolution of the method. Secondly, it may be necessary to study the effects of hormones on brain cells in culture, that is, brain slices containing an essentially normal population of cells (although many cells are isolated from their inputs or targets), as well as on cultures of neurons only or pure cultures of glial cells. Now that such relatively pure cultures of neurons or glial cells can be prepared (McCarthy and Partlow, 1976*a*), the binding of hormones to identified types of nerve cells and the consequent cellular changes may be studied with greater rigor than is possible in the intact organism.

The protean effects of hormones on the developing nervous system are more common but more difficult to understand than the specific effects on identified neurons that subserve particular forms of behavior. The chain of causality from hormone to neuron to behavior can rarely be delineated. However, familiarity with developing systems leads one to the realization that simple chains of cause and effect are rarely found in complex multicellular systems or in the whole animal. When the intact organism is considered, the chains of causality branch into trees and link with others to form causal networks (see Section 7.1). In such complex systems the causal relationships among a hormone, its targets in the brain, and the final functional effects that it produces form an intricate network of cause and effect that may be better studied *in vitro* than in the intact organism.

6.3. Thyroid Hormone Actions on Neural Development

While there are numerous reports of the effects of a deficit or an excess of thyroid hormones on nerve cell proliferation, cell death, neuronal differentiation,synaptogenesis, and myelination, the mechanisms of action of thyroid hormones on the nervous system are not well understood. Pitot and Yatvin (1973), in reviewing the effects of thyroid hormones on enzyme levels, concluded that the present evidence leads to the generalization that thyroid hormones affect many enzyme systems in different ways in different cells. Thyroxine binds to a nuclear receptor and acts at the transcriptional level, probably by increasing RNA polymerase activity. Thyroxine increases the level of thymidine kinase prior to its stimulating effect on DNA synthesis and cell proliferation in the cerebellum of the newborn rat (Weichsel, 1974). These metabolic effects are consistent with the facts that thyroxine accelerates development in the amphibian nervous system (Hambergh, 1969, review) as well as in the mammalian cerebral and cerebellar cortex and that thyroxine stimulates myelination in the central nervous system as well as in peripheral nerves (Balázs, 1974, review). The effect of thyroxine on the nervous system depends on the species, stage of development, and types of target cells.

Thyroid hormones control metamorphosis in the amphibians and thus play a special role in the developmental changes that the nervous system undergoes during metamorphosis. The change from an aquatic to a terrestrial mode of living requires remodeling of many parts of the nervous system correlated with the changes in behavior that are entailed by emergence from water onto land. Studies of these changes can give unparalleled opportunities for enlarging our knowledge of the neuroanatomical and neurophysiological foundations of behavior. The change from a sluggish aquatic browser to a voracious terrestrial predator that occurs when the tadpole changes into a frog involves changes in all the sense organs and sensory systems and development of the central nervous mechanisms controlling posture and locomotion on land. These changes require modification or elimination of some of the nervous structures used by the tadpole, for example, the Mauthner's neuron (Stefanelli, 1950) and the neurons supplying the tail (M. E. Brown, 1946). New structures arising during metamorphosis include addition of the major part of the retina (Pomeranz, 1972; M. Jacobson, 1976*a*, 1977) and the associated visual central projection neurons in the diencephalon and mesencephalon (Currie and Cowan, 1974*a*; M. Jacobson, 1977), development of the cerebellum (Gona, 1972, 1973, 1975, 1976) and the mesencephalic nucleus of the trigeminal nerve (Kollros and McMurray, 1956), and changes in the sensory innervation of the skin (M. Jacobson and Baker, 1969). Thyroid hormones play a part in regulating all these changes. In no other case can the effects of a hormone on nerve cell production, differentiation, and death be correlated with the changes in behavior so effectively as they can during amphibian metamorphosis.

Administration of thyroxine to amphibian larvae results in precocious maturation of the nervous system. Thyroxine applied locally to various parts of the nervous system of amphibians hastens the development of the neurons that are directly affected by the hormone. A direct effect of thyroxine has been shown on the corneal reflex center (Kollros, 1943*a*), the mesencephalic V nucleus (Kollros and Pepernik, 1952; Kollros and McMurray, 1956), and Mauthner's neuron (Weiss and Rossetti, 1951; Pesetsky and Kollros, 1956; Pesetsky, 1960, 1962).

Thyroxine applied to the medulla of the frog tadpole causes precocious development of the corneal reflex on that side compared with the opposite side (Kollros, 1942, 1943*a*). The corneal reflex consists of retraction of the eye in response to mechanical stimulation of the cornea. It starts during metamorphosis and is not present in younger tadpoles, although all the peripheral mechanisms are present, presumably because the central reflex mechanisms mature only during metamorphosis (Kollros, 1958).

Kollros and McMurray (1956) showed that thyroxine implanted in the midbrain of the frog tadpole results in a graded increase in size of the neurons of the mesencephalic V nucleus. Increase in size of the neuron perikarya varies inversely with the distance from the source of the hormone. Hypophysectomy or administration of thiourea to frog tadpoles results in a reduction in size of neurons of the mesencephalic V nucleus, which indicates that the growth of the neurons depends on continuous stimulation by thyroxine (Kollros and McMurray, 1956).

The effects of thyroxine on mitosis in the central nervous system of amphibians have been described by Baffoni (1957*b*, 1959, 1960). After administration of thyroxine to frog tadpoles, he observed an initial increase, followed by a decrease, in the number of mitotic figures in various parts of the brain. No increase in the final size of the brain appears to result from treatment with thyroxine. Although thyroidectomized tadpoles may attain giant size, they have brains smaller than normal controls (B. M. Allen, 1924). It is not known whether the reduction in brain size is due to a reduction in cell number, cell size, or myelin formation. Ferguson (1966) found that after unilateral excision of the medulla of frog tadpoles, thyroxine increases the mitotic activity that occurs during regeneration of the medulla. However, the extent of restitution of the excised half is the same in animals treated with thyroxine as in untreated frogs. He concluded: "exogenous thyroxine merely accelerates mitotic activity in neurons ready or nearly ready to divide and . . . upon termination of division an overall decline in proliferation occurs."

The effects of thyroxine on neurons in the spinal cord and spinal ganglia are complicated by the fact that thyroxine directly stimulates growth of the limbs and resorption of the tail, and this in turn results in an increase in the size and number of neurons in the spinal cord and ganglia supplying the limbs, and in degeneration of the neurons supplying the tail. During metamorphosis the neurons that supply the tadpole tail degenerate. There is some evidence that the primary action of thyroxine is on the tail (R. Weber, 1962), whereas the degeneration of neurons in the tail occurs secondarily as a result of the loss of their peripheral connections (M. E. Brown, 1946). Histolysis of muscles of the tadpole tail is well advanced before degenerative changes appear in the neurons of the spinal cord that supply the tail. Moreover, nerve degeneration starts peripherally, and retrograde degeneration proceeds slowly toward the cell bodies, which suggests that the primary cause of degeneration is the loss of peripheral connections in the tail rather than a direct effect of thyroxine on the spinal neurons during metamorphosis (M. E. Brown, 1946).

Beaudoin (1955) observed that the cells of the lateral motor column of the spinal cord of *Rana pipiens* are generated, migrate, and grow steadily until midlarval stages, but at the time when thyroxine causes rapid growth of the hindlimbs, more than two-thirds of the lateral motor neurons degenerate while the surviving neurons increase in size. Beaudoin (1956) showed that thyroxine can influence the development of the spinal motor neurons of the frog, directly or indirectly, by stimulating limb growth. Implantation of thyroxine into one hindlimb of a frog tadpole causes precocious growth of the limb and an increase in the size of the neurons of the lateral motor column on that side. However, thyroxine also has a direct effect on the frog spinal motor neurons, as was shown in two ways by Beaudoin (1956). First, amputation of the limb bud at early larval stages, followed later by immersion of the tadpole in thyroxine solutions, results in more rapid loss of motor neurons on the operated side than that occurring without the influence of thyroxine. Second, thyroxine implanted adjacent to the spinal cord results in an increase in the size of the lateral motor neurons on that side.

Hypophysectomy arrests the differentiation of neurons of the lateral motor column of the spinal cord of *Rana pipiens* (Race, 1961), whereas immersion of *Rana pipiens* embryos or early larvae in thyroxine solutions results in precocious maturation of the lateral motor column neurons (Reynolds, 1963). Thyroxine is not necessary for the initial formation, migration, and early differentiation of lateral motor column neurons, as a typical column forms in hypophysectomized tadpoles (Race, 1961). Reynolds (1963) concluded that the capacity of the lateral column neurons to respond to thyroxine is not present before late embryonic stages (Stage 25 of Shumway, 1940, 1942). A. F. Hughes (1966) showed that differentiation of lateral motor neurons in *Eleutherodactylus* is accelerated by thyroxine and retarded by treatment with thiourea. However, thyroidectomy or hypophysectomy in *Eleutherodactylus* does not prevent the loss of lateral motor neurons, while hypophysectomy prevents the reduction in the number of lateral motor neurons in *Rana pipiens* (Race, 1961).

In summary: The effects of thyroxine on neurons of the lateral motor column in anurans are acceleration of cytodifferentiation of neurons and perhaps hastening of the degeneration of the motor neurons that have failed to make peripheral connections. There is little evidence that thyroxine affects proliferation or migration of neurons (Kollros, 1968*a,b,* reviews), but adequate experiments using tritiated thymidine autoradiography have not yet been performed.

The difficulty of distinguishing local or primary effects of thyroxine from its general or secondary effects on neurons is illustrated by the conflicting reports of the hormone's effects on the Mauthner's neurons in the medulla of larval anurans. During normal metamorphosis the level of thyroxine increases to a climax and declines thereafter. Mauthner's neurons increase in size during normal metamorphosis and then slowly degenerate after normal metamorphosis (Fig. 6.3) or after precocious metamorphosis induced experimentally with thyroxine (Baffoni and

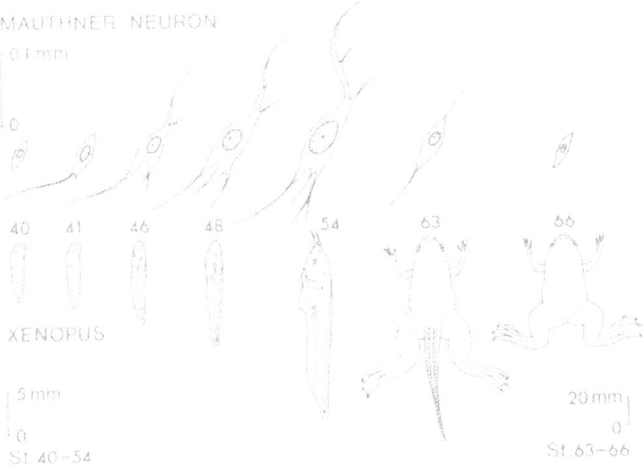

Figure 6.3. Mauthner's neuron in *Xenopus* during larval development at Stages 40–54 of the normal series of Nieuwkoop and Faber (1956), showing their differentiation and growth during larval stages, the atrophy of the neuron during metamorphosis, and degeneration in the adult.

Catte, 1950, 1951; Baffoni, 1953; Stefanelli, 1950, 1951; H. Fox and Moulton, 1968; Moulton *et al.,* 1968). Stefanelli (1950) concluded that degeneration of Mauthner's neurons is a secondary effect of degeneration of the motor neurons in the tail and the lateral lines. However, there is evidence that Mauthner's neurons do not depend for their growth and maintenance on the size of their peripheral field. The size of Mauthner's neurons in the frog tadpole is not affected by removal of the tail (Weiss and Rossetti, 1951) or by unilateral ablation of posterior lateralis nerves (Pesetsky, 1960). Mauthner's neurons also develop normally in grafts of rhombencephalic portions of embryonic *Rana pipiens* heads in which the Mauthner's neurons are isolated from motor centers and are connected with a reduced number of lateral line organs (Pesetsky, 1960).

Since the regression of Mauthner's neurons following amphibian metamorphosis cannot be attributed to a reduction of their axonal load, one has to consider whether it may be due to direct action of thyroxine on the neurons, or whether death of Mauthner's neurons is predetermined by a mechanism like that of the "death clock," which results in cell death in the developing limb (Saunders, 1966; Saunders and Fallon, 1966). That the death of Mauthner's neurons is not preordained is indicated by the fact that the neurons survive indefinitely if metamorphosis is delayed with thiourea. Evidence that Mauthner's neurons respond directly to thyroxine is that implantation of thyroxine pellets on one side of the medulla results in decrease in the size of Mauthner's neuron and increase in the size of the surrounding medullary neurons on the side of the thyroxine implant (Weiss and Rossetti, 1951; Pesetsky and Kollros, 1956). Pesetsky (1962) has suggested that the decrease in size of Mauthner's neurons observed after implantation of thyroid pellets is due to withdrawal of the hormone when the implanted pellet becomes depleted of thyroxine. He found that Mauthner's neurons increase in size when tadpoles are immersed in high concentrations of thyroxine (Pesetsky, 1962) and diminish in size in thyroidectomized tadpoles (Pesetsky, 1966). Pesetsky proposed that the growth of Mauthner's neurons is stimulated by thyroxine during the late larval stages and that the neurons develop a dependence on the hormone; therefore, he thought, the reduction in the level of thyroxine in the blood that occurs at the climax of metamorphosis (Etkin, 1964) may result in involution of Mauthner's neurons. The Rohon-Beard neurons in the spinal cord of frog tadpoles also increase in size in response to thyroxine (L. B. Stephens, 1965). In both these cases, the initial increase in size of the neuron may merely be due to increased water content, not to growth, and is thus an early change leading to cell death.

Tissue culture offers a method of resolving the difficulties of determining whether thyroxine has a direct or indirect effect on the nervous system. Hamburgh and Bunge (1964) have shown that thyroxine has a direct effect, accelerating the growth and maturation of rat cerebellar neurons in tissue culture. Thyroxine greatly increases the myelination of axons of rat cerebellar neurons *in vitro* (Hamburgh and Bunge, 1964; Hamburgh, 1968). By the application of [^{125}I]thyroxine and [^{125}I]triiodothyronine to tissue culture of mammalian nervous tissue, Manuelidis and Bornstein (1970) showed that the labeled thyroid hormones are located mainly on neurons, and particularly over the nucleolus.

In mammals, thyroxine deprivation during intrauterine development does not affect the development of the fetal brain (Hamburgh, 1968). However, thyroidectomy or the administration of antithyroid drugs to mammals during the postnatal period results in failure of growth and maturation of the cerebral cortex

(Eayrs, 1955, 1960; Gomez *et al.,* 1966) and in a delay in the maturation of the cerebellar cortex (Legrand, 1963; Legrand *et al.,* 1961; Hamburgh, 1968).

Neonatal thyroidectomy of rats results in marked reduction in the growth of the brain after 14 days of age. This is due to a decrease in myelination (Balázs *et al.,* 1969) and a reduction in volume of neurons, but not to a reduction in the number of cells (Geel and Timiras, 1967; J. M. Pasquini *et al.,* 1967; Balázs *et al.,* 1968). The development of dendrites is retarded and the degree of dendritic branching is reduced in the cerebral cortex of hypothyroid mammals (Eayrs, 1955). The number of axodendritic synapses in the cerebral cortex also seems to be reduced in rats after neonatal thyroidectomy (Balźs *et al.,* 1968). These changes are associated with behavioral changes (Eayrs and Lishman, 1953; Eayrs, 1960) and changes in the electroencephalogram (P. B. Bradley *et al.,* 1960*a,b*).

Reduction in the number of synapses in the molecular layer of the cerebellum of hypothyroid rats, as seen by electron microscopy (Nicholson and Altman, 1972) or as shown by assay of the synaptosomal fraction of cerebellar homogenates (Rabié and Legrand, 1973), has been considered to indicate a direct effect of thyroid hormones on synaptogenesis. However, evidence to the contrary is that cerebellar axodendritic synapses appear normal in hypothyroid rats (M. C. Brown *et al.,* 1976) and that the primary effect of hypothyroidism seems to be on dendritic growth. This illustrates the difficulty of distinguishing between primary and secondary effects of the hormone on synaptogenesis.

The effect of thyroid hormone on cell proliferation in the cerebellar external granule layer is now fairly clear. Thyroidectomy of newborn rats results in a 25 percent reduction in the cerebellar DNA content by the end of the second week, but the external granule layer persists for longer in hypothyroid rats and the normal DNA content of the cerebellum is ultimately reached in the fourth or fifth postnatal week (Legrand, 1967*a,b;* Balázs *et al.,* 1968; Patel *et al.,* 1976). Nicholson and Altman (1972) suggested that lack of thyroxine results in a reduced rate of cell proliferation, but more careful observations have shown no changes in the length of the cell cycle and duration of phases of the cell cycle (P. D. Lewis *et al.,* 1976). The retardation is due to death of granule cells that fail to make adequate connections with Purkinje cell dendritic spines. The primary effect of hypothyroidism on the neonatal cerebellum is to produce stunting of dendrite development, and the secondary consequences are failure of synaptogenesis, death of some granule cells, and probably some reactive hypertrophy of astrocytes.

The effect of neonatal thyroid deficiency on development of the cerebrum is primarily on differentiation and growth, resulting in a reduction of dendritic growth and synaptogenesis. Thyroid deficiency produces no changes in the length of the cell cycle, the phases of the cycle, or DNA synthesis in the subependymal layer of the lateral ventricle (P. D. Lewis *et al.,* 1976). Cell proliferation in the subependymal layer mainly or exclusively produces glial cells (see Section 3.2), so that lack of thyroid apparently does not impair neuron production in the forebrain. This is also consistent with the observation that postnatal increase in DNA content of the forebrain is not altered by thyroid deficiency (Patel *et al.,* 1976). However, the DNA content of the olfactory bulb is reduced after neonatal hypothyroidism, indicating that some loss of neurons, probably granule cells, occurs there.

Postnatal treatment of rats with thyroxine results in a decrease in brain weight and body weight, accelerates the histogenesis and morphogenesis of the cerebellar cortex (Nicholson and Altman, 1972; Clos *et al.,* 1974), and increases the number of dendritic spines in layer IV of the visual cortex (Schapiro *et al.,* 1973). Thyroxine stimulates DNA synthesis in the cerebellum of the rat 2–6 days postnatally, but by 12 days of age the cerebellar DNA content is reduced below normal levels (Weichsel, 1974). A similar early increase by 6 days of age, before a later decline in DNA content of the cerebellum, was noted by Gourdon *et al.* (1973). The ultimate decrease has also been found by Balázs *et al.* (1971), who administered large doses of triiodothyronine to newborn rats and recorded a 20–30 percent reduction in the body weight and brain weight at 50 days of age. The reduced brain weight was found to be due to a 30–40 percent reduction in the number of brain cells formed after birth. They concluded, erroneously as it now seems, that the effect is probably on cell formation rather than cell death, and that the growth of brain cells and their size are not affected by triiodothyronine. Other evidence, however, shows that the loss of cerebral DNA following thyroxine treatment of neonatal rats is the result of reduced Purkinje cell dendritic growth, which, in turn, results in death of granule cells deprived of their synaptic targets on the Purkinje cell dendritic spines (P. D. Lewis *et al.,* 1976).

6.4. Sex Hormones in Brain Development

The concept of sexual dimorphism of the nervous system arises from observations of differences in behavior, brain function, and structure between males and females. How, then, do such differences develop: how much is due to genetic differences, and how much is organized and activated by hormones? Ancillary questions are concerned with the age at which the hormonal effects normally occur or can be produced experimentally, and with the target areas of the brain and cellular mechanisms of action of the hormones.

Sex determination is primarily genetic in that the development of the gronads is under genetic control, as is the subsequent gonadal secretion of hormones (J. L. Goldstein and Wilson, 1975). The sex steroids, testosterone and estradiol, enter the cells of the target tissues and bind to specific receptors in the cytoplasm of the target tissues, where their effects are to increase RNA and protein synthesis (O'Malley and Means, 1974; Liao, 1975, reviews). Testosterone is the only androgen formed by the fetal testes in rabbit and man, and it is enzymatically converted to dihydrotestosterone. These two androgens have different peripheral and nervous target tissues both prenatally and postnatally. In the fetus, testosterone promotes virilization of the urogenital tract by acting on the Wolffian duct to induce the development of the epididymis, vas deferens, and seminal vesicle. Its action on the nervous system will be discussed below. Dihydrotestosterone acts on the urogenital sinus to induce the formation of the prostate and on the urogenital tubercle to induce development of the male external genitalia. Dihydrotestosterone has no effect on sexual behavior, although it can stimulate gonadotropin release in adult rats.

The secondary sexual characteristics that are organized by gonadal hormones include not only those of the genitalia and secondary sexual organs but also the appropriate brain functions that subserve sexually dimorphic behavior (Money and Ehrhardt, 1972, review). The subsequent development of sexual behavior in mammals is determined by or modified by sex hormones that bind to specific receptors in the brain regions which subserve sexual behavior and gonadotropin release from the pituitary. Adult male and female mammals differ in their phenotype as well as in their sexual behavior and in the pattern of their gonadotropin secretion. Females have a cyclic pattern whereas males have a tonic pattern of gonadotropin secretion, gonadal hormone secretion, and sexual activity. The patterns are largely under the control of the hypothalamus. All mammals have, to a degree which varies with species, the potential for both male and female patterns of behavior, and the behavior pattern that eventually develops is the outcome of hormonal stimulation of the brain at the appropriate time. The neurons subserving male sexual behavior differentiate in some unknown manner under the influence of testosterone. It is not known whether the effect of testosterone is to alter the electrical activity of these neurons, producing changes in synthesis, secretion, or uptake of neurotransmitters, or whether changes in their connections are produced by the hormone. This problem is not likely to be elucidated until the neuronal circuits mediating sexual behavior are more adequately characterized. The evidence is scanty showing an effect of sex hormones on synaptogenesis. Androgenization of female rats results in changes in the morphology of synaptic endings in the arcuate nucleus (Ratner and Adamo, 1971). Sexual dimorphism in the number of nonamygdaloid synapses on the dendritic spines of neurons in the preoptic nucleus of the adult rat has been found by Raisman and Field (1973*a*), the male having fewer synapses than the female. They reported that the number of synapses in the androgenized female is as low as in the male and that in males castrated shortly after birth the number of synapses increases to the female level.

A single injection of testosterone given to a female or castrated male rat within the first few days after birth results in male sexual behavior at maturity (Segal and Johnson, 1959; G. W. Harris and Levine, 1962, 1965; Grady *et al.,* 1965; S. Levine and Mullins, 1966). There is considerable evidence that prior to a critical period the central nervous structures controlling sexual behavior in mammals of both sexes are undifferentiated (G. W. Harris, 1964; G. W. Harris and Levine, 1965; Gorski, 1966). During this critical period, sexual differentiation of the neural tissues mediating masculine sexual behavior occurs under the influence of testosterone, while feminine sexual behavior ensues in the absence of testosterone. Female or male rats castrated at birth will develop male sexual behavior at maturity if they are given a single injection of testosterone in the first 10 days after birth (Grady *et al.,* 1965; Adams Smith, 1967).

In the male, the level of testosterone in the blood increases during the perinatal period, declines after birth, and rises again at puberty. The perinatal rise in testosterone levels is required for the *organization* of neural mechanisms subserving male sexual behavior, while the increased testosterone at puberty is required for *activation* of some of the neural mechanisms resulting in masculine behavior. The perinatal testosterone has a priming effect on tissues whose full expression of male function is triggered by the increased testosterone normally secreted at puberty. Thus it is customary to distinguish between the *organizing action* of the hormone on the brain during development and the *activating action* of the hormone in the adult. Some types of behavior require an action of the hormone only during development, for example, the leg-lifting during micturition in male dogs or mounting in male monkeys. These forms of behavior are displayed by females that are masculinized by testosterone given prenatally or neonatally. Other types of behavior require hormonal activation as well as organization, for example, mounting in the rat. Thus females that are masculinized by testosterone at birth exhibit male mating behavior only when it is activated by hormones. Yet other kinds of sexually dimorphic behavior, such as the masculine "yawn" in the monkey, require activation but not organization, and therefore can be produced in normal adult females treated with androgens (F. A. Beach, 1975, review).

One difficulty of studying the effects of neonatal castration arises from species differences in the effects of prenatal androgens, because the duration of exposure of the fetus to androgens varies with the length of gestation. In hamsters, in which gestation lasts only 16 days, castration of males on the day of birth results in abolition of the activating effect of testosterone given to the adult (Noble, 1973). By contrast, castration of male rats (gestation 22 days) on the day of birth does not abolish the mounting that results from testosterone treatment in adults (Grady *et al.*, 1965). Conversely, in the female rat, administration of testosterone prenatally and postnatally results in a marked increase in mounting behavior. Even a single injection of testosterone given to female rats on the fourth day of life can result in increased mounting under certain conditions (Södersten, 1973), whereas dihydrotestosterone given prenatally or postnatally has no such effect on female rats (Whalen and Luttge, 1971*a,b*). This difference has been attributed to the fact that testosterone is converted to estradiol, whereas dihydrotestosterone is not. The conversion of testosterone to estradiol occurs *in vitro* in brain tissue incubated with some androgens (Reddy *et al.*, 1974), as well as in the intact perfused brain (Flores *et al.*, 1973). Estradiol accumulates in neonatal rat brain cell nuclei after administration of testosterone, indicating that estradiol is a normal metabolite of testosterone (Lieberburg and McEwen, 1975).

The uptake of [^{3}H]testosterone from the bloodstream by the brains of male rats and of [^{3}H]estradiol by the brains of female rats was first shown by scintillation counting of extracts of brain, and these studies indicate that the hormones are concentrated in the anterior hypothalamus and preoptic region (Eisenfeld and Axelrod, 1965; Kato and Villee, 1967; Resko *et al.*, 1967). Binding of sex steroids also occurs in the septum, amygdala, and hippocampus (McEwen and Pfaff, 1970). Although binding of tritiated testosterone has been shown by autoradiography as will be discussed below, there has been no success in isolating the testosterone receptor from prenatal and neonatal brain tissue, and only limited success in the biochemical identification of specific testosterone receptors in the adult mammalian brain (Jouan *et al.*, 1971, 1973). A component of the adult rat hypothalamus that binds dihydrotestosterone has been isolated (Kato and Onouchi, 1973). Evidence of more precisely localized nervous uptake of sex hormones has been obtained by autoradiography of sections of brain following intravenous injection of [^{3}H]testosterone or [^{3}H]estradiol (Pfaff, 1968*a,b,c;* Pfaff and Keiner, 1973; Morrell *et al.*, 1975, review).

Failure of the initial attempts to detect brain cells that bind to hormones occurred because of limitations of the autoradiographic technique for detecting tritiated hormones bound to brain cells. In all such studies published before 1968, movement of radioactive molecules in the tissues occurred because liquid fixatives were used, thus greatly reducing the accuracy of localization of the hormone in the nervous system. Only after introduction of the dry-mount autoradiographic technique (W. E. Stumpf, 1971*a*, review) could accurate mapping of hormone target cells be achieved.

There is a remarkable similarity in the anatomical distribution of sex hormone binding sites in males and females and in all vertebrate orders, and where species specializations have been found the brain sites of sex hormone accumulation are also implicated in species-specific sexual behavior. For example, mating behavior, song, and other vocalizations in the male chaffinch are dependent on testosterone, and there is testosterone binding to neurons in the midbrain and other regions that are implicated in the hormone-dependent behavior (R. E. Zigmond *et al.,* 1973). The pattern of labeling of the male brain with [^{3}H]testosterone (Morrell *et al.,* 1975) is quite similar but not identical to that of the female brain with [^{3}H]estradiol. Most if not all the label seems to be associated with the nuclei of neurons, although some glial cells are also labeled (Pfaff and Keiner, 1973). The preoptic region, tuberal region of the hypothalamus, rostral regions of the limbic system and hypothalamus, and the mesencephalon underneath the tectum are sites of sex steroid binding in all vertebrates, and these are also regions that have been implicated in sexual behavior and in gonadotropin release (Fig. 6.4).

It has long been known that a small percentage of normal female mammals of many different species will exhibit male sexual behavior, while the spontaneous display of female sexual behavior by male mammals is much rarer (F. A. Beach, 1975). It now appears that such "atypical behavior" may be due to the fact that, in both sexes, the hormone which alters sexual behavior is estradiol and the effect of estradiol on the developing brain is to produce male sexual behavior. Naftolin *et al.* (1971*a,b,* 1972) have proposed that testosterone is converted to estradiol in the brain and that the masculinizing effect of testosterone is mediated by estradiol.

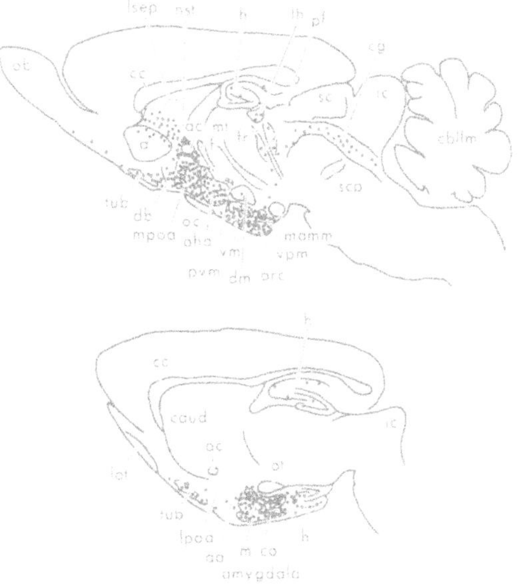

Figure 6.4. Distribution of estrogen-concentrating neurons in the brain of the female rat represented schematically in two sagittal sections. Most labeled neurons could be represented in a medial plane (bottom drawing). Estradiol-concentrating neurons in the amygdala and hippocampus are represented in a more lateral plane (top drawing). Locations of estradiol-concentrating neurons are represented by black dots. a, Nucleus accumbens; aa, anterior amygdaloid area; ac, anterior commissure; aha, anterior hypothalamic area; arc, arcuate nucleus; caud, caudate nucleus; cbllm, cerebellum; cc, corpus callosum; cg, central gray; co, cortical nucleus of the amygdala; db, diagonal band of Broca; dm, dorsomedial nucleus of the hypothalamus; f, fornix; fr, fasciculus retroflexus; h, hippocampus; ic, inferior colliculus; lh, lateral habenula; lot, lateral olfactory tract; lpoa, lateral preoptic area; lsep, lateral septum; m, medial nucleus of the amygdala; mamm, mammillary bodies; mpoa, medial preoptic area; mt, mammillothalamic tract; nst, bed nucleus of the stria terminalis; ob, olfactory bulb; oc, optic chiasm; ot, optic tract; pf, nucleus parafascicularis; pvm, paraventricular nucleus (magnocellular); sc, superior colliculus; scp, superior cerebellar peduncle; tub, olfactory tubercle; vm, ventral premammillary nucleus. From D. W. Pfaff and M. Keiner, *J. Comp Neurol.* *151:*121–158 [1973].

Fetal and neonatal blood contains an estrogen binding protein, that is identical to the α-fetoprotein, that prevents the estrogen from entering the developing brain (Raynaud *et al.,* 1971; B. Attardi and Ruoslahti, 1976). Testosterone, or synthetic estrogen such as diethylstilbestrol, does not bind to this protein and is free to enter the developing brain (McEwen *et al.,* 1975). In the brain, testosterone is converted to estradiol particularly well in the hypothalamus, amygdala, and preoptic area, but not in the cerebral cortex, which nevertheless contains specific nuclear estrogen receptors (Lieberburg and McEwen, 1975; McEwen *et al.,* 1976). The masculinizing effects of testosterone as well as estrogen in the fetus and neonate are apparently mediated by the brain estrogen receptors. These effects refer to the developing brain only. In the adult, testosterone is preferentially bound by the hypothalamus in the male whereas estradiol is preferentially bound by the female hypothalamus (Plapinger and McEwen 1973; Plapinger *et al.,* 1973). This selectivity is not present in prenatal and neonatal rats before sexual differentiation of the hypothalamus occurs (Tuohimaa and Niemi, 1972). Experimental androgenization of female rats as well as the normal masculinization of the brain of male rats results in loss of the capacity of the hypothalamus to accumulate estradiol (Tuohimaa and Johansson, 1971; Vertes *et al.,* 1973).

Whereas in animals androgenized females exhibit masculine sexual behavior, in human females who have been androgenized *in utero* the suppression of feminine behavior is minimal, although there is some behavioral masculinization. The remarkable observation on such human females who have been exposed to androgens prenatally and also female pseudohermaphrodites with the adrenogenital syndrome is that they have unusually high IQ (Ehrhardt and Money, 1967; V. G. Lewis *et al.,* 1968; Money, 1971; P. A. Walker and Money, 1972; Money and Ehrhardt, 1972, review). In a sample of 70 boys and girls with the adrenogenital syndrome, Money and Lewis (1966) reported a slightly increased mean IQ (mean full IQ 109.9), indicating that prenatal androgens have an elevating effect on the ultimate IQ. The effect is greater in girls exposed to androgens prenatally as a result of administration to the mother of steroids with an androgenic action, to prevent miscarriage. Ehrhardt and Money (1967) reported that in ten such girls the mean full IQ was 125 (S.D. 11.8), and six had an IQ above 130. A similar increase in IQ is found in males exposed to excess androgen *in utero* (Money and Ehrhardt, 1972, p. 102). Such findings raise virtually insoluble questions about the relationships between human intelligence and the brain structures and functions sensitive to hormone stimulation. Are there specific structures stimulated by hormones that increase IQ, or is the effect a general one, resulting in an increase in the total number of neurons or total number of synaptic connections, or merely in the efficiency of functions of neurons responsible for the elevated IQ?

6.5. Effects of Adrenal Glucocorticoids on Brain Development

Adrenal glucocorticoids bind to proteins in the nucleus and cytoplasm of brain cells. After injection of [^{3}H]cortisol to rats, a stereotyped pattern of labeling is seen in autoradiographs (W. E. Stumpf, 1971*a*; McEwen *et al.,* 1974; Pfaff *et al.,* 1976). The most heavily labeled cells are the granule cells of the hippocampal dentate gyrus. Lighter labeling is seen over large portions of the hippocampal formation, indusium griseum, septal nuclei, pyriform cortex, and portions of the amygdala. This localization of glucocorticoid target cells is in marked contrast to the distribution of cells that bind sex steroids, which are mainly localized to the hypothalamus in the preoptic, septal, and parolfactory areas and in the amygdala.

There is also evidence that glial cells have glucocorticoid receptors. The evidence has been summarized by de Vellis and Kukes (1973) that the enzyme glycerophosphate dehydrogenase, localized in glial cells, is specifically induced by cortisol in developing rat brain as well as in cultured glial cells. Hydrocortisone also induces the synthesis of glutamine synthetase in the neural retina of the chick embryo and in cultured chick embryo cerebral cells (Piddington, 1967). The effect of corticosteroids on glial cells is significant because these hormones are not secreted in the embryo during the period of neuron production but only during the period of glial cell production. In the chick embryo, the pituitary–adrenal axis develops in the last third of incubation (Woods *et al.,* 1971).

The effects of corticosterone administered to newborn mice are to reduce DNA synthesis (Cotterrell *et al.,* 1972) and to reduce brain weight (E. Howard, 1965, 1968). The effect is, as expected, on the cerebellar cortex, where DNA content is diminished by 15 percent below control values, and on the cerebral cortex, where the DNA content is reduced 18 percent below control values at 14 days of age (E. Howard, 1968). In the cerebrum, where no addition of neurons occurs postnatally, the reduction of DNA content is probably due to reduction of glial cells. An effect on neuronal growth has been shown, namely retardation of growth of dendritic spines in the cerebral cortex of rats treated postnatally with corticosteroids. The interpretation of these results is complicated by the fact that corticosteroids administered to newborn mammals result in a loss of body weight of about the same magnitude as the loss of brain weight. We know that nutritional deprivation, with resulting loss of body weight, also results in loss of brain weight and brain DNA content (see Section 6.1). Therefore, the present evidence does not allow us to ascribe the loss of brain DNA content and brain weight to the direct effect of corticosteroids on the brain rather than to an indirect effect on nutrition and body weight.

6.6. Role of Growth Hormone in Neural Ontogeny

Studies of the effects of growth hormone on the developing nervous system have been limited not only by technical difficulties such as contamination of the growth hormone with other trophic hormones of the anterior pituitary but also by uncertainties regarding the site and mode of action of the hormone on the nervous system. Some of these limitations are apparent in the study of the effects of growth hormone on *Rana pipiens* tadpoles (Zamenhof, 1941). A preparation of growth hormone was injected for 12–22 days on alternate days into tadpoles at the stages of limb growth. The treated animals showed a 44–126 percent increase in the number of cells (neurons and glia) in the cerebral hemispheres, in comparison with normal controls. It was concluded that the growth hormone stimulates cellular proliferation in the brain. However, the alternative, that the hormone might reduce cell death, was not considered. Moreover, an impure preparation of growth hormone was used, and the increase in cells might have been produced by adrenocorticotropin, thyrotropin, and prolactin that were probably present in the injections. The effects of purified prolactin or growth hormone on the brain of *Rana pipiens* during development were studied by R. K. Hunt and Jacobson (1970, 1971). They found that six injections of prolactin (5 μg) administered to early larvae produced a 20–25 percent increase in brain weight and a 35–43 percent increase in total brain DNA at metamorphosis. In contrast, six injections of growth hormone (25 μg) increased brain weight by 12–20 percent and brain DNA by 10–15 percent. Additional studies with [^{3}H]thymidine suggest that the effects of both hormones are at least partially due to increased cellular proliferation, although the patterns of precursor incorporation are quite different in the two cases. The rate of incorporation of [^{3}H]thymidine into DNA in the brain nearly doubles during the period of growth hormone injections, but returns to the control rate shortly thereafter. Conversely, prolactin only slightly increases the rate of DNA synthesis in the brain during the injection period, but the rate of DNA synthesis is markedly increased during the following 10-day period when it normally declines.

Growth hormone administered to rats after birth does not increase the size or weight of the nervous system (Rubenstein, 1936; Zamenhof, 1942; M. C. Diamond *et al.*, 1969). Hypophysectomy of rats a few days after birth does not alter brain weight, brain protein content, thickness of the cerebral cortex, or branching of basal dendrites of cortical pyramidal cells (M. C. Diamond *et al.*, 1964, 1969; Gregory and Diamond, 1968*a,b*). This shows either that growth hormone secreted after birth is not important in the postnatal development of the rat brain or that growth hormone and other pituitary trophic hormones persist or are able to continue acting in the brain after hypophysectomy.

By contrast with the negative results of injecting growth hormone postnatally, administration of growth hormone to pregnant female rats has been shown to affect the nervous system of the offspring. Zamenhof (1942) injected pregnant female rats with an impure preparation of growth hormone (Antuitrin G) daily from days 7 to 20 of gestation, and examined the brain of the fetuses at birth (delivered by caesarian section at term) or after reaching maturity. Compared with control rats, the offspring of the treated females had an increase of 18.7 percent in body weight, 36 percent in cerebral hemisphere weight, 21 percent in the thickness of the cerebral cortex, and 86 percent in the number of cells in the entire cortex. The rats that developed to adults had an increase of 15–28 percent in cell density and 38–41 percent in the total number of cells in the cerebral cortex as compared with counts in untreated rats. The accuracy of these cell counts is questionable because no corrections were made for shrinkage of the brains during fixation or for the increase in cell size in the treated animals, which are sources of serious error (Abercrombie, 1946; Hendry, 1976). Moreover, the preparation of growth hormone used in the experiments was contaminated by detectable amounts of other hormones of the anterior pituitary (footnote in Clendinnen and Eayrs, 1961).

In a later series of experiments, Zamenhof *et al.* (1966) reported that purified growth hormone administered to pregnant rats resulted in a 10–20 percent increase in the weight and DNA content of the brain of the offspring and comparable increases in density of cells in the cerebral cortex, in number and length of dendrites of cortical pyramidal cells, and in the ratio of neurons to glia. Therefore, they concluded that prenatally administered growth hormone primarily affects the neurons and results in a relatively greater increase in the number rather than the size of neurons. This conclusion is not supported by the results of Clendinnen and Eayrs (1961), who studied the offspring of rats given daily injections of purified growth hormone from day 7 to day 20 of gestation. These offspring are slightly heavier at birth, and their motor activity matures somewhat earlier than normal controls. At 33 and 60 days of age, the cell–gray coefficient (the proportion of cortex occupied by cell bodies) was found to be increased by 20 percent above the normal value in the treated rats. There was a 22 percent increase in the mean length of dendrites and a 23 percent increase in the mean number of dendritic branches of cerebral cortical neurons (Fig. 6.5). These observations indicate that an increase in neuronal size and probably of connectivity occurs, but there is no evidence of an increase in the number of neurons. Because the histology of the cerebral cortex was studied at 33 and 60 days, after the growth of dendrites and the formation of synapses in the cerebral cortex are virtually completed in normal rats, these observations do not show whether the maturation of the cortex occurs earlier in rats treated prenatally with growth hormone or whether maturation occurs at the usual time postnatally, with a time lag after prenatal administration.

Whether the effects represent the primary response to the hormone or a secondary response is often impossible to decide. Secondary effects may be on the general metabolism or nutrition of the animal or on the hypothalamopituitary axis, resulting in changes in other hormones. Interactions between thyroid hormone and growth hormone have been demonstrated in rats in the control of skeletal growth, and in the control of RNA content in the cerebral cortex (Geel and Timiras, 1970). Growth hormone (400 μg/100 g body weight per day) produces no increase in body or brain growth in hypothyroid rats in the first 25 days after birth. A similar problem regarding the mode of action of the hormone arises in connection with reports of stimulation of brain development in the fetus after administration of growth hormone to the mother (Zamenhof *et al.*, 1966, 1971*c*; Sara and Lazarus, 1974; Sara *et al.*, 1974). The problem with these results is that growth hormone does not cross the placenta from mother to fetus (Gitlin *et al.*, 1965; Laron *et al.*, 1966). The growth hormone may affect the fetus indirectly by mobilizing maternal nutrient supplies, may increase uterine size and blood

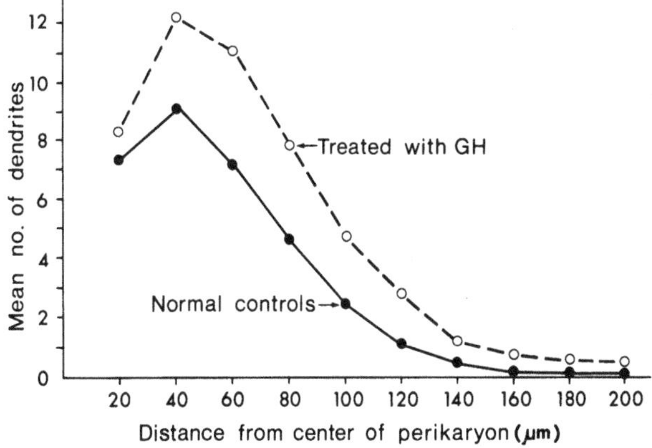

Figure 6.5. Distribution of basal dendrites of pyramidal cells in layer IIIc of the sensorimotor cortex of rats at 33 and 60 days of age, treated prenatally with growth hormones, compared with normal controls. From B. G. Clendinnen and J. T. Eayrs, *J. Endocrinol. 22:*183–193 (1961).

supply, may increase placental size, or may enhance maternal hormonal mechanisms that stimulate fetal growth.

Another factor that may confound the assessment of the prenatal action of growth hormone is the fact that the hormone prolongs gestation (Croskerry and Smith, 1975). In many of the reports of increased brain weight at birth, the animals may well have been postmature. No increase in body or brain weight is found in rats after prenatal treatment with growth hormone when the fetuses are delivered by caesarian section near term (Croskerry *et al.,* 1973).

The conflicting results obtained by different investigators are indicative of the uncertainties and sources of error in such experiments in which there are many uncontrolled variables. Variables such as the length of gestation and the size of the litter may be controllable. More difficult to control are the effects of the hormone on the mother's nutrition, metabolism, hormonal function, and placental function. These may have much greater indirect effects on the fetus than any direct effect of the hormone on fetal brain development.

6.7. Effects of Nerve Growth Factor on Development of the Nervous System

6.7.1. Discovery of NGF

The history of the discovery of a factor in mouse sarcoma and salivary glands that dramatically increases metabolism and growth of neurons in sensory and sympathetic ganglia has frequently been reviewed (Levi-Montalcini, 1964*d,* 1965, 1966; Levi-Montalcini and Angeletti, 1968). The nerve growth factor, or NGF as it has come to be called, has, from the time of the discovery of its effect in 1948, emerged as a very potent agent for promoting growth of spinal sensory and sympathetic adrenergic neurons during normal development, and its maintenance role in the adult is now becoming evident.

In 1948, Bueker reported that mouse sarcoma 180 grafted into the body wall of 3-day chick embryos resulted in a 20–40 percent increase in the size of spinal sensory ganglia and the sympathetic ganglia that innervated the tumor. Bueker's experiment was repeated by Levi-Montalcini and Hamburger (1951), who found that implantation of a mouse sarcoma into 3-day chick embryos results in a two- to threefold increase in the size of the spinal sensory ganglia and a five- to sixfold increase in the sympathetic ganglia supplying the sarcoma, as well as in those not supplying the sarcoma. Increased size of the ganglia is first seen on day 6 of incubation, shortly after the nerves have grown into the sarcoma. The nerve fibers do not make synaptic connections with the sarcoma, but branch profusely between the sarcoma cells. Although all the sympathetic ganglion cells appear to increase in size, only the small mediodorsal cells and not the large ventrolateral cells of the sensory ganglia respond to stimulation by the tumor. The mediodorsal (MD) cells are largely or entirely connected to muscle spindles, whereas the ventrolateral (VL) cells are connected to cutaneous sense organs (see Section 7.10). The response of sensory ganglia of the chick embryo to stimulation by the sarcoma is maximal between days 7 and 9 of incubation, declines thereafter, and is no longer apparent after day 15. A similar period of responsiveness of explanted chick sensory ganglia *in vitro* to purified nerve growth factor has been reported by Winick and Greenberg (1965*a,b*). It is important to note that production of neurons ceases between days 7 and 9 of incubation in the chick embryo spinal cord, spinal sensory ganglia, and sympathetic ganglia, whereas proliferation of glia starts only after the production of neurons has ceased, and continues until hatching (Brizzee, 1949; Bensted *et al.,* 1957). The period of responsiveness to NGF corresponds with the period of glial proliferation and outgrowth of neurites from the neurons. Levi-Montalcini and Hamburger (1951) concluded that the increase in size of the ganglia is due to an increase in mitotic activity, to acceleration of the differentiation of young neurons, and to hypertrophy of differentiated nerve cells. The same conclusions were reached by Levi-Montalcini and Booker (1960*a*) regarding the effects of NGF on sympathetic ganglia of newborn mice in tissue culture. These conclusions will be discussed more critically below.

Levi-Montalcini (1952) discovered that a diffusible agent released from the sarcoma resulted in overgrowth of sensory and sympathetic ganglia. Using 4- to 6-day chick embryos, she demonstrated that the sarcoma produces its effects on the ganglia even when it is implanted on the chorioallantoic membrane so that the sarcoma and the embryo are in communication only through the bloodstream. When sarcoma and ganglion are cultured in the same hanging drop of plasma clot, the sarcoma produces a halo of nerve fibers growing out of the ganglion, but no fiber outgrowth occurs from a ganglion cultured in the absence of a source of nerve growth factor, as Fig. 6.6 shows (Levi-Montalcini *et al.,* 1954). The nerve growth factor appears to be an absolute requirement for the outgrowth of nerve fibers from explanted sensory and sympathetic ganglia in tissue culture. The size and density of the halo of fibers growing out of ganglia at 37°C *in vitro* 18–24 hours after the addition of serial dilutions of NGF have become the standard tests of the presence and potency of NGF in tissue extracts (Levi-Montalcini, 1964*d,* 1966). The biological unit of NGF is defined by this assay as the concentration of NGF (units per milliliter) required to produce maximum outgrowth of fibers from the explanted ganglion. One biological unit corresponds to about 10 ng of NGF. In tissue culture of explanted ganglia the axons have been cut, and the fiber halo may be reasonably assumed to consist of regenerating axons as well as axons that have sprouted *ab initio* in culture. Although the ratio of the two kinds of axons has not been determined, it is probable that the later in development the ganglia are excised the larger the proportion of fibers that are cut and must be regenerated.

The nerve growth factor was found in a nucleoprotein fraction of the mouse sarcoma (S. Cohen *et al.,* 1954). Phosphodiesterase in the form of snake venom was added to the sarcoma extract in order to break down the nucleic acid, with the unexpected result that growth of nerve fibers was increased. The snake venom yields preparations of NGF about a thousand times more potent than the crude extract from mouse sarcoma (S. Cohen and Levi-Montalcini, 1956; Levi-Montalcini and Cohen, 1956; S. Cohen, 1958, 1959). Because the snake venom gland is homologous with a salivary gland in mammals, a search was made for NGF in salivary glands. A protein nerve growth factor 10,000 times more potent than the sarcoma extract can be prepared from mouse submaxillary glands (S. Cohen, 1960), in which the concentration of NGF is about 400 ng per milligram of tissue in adult male mice.

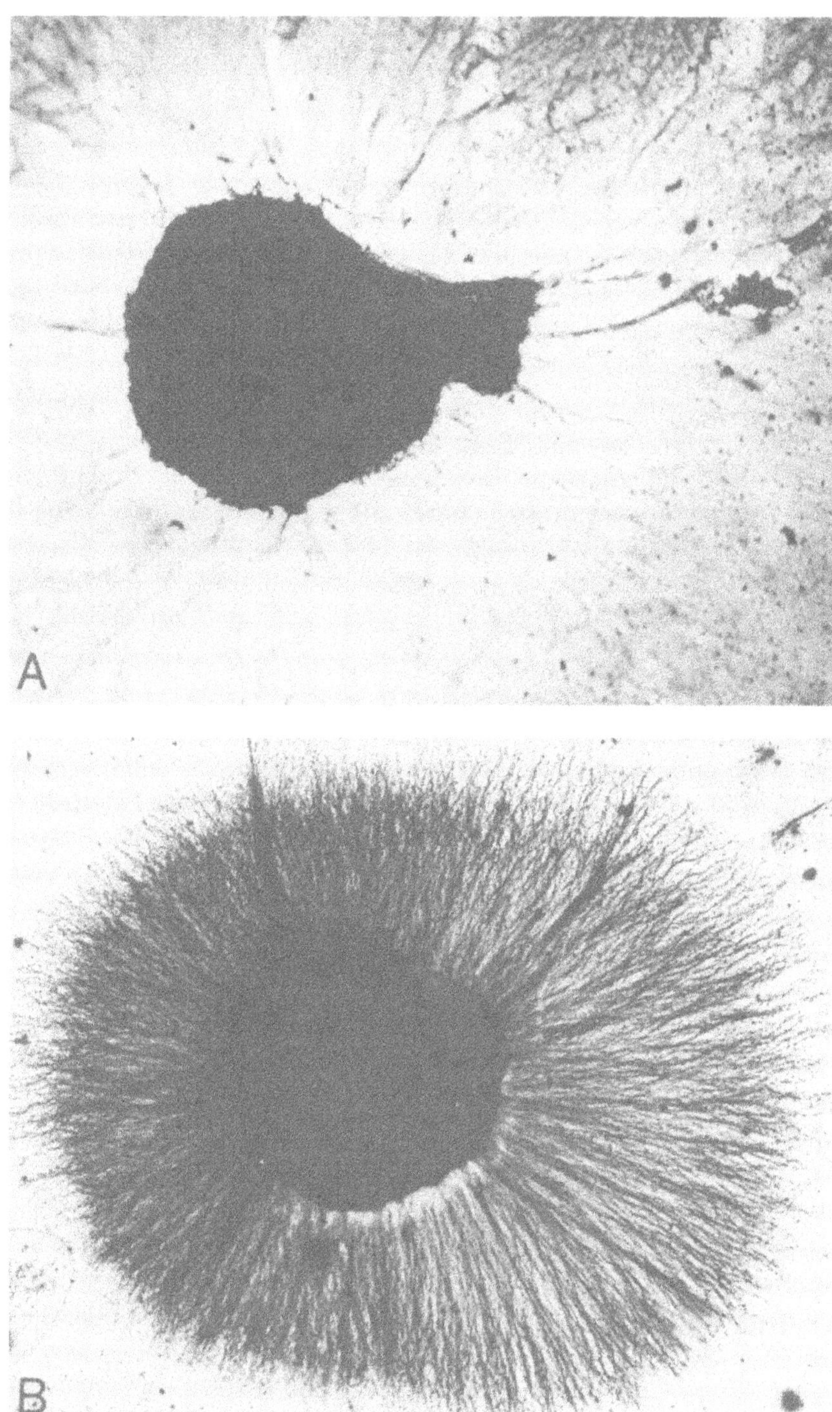

Figure 6.6. Photomicrographs of sensory ganglia of a 7-day chick embryo cultured in a control medium (A) and in the same medium supplemented with nerve growth factor (0.01 μg/ml) for 24 hr (B). Silver impregnation. From R. Levi-Montalcini, *Science 143:* 105–110 (1964), copyright American Association for the Advancement of Science.

6.7.2. Characteristics and Distribution of NGF

The nerve growth factor extracted from mouse submaxillary glands occurs in a high molecular weight complex known as 7S NGF. This contains the nerve growth factor itself, known as βNGF, and two other subunits, α and γ, which do not stimulate nerve growth (Varon *et al.,* 1968). The βNGF alone has all the nerve growth activity of the material first prepared by S. Cohen (1960) and used in the original experiments by Levi-Montalcini's group. The purified NGF is a dimer consisting of two identical polypeptides which are not covalently linked. Each polypeptide contains 118 amino acids and has a molecular weight of 13,259 (L. A. Greene *et al.,* 1971). The amino acid sequence of NGF resembles that of proinsulin, which is the protein precursor of insulin, but NGF and insulin have different membrane receptors and different actions (Angeletti and Bradshaw, 1971; Frazier *et al.,* 1972).

NGF is found in all vertebrates except the elasmobranchs (Winick and Greenberg, 1965*b*), which suggests that it first appeared in evolution in the teleosts. That it is not species specific is apparent from the growth effects of snake venom NGF or mouse submaxillary gland NGF on chick ganglia. NGF is found in many different tissues. It is present in the blood serum of all mammals (Levi-Montalcini and Angeletti, 1968), in extracts of normal sensory and sympathetic ganglia of embryos and adults (Bueker *et al.,* 1960; Levi-Montalcini and Angeletti, 1968), and in the urine and saliva of mice (Levi-Montalcini and Booker, 1960*a*). Its presence in normal tissues suggests that it may play a role in the normal animal. The nerve growth factor is present in high concentration in the convoluted tubules, but not in the acini, of the submaxillary salivary gland of the mouse. It has been localized to the tubules by means of fluorescent antibodies to NGF (M. N. Goldstein and Burdman, 1965). Secretion of saliva containing high concentrations of NGF is induced in male mice by injection of epinephrine or norepinephrine (L. J. Wallace and Partlow, 1976). Nerve growth factor has not been detected in the salivary glands of the rat; it develops in the salivary glands of mice only in the adult. The concentration of NGF in submaxillary glands of adult male mice (about 400 ng per milligram of tissue) is 10 times greater than the concentration in adult female submaxillary glands and about 1000 times greater than in other tissues. Excision of the submaxillary salivary glands of adult mice does not result in any adverse effects (Levi-Montalcini and Cohen, 1960). Levi-Montalcini and Angeletti (1968), in discussing the origin of NGF, reached the conclusion that although there was some evidence that NGF can be synthesized in the submaxillary salivary glands, these are not the only source of the factor. After removal of the submaxillary glands from adult mice, there is a temporary decline in concentration of NGF in the blood plasma to about 15 percent of the normal value, but the concentration increases to normal levels after about 4 months, although no regeneration of the submaxillary gland occurs (Hendry and Iverson, 1973).

There have been several reports showing that a variety of tissues may produce NGF or a material with a similar stimulating action on outgrowing axons from sympathetic and sensory ganglia. Levi-Montalcini (1966) noted that NGF may be produced by fast-growing mesodermal tissues, and this is consistent with the large body of evidence that mesenchyme exerts a strong attraction on growing axons (Ramón y Cajal, 1910, 1928, p. 358). Malignant cells of mesenchymal origin secrete NGF (Levi-Montalcini, 1952; Oger *et al.*, 1974), as do fibroblasts *in vitro* (M. Young *et al.*, 1975), neuroblastoma cells (R. A. Murphy *et al.*, 1975), and glioma cells (Longo and Penhoet, 1974). The fact that glial cells can be substituted for NGF to maintain neuronal growth *in vitro* also indicates that glia are a source of NGF or a similar substance (Burnham *et al.*, 1972; Varon *et al.*, 1974*a*). Neuronal growth can be supported by glia without the addition of NGF to the tissue culture medium, but NGF alone is unable to sustain the growth of neurons cultured in the absence of glial cells (Varon *et al.*, 1974*a*; Monard *et al.*, 1975). That NGF antiserum inhibits the effect of glial cells on neuronal outgrowth indicates that the effect is mediated by NGF (Varon *et al.*, 1974*b*).

6.7.3. Growth Effects of NGF

Injection of NGF into chick or mouse embryos results in hyperplasia of sympathetic ganglia, which can increase their weight 5–12 times above control values (Levi-Montalcini and Booker, 1960*a*). Profuse overgrowth occurs of cutaneous sensory nerve fibers, and overgrowth of sympathetic nerve fibers is seen in meso- and metanephros, ovaries, testes, thyroid, spleen, liver, pancreas, and feather bulbs. No increase of nerve fibers occurs in the skeletal muscles, heart, gut, or respiratory tract (Levi-Montalcini, 1952; Levi-Montalcini and Hamburger, 1953). It is not known whether the nerves that supply the latter organs do not respond to NGF at all stages of development or whether they had merely lost their responsiveness at the stages when the experiments were performed.

Although NGF does not have an effect on spinal sensory ganglia in adults, the effects on sympathetic adrenergic neurons persist in the adult. Administration of NGF to adult rats results in hypertrophy of sympathetic adrenergic neurons (Angeletti *et al.*, 1971*b*) and increased density of adrenergic nerve terminal plexuses in the iris, salivary glands, heart, intestine, spleen, and pancreas, as well as increased levels of norepinephrine in those organs (Bjerre *et al.*, 1975*a*). However, those increases require continued administration of NGF, and they subside to normal levels in about 2 months after NGF treatment ceases.

The sensory and sympathetic ganglion cells respond maximally to NGF for a relatively short period in their development, which coincides with the period during which outgrowth of their axons normally occurs (Fig. 6.7). In the spinal sensory ganglia of the chick embryo, there are two types of cells, mediodorsal and ventrolateral (see Section 7.10). The ventrolateral cells, which innervate the skin, differentiate before E7 and apparently do not respond to NGF, while the mediodorsal cells, which innervate muscle spindles, differentiate after E7 and respond to NGF administered during that time (Weis, 1970, 1971). In the trigeminal ganglion of the 8-day chick embryo in culture, only the small and less differentiated MD neurons grow much larger in response to NGF, while the VL neurons, which are large and well differentiated before day 8, show no growth response (Ebendal and Hedlund, 1975). It is not known when the effect of NGF on chick embryo spinal ganglia begins, but it first becomes detectable at 6 days of incubation, reaches a maximum at 7–9 days, and is no longer detectable after 16 days of incubation (Levi-Montalcini and Hamburger, 1951; Winick and Greenberg, 1965*a*). In sympathetic ganglia 23–30 of the chick embryo, nerve growth factor first produces a detectable effect at 9 days; its effect is maximal at 13–15 days and then gradually declines until it is no longer detectable at 4–17 days after hatching (W. T. Brown, L. M. Partlow, and M. G. Larrabee, personal communication). In the mouse superior cervical ganglion, the effect of NGF is maximal during the first 4 postnatal days and then declines until it is no longer apparent after postnatal day 16 (Halstead and Larrabee, 1972). These periods refer to the outgrowth of axons in response to nerve growth factor. The hypertrophic effect on adrenergic nerve cell bodies and the stimulation of sprouting at adrenergic axon terminals continue in the adult. The duration of the effect on the number of surviving neurons has not been investigated systematically, but it need not of necessity parallel the effect on metabolism and growth. NGF acts only on spinal sensory and sympathetic ganglia (Levi-Montalcini, 1966; Levi-Montalcini and Angeletti, 1968, reviews), trigeminal cells (Rieske, 1969; Ebendal and Hedlund, 1975), central aminergic neurons (Björklund and Stenevi, 1972; Stenevi *et al.*, 1974), and adrenal medulla (Angeletti *et al.*, 1972).

Four- to sixfold increase in the total volume of sympathetic ganglia of newborn mice treated with NGF, compared with that of untreated ganglia, has been reported (Levi-Montalcini and Booker, 1960*a*). The nuclei and cell bodies of the affected cells are appreciably increased in volume. The total number of cells in sympathetic ganglia of newborn mice treated with NGF ranges from 1.03 to 2.5 times the total number of cells in untreated ganglia (Levi-Montalcini and Booker, 1960*a*). Unfortunately, these authors do not seem to have applied any correction for increase in nuclear and cell size (Abercrombie, 1946) when cell counts in ganglia treated with nerve growth factor are compared with those of untreated ganglia. The same criticism may apply to the report that the superior cervical ganglion of the normal 5-day-old rat contains 29,800 neurons, while after NGF treatment the count increases to 74,000 neurons at 5 days of age (Thoenen *et al.*, 1971). When appropriate corrections are made for increase in volume of the

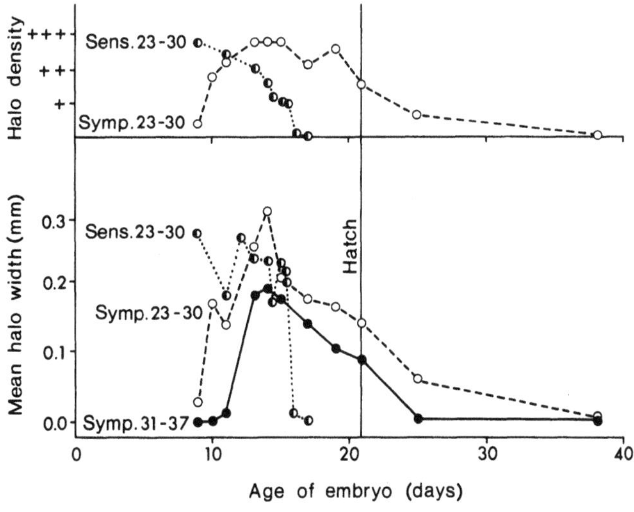

Figure 6.7. Growth response of sensory and sympathetic ganglia of the chick embryo at different ages, incubated in tissue culture for 24 hr in the presence of nerve growth factor (0.5 μg/ml culture medium). The growth response was measured as the mean width and density of the halo of nerve fibers growing from the ganglia. By courtesy of W. T. Brown, M. G. Larrabee, and L. M. Partlow, unpublished data.

nucleus and cell body after NGF treatment (Hendry and Campbell, 1976), the neuron count in the 5-day-old rat superior cervical ganglion is 19,186 ± 539, and after NGF treatment there is an increase to 24,720 ± 885 (Hendry, 1976). Thus the count of 32,000 neurons in the superior cervical ganglion of normal 7-day-old rats and the increase to double that number after NGF treatment are considerable overestimates (Levi-Montalcini and Booker, 1960*a*). Counts of mitotic figures are also liable to the errors mentioned in Section 2.3, and, after NGF treatment, counts of mitotic figures in ganglia have to be corrected for increases in cell size as well as for changes in the length of the M phase and of the duration of the cell cycle. For example, the number of mitotic figures in mouse sympathetic ganglia treated *in vitro* with NGF is reported to increase to a maximum of twice that in untreated ganglia (Levi-Montalcini and Booker, 1960*a*). No corrections for changes in cell cycle time or for increase in cell size appear to have been made, nor is it clear whether the mitotic figures are in neuron or glial precursors. Therefore, the conclusion that NGF increases mitosis of neuronal precursors as well as the estimates of magnitude of increased mitotic activity (Levi-Montalcini and Hamburger, 1951; Levi-Montalcini, 1965, 1966; Levi-Montalcini and Booker, 1960*a*; Levi-Montalcini and Angeletti, 1968; Thoenen *et al.*, 1971) should be treated with the proper reservations.

The extent of the apparent increase in cell numbers in ganglia treated with NGF is not certain, nor is it clear whether changes in neuron-to-glia ratio also occur, as might be expected, as a result of neuronal hypertrophy. An increase in the number of neurons (resulting from diminished cell death rather than increased proliferation) and hypertrophy of the surviving neurons would be expected to result in a glioblastic response. Increased proliferation of the supporting cells, which Brizzee (1949) has shown are identical or very similar to oligodendroglia, could account for the increase in mitotic activity in ganglia treated with nerve growth factor. Another indication that the mitotic activity observed in ganglia treated with NGF may be glial is that NGF exerts its maximal action after the time when neuron production normally ceases and during the period of increasing production of glial cells. The mitogenic effect of neurons on glial cells, both obtained from 11-day chick embryo sympathetic ganglia, has been assayed *in vitro* by McCarthy and Partlow (1976*b*). Addition of nondividing neurons to an equal number of proliferating glial cells results in an increase in the incorporation of [^{3}H]thymidine to 370 percent above that incorporated by the glial cells alone. The stimulation of glial cell DNA synthesis requires contact between neurons and glial cells and does not occur when the glial cells and neurons are allowed to communicate only through the culture medium. The sympathetic ganglion glial cells do not require NGF for their survival *in vitro* (Levi-Montalcini and Angeletti, 1963). However, addition of NGF significantly increases the incorporation of [^{3}H]thymidine when added to 99 percent glial cultures but not when added to 100 percent glial cultures (McCarthy and Partlow, 1976*b*). This indicates that NGF stimulates the neurons directly, and the mitogenic effect of NGF on glial cells is indirect, mediated by the neurons.

It is very likely that NGF results in the survival of neurons that might have degenerated *in vivo*. There is good evidence that a large percentage of the young neurons that are generated in spinal and sympathetic ganglia die in the course of normal development (Levi-Montalcini and Levi, 1943; Hamburger and Levi-Montalcini, 1949; Prestige, 1965, 1967*a*). Moreover, axotomy would be expected to result in degeneration and death of neurons in ganglia explanted into tissue culture. By increasing the synthesis of RNA, proteins, and lipids, NGF may preserve many neurons from the death that might have occurred in its absence.

The young neurons appear to be able to develop normally in the absence of NGF until they start sprouting axons, and then they become highly dependent on the factor for further growth. During this period there is a great increase in the synthesis of proteins that are transported into the growing axon. The ultrastructural changes that normally occur in neurons at that stage of differentiation are an increase in the cisternae of rough endoplasmic reticulum that compose the Nissl substance, an increase in the size of the Golgi apparatus, an increase in the number of neurotubules and neurofilaments, and an increase in the number of synaptic vesicles and of dense-cored vesicles at the presynaptic endings of adrenergic neurons. An exaggeration of these appearances has been observed in embryonic sensory ganglia cultured with NGF: increase in cisternae of rough endoplasmic reticulum, increase in the number and size of the vesicles of the Golgi apparatus, and increase in neurofilaments have been observed with the electron microscope (S. M. Crain *et al.*, 1964*a*; Levi-Montalcini *et al.*, 1968; Angeletti *et al.*, 1971*a*). It is of interest that the electron microscope has revealed similar appearances in neurons of spinal sensory ganglia during regeneration of their axons (Pannese, 1963*a*) and in spinal sensory neurons undergoing hypertrophy as a result of peripheral overloading following regeneration of the tail of the lizard (Pannese, 1963*b*).

6.7.4. Effects of NGF Antiserum

One of the strongest lines of evidence that NGF is essential for growth and survival of sympathetic adrenergic neurons is that NGF antibodies totally inhibit outgrowth of nerve fibers from chick embryo ganglia cultured in optimal concentrations of NGF and that injection of NGF antiserum to newborn mammals results in selective destruction of sympathetic adrenergic neurons (S. Cohen, 1960; Levi-Montalcini and Booker, 1960*b*; Levi-Montalcini and Angeletti, 1966; Zaimis, 1964; Zaimis *et al.*, 1965; Zanini *et al.*, 1968). Injections of NGF antiserum into pregnant mice on days 15–17 of gestation result in almost total destruction of the sympathetic nervous system of the offspring at birth (Klingman and Klingman, 1967). Daily injections of NGF antiserum into newborn mammals produce almost complete destruction of the prevertebral and paravertebral ganglia of the sympathetic nervous system (Fig. 6.8), an effect that is termed *immunosympathectomy*. Antiserum from rabbits injected with NGF from mouse submaxillary glands (rabbit antimouse NGF) produces immunosympathectomy when administered to newborn mice, rats, rabbits, cats, and monkeys (Levi-Montalcini and Booker, 1960*b*), which shows that NGF antibody is not species specific. The adrenergic neurons in the prevertebral ganglia which innervate the male and female reproductive organs are relatively unaffected by NGF antiserum (Klingman and Klingman, 1967), and they also fail to respond to injected NGF (Levi-Montalcini, 1966).

The first effects of NGF antiserum are observed within a few hours after injection. Synaptic transmission in sympathetic ganglia fails (Larrabee, 1969; Halstead and Larrabee, 1972), and the first cytological abnormalities can be detected (Levi-Montalcini and Booker, 1960*b*; Sabatini *et al.*, 1965; Levi-Montal-

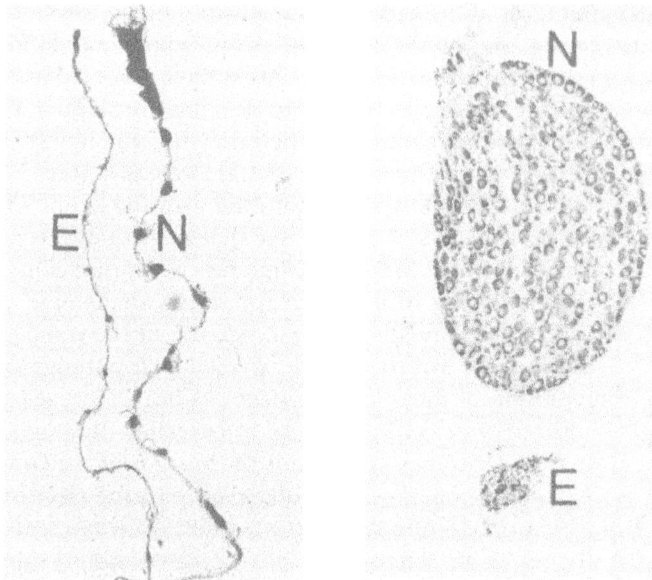

Figure 6.8. Left: Normal sympathetic chain (N) of 1-month-old mouse compared with sympathetic chain (E) of 1-month-old mouse treated for 5 days after birth with antiserum to nerve growth factor. From R. Levi-Montalcini and S. Cohen, *Ann. N.Y. Acad Sci. 85:*324–341 (1960). Right: Transverse section through the superior cervical ganglion of a normal 9-day-old mouse (N) and the superior cervical ganglion (E) of a 9-day-old mouse treated for 3 days after birth with antiserum to nerve growth factor. From R. Levi-Montalcini, *Science 143:*105–110 (1964), copyright American Association for the Advancement of Science.

cini *et al.,* 1969) within a few hours after injection of antiserum. Degenerative changes in sympathetic nerve cells are seen with the electron microscope 2 hours after antiserum injection, and 12 hours later there are obvious signs of degeneration such as condensation of chromatin, folding of the nuclear membrane, loss of neurofilaments and neurotubules, reduction of endoplasmic reticulum, and reduction in size of the adrenergic nerve cells. After 2 days many dead cells can be seen, and the number of mitotic figures is reduced to zero 3 days after antiserum administration. By the end of the first week most of the neurons have disappeared, but the satellite cells are apparently unaffected. After a month almost all the satellite cells have disappeared, leaving only a few neurons, including the SIF cells, which are not affected by NGF, and nonneuronal cells (Levi-Montalcini, 1972). Functional changes that follow injection of NGF antiserum include loss of synaptic transmission in sympathetic ganglia (Larrabee, 1969), impaired uptake of [^{3}H]norepinephrine into the ganglia (Angeletti *et al.,* 1971*a*), and rapid depletion of catecholamines from the adrenergic nerve terminals in the organs innervated by sympathetic ganglia as well as in central catecholaminergic neurons. There is a parallel decline in the catecholamine-synthesizing enzymes, tyrosine hydroxylase and dopamine β-hydroxylase, whose activity is reduced by 40 percent after a single injection of NGF antiserum (Angeletti *et al.,* 1971*a*; Hendry and Iversen, 1971). Whereas an adequate dose of NGF antiserum produces permanent immunosympathectomy in newborn mammals, administration of antiserum to adults does not result in death of adrenergic neurons, and the depletion of catecholamines and other metabolic effects of the antiserum are reversible (Angeletti *et al.*, 1971*a*).

6.7.5. Mechanism of Action of NGF

Several converging lines of evidence show that NGF plays a role during normal embryonic development and probably in the subsequent maintenance of spinal sensory ganglion neurons and sympathetic adrenergic neurons. First, the fact that maximum outgrowth of fibers from cultured chick embryo sympathetic ganglia occurs at a NGF concentration of 4×10^{-10} M suggests that it has a normal physiological role in promoting nerve fiber outgrowth.

NGF is selectively taken up at nerve endings of sympathetic adrenergic and spinal sensory neurons when it is injected in the vicinity of the nerve terminals or when it is injected intravenously (Hendry *et al.*, 1974*a,b*; Stoeckel *et al.*, 1976). The NGF is transported to the cell body by peripheral adrenergic nerve fibers at a rate of 2.5–3 mm per hour. This transport is specific for NGF and for postganglionic sympathetic neurons: NGF uptake does not occur at the nerve terminals of motoneurons, and a number of other proteins fail to be taken up by adrenergic nerve terminals (Stoeckel *et al.*, 1974). However, uptake of ferritin by pinocytosis into sympathetic postganglionic nerve terminals has been observed in tissue culture (Birks *et al.*, 1972). It is not clear whether NGF is transported in the axoplasm, possibly after entry by pinocytosis (Norr and Varon, 1975), or whether NGF remains attached at the cell surface and is transported with other membrane components (Koda and Partlow, 1976). A way of reconciling these apparent contradictions is to assume that high-affinity binding of NGF to specific receptors occurs at the cell surface, especially at the axonal terminals, and that the bound NGF is transported on the cell surface to the perikaryon where pinocytosis or some other mechanism transfers membrane components, including the NGF–receptor complex, into the interior of the cell. The increased uptake of NGF at nerve terminals occurs because the surface area of the terminal branches of the axon is 1–2 orders of magnitude greater than the surface area of the cell body, and also perhaps because the investment by glial cells makes the cell body less accessible to blood-borne substances.

Because NGF and proinsulin have similar amino acid sequences, and because insulin exerts its effects by first binding to a specific receptor on the cell membrane (Cuatrecasas, 1969), it seems likely that NGF also binds to a receptor on the cell surface. Proof that NGF acts on the cell surface was obtained by showing that NGF insolubilized by covalent attachment to Sepharose beads is able to stimulate outgrowth of nerve fibers from sympathetic and sensory ganglia in culture (Frazier *et al.*, 1973*a*). The properties of the NGF receptors have been studied by measuring the binding of NGF, labeled with radioactive iodine, to sensory ganglion cells (Banerjee *et al.*, 1973; Herrup and Shooter, 1973). That the labeled NGF can be displaced from the cells by unlabeled NGF but not by proinsulin or other proteins indicates that the NGF binds to specific receptors. Receptors for NGF are not present on cells of chick embryo brain or on liver or kidney cells. The rate of binding to the embryonic chick spinal ganglion cell is rapid, with a half-time of 1 minute, whereas the half-time of dissociation is about 10 minutes. The binding sites can be saturated at an NGF concentration of 50 ng/ml, and are at half saturation at 7–8 ng/ml, a concentration which produces maximal outgrowth of neurites from neurons *in vitro.* The number of receptors, assuming that they are all on the neurons, is about 20,000 per neuron of the chick spinal sensory ganglion. The mechanism of action of the NGF–receptor complex is not known. That its action does not seem to be linked to adenylyl cyclase is shown by failure to find increased intracellular levels of cyclic AMP in response to NGF (Frazier *et al.,* 1973*b*). However, dibutyryl cyclic AMP, at a concentration of 10^{-3} M added to the culture medium, stimulates fiber outgrowth from chick spinal ganglia (Roisen *et al.,* 1972*a,b*), but not from sympathetic ganglia, and the fiber outgrowth is considerably less when stimulated by dibutyryl cyclic AMP than by NGF (Frazier *et al.,* 1973*a*).

The effect of NGF on RNA and protein synthesis has been the subject of considerable research, but the results and conclusions have often been conflicting and difficult to evaluate. The initial conclusion—that NGF stimulates transcription of messenger RNA, and that as a result there is an increased synthesis of proteins and lipids and increased glucose utilization (Angeletti *et al.,* 1965, 1968)—has been serously criticized. For example, Partlow and Larrabee (1969) showed that following pretreatment with actinomycin D, and in its presence in concentrations that virtually stop uridine incorporation into RNA, NGF still produces axonal outgrowth that is almost as great as the outgrowth from control ganglia treated with NGF alone. Further evidence that NGF does not alter the base ratios of RNA in ganglia (Toschi *et al.,* 1965) or in isolated ganglion cells (Burdman, 1967), compared with those of untreated ganglia, argues against an action of NGF on transcription. It is possible that NGF acts, in part or in whole, on translation, but there is no evidence of this. The epidermal growth factor—which, like nerve growth factor, is a protein obtained from mouse submaxillary glands—increases protein synthesis, possibly by acting on translation (S. Cohen, 1964, 1965; Hoober and Cohen, 1967; S. Cohen and Stastny, 1968; S. Cohen and Taylor, 1974). However, the epidermal growth factor is a small polypeptide of molecular weight 6045, and, unlike NGF, it markedly stimulates mitosis of fibroblasts (S. Cohen and Taylor, 1974). Other protein hormones with anabolic actions, such as insulin, glucagon, ACTH, and STH, act at least in part at the level of translation, but they also increase the transport of substrates into the cell (Stirewalt *et al.,* 1967; Korner, 1968, 1970; O'Malley, 1969; Sutherland, 1972).

Reports that the outgrowth of axons, stimulated by NGF, requires protein synthesis are misleading because, although maintained axonal outgrowth requires protein synthesis (Mizel and Bamburg, 1976), the initial outgrowth of axons from explanted ganglia in response to NGF can occur after virtually complete inhibition of protein synthesis (Partlow and Larrabee, 1971; K. M. Yamada and Wessells, 1971; Burnham and Varon, 1974). In the latter experiments, the outgrowth of axons occurred on a semisolid agar medium or plasma clot, whereas in a liquid medium both RNA and protein synthesis are required for outgrowth of nerve fiber (Angeletti *et al.,* 1965, 1968; Mizel and Bamburg, 1976).

Neurons treated with NGF contain more neurotubules than untreated ganglia, and one of the effects of NGF antiserum is to reduce the number of neurotubules (Angeletti *et al.,* 1971*a,b*). NGF produces a rapid increase in neurotubule protein in chick embryo sensory ganglia, which is reported to be due to increased synthesis of tubulin (Hier *et al.,* 1972). This effect is not specific, for the increase in tubulin parallels that of other proteins in response to NGF (Stoeckel *et al.,* 1974). Moreover, the outgrowth of nerve fibers in response to NGF occurs after virtually total inhibition of protein synthesis (Partlow and Larrabee, 1971). This indicates that NGF does not specifically increase tubulin synthesis but may enhance its assembly into neurotubules.

One of the indubitable effects of NGF is to induce the synthesis of tyrosine hydroxylase and dopamine β-hydroxylase in sympathetic adrenergic neurons (Hendry and Iversen, 1971; Thoenen *et al.,* 1971). These enzymes are found specifically in adrenergic neurons and in the chromaffin cells of the adrenal medulla, where they catalyze the synthesis of epinephrine and norepinephrine. By contrast, dopa decarboxylase, the third enzyme in the biosynthetic pathway to norepinephrine, has a wider cellular distribution and is unaffected by NGF.

The present evidence shows that NGF plays an essential role in stimulating the growth of developing axons from neurons of the spinal sensory ganglia and sympathetic ganglia. NGF may be secreted by the tissues along the route of growth of these axons as well as by the target tissues normally supplied by these neurons. Stimulation of axonal growth toward a source of NGF has been demonstrated in tissue culture (Chamley *et al.,* 1973; Ebendal and C. O. Jacobson, 1976). This suggests that NGF may lure axons toward their targets during normal development.

The fact that neural crest cells require an interaction with somitic mesenchyme in order to differentiate into sympathetic ganglia suggests that NGF, secreted by somitic mesenchyme, stimulates the expression of sympathetic neuron phenotypes in neural crest cells (A. M. Cohen, 1972). NGF stimulates regeneration of peripheral and central adrenergic nerve fibers and may be required for the regeneration and maintenance of those fibers throughout life (Bjerre *et al.,* 1973, 1974). The presence of NGF in the tissues of adult mammals and the persistence of NGF receptors in adult sympathetic adrenergic neurons imply that NGF has a continued role in the adult.

In summary, NGF has the function of stimulating axonal outgrowth and probably attracting nerve fibers to their targets during development. It probably continues to regulate the number of terminal branches of adrenergic nerve fibers throughout life. This appears to involve a tissue homeostatic mechanism in which increased NGF production by the target organs stimulates sprouting of adrenergic nerve terminals, while reduced synthesis of NGF results in a reduced density of the terminal plexuses of adrenergic neurons.

7

Cellular Interactions and Interdependence during Development of the Nervous System

7.1. Introduction

It will have become clear from the preceding chapters of this book that the manifold and diverse components of the developing nervous system provide each other with a mutual environment and produce reciprocal effects as a result of their competitive and their cooperative interactions. Nothing in the organism is completely autonomous: every part, however free and fundamental it may seem to those with a limited point of view, is dependent on its mutual relations with other parts of the organism. As Claude Bernard, in his *Introduction to the Study of Experimental Medicine,* (1865) puts it, "The properties of living bodies are revealed only through reciprocal organic relations. A salivary gland, for instance, exists only because it is in relation with the digestive system, and because its histological units are in certain relations one with another and with the blood. Destroy these relations by isolating the units of the organism, one from another in thought, and the salivary gland ceases to be." But later in the same work he says, "It is doubtless correct to say that the constituent parts of an organism are physiologically inseparable from one another, and that they all contribute to a common vital result; but we may not conclude from this that the living machine must not be analyzed as we analyze a crude machine whose parts also have their role to play in a whole. With the help of experimental analysis we must transfer physiological functions as much as possible outside the organism; segregation allows us to see and to grasp hidden conditions of the phenomena, so as to follow them later inside the organism and to interpret their vital role." Every experiment on living matter presents this dilemma. We are forced to choose between two alternatives, both unfavorable: either to be overwhelmed by complexity or, by reduction of the developing organism to its cellular and subcellular components, to risk the elimination of those vital qualities which are found only in the organized system.

It is obvious that development of the organism generates new qualities that are more than the sum of the isolated parts. Many examples will be given in this and the following chapter of interactions between two or more types of cells that result in qualitative changes that cannot occur in the isolated cellular components. Such cellular interactions have been considered in the first chapter under the rubric of *neural induction.* Other inductive or trophic influences of nerves on their target organs, of neurons on one another, and, in the reverse direction, trophic influences from the target organ on the nerve, will be considered in this chapter. At the outset, it must be admitted that the terms "inductive" and "trophic" are merely convenient ways of distinguishing these apparently nutritive effects of nerves from the electrical activities of neurons. But we have to admit that these terms are no more than an *asylum ignorantiae.*

The history of embryonic induction as well as of trophic interactions shows how easily the mind is beguiled into the belief that a specific agent, an inductor or a trophic factor, necessarily mediates the transmission from one type of cell to another. The history of the trophic effect of nerve on muscle is an instructive example. Although Brown-Séquard had claimed as early as 1853 that daily electrical stimulation of denervated limb muscles of mammals and birds produces a gradual but complete restoration of the bulk of the muscle, and others had also shown that direct electrical stimulation of denervated muscle retards its atrophy (Gutmann and Gutmann, 1942; Steinberger and Smith, 1968), the strength of the conviction that a specific trophic agent must mediate the effect prevented any other concept from being entertained seriously. The hypothesis that a specific trophic agent is transmitted from the nerve to the muscle, introduced in the 1930s (Parker, 1932; Parker and Paine, 1934), continued to be the idea that dominated research, as is shown in recent reviews on the subject (Guth, 1968; A. J. Harris, 1974). Conviction was apparently unshaken by failure to identify the trophic factor, until the belief in its existence became untenable in the face of the evidence that cessation of muscle contraction is in itself largely, if not entirely, responsible for the atrophic effects of denervation (see Chapter 8). Changes of this type have occurred quite frequently in the history of science: hypotheses continue to be held, not because they are strongly supported by evidence, but because evidence against them accumulates very slowly. Lack of evidence against a hypothesis is not a good reason for holding it, but that seems to be the main reason for the persistence of hypotheses regarding control of development by agents directly transmitted through intercellular junctions (Loewenstein, 1968*a,b,* 1973) or by trophic agents that diffuse across the intercellular or synaptic cleft (A. J. Harris, 1974). Nevertheless, I would be the last person to support the dictum that "a little knowledge is a dangerous thing," for if that is true nobody would ever be out of danger. Our "little knowledge" of development of the nervous system would seem to Claude Bernard or Ramón y Cajal to be an undreamed-of vision of scientific truth.

A tentative classification of phenomena that involve cellular interactions during neurogenesis is given below, with references to selected papers in which the various interactions and interdependencies have been demonstrated or postulated. This classification will be necessarily superseded by one based on fundamental mechanisms when these are discovered.

1. Influences of peripheral organs on the neurons with which they connect.
   a. Connection with the peripheral organs promotes differentiation of the young neuron and maintains it (Detwiler, 1936; Barron, 1948; A. F. Hughes, 1968*a;* Prestige, 1970; A. F. Hughes and Carr, 1978).
   b. Central connections of sensory and motoneurons are regulated by the peripheral organs (Weiss, 1936, 1942, 1952, review; Miner, 1956; M. Jacobson and Baker, 1969; Hollyday and Mendell, 1975).
2. Transsynaptic trophic influences of one neuron on another.
   a. Presynaptic neuron stimulates growth and maintains the vitality of the postsynaptic neuron: anterograde transsynaptic trophic effect (Piatt, 1947; Cowan, 1970, review).
   b. Postsynaptic neuron maintains the vitality of the presynaptic neuron: retrograde transsynaptic trophic effect (Torvik, 1956; Cowan, 1970; Landmesser and Pilar, 1974).
3. Trophic influences of neurons on their target organs.
   a. Neurotrophic effects of spinal ganglion neurons on sensory cells (M. Jacobson, 1971*a,* review; Saxod, 1978, review).
   b. Neurotrophic effects of motoneurons on muscle (Guth, 1968).
   c. Neurotrophic influences of autonomic postganglionic neurons on their target organs (M. R. Bennett, 1972; Fleming, 1975).
   d. Neurotrophic influences on tissue and organ regeneration (M. Singer, 1952, 1965; H. Wallace, 1972).
4. Interactions between glial cells and neurons.
   a. Neurons stimulate production of glial cells (Sjöstrand, 1966*a,b,;* McCarthy and Partlow, 1976*a,b*).
   b. Glial cells "nourish" neurons (W. E. Watson, 1974*b,* review).
   c. Glial cells guide neurons migrating from the germinal zone (Sidman and Rakic, 1973, review).
   d. Glial cells guide axons to their destinations either mechanically or by releasing substances that promote nerve growth (Burnham *et al.,* 1972; Longo and Penhoet, 1974; Varon *et al.,* 1974*a;* Monard *et al.,* 1975; Ebendal and C.-O. Jacobson, 1975).
   e. Glial cells ensheath and myelinate axons (R. P. Bunge, 1968, review).

7.2. Role of Transsynaptic Stimulation on Developing Neurons

As connections develop between neurons, the possibility arises of one neuron stimulating the development of another across the synapse. As a result of such transsynaptic stimulation, neurons may exercise an influence on others, either directly across a single synapse or indirectly via interneurons in a chain or circuit. Although transsynaptic stimulation of neuronal development has been amply demonstrated, its fundamental mechanisms are still unknown. According to the theories of neurobiotaxis and stimulogenous fibrillation (Bok, 1915; Ariëns Kappers, 1917, 1921), the impulse traffic in the intracentral fiber tracts and the consequent release of synaptic transmitters stimulate cellular proliferation and differentiation in various nuclei with which the fibers connect in the brain and spinal cord. In the extreme form in which it was adopted by Holt (1931), the theory of neurobiotaxis became the basis of a theory of the sovereign role of sensory stimulation in the development of neuronal connections during development as well as during learning. According to Holt, the "growth of dendrites under the stimulus of nerve impulses is the sole basis of learning" and this leads to the absurd conclusion "that the possibility is open for any sense-organ to acquire functional connection with any muscle" (Holt, 1931, pp. 27 and 33). Those theories are now mainly of historical interest. However, the observations themselves need not be discarded. Several curious phenomena of neuronal hypertrophy and hyperplasia that originally found an explanation in terms of the theory of neurobiotaxis now require reassessment. For example, Detwiler (1936) thought that the motor neuron hyperplasia that occurs after segments of spinal cord have been grafted to more rostral levels is due to stimulation by the descending fiber tracts: the medial longitudinal fasciculus and the bulbospinal tract. However, this does not appear to be the correct explanation, because the hyperplasia also occurs in the spinal cord caudal to the graft, in the absence of the bulbospinal tract, after a segment of spinal cord has been grafted in place of the medulla (Detwiler, 1937*b*). Moreover, hyperplasia occurs in segments of the spinal cord transplanted with adjacent notochord and myotomes to the body wall of *Ambystoma* embryos before the descending tracts have developed, as is shown in Fig. 7.1 (Severinghaus, 1930; Detwiler, 1933*c;* Zacharias, 1938). It has not been ascertained whether the hyperplasia includes glial cells as well as neurons. The nature of such hyperplasia and the causes of its development in transplanted segments of spinal cord are still unknown.

Transsynaptic stimulation is required by many types of neurons to complete their development. If the direction of this effect is from the presynaptic to the postsynaptic neuron, it is referred to as *anterograde transsynaptic* or anterograde transneuronal stimulation, whereas if the stimulation is in the reverse direction, it is termed *retrograde transsynaptic* or retrograde transneuronal stimulation. The evidence given above shows that cellular proliferation and the initial stages of cellular differentiation in the nervous system can occur in the absence of intracentral, afferent or efferent connections, but the final maturation and continued vitality of neurons depend on transsynaptic stimulation. The transsynaptic effects continue throughout life, and can be demonstrated in adult mammals by showing that some neurons atrophy after removal of their afferent nerves or their postsynaptic targets. Where the targets of one set of neurons are the presynaptic inputs to another set, the transsynaptic degeneration may extend across more than one synapse, and the effect is then called primary, secondary, tertiary, etc. Thus, after removal of an eye, the atrophy of cells in the lateral geniculate nucleus which occurs across one synapse is called primary anterograde transsynaptic degeneration (W. H. Cook *et al.*, 1951; Kupfer and Palmer, 1964), while the loss of dendritic spines in the visual cortex, which occurs across two synapses, is an example of secondary anterograde transsynaptic degeneration (A. Globus and Scheibel, 1966, 1967*b;* Valverde, 1967). The effect in the reverse direction is known as retrograde transsynaptic degeneration. It is seen, for example, in the retinal ganglion cells after removal of the striate cortex in primates (Van Buren, 1963).

The fact that transsynaptic effects occur in a direction opposite to that of impulse traffic and synaptic transmission makes it unlikely that the stimulus is entirely due to synaptic transmission. However, even a retrograde transsynaptic effect may be coupled to anterograde synaptic transmission. There is strong evidence that the normal synaptic transmitter, acetylcholine, is entirely responsible for mediating the trophic effects of motoneurons on skeletal muscle (see Section 8.3). Thus botulinum toxin, whose only known effect is to block the presynaptic release of acetylcholine at the neuromuscular junction, results in atrophy of the muscle to which the toxin is applied. Similarly, administration of a ganglionic blocking agent, chlorisondamine, which prevents postsynaptic depolarization by

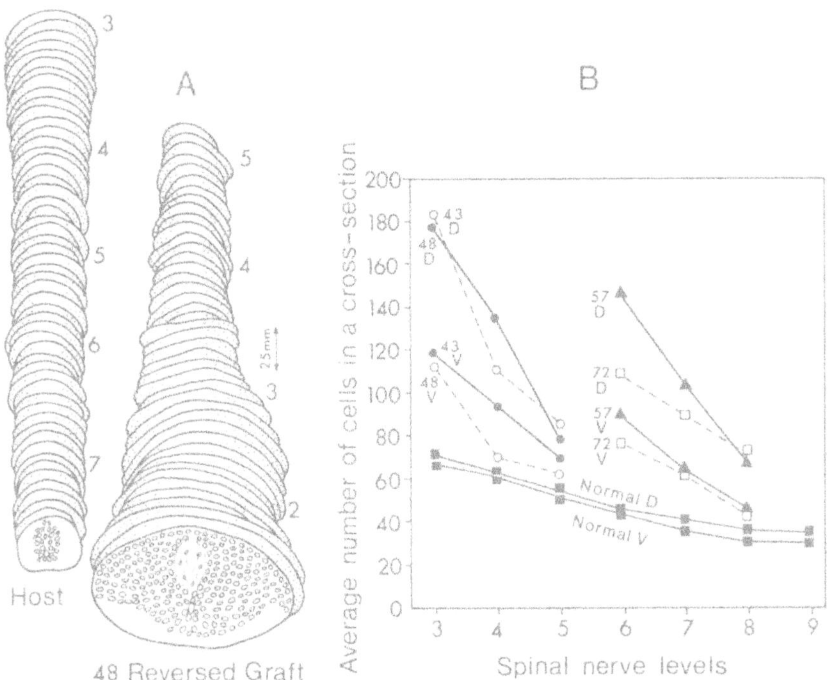

Figure 7.1. A: Reconstructions of the spinal cord of the salamander. The spinal cord of the host is to the left and the grafted cord to the right. The graft had been excised from another salamander and transplanted with adjacent myotomes and notochord to a position lateral to the cord of the host in the tail bud stage of embryonic development. The graft was rostrocaudally inverted. The numbers refer to the levels of the spinal nerves. B: Increase in the number of cells in the dorsal, D, and ventral, V, halves of four spinal cord grafts and in the average of five normal cords. Grafts 48 and 72, with rostrocaudal axis reversed, are shown with broken lines; grafts 43 and 57 were transplanted in the normal orientation. All animals were killed 50–65 days after the operation. In all cases, the number of cells in the graft was greater than in the spinal cord of the host, but the size of the cells and the intercellular distances were not different. Graft 48, shown in A, had the smallest increase of the four cases. From A. E. Severinghaus, *J. Comp. Neurol. 51:*237–270 (1930).

competing with acetylcholine for receptor sites, results in atrophy of postganglionic sympathetic neurons (Black and Green, 1974). The fact that secondary anterograde transsynaptic degeneration may occur in the presence of the presynaptic cells (for example, in the second- and third-order neurons of the olfactory bulb after destruction of the olfactory epithelium) suggests that the mere physical presence of the presynaptic endings is not sufficient to stimulate the postsynaptic cell. In fact, transsynaptic degeneration occurs in neurons that have never been in contact with their normal presynaptic neurons if the latter are removed early in development. Degeneration is delayed in such cases until the stage at which the presynaptic inputs would normally have started functioning, and this, too, suggests that the trophic effect is mediated by the synaptic transmitter or is coupled with the synaptic transmission mechanism.

Returning to the phenomenon of secondary anterograde transsynaptic degeneration, it should be noted that it occurs in those relay nuclei which form a closed system, that is, in which the relay nuclei are exclusively or nearly totally limited to connecting with one another. The retinogeniculostriate system has already been mentioned. Other systems in which secondary and tertiary transsynaptic degeneration is seen are the secondary auditory relay nuclei, such as the lateral superior olive, which degenerate after destruction of the cochlea in newborn mammals (Powell and Erulkar, 1962), and the mammalian olfactory bulb after destruction of the olfactory mucosa (Graziadei and Graziadei, 1978). Other examples are given in the review by Cowan (1970), which leaves little more to be said on the subject of transsynaptic *degeneration.* However, some further remarks are needed on the role of transsynaptic *stimulation* during development.

It will have occurred to the reader that the studies on adults show only the degenerative effects on neurons after removal of their afferents or target cells, that this constitutes no more than indirect evidence of a stimulating effect, and that such studies preclude any possibility of investigating the mechanisms of transsynaptic stimulation directly or of identifying the trophic agents that are presumed to mediate the effects. The advantage of studying transsynaptic effects in developing organisms is that, in some organisms, additional afferents or target organs can be grafted and the additional transsynaptic stimulus can be observed directly.

For all practical purposes, grafting central nervous tissue is restricted to amphibians, but, notwithstanding this limitation, full advantage has not been taken of the possibility of such a direct approach to the mechanisms of transsynaptic stimulation. The classical experiments, particularly those of Burr (1920, 1924, 1930, 1932) and of R. M. May and Detwiler (1925), show that when additional olfactory organs or eyes are grafted on salamander embryos, the ingrowing nerves from the grafts apparently stimulate cell proliferation in the brain. Burr's experiments also indicate that the nerves from the grafts are inclined to enter regions of high proliferative activity in the brain. Apparently, then, these experiments indicate anterograde transsynaptic stimulation of cell proliferation as well as a regrograde stimulation of axonal growth, but the experiments were done at a time when the distinction between neuronal and glial cell proliferation was not clearly made. The history of this subject has shown that what was originally thought to be neuronal hyperplasia has later proved to be glial cell proliferation (Carr, 1975, 1976; also see Section 2.6). There are also technical limitations that may reduce the validity of the observations, for example, the possibility that parts of the central nervous system were grafted in addition to the sensory organs. This appears to have been the case in experiments by R. M. May (1927*a,b*) in which an eye grafted to the position of the otic vesicle of the frog embryo apparently produced marked hyperplasia at the point of entrance of the optic nerve into the medulla. These and other such experiments (for example, those on grafted eyes, discussed in Section 7.3) should be repeated, using electron microscopy, autoradiography, physiological recording, and biochemical assays of the transsynaptic stimulating effects.

Another advantage of studying transsynaptic effects during development is that they occur more rapidly and more severely in the developing than in the mature nervous system. Developing neurons are much more sensitive than mature neurons to direct injury as well as to deafferentation and to removal of their targets. Although the time course of transsynaptic degeneration varies in different organisms and in different neuronal systems in the same organism, for any given system the latency is less and the severity of degeneration is greater in younger than in older animals. Thus anterograde transsynaptic atrophy that occurs after deafferentation, for example, of the lateral geniculate nucleus is slow in adult cats: after an initial period of a few weeks during which little atrophy is apparent, the degeneration reaches a peak in the second month and then levels off by about 60–90 days. By contrast, in newborn cats, degeneration of deafferented neurons occurs within a few days and results in death of a considerable percentage of the affected neurons within a few weeks (Torvik, 1956; Kupfer and Palmer, 1964). The reasons for these differences between younger and older animals can only be surmised. First, older neurons may have a larger store of the supposed "trophic agent," or younger neurons may have a greater rate of utilization of the putative agent. A reservoir of the "trophic agent" may be larger in mature than in developing neurons because a longer segment of afferent axon is left in connection with the mature than the immature neurons. This, however, could hardly account for the large differences in the latent period before onset of degeneration in young neurons compared with mature neurons. For example, after eye enucleation in the adult cat, degeneration of cells in the lateral geniculate nucleus is not appreciable for several weeks, whereas in newborn cats the lateral geniculate neurons degenerate within a few days of enucleation (Kupfer and Palmer, 1964). Second, older neurons may have sustaining axonal collaterals which protect them from retrograde transsynaptic degeneration, and multiple sources of afferents may protect older neurons from the effects of removal of one afferent system. These protections might not have developed in the younger neurons. Third, the completeness of the deprivation, either of afferents or of target organs, appears to be an important factor: the severity of the degeneration tends to be directly proportional to the number of afferents that are removed. This is best exemplified in the various auditory relay nuclei in the chick embryo, which will be discussed below. However, the rule does not appear to apply to some other cases. For example, in young kittens, unilateral lesions in the brain stem result in virtually complete loss of cells in the inferior olive on both sides, indicating that some cells die after deprivation of only half their afferents (Torvik, 1956). Another apparent exception to the rule is the relatively mild effect of complete deafferentation of cells of the superior cervical ganglion. The postganglionic cells do not die even after they are deafferented during development, but they are reduced in size and have reduced levels of tyrosine hydroxylase and a reduced number of axonal terminals in the iris (Black *et al.*, 1976; Black and

Mytilineou, 1976*a*). These cells may survive because they are maintained by NGF. Although NGF and transsynaptic stimulation appear to have different mechanisms of sustaining the superior cervical ganglion cells, they are able to survive after total deprivation of their afferents because NGF functions as a residual maintenance factor (Thoenen *et al.,* 1972; Black and Mytilineou, 1976*b*).

The most thorough studies yet made of transsynaptic degeneration during development have been on the auditory relay nuclei of the chick embryo (Levi-Montalcini, 1949; Rubel *et al.,* 1976). After removal of the otocyst in the 2-day chick embryo, Levi-Montalcini (1949) found that neuron production and differentiation are unaffected in the primary auditory relay nuclei, known as the nucleus angularis and the nucleus magnocellularis. However, cell degeneration becomes evident at 11 days of incubation after deafferentation in both the latter nuclei after all their neurons are produced and are well differentiated. Neuron production and death have been carefully studied in the nucleus magnocellularis and in the secondary auditory relay nucleus, known as n. laminaris (Rubel *et al.,* 1976). The neurons of n. magnocellularis are all produced between 48 and 72 hours of incubation, with a peak at 60 hours. Nucleus laminaris neurons are produced in the period from 72 to 108 hours, with a peak at 84 hours. By 7 days of incubation the neurons have migrated from their germinal zone in the rhombic lip to their positions in the brain stem. By day 9 a total of about 5400 magnocellularis neurons and about 4500 laminaris neurons are present, but during the following 4 days the number of neurons decreases by 18 percent in n. magnocellularis and by 84 percent in n. laminaris (Rubel *et al.,* 1976), as shown in Fig. 7.2. After removal of the otic vesicle there is a further cell loss of 30 percent in n. magnocellularis and of 80 percent in n. angularis, compared with the normal side, according to Levi-Montalcini (1949). She also found that removal of various intracentral afferents to the primary auditory relay nuclei has little or no effect on

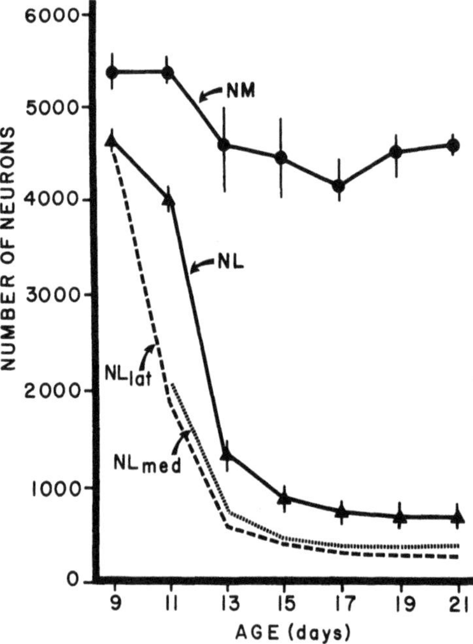

Figure 7.2. Cell counts in nucleus magnocellularis and nucleus laminaris in the chick embryo from 9 days to hatching. Points are means for each time, and vertical bars show ranges. Lines showing counts for the divisions of nucleus laminaris are mean values. NM, Nucleus magnocellularis; NL, n. laminaris (total); NL_{lat}, lateral division of n. laminaris; NL_{med}, medial division of n. laminaris. From E. W. Rubel, D. J. Smith, and L. C. Miller, *J. Comp. Neurol. 166:*469–490 (1976).

their development and survival, provided that the primary afferents from the same organs are intact. The secondary auditory relay nucleus, n. laminaris, receives its afferents from two sources: the dorsal dendrites receive afferents from the ipsilateral n. magnocellularis, while the ventral dendrites receive input exclusively from the contralateral n. magnocellularis (Rubel and Parks, 1975). The fact that no loss of cells of n. laminaris was observed by Levi-Montalcini (1949) after removal of the primary auditory neurons is probably due to the sustaining effect of the remaining input via the crossed dorsal cochlear tract from the contralateral n. magnocellularis. Cutting the crossed dorsal cochlear tract of 5- to 7-day-old chicks results, within 96 hours, in virtually complete atrophy of the ventral dendrites of n. laminaris cells (Benes *et al.,* 1975). The importance of this observation is that it shows that the transsynaptic degeneration is localized to the dendritic branches from which the presynaptic terminals have been removed.

Mauthner's neuron in amphibian embryos should provide an unparalleled situation for studying transsynaptic effects during development: the Mauthner's neuron is produced and starts it differentiation before its afferents develop and before its axon makes synaptic connections in the spinal cord. However, the development of the lateral dendrite of Mauthner's neuron requires transsynaptic stimulation from the vestibular nerve: excision of the vestibular apparatus in *Ambystoma* larvae results in failure of development of Mauthner's neuron on the affected side (Piatt, 1947). When the vestibular apparatus is grafted to the region of the eye, an additional Mauther's neuron frequently develops at the point of entrance of the vestibular nerve into the midbrain (Piatt, 1947, 1969). This might occur if part of the hindbrain is included in the graft, or it might show that either the vestibular input induces the formation of Mauthner's neuron *de novo* (which would be the only known instance of induction of a neuronal type by axonal endings) or the vestibular afferents prevent the death of a Mauthner's neuron precursor that would otherwise have died in the absence of adequate vestibular input. That the vestibular input is not absolutely necessary is shown by the fact that Mauthner's neuron may develop and sprout an axon in the isolated medulla grafted to the flank of *Ambystoma* (Piatt, 1944).

An effect of the periphery on the development of the organization in the somatosensory cerebral cortex is shown by the "barrels," each of which represents one vibrissa and which depends on the vibrissa for its normal development. A single barrel is composed of many neurons which are arranged to form a cylindrical structure. In the mouse there are five rows of barrels in an area of the somatosensory cortex known as the barrel field. They are arranged in a pattern that mirrors the pattern of arrangement of the whiskers, known as mystacial vibrissae (Woolsey and Van der Loos, 1970). Similar patterns of barrels, homeomorphic with the pattern of vibrissae, are found in other rodents (Welker and Woolsey, 1974; Woolsey *et al.,* 1975). Destruction of vibrissae at birth results in failure of development of the corresponding barrels, as shown in Fig. 9.11 (Van der Loos and Woolsey, 1973), whereas a similar lesion 5 days after birth has no effect (Welker and Johnson, 1975). The time at which a lesion of the vibrissal follicle no longer results in failure of development of the barrel is correlated with the earliest appearance of the barrels on the third or early fourth day after birth (Rice and Van der Loos, 1977). At that time, all the barrels first appear simultaneously in presumptive layer IV of the cortex, in the deepest layer of the cortical plate. The walls of the barrels are formed by increased packing of the neurons relative to the core of the barrel. Displacement of the cell bodies to the walls is probably the result of ingrowth of thalamocortical axons and the concomitant growth of dendrites into the core of the barrel (Pasternak and Woólsey, 1975). The failure of development of the barrel after destruction of the vibrissal follicle is a transsynaptic effect on the cortical neurons involving the thalamic relay neurons as well as their cortical targets. Although it has not yet been demonstrated, sensory stimulation of the vibrissae may play a role in the development of the barrel. However, such an effect may be expected to be on the final phase of development of synaptic connections rather than on the morphogenetic mechanisms that result in formation of the barrels. Effects of sensory stimulation, and the failure of development as a result of sensory deprivation, are discussed in Section 9.12. One case that appears to have relevance to this discussion is the pair of abdominal sensory appendages called cerci in the cricket. In this insect the cerci are connected to two giant interneurons so that each cercus makes an excitatory connection with the ipsilateral giant interneuron and an inhibitory connection with the contralateral interneuron. Removal of one or both cerci during development results in transsynaptic atrophy of the interneurons (J. S. Edwards and Palka, 1974), while covering one cercus with a cream which reduces sensory stimulation during development also results in transsynaptic changes in the interneurons (S. G. Matsumoto and Murphey, 1977).

Sensory stimulation is undoubtedly required for the maturation of some neuronal circuits, and in those cases failure of neural maturation may occur after sensory deprivation. Although the neurons originate and form connections according to a developmental timetable that is not contingent on stimulation or experience, the connections may break down or fail to become fully mature in the absence of the appropriate sensory stimulation. This final phase of development of connections has been termed *functional validation* (M. Jacobson, 1969, 1970*a;* Hirsch and Jacobson, 1975). The effects of early sensory stimulation on the development of neuronal connections and on the development of behavior will be discussed at length in Chapter 9. Here, it is pertinent to note that some neuronal circuits can apparently develop normally when electrical activity in their afferent nerve is either absent or greatly reduced. For example, amphibian embryos develop normally while anesthetized with chloretone and show normal behavior and reflex activity immediately after they are removed from the anesthetic (Harrison, 1904; S. A. Matthews and Detwiler, 1926; Carmichael, 1926, 1927). Salamander larvae develop normally while impulse traffic in their nerves is inhibited with tetrodotoxin (Piatt, personal communication). Development of synaptic connections between neurons in tissue culture occurs in the presence of xylocaine applied for 5–30 days (S. M. Crain *et al.,* 1968; S. M. Crain, 1976, p. 210). Xylocaine inhibits all bioelectrical activity, but the synapses that develop in the absence of electrical activity are normal, as seen with the electron microscope, and recover normal electrical activity within a few minutes of removal of the inhibitor (Model *et al.,* 1971).

The following examples show that isolated parts of the central nervous system may develop normally and that cutting intracentral fiber tracts may have little or no immediate effect on the development of their postsynaptic neurons. Hamburger (1946) showed that proliferation and differentiation of neurons continue normally after the brachial part of the spinal cord of the chick embryo is isolated *in situ,* by means of tantalum foil, from the rest of the central nervous system.

After half of the brachial region of the spinal cord of the chick embryo has been cut out, the remaining parts develop normally after having been disconnected from commissural fibers that join right and left halves of the cord or from association fibers that connect cells in the alar plate with those in the basal plate (Wenger, 1950). After removal of the dorsal part of the chick embryo spinal cord, the motoneurons develop normally in the absence of sensory input to the spinal cord and form functional connections with muscles (Hamburger *et al.*, 1966; Burt and Narayanan, 1970). Nor do longitudinal fiber tracts within the spinal cord exert any effect on the proliferation and differentiation of the spinal motoneurons in the chick embryo (Bueker, 1943; Levi-Montalcini, 1949). The hippocampal cells of the urodele pallium migrate outward in the usual manner after removal of the olfactory and diencephalic fibers with which they normally connect (Piatt, 1951). Transplantation of the medulla to the flank in *Ambystoma* does not affect the normal direction and course of outgrowth of the axon of Mauthner's neuron in the transplant (Piatt, 1944). The acoustic and vestibular centers of the chick embryo undergo normal cell production and differentiation in the absence of either afferent nerve fibers or descending fiber tracts (Levi-Montalcini, 1949), but a large percentage of neurons in these centers fail to survive in the absence of their afferents. Their death is an example of anterograde transsynaptic degeneration, and shows that young neurons require presynaptic connections for their survival. The reciprocal dependence, namely of the presynaptic neuron on the postsynaptic cell, is illustrated in the next example. The neurons of the inferior olive are generated normally, migrate to their positions in the olive, and sprout axons in the absence of the cerebellum, which is the central projection field of the olivocerebellar axons. The neurons of the inferior olive project in somatotopic order onto cells of the cerebellum. The olivary neurons in the chick originate and migrate from the rhombic lip on the 5th–11th days of incubation (Harkmark, 1954). Destruction of the cerebellum of the chick embryo before the 13th day of incubation has no effect on the production, migration, and early differentiation of neurons of the inferior olive (Harkmark, 1956). However, the olivary neurons degenerate between the 16th and 19th days of incubation, after their axons fail to form connections with neurons in the cerebellum. This is an example of retrograde transsynaptic degeneration, and shows that there is a reciprocal interdependence between the presynaptic and postsynaptic neurons. The strength of this interdependence is proportional to the exclusivity of their association. In both of the examples cited above, the neurons form an exclusive linkage.

These examples suffice to show that the ultimate health and **survival of neurons may require transsynaptic stimulation, but the production, migration, initial differentiation, and outgrowth of axons depend on a developmental timetable that is intrinsic to the developing neurons and is unaffected by sensory input or by retrograde or anterograde transsynaptic stimulation.** The basic patterns of reflex activity develop without reference to sensory stimulation, experience, or adequacy of the reflexes for survival of the animal. The experiments of Weiss (1941*b*) show that limb buds transplanted in reverse orientation in salamanders move in reverse, and the experiments by Sperry and others, which are discussed fully in Chapter 9, show that the neuronal connections that develop after excision and inversion of the eyes of amphibians result in permanent inversion of visual reflexes. These maladaptive reflexes are not changed by experience or learning. In these cases, the genetic and developmental programs have a sovereign role in controlling the basic patterns of reflex behavior, and functional adaptations are subordinate or absent. The evidence that anatomical development of a part of the nervous system can occur in the absence of sensory stimulation does not necessarily mean that normal functional maturation occurs. Where sensory stimulation is deficient or absent during development, motor patterns develop in accordance with genetically determined potentialities and restrictions. These do not guarantee the development of fully integrated behavior. "Nature" and "nurture" will have different relative importance in different species and in the development of different kinds of behavior. As the evidence presented in Chapter 9 shows, genetic and developmental mechanisms are necessary for the formation of organized motor circuits, but in the absence of sensory input they are not always sufficient to result in maturation of adaptive motor behavior.

7.3. Transsynaptic Influence of the Eye on Development of Visual Centers

The eye exerts a twofold influence on the development of the neurons with which it connects in the brain, namely a transsynaptic trophic stimulating effect and an effect that depends on visual experience. The main function of the latter is to organize the functional operations of neurons in the visual centers so that inputs from the two eyes are congruent. Removal of one eye creates an imbalance in the functional drive to the visual centers, which results in various defects that are considered in Sections 9.11 and 9.12. The effect of the optic nerve fibers that will be considered here is their transsynaptic stimulation of differentiation and growth of neurons in the visual centers. Withdrawal of this trophic influence has harmful effects in all cases. However, the precise effects of removal of the retinal axons, in part or whole, depend on the stage of development of the operation and on the phylogenetic status of the experimental animal. To generalize, it can be said that the operation has its most catastrophic effects earlier in development and in animals higher on the phylogenetic scale. In no case has any effect of optic afferents been found on the production of cells in the visual centers. This is what may be predicted from the fact that production of neurons in the visual centers is virtually complete in all vertebrates before the arrival of optic nerve fibers. In the frog and other submammalian vertebrates in which neuron production in the retina and visual centers is protracted over several weeks, it can be seen that the optic axons reach only as far as the postmitotic neurons and do not extend into the ventricular germinal zone in which the neurons of the visual centers arise (M. Jacobson, 1977).

The debate regarding the effect of afferent axons on cell proliferation in the brain was already settled at the time of writing the first edition of this book (pp. 257–260) on the logical grounds given above and also on the evidence that removal of the eye affects mitosis only during the phase of glial production. This issue has now been conclusively settled in the frog (Currie and Cowan, 1974*b*) and the chick (Cowan *et al.*, 1968; Kelly and Cowan, 1972), and there are no reasons to believe that other vertebrates behave differently in regard to the lack of influence of afferent nerve fibers on production of neurons in the central nervous system.

The result of removing the eye has been shown to be on neuron differentiation and growth and on gliogenesis. The effect on glial cell production is secondary to reduced growth of the deafferented neurons and to absence of the axons which would normally be ensheathed by neuroglia. The opposite effect appears to result from increasing the afferent supply to the visual centers, either by grafting an additional eye or as a result of deflecting optic afferents from one side to superinnervate the visual centers on the other side.

The effects on the visual centers of removal of an eye during embryonic development have been described in all the vertebrate classes, although most often in the submammals. In the submammalian vertebrates, the majority of optic nerve fibers terminate in the contralateral optic tectum, although some end in the contralateral diencephalon and mesencephalic tegmentum, and a small percentage terminate in the ipsilateral thalamus. There is also a projection from the retina to the ipsilateral optic tectum in the frog, but the pathway to the ipsilateral tectum is an indirect one through the contralateral tectum and via a tegmental commissure. All modalities of visual perception—such as the sense of direction and location in visual space, the perception of patterns, and the detection of movement—are functions of the optic tectum in the submammals, and its homologue in mammals, the superior colliculus, also subserves many of these functions. Electrophysiological experiments have shown that there is a point-to-point (or area-to-area) projection of the retina on the optic tectum, thus confirming the older anatomical evidence for a retinotopic projection onto the tectum.

The map of the retinal projection to the frog's tectum, both ipsi- and contralateral, is shown in Fig. 9.9. With minor variations, a similar retinotectal map has been found in all vertebrates. The differences have to do with the presence and size of the retinal area centralis or fovea, the degree of binocularity, and the amount of visual processing that is performed in the tectum rather than in other visual centers, which differ in various animals. The development and regeneration of the retinotectal projection are discussed in Chapter 9.

The complexity of tectal architectonics has thwarted all attempts to follow individual axons from the retina to their tectal terminations or to determine the ways in which various classes of optic axons synapse on tectal neurons. The only definite knowledge is that optic axons terminate in retinotopic order in the tectum and that axons conveying information about different functional attributes of the visual stimulus terminate at different depths in the superficial tectal laminae (Fig. 7.3).

In the frog (*Rana pipiens*) there are about 450,000 retinal ganglion cells, more than 90 percent giving rise to unmyelinated optic nerve fibers (Maturana, 1959). The number of cells in one side of the frog's optic tectum has been estimated as 250,000 by Maturana *et al.* (1960) and as about 500,000 by Lázár and Székely (1967) and Kemali and Braitenberg (1969). The packing density of ganglion cells in the area centralis of the frog's retina (*Rana temporaria*) is about 3 times as great as in the peripheral retina (M. Jacobson, 1962), and about 3 times as many cells in the tectum connect with the area centralis as in tectal regions that connect with the peripheral retina (M. Jacobson, unpublished). Assuming that all the tectal cells receive primary visual input, each optic nerve fiber may connect, on average, with several tectal cells, and each tectal cell may connect with several optic afferents (George and Marks, 1974). However, the manner in which optic nerve fibers terminate in the frog tectum is still uncertain, as Fig. 7.3 shows.

There is a modicum of information concerning the identity of tectal neurons that synapse directly with afferent nerve fibers from the retina and of those that also synapse with other afferents. It is known that the optic tectum receives other afferent fiber projections in addition to the visual projection (Huber and Crosby, 1933; Ariëns Kappers *et al.*, 1936; Bücher and Bürgi, 1950; Bürgi, 1957; Altman, 1962*b*). Responses to auditory and somatosensory stimulation have been recorded in the tectum of the frog (Samsonova, 1965; Fite, 1969). This has to be taken into consideration in experiments designed to clarify the effect of the eye on the developing tectum. Removal of an eye in the embryo would not be expected to result in transneuronal degeneration of tectal neurons that also receive afferent connections from other systems.

There are several reports of reduction in volume of the contralateral optic tectum in fish after removal of an eye during embryonic development (E. L. White, 1948; Leghissa, 1951; Pflugfelder, 1952; Schmatolla, 1972), but the causes of the hypoplasia of the affected tectum cannot be determined from those reports.

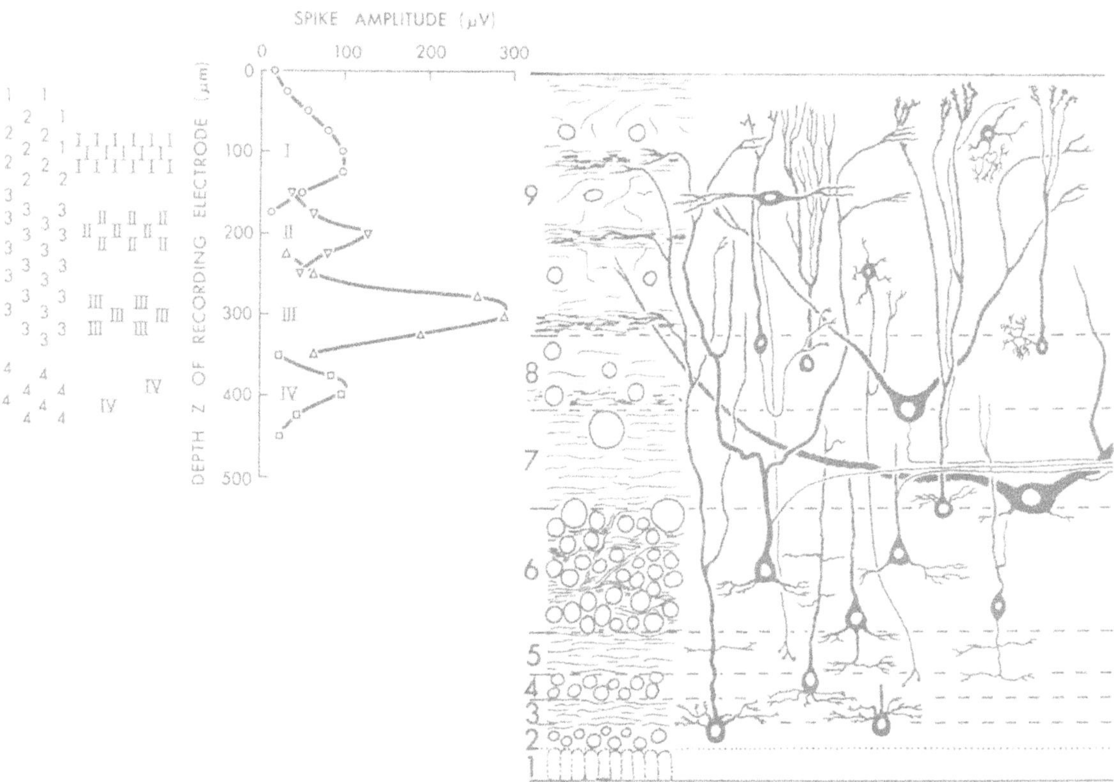

Figure 7.3. Correspondence between function and structure in the optic tectum of the frog. Classes of visually evoked responses recorded in the tectum at different depths are shown according to Lettvin *et al.* (1959). 1, Sustained edge detectors; 2, convexity detectors; 3, moving edge detectors; 4, dimming detectors. According to Witpaard and ter Keurs (1975), there are four types: I, contrast; II, slow on–off; III, fast on–off; IV, off. The depths at which these types of responses are recorded are shown in relation to fiber and cellular layers (1–9, after Larsell, 1931) and some types of tectal cells described by Székely *et al.* (1973).

The effects of removing an eye in frog embryos and larvae have been studied by Dürken (1913, 1930), Larsell (1929, 1931), and Kollros (1953). After ablation of one eye in the embryo of the frog *Rana fusca,* Dürken (1913, 1930) reported that the contralateral optic tectum fails to develop fully: there is virtual absence of the superficial layer in which the optic nerve fibers run, and a slight thinning of the deeper layers. Larsell (1929, 1931) removed one eye in larvae of the tree frog *Hyla regilla* and observed a reduction in size and thickness of the contralateral optic tectum after metamorphosis. He distinguished nine tectal layers, numbered 1 to 9 from the periventricular cell layer to the superficial layer, in which the optic nerve fibers run (Fig. 7.3). He reported that the number of cells in layer 9 of the deafferented tectum hardly increases between the time of eye removal and metamorphosis, whereas the number of cells in layer 9 of the control tectum almost doubles in the same time. The deep layers of cells surrounding the ventricle are virtually unaffected. In addition to the absence of optic nerve fibers from the affected tectum, the growth of dendrites in the superficial tectal layers is greatly reduced (Larsell, 1931), thus providing yet another example of the failure of dendrites to develop in the absence of the axons that synapse on them. Other examples are discussed in Chapter 5.

Kollros (1953) removed one eye from embryos of the frog *Rana pipiens* and found a reduction of 50 percent in the volume and number of cells in the superficial layers (7, 8, and 9) and a reduction of 25 percent in the deep cellular layers of the affected tectum when compared with the control side at the end of metamorphosis. There are fewer mitotic figures in the affected tectum than in the normal tectum. The difference in the number of mitotic figures amounts to 10 percent by early larval stages and to 60 percent by the end of metamorphosis. Kollros attributed the hypoplasia of the tectum to a reduction in proliferation and migration of neurons. This is unconvincing, not only because of the large individual variations in the counts of mitotic figures reported by Kollros, but also because no distinction was made between mitoses giving rise to neurons or to glial cells. The main effect was found in the rostral half of the tectum at late larval stages when production of tectal neurons has virtually ceased in that part of the tectum but when gliogenesis is probably at its maximum. Moreover, it is difficult to imagine how the optic axons, which terminate in the superficial layers of the tectum and do not extend as far as the ventricular germinal zone, can influence production of neurons. What Kollros (1953) and later investigators (McMurray, 1954; Terry and Gordon, 1960; Eichler, 1971) seem to have demonstrated is that removal of the optic afferents has a transsynaptic effect on tectal neurons, almost certainly resulting in slowing of their growth, and so removing a potent stimulus for glial cells to divide, namely their associations with growing neurons (McCarthy and Partlow, 1976*b*).

Currie and Cowan (1974*b*) have shown that removal of an eye during embryonic stages has no effect on the subsequent production and migration of tectal neurons in the frog. However, a reduction in the number of mitoses in the tectum starts at the beginning of metamorphosis. Most of the reduction in mitotic activity, amounting to about 16 percent, is seen in the rostral part of the tectum, whereas proliferation continues at the caudomedial margin of the tectum. Most or all of the cells that are formed in the rostral part of the tectum after the onset of metamorphosis are glial cells.

Increase in volume of the amphibian optic tectum occurs after the tectum has formed connections with an additional eye or with a large eye transplanted in place of a small one. P. Pasquini (1927) transplanted an additional eye to the embryo of the salamander *Pleurodeles waltlii* and found cellular hyperplasia of the tectum roughly proportional to the increase in the additional visual input to the tectum. An increase in tectal size has also been seen after both optic nerves have grown into the tectum on one side in the frog (Hirsch and Jacobson, 1973) and in the goldfish (R. Levine and Jacobson, 1975). An increase in tectal size also occurs in the frog when an additional eye is grafted into the eye socket and superinnervates the contralateral tectum (M. Jacobson and Hunt, 1973). Heteroplastic grafting of eyes between the salamanders *Ambystoma tigrinum,* which has large eyes, and *Ambystoma punctatum,* which has small eyes, shows that the size of the tectum is proportional to the size of the eye that connects with it (Harrison, 1929; Twitty, 1932; L. S. Stone, 1930, 1953). It is not known whether the hyperplasia in these cases consists of an increase in the number or size of cells or is the result of a combination of factors.

There have been several studies of the development of the optic tectum in the chick embryo and of the effects of removing an eye during development. Filogamo (1950) removed the optic vesicle of the chick embryo during the first 3 days of incubation and detected no changes in the differentiation and growth of neurons in the optic tectum until embryonic day 12. Then the dendrites of the deafferented tectal neurons fail to develop, and this is followed by degeneration of a large but undetermined number of tectal neurons. After removal of the optic vesicle at E3, the acetylcholinesterase (AChE), which is detected histochemically, develops normally in all layers of the tectum until E12 (Filogamo, 1960). However, there is a failure of development of AChE in the layer into which optic nerve fibers normally grow on E12–E14. Subsequently, the AChE diminishes during the period when the synaptic connections develop in the tectum (Marchisio, 1969). Electrical potentials in the optic tectum, evoked by photic stimulation of the eye, are first detectable on day 18 of incubation in the chick embryo (Sedlaček, 1967; Corner *et al.,* 1967). However, optic nerve fibers first reach the tectum on days 6–12, as shown by staining (Cowan *et al.,* 1968). On day 13, optic nerve fibers in the tectum can be demonstrated by autoradiography of materials that have entered the tectum as a result of of axonal transport from the eye (Bondy and Madsen, 1971).

Several investigators have observed no changes in cellular proliferation after removal of the optic vesicle in the early chick embryo (Filogamo, 1950; Leghissa, 1951, 1959; Pflugfelder, 1952; Cowan *et al.,* 1968). The first changes in the number of tectal cells are found after E12, whereas mitoses have virtually ceased after E10 (Cowan *et al.,* 1968). S. Fujita (1964) has shown by means of autoradiography after the injection of [^{3}H]thymidine that neurons of the chick embryo tectum originate before E9, the deep cellular layers being formed before the superficial cellular layers. After day 9 of incubation, only glial cells are produced in the tectum.

Cellular proliferation in the optic tectum of the chick embryo is completely independent of the developing eye (Cowan *et al.,* 1968; Currie and Cowan, 1974*b*). No change in either the total number of mitotic figures in the tectum or in their spatial distribution is found after removal of the optic vesicle at the end of day 2 of incubation. The total number of mitotic figures in the optic tectum of the chick embryo increases from about 20,000 on E4 to a maximum of about 45,000 on days 5 and 6, and then declines to 2000 on E9 and to about 18 on E12 (Fig. 7.4). The number of mitotic figures in the caudal part of the optic tectum exceeds the number in the rostral part at all stages of incubation. The number of mitotic figures in the ventrolateral half of the tectum exceeds that in the dorsomedial half between days 4 and 7 of incubation. This proliferative gradient is reversed during E8–E12, while neuron production declines and glial cell production increases.

Gradients of time of origin of tectal neurons in the chick embryo were demonstrated by Cowan *et al.* (1968) by labeling with tritiated thymidine. These studies indicate that tectal neurons originate in the rostral and ventrolateral pole of the tectum on E3–E7, and at progressively later times from days 7 to 12 the cells originate in a gradient extending caudally and dorsomedially (Fig. 7.5). These gradients of cellular proliferation are unaffected by removal of the optic vesicle.

Removal of the eye in mammalian embryos has no discernible effect on the proliferation, migration, and differentiation of neurons in the superior colliculus, which is homologous with the optic tectum. In a strain of mice in which the eyes fail to develop at an early embryonic stage, H. B. Chase (1945) found that the superior colliculi atrophy later.

In an experimental study using the technique of tritiated thymidine autoradiography, DeLong and Sidman (1962) elucidated how removal of the eye of the mouse at birth affects the superior colliculus. They showed that cells of the superior colliculus originate in two bursts: Almost all the neurons originate on the 11th through the 13th days of gestation. Neurons of all layers originate during this period; however, the temporal resolution of their experiments was not good

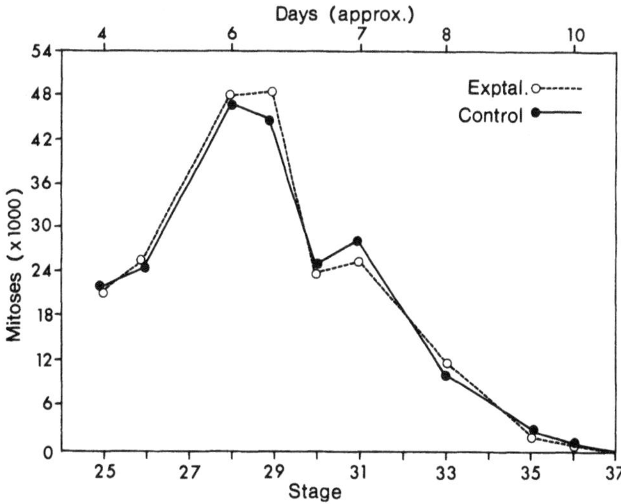

Figure 7.4. Total number of mitotic figures in the optic tectum of chick embryos at different embryonic stages following removal of the optic vesicle on one side at Stages 10–13 of the Hamburger and Hamilton (1951) series, that is, between 34 and 50 hr of incubation. There were no significant differences between the experimental and control sides of the tectum. From W. M. Cowan *et al., J. Exp. Zool. 169:* 71–92 (1968).

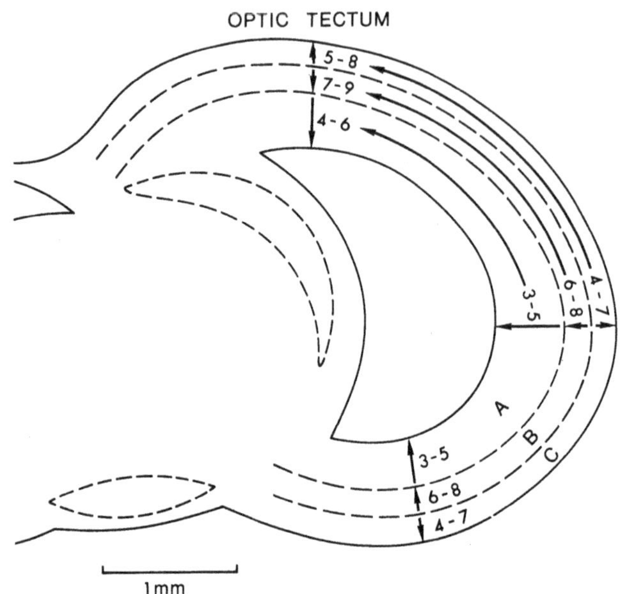

Figure 7.5. Time of origin of cells in the three major developmental strata of the optic tectum (A, B, C) of the chick embryo, determined autoradiographically. The times are given for the rostral part of the tectum: cells originate 1–2 days later in the equivalent parts of the caudal part of the tectum. Arrows indicate the ventrolateral to dorsomedial gradient of time of cell origin in each stratum, and the apparent inside-out gradient in stratum C, and the outside-in gradients in strata A and B. Modified from J. H. LaVail and W. M. Cowan, *Brain Res.* *28*:421–441 (1971).

enough to disclose any spatial or temporal order. A small percentage of neurons originate in the first week after birth. Most of the cells originating postnatally are neuroglia. Therefore, removal of the eye at birth cannot affect the production of neurons, but might affect glial cell production.

The optic nerve fibers first reach the colliculus of the mouse at about day 14 of gestation. Therefore, removal of the eye at birth involves transection of the optic nerve. DeLong and Sidman (1962) found that this results in severe transneuronal atrophy and degeneration of about 40 percent of the cells in the contralateral colliculus between 4 and 7 days after birth. In addition, there is a large reduction in the production of glial cells of the colliculus 4 days after birth. Thereafter, there is an increase in the production of glial cells which results in restoration of the number of cells in the colliculus to 86 percent of normal in the adult.

The experiments with eye–brain connections show that the neurons of the visual centers are dependent on adequate connections from the eye. In considering these experiments some attention should be given to their shortcomings. First, it has often been impossible to identify the neurons in the visual centers that are directly connected to optic afferent nerve fibers. Second, the dual effects of removal of an eye should be noted: a combination of anatomical deafferentation and functional deprivation. There is evidence, discussed in Chapter 9, that deprivation of vision alone, without disruption of anatomical connections between the eye and the brain, during development, results in profound physiological and anatomical changes in the neurons of the visual centers.

Cutting the axon not only injures the cell but also isolates it from its postsynaptic neighbors. The injured cell eventually becomes totally isolated because axotomy also leads to disconnection of the presynaptic endings from the injured cell. The disconnected, isolated neuron cannot survive long, and it is the axonal connection which is evidently crucial for the survival of the entire cell. There is abundant evidence that the young neuron dies if its axon fails to make synaptic connections. Why and how the cell depends on its postsynaptic target are not known. This dependence persists in the adult, and can be studied with relative ease by separating neurons from their end organs or from their postsynaptic neurons in adult animals. This has generally been done by crushing or cutting the axon, but functional disconnection of the axon terminals from the cell body without injuring the axon can also be achieved by blocking axonal transport by means of colchicine (Pilar and Landmesser, 1972) and by preventing exocytosis and pinocytosis at motor nerve endings by means of botulinum toxin (W. E. Watson, 1969). Disconnection of adrenergic neurons from their postsynaptic targets can be achieved without surgery by administration of 6-hydroxydopamine, which is selectively taken up by adrenergic nerve terminals and rapidly results in their degeneration (Angeletti and Levi-Montalcini, 1970).

Cutting the axon results in a train of events that extend in both directions from the cut, and also extend across the synapses in both directions. The anterograde effects are, first, degeneration of the distal axonal segment, which is deprived of vital materials necessarily supplied by axonal flow from the cell body, and, second, anterograde transsynaptic effects on the end organ or postsynaptic neuron as described in Chapter 8. The retrograde effects are, first, increased RNA and protein synthesis in the cell body, manifested as chromatolysis; second, swelling of the neuron; third, dendritic retraction associated with stripping of some or all of the boutons from the injured neuron, depending on the severity of the chromatolysis; and, fourth, proliferation of glial cells and growth of their processes around the injured neuron, effectively isolating it from presynaptic input.

Degeneration of the distal or peripheral section of the axon severed from its cell body was first described in the glossopharyngeal and hypoglossal nerve of the frog by Waller (1851), and is called *anterograde degeneration* or *Wallerian degeneration* (Ramón y Cajal, 1928). This invariably occurs rapidly, within days to weeks, in all vertebrates and insects (J. S. Edwards and Palka, 1973; D. Young, 1973), and occurs very slowly, over a period of months, in central neurons of crustaceans (Wine, 1973). It shows that the survival of the axon depends on its continuity with the perikaryon of the neuron. But in the giant axons of annelids, which are septate, with cell bodies at intervals, fusion of the cut ends can occur (Yolton, 1923; Stough, 1930; Birse and Bittner, 1976). In some axons of the crayfish (Hoy *et al.*, 1967; Hoy, 1973; Bittner, 1973) and leech (Van Essen and Jansen, 1977), the distal part of the axon when isolated from its cell body can survive for a long time, and the cut ends of the axon can heal together. Restoration of function may occur after regeneration of the axon to form connections with its target cells as well as after axonal fusion.

Wallerian degeneration of axons of vertebrates can first be seen histologically close to the site of axotomy. By conventional histological methods axons are seen to start fragmenting by the third or fourth day after axotomy, but observations of living nerve fibers have revealed changes up to several millimeters distal to a crush occurring within minutes of the injury (Williams and Hall, 1971). Degeneration then progresses in a centrifugal direction in the distal segment of the axon and the loss of axons is completed in 3 or 4 weeks. The large-diameter axons degenerate more rapidly than the finer axons. The cellular debris is removed by macrophages which invade the degenerating nerve from the blood and are usually seen in large numbers approximately 5–7 days after axotomy (Olsson and Sjöstrand, 1969). Proliferation of Schwann cells in the degenerating nerve occurs within a few days of axotomy (Ramón y Cajal, 1928; Abercrombie and Johnson, 1946; J. Joseph, 1948; G. A. Thomas, 1948). Nerves undergoing Wallerian degeneration maintain essentially normal conduction velocity until late in the process, whereas the conduction velocity is diminished relatively early as a result of degeneration due to disease (Erlanger and Schoepfle, 1946; Gilliatt, 1961).

Changes in the proximal stump of the axon are called *retrograde degeneration,* and are not evident until days 10–20 after axotomy in adult animals, although they can occur earlier in newborn animals (Ranson, 1906, 1912; Brodal, 1940*a;* Torvik, 1956; Cole, 1968). The intensity of retrograde degeneration of the axon decreases centrally and usually does not extend more than a few centimeters proximal to the lesion (Ranson, 1906, 1912; Ramón y Cajal, 1928). Except for this short segment, the central end of the axon does not degenerate unless degeneration of the cell body occurs. The large-caliber axons are affected before the fibers of smaller diameter in both Wallerian and retrograde degeneration.

Chromatolysis is a characteristic sequence of changes that occur in the nerve cell body after its axon has been cut. Chromatolysis occurs in motor and sensory nerves in both vertebrates and invertebrates. After an axon has been cut, chromatolysis may occur without any changes being visible in the proximal segment of the axon except for a short length of axon close to the site of injury. Nissl (1892, 1894) first described changes in basophilic granules in the nerve cell body after severing its axon, and these have since been called *Nissl granules.* An excellent review of the literature on Nissl granules and an account of the changes in Nissl granules during development of the neuron has been given by Lavelle (1951, 1956). The lucid and thorough reviews by Lieberman (1971, 1974) make additional comments largely redundant here, and only a brief description of chromatolysis and its relevance to development will be given.

The most characteristic change that occurs during chromatolysis of vertebrate neurons is a dissolution of the Nissl granules. Evidence that the Nissl granules contain nucleic acid was obtained as long ago as 1895 by Hans Held from their staining properties and high phosphorus content. Ribonucleic acid was finally demonstrated in the Nissl granules and in the nucleolus by means of ultraviolet microspectrophotometry (Caspersson, 1940, 1950; H. Landström *et al.,* 1941). Electron microscopy has revealed that Nissl granules consist of arrays of flattened cisternae of endoplasmic reticulum with attached ribosomes (Palay and Palade, 1955; Deitch and Murray, 1956; A. Peters *et al.,* 1970). During chromatolysis in neurons of vertebrates, the long parallel cisternae of endoplasmic reticulum disperse and are replaced by randomly oriented small cisternae which are displaced toward the periphery of the cell. An increase in the number of free ribosomes occurs at the same time as an increase in volume of the nucleolus (Barr and Bertram, 1951; H. A. Lindsay and Barr, 1955; Haggar, 1957; Porter and Bowers, 1963). Haggar (1957) observed 31 percent increase in volume of the nucleolus 7 days after axotomy and a return to normal by 41 days. Increase in RNA synthesis in the nucleolus and increased ribosomal synthesis also occur (Hydén, 1943, 1960; Brattgard *et al.,* 1957; Eckholm and Hydén, 1965). The uptake of tritiated uridine into RNA first increases in the nucleus and nucleolus and then in the cytoplasm (Porter and Bowers, 1963; W. E. Watson, 1968). The closer the site of axotomy is to the cell body, the sooner the onset of chromatolysis (Geist, 1933; Bodian, 1947). W. E. Watson (1968) showed that the nucleolar RNA content of hypoglossal neurons reaches a maximum about 3 days after crushing of the hypoglossal nerve as it emerges from skull, 5 days after its crushing at the level of the carotid bifurcation, and about 9 days after its crushing in the tongue (Fig. 7.6). This indicates that the latent period increases by about 1 day per millimeter distance between the cell nucleus and site of axotomy.

In addition to changes in the quantities, distribution, and activities of endoplasmic reticulum and ribosomes during chromatolysis, many other changes have been observed. An increase in the volume of the cell body usually occurs during chromatolysis. For example, 3–12 days after cutting the hypoglossal nerve, Brattgard *et al.* (1957) observed almost a threefold increase in the volume of hypoglossal neurons. The nucleus is usually displaced from the center of the cell body toward the base of one of the dendrites (Ramón y Cajal, 1928). The Golgi apparatus may undergo displacement to the periphery of the cell, and dispersion of the Golgi apparatus has been reported by investigators using classical methods of impregnation (Penfield, 1920; Ramón y Cajal, 1928, Fig. 204; Moussa, 1955–1956) or histochemical methods of detecting enzymes in the Golgi apparatus (Barron and Tuncbay, 1962, 1964; Söderholm, 1965; Watanabe, 1965). However, as seen with the electron microscope, the changes in the Golgi apparatus during chromatolysis are minimal, at most consisting of dilatation of the cisternae (reviewed by Lieberman, 1969).

Changes in the enzymes of neurons undergoing chromatolysis and during recovery, as well as in the associated glial cells, have been shown by means of histochemical techniques. The increase in acid phosphatase, an enzyme character-

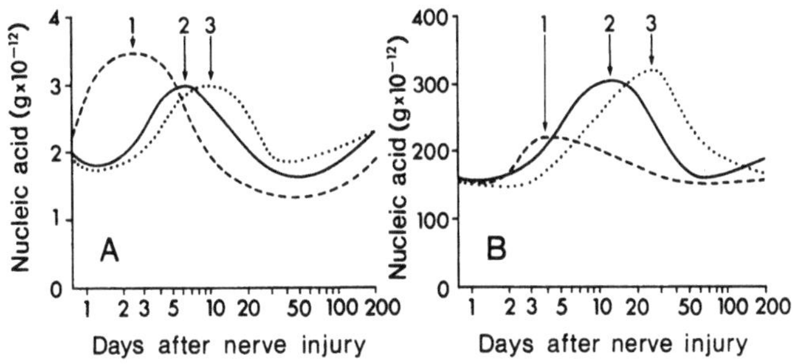

Figure 7.6. Changes in nucleolar nucleic acid (A) and in total cell-body nucleic acid (B) in neurons of the hypoglossal nucleus of the rat after crushing of the hypoglossal nerve at different distances from the hypoglossal nucleus. The different levels at which the nerve was crushed were as follows: at the base of the skull (curve 1), at the carotid bifurcation (curve 2), and distally in the tongue (curve 3). The closer to the nerve cell body that the axon was injured, the earlier the onset and decline of the increase in nucleic acid. From W. E. Watson, *J. Physiol. (London) 196:*655–676 (1968).

istic of lysosomes (Bodian and Mellows, 1945; Cerf and Chacko, 1958; Barron and Tuncbay, 1964; Holtzman *et al.*, 1967), as well as in various forms of lysosomes (Barron and Tuncbay, 1964; Holtzman *et al.*, 1967; M. R. Matthews and Raisman, 1972) is an indication of increased intercellular catabolism in neurons undergoing chromatolysis.

Proliferation and other changes in glial cells accompanying those in chromatolyzed neurons are seen within a few days after axotomy (Brodal, 1940*a;* Torvik, 1956; Cammermeyer, 1965*a,* 1970, review). Using the light microscope, these glial cells have been variously identified as oligodendrocytes (W. E. Watson, 1965) or microglia (Sjöstrand, 1965, 1966*a,b,* 1971; Kreutzberg, 1966). With the electron microscope, these proliferating cells have been classified as multipotential glia (Vaughn and Peters, 1968, 1971; Vaughn *et al.*, 1970). The term "multipotential glia" is meant to refer to a cell type that can develop into either microglia, astrocytes, or oligodendrocytes, but although the existence of such cells was first postulated by Schaper (1897*a,b*), there is still no definitive evidence. The proliferation of microglia around axotomized neurons has been observed with the electron microscope after sciatic nerve transection in adult rats (Kerns and Hinsman, 1973*b*), after hypoglossal nerve section in adult rats and rabbits (Fernando, 1971; Hamberger *et al.*, 1970*b;* Sumner and Sutherland, 1973), after facial nerve section in adult mice (Blinzinger and Kreutzberg, 1968; Torvik and Skjörten, 1971*b*) or newborn rabbits (Torvik, 1972), and after spinal nerve transection in frogs (D. L. Price, 1972). The glial reaction is prevented by injection of actinomycin D before axotomy, but as the drug also prevents chromatolysis it is not known whether the effect on glia is direct or indirect (Torvik and Heding, 1969; Torvik and Skjörten, 1974). In all these studies, there was no visible response of the oligodendrocytes, and the reaction in the astrocytes was limited to changes in ultrastructure and rarely to duplication of the chromosomes without cytoplasmic division (so-called amitosis, see Section 2.6). The proliferating cells, which will be simply termed *microglia* in the absence of more definitive identification, do not appear to arise from pericytes (Kerns and Hinsman, 1973*a*. There is considerable evidence that they are not derived from the blood (W. E. Watson, 1974*b,c,* reviews). They do not act as macrophages. They surround the injured neurons, become inserted into the synaptic clefts, and only rarely are seen to have engulfed the displaced boutons (Blinzinger and Kreutzberg, 1968; Hamberger *et al.*, 1970*b;* Sumner and Sutherland, 1973; Sumner, 1975).

Starting a few days after axotomy and reaching a maximum during the second week, the glial response is accompanied by dendritic retraction (Grant, 1965; Grant and Westman, 1968; Sumner and Watson, 1971) and by stripping of some presynaptic terminals from the dendrites and soma. The degree of presynaptic disconnection apparently depends on age; the boutons are almost completely lost in newborn rabbits (Torvik and Söreide, 1972), but are reduced to about 50 percent in adult rats (Cull, 1974; Sumner, 1975). There is evidence that excitatory synapses only are disconnected (Sumner, 1975). The disconnected presynaptic terminals withdraw a short distance but are not destroyed. They can reconnect after the injured axon has restored its contact with its end organ (Sumner and Watson, 1971; W. E. Watson, 1974*c*), but the boutons remain disconnected if nerve regeneration is delayed (Sumner, 1976).

It should be noted that chromatolysis is not a lysis but a change of the protein synthesis of the neuron. The arrays of parallel cisternae of rough endoplasmic reticulum in the normal, mature neurons of vertebrates are an indication that the cell body is synthesizing protein for export into the axon, some of which forms the packaging for synaptic transmitters that are secreted at the axon terminals. This may be called the *secreting* mode of synthesis. By contrast, the growing neuron, or the neuron that is regenerating an axon and is synthesizing enzymes and proteins for growth, has few parallel long cisternae of rough endoplasmic reticulum but has an abundance of free polyribosomes. This may be called the *growing* mode of synthesis (Eckholm and Hydén, 1965; M. J. Cohen, 1967).

The changes summarized above occur in the neurons of vertebrates during chromatolysis. Different changes are seen in the neuron of invertebrates, where the cytoplasm has a uniform basophilia due to the uniform distribution of free ribosomes and the paucity of endoplasmic reticulum (Malhotra, 1960; Trujillo-Cenóz, 1962; Rosenbluth, 1963; Coggeshall, 1967). The response of invertebrate neurons to axotomy consists of aggregation of ribosomes onto endoplasmic reticulum in the perinuclear region to form arrays of rough endoplasmic recticulum that look rather like Nissl granules in neurons of vertebrates. This aggregation is maximal about 3 days after axotomy in the cockroach, then begins to disperse, and has disappeared after about 2 weeks (M. J. Cohen and Jacklet, 1965, 1967; M. J. Cohen, 1967; Jacklet and M. J. Cohen, 1967*b*). Chromatolysis in the neurons of cephalopod molluscs seems to be similar to that in vertebrate neurons (J. Z. Young, 1932).

The severity of chromatolysis, the latency of onset after axotomy, and the delay before recovery vary according to the severity of the injury as well as the distance of the axotomy from the cell body. Chromatolysis occurs more rapidly, is severer, and has a longer duration and slower recovery the nearer the site of axotomy to the nerve cell body. The type of neuron, morphological characteristics of the affected neurons, and the age and species of the animal also play a part in determining the severity of chromatolysis. Von Gudden (1869) discovered that retrograde degeneration of the proximal stump of an axon and chromatolysis are much more rapid and severe in newborn animals. This is the basis of the Gudden method of mapping the distribution of degenerating neuron perikarya after cutting of their axons (for examples, see Brodal, 1940*a;* Romanes, 1946; Torvik, 1956).

The effect of age on the time course and severity of chromatolysis may be a reflection of the state of maturity of the neuron and of its state of synthesis at different ages. If the peripheral nerve axon is cut during the period when synthesis is directed to dendritic growth and synaptogenesis, little or no chromatolysis is seen, because the neuron is already in a state of maximal protein synthesis. At a later age, when synthesis is largely directed at production of materials to be transported to the axonal endings, cutting the axon results in a change of protein synthesis from a secreting to a growing mode of synthesis, and in a sense that is a reversion to a mode of synthesis found at an earlier stage of development. That may be why young neurons show less marked chromatolysis, and very young neurons may show none of the classical changes after their axons are cut during the period of maximal dendritic growth because they are already in the growing mode at the time of axotomy. Why young neurons are more likely than old neurons to die after axotomy is an old problem that continues to remain unsolved. Young neurons have a greater susceptibility than older neurons to toxins, anoxia, and transsynaptic degeneration, both retrograde and orthograde. Much more information is required about the basic cellular processes in developing neurons before the susceptibility of young neurons to axotomy can be attributed to a specific mechanism. The literature shows that the change in vulnerability to axotomy occurs rapidly as the neuron matures. Thus Romanes (1946) found that axotomy produces rapid and almost total loss of motoneurons supplying the hindlimb in the newborn mouse, but by 1 week of age the motoneurons recover completely after axotomy. The transition to greater resistance to axonal section is seen in a single animal in relation to the time of origin of the motoneurons supplying the hindlimb—those that supply the more proximal muscles are situated most ventrally in the ventral horn of the spinal cord, are the first in the field, and are more resistant to axotomy than those that are born later and supply distal leg muscles (Romanes, 1946). A similar reduction in vulnerability to axotomy of hypoglossal neurons is seen in the cat: dendritic degeneration of hypoglossal neurons can be seen with silver impregnation only when axotomy is performed in kittens less than 11 days old but not in kittens at 20 days of age or in adult cats (G. Grant, 1970).

Lavelle (1973, review) has shown that the strength of the chromatolytic reaction at different stages of development is related to the maturity of the nucleolus (Fig. 4.2). In the hamster, the nucleolus has not developed fully before birth, and facial nerve section results in death of the facial neurons with little or no chromatolysis. After birth, as the nucleolus matures, the strength of chromatolysis increases. The survival of axotomized facial neurons also increases from complete degeneration of all the facial neurons within 6 days after axotomy at birth, to nearly 90 percent survival 30 days after axotomy at 15 days of age (Lavelle and Lavelle, 1958). The evidence also shows that the increasing ability with age of neurons to survive is correlated with the maturation of their capacity for RNA and protein synthesis.

Chromatolysis is a complex of changes representing repair activities rather than the direct response to injury. Chromatolysis is a consequence of disconnecting the cell body from the terminal connections of the axon, be they sense organs or muscles, rather than the result of injury *per se.* That chromatolysis is due to a break in the continuity of the axoplasm between the cell body and peripheral terminals of the axon, rather than to the effects of injury, is shown directly by the fact that blocking axonal flow with colchicine produces chromatolysis without either blocking impulse conduction or overtly damaging the neuron (Pilar and Landmesser, 1972). Chromatolysis occurs in peripheral adrenergic neurons after treatment with 6-hydroxydopamine, which is selectively taken up at adrenergic nerve endings, and results in their degeneration (Angeletti and Levi-Montalcini, 1970). Additional evidence is that botulinum toxin injected into the tongue muscle results in chromatolysis of the hypoglossal neurons without damaging them (W. E. Watson, 1969). Chromatolysis occurs rapidly in primary sensory neurons of all sizes in cranial and spinal sensory ganglia of mammals after their peripherally directed axons have been cut, but it does not occur, even after years, following section of their centrally directed axons (Hinsey *et al.,* 1937; Tower, 1937*a;* Hare and Hinsey, 1940; Lassek and Perry, 1944; Lieberman, 1968; Carmel and Stein, 1969). This is indirect evidence that chromatolysis is caused by disconnection of the cell body from the end organ rather than by injury itself. It should be noted that in submammalian vertebrates the neurons of the spinal dorsal root ganglia are among the most resistant to injury of their peripheral as well as their central neurites, and survive transplantation very successfully.

Two hypotheses have been advanced to account for the relative lack of chromatolysis after axotomy within the central nervous system. That neurons in the central nervous system can survive after axotomy at some distance from the cell body has long been thought to be due to the presence of intact axonal branches proximal to the point of axon section. This has come to be known as the hypothesis of the *sustaining collaterals,* initially propounded by Ramón y Cajal (1928). Evidence in favor of this hypothesis was obtained by Fry and Cowan (1972). They studied the response of neurons in the lateral mammillary nucleus, which has one tract connected to the thalamus (mammillothalamic tract) and another tract connected to the tegmentum (mammillotegmental tract). A slight loss of cells in the nucleus occurs when the former tract is cut, and no cell loss results from section of the latter tract, but after cutting of both tracts 60 percent of the cells of the nucleus die and the remainder are shrunken. The authors concluded that at least 60 percent of the neurons have axonal branches in both tracts, and that cutting one branch is insufficient to cause the cells to die. Another hypothesis that might account for the lack of chromatolysis after central nervous system lesions is that injury to the central nervous system exposes brain autoantigens that are normally sequestered by the blood–brain barrier; therefore autoantibodies as well as sensitized cells enter the injured area, prevent an increase in protein synthesis in the injured neurons, and thus prevent axonal regeneration (M. Berry and Riches, 1974).

An intriguing and unsolved problem is the nature of the signal that initiates the changes in the nerve cell body after axonal transection located at a relatively great distance from the perikaryon (Cragg, 1970). The stimulus that initiates chromatolysis must be transmitted to the cell body from the point of axonal injury. The signal must be associated with the injured neurons because the chromatolysis is confined to them and does not affect adjacent, uninjured neurons. Therefore, the signal cannot be some product of injury that is released into the extracellular fluids, but must travel centripetally in some component of the axon or be transmitted centrally by the Schwann cells. The message that starts chromatolysis is also unlikely to be electrical. Antidromically conducted action potentials arising from injury currents might have some effect on motoneurons but not on sensory neurons, in which the impulse traffic is normally in the direction of the cell body.

The possibility that chromatolysis is started by material that enters the axons at the site of the lesion and is transported to the cell body is rendered more plausible since the demonstration that horseradish peroxidase, applied to the cut or crushed region of the facial nerve of mice, is transported in 6 hours to the perikarya in the facial nucleus (Kristensson and Olsson, 1974). Chromatolysis is seen in those neurons 12 hours after axotomy. It remains to be seen whether horseradish peroxidase or other tracers can enter the axon at the site of application of colchicine or botulinum toxin, which has been shown to result in chromatolysis without apparent damage to the axon. The signal for chromatolysis in motoneurons seems to be linked with acetylcholine release at the motor nerve ending because botulinum toxin injected into the tongue muscle results in chromatolysis of the hypoglossal neurons (W. E. Watson, 1969). A plausible model is that a substance is taken into the nerve endings when acetylcholine is released. In fact, electrical stimulation of nerves increases uptake of horseradish peroxidase into their endings at the neuromuscular junction (Holtzman *et al.,* 1971; Heuser and Reese, 1973; Heuser *et al.,* 1974). The hypothetical signal could then flow in the axon to the cell body where it could regulate the synthesis of materials required for growth and maintenance of the axon. Another route which the signal for chromatolysis might take is the plasma membrane, in or on which materials have been shown to be transported at a rate of a few millimeters per day from the nerve ending to the cell body (Koda and Partlow, 1976). The latter hypothesis is consistent with the observation that the duration of the latent period before onset of chromatolysis is related to the distance of axotomy from the cell body; the longer the axonal stump, the greater the reservoir of the essential material. These observations imply that the signal for chromatolysis travels up the axon at a rate of about 4–5 mm per day.

The present evidence is consistent with a model in which axotomy cuts off the return of material that is recirculated in the neuron, but it is not consistent with a model in which flow is interrupted of material that is transmitted from the end organ. The latter model is not consistent with evidence that chromatolysis occurs in embryonic neurons in culture after their axons, which lack connections with end organs, have been cut (Levi and Meyer, 1945). The hypothesis that loss of a substance transported from the target organ initiates chromatolysis is also not consistent with the evidence that RNA synthesis is further increased by a second axotomy proximal to the first or by repeated crushing of the axon (W. E. Watson, 1968). These latter observations are also consistent with the hypothesis that material entering the axon at the site of injury starts chromatolysis (Kristensson and Olsson, 1974).

The question that always arises when the effects of surgery on the developing nervous system have to be evaluated is how they can be related to normal development. The critical remarks that were made at the end of Chapter 5 in relation to the phenomena of axonal sprouting after surgical operations also apply to the effects of cutting the axon. It is reasonable to assume that axotomy puts into effect a number of processes in an exaggerated form that are hidden during normal development, and that the transsynaptic effect and the neuroglial reaction may also give some indications of the interactions that the developing neuron has with neighboring neurons and glial cells during normal development. In this case, the evidence that has been obtained from the relatively undisturbed developing nervous system can be freely used to understand the mechanisms of chromatolysis, but the freedom of extrapolation is much more restricted in the reverse direction, that is, from the pathological to the normal. In general, it can be shown that knowledge of normal mechanisms can be used to infer or deduce the effects of various perturbations, but information about pathological processes can rarely throw light on normal developmental mechanisms, as the meager contribution of neuropathology to developmental neurobiology has demonstrated. In this case, the effects of axotomy can be inferred from information about normal processes of synthesis and transport of materials in the neuron. However, the reverse does not hold: knowledge of the effects of axotomy, in the absence of other information, permits only weak inferences to be made about normal development. Such inferences can be strengthened if they are found to be consistent with information obtained from other systems or from the same system using different techniques. However, consistency of results, all obtained from abnormal systems, is not sufficient: these results must also be consistent with those obtained from normal developing systems if the latter are what we want to understand.

7.5. Influence of Peripheral Organs on the Neurons with Which They Connect

Striking changes are produced in developing neurons by increasing or diminishing the size of their peripheral innervation zones. These changes are usually discussed under the rubric *center and periphery* and are best considered in terms of reciprocal cellular interactions between the peripheral nerves and the organs with which they connect in the periphery (A. F. Hughes, 1968*a;* A. F. Hughes and Carr, 1978, review). Not only are the neurons in the centers dependent on making connections with their peripheral organs, but also the peripheral organs are dependent on their nerves (see Chapter 8). Muscles and sense organs differentiate fully only after they have been innervated, and they degenerate after denervation. There is thus a mutual dependency of nerve and end organ. Physical contact is necessary for the interaction between nerve and end organ, but may not be sufficient. Their mutual dependence may be based on an exchange of essential molecules. If this is correct, the interaction between nerve and end organ should be considered within the broader context of cellular interactions during embryonic development, and should be related to some other cases in which intercellular transfer of molecules may occur. This was discussed more fully in connection with embryonic induction (Chapter 1) and will be related to the innervation of muscle and sense organs in Chapter 8.

The total number of neurons that survive to maturity is greatly influenced by the size of the peripheral area that they are destined to innervate. The experimental analysis of this dependence has been concentrated on amphibian and chick embryos, to the relative neglect of other vertebrates and the invertebrates. The usual strategy, which was first used by Shorey (1909), has been to note the effects on the spinal sensory and motoneurons after amputation of a developing limb, after grafting of a supernumerary limb, or after transplantation of a limb to a new position. In other cases, the effects of extirpation, grafting, or transplantation of developing sense organs have been observed. The general conclusions from these experiments are that reducing the peripheral field of developing sensory, motor, or autonomic neurons results in a reduction of the number of neurons (hypoplasia) that survive to maturity. Conversely, an increase in the size of the peripheral field usually results in an increase in the number of neurons (hyperplasia) that survive to maturity.

It is evident that such changes in the final cell population can come about as a result of changes in the number of cells that are produced as well as in the number of cells that migrate out of the population or that die before development has been completed. The actual factors that result in the final total number of cells must be determined empirically in each case. There is no doubt that neuronal death is one of the mechanisms of controlling the number of cells in a given set and of achieving the constancy of cell numbers of many cellular populations in the nervous system (Cowan, 1973, review). It should be emphasized that if the number of cells in a given neuronal population is controlled by death of those cells whose presynaptic endings fail to make adequate connections with another neuronal population (the target cells) then the actual control is exerted by the target cells, and that the genetic control of the postsynaptic target cells is the ultimate mechanism of control of the number of cells in the presynaptic set. One can conceive of two mechanisms of control of the number of presynaptic neurons which may be exerted by the postsynaptic neurons. The postsynaptic target cells may provide the presynaptic cells with a limiting quantity of a trophic agent and limitations of the postsynaptic space may put constraints on the number of synaptic terminals that can be accommodated. Further consideration of the significance of the "survival of the fittest" in the competition for nutrients or space is given in Section 7.11.

Reduction in the number of motoneurons in the developing spinal cord occurs after removal of a developing limb in urodele amphibians (Stultz, 1942), in anuran amphibians (R. M. May, 1930, 1933; Beaudoin, 1955; A. F. Hughes and Tschumi, 1958; A. F. Hughes, 1961; Prestige, 1967*a,b*), in the chick embryo (Hamburger, 1934, 1958; Hamburger and Keefe, 1944; Bueker, 1944, 1945*a;* Barron, 1946, 1948; Mottet, 1952; Mottet and Barron, 1954), and in the mammalian fetus (Barron and Barcroft, 1938; Hall and Schneiderhan, 1945).

Increase in the number of spinal motoneurons results from grafting an additional limb adjacent to a normal limb in amphibians (R. M. May, 1933, Bueker, 1945*b;* Hollyday and Mendell, 1976), and in the chick embryo (Hamburger, 1939; Hamburger and Keefe, 1944; Bueker, 1945*a;* Hollyday and Hamburger, 1976), and has been found in mice with supernumerary fingers (Tsang, 1939).

Decrease in the number of sensory neurons in the spinal ganglia occurs after removal of a developing limb in amphibians (Detwiler, 1933*a,b,* 1936; R. M. May, 1930, 1933; Prestige, 1965, 1970) and chick embryos (Shorey, 1909; Hamburger, 1934, 1958; Hamburger and Levi-Montalcini, 1949; Carr and Simpson, 1975), rat embryos (Hall and Schneiderhan, 1945; Lawson *et al.,* 1974), and rabbit embryos (McBride, 1974).

Increase in the number of sensory neurons in the spinal ganglia occurs after grafting an additional limb in *Ambystoma* (Detwiler, 1920*a,b,* 1933*a,* 1936, review), frogs (R. M. May, 1933; Bueker, 1945*b;* Hollyday and Mendell, 1976), and chick embryos (Hamburger, 1939; Hamburger and Levi-Montalcini, 1949). Hyperplasia of cranial sensory ganglia occurs after grafting of a limb to the head of *Ambystoma* (Detwiler, 1930*a*).

The analysis of the influence of the periphery is complicated by the fact that normally there is considerable overproduction of many types of neurons, including all types that innervate peripheral organs. Many of these neurons die during normal development at the stage when their axons reach the peripheral organs. We would like to know whether peripheral changes that result in changes in the final number of neurons are the result of changes in cell proliferation, migration, or death of immature neurons, and whether there is also an effect on glial cells.

7.6. Cell Death during Development of the Nervous System

Death of young nerve cells in the developing nervous system of vertebrates occurs as part of the normal program of development of certain types of neurons. Since cell death in the developing nervous system was first reported (Collin, 1906), and since Hamburger and Levi-Montalcini (1949) first drew attention to the general importance of neuronal death during development, it has become apparent that neuronal death serves constructive purposes. Its primary function is to reduce the number of young neurons, by a process of selective depletion, in order to match the number of presynaptic neurons with the number of postsynaptic targets with which they form connections. That view has now become generally accepted (M. Jacobson, 1970*b;* Cowan, 1973). Another advantage of producing more neurons than are finally needed may be to reduce the genetic load that would be required to preprogram an exact fit between presynaptic neurons and their postsynaptic targets (M. Jacobson, 1969). The initial set of neurons is not only larger than the final set but also may have greater phenotypic variability than the final surviving set of neurons. Selective death occurs of those neurons that are least capable of competing for the limited number of available postsynaptic targets. Cell death of this kind is a means of developmental regulation, and it has an adaptive role in development. This type of cell death may be regarded as a form of adaptive plasticity. It is usually referred to as "histogenetic" cell death.

Glücksmann (1951, 1965) defined three types of cell death during development: histogenetic, morphogenetic, and phylogenetic. These terms serve, at present, to make distinctions that appear to be significant in the present state of our ignorance about the mechanisms of cell death during development. We should be prepared to abandon such terms with no compunction when the basic mechanisms and functions of nerve cell death during development are more completely known. These terms are conveniences that appear to have some validity in the dim light of our present understanding. Death of Rohon-Beard cells shows that the categories of cell death may not be sufficient. Rohon-Beard cells are derived from the neural crest and form a transent primary sensory system linking the ectoderm and neural tube in amphibian embryos. The Rohon-Beard cells degenerate as their place is taken by spinal dorsal root ganglia (Hughes, 1957). The cause of their degeneration is unknown. It is unlikely to be due to thyroxine (Stephens, 1965). The number of Rohon-Beard cells is diminished by removal of the ectoderm with which they connect, but it is not clear whether this is caused by injury of the cells or whether this shows that they are maintained by contact with their peripheral targets (Stephens, 1965; Bacher, 1973). Death of Rohon-Beard cells appears to be inevitable, that is, of the phylogenetic or morphogenetic type, but the possibility that it may be histogenetic, resulting from removal of conditions that are necessary for its survival, has not been adequately studied.

Phylogenetic cell death occurs during the regression of vestigial organs. Thus the paraphysis is present in all vertebrate embryos, and persists in the submammalian species, but degenerates in the mammalian embryo (Ernst, 1926). Death of nerve cells which occurs in the caudal end of the spinal cord of vertebrate embryos, leaving only glial cells in the filum terminale, is another such case.

Morphogenetic cell death occurs during folding and bending of the neural plate and neural tube during the stages when the main regions of the central nervous system are laid down (see Section 1.3). A considerable number of cells die during reduction in thickness of the dorsal part of the neural tube which accompanies the formation of the dorsal raphe in the mesencephalon and the choroid plexuses of the third and fourth ventricles (Källén, 1955; Maruyama and D'Agostino, 1967; Mattanza, 1973). Morphogenetic cell death also occurs during formation of the optic vesicle and choroid fissure. A localized zone of cell death, termed the "suboptic death center" by Källén (1955, 1965), is seen ventral to the emergence of the optic stalk from the forebrain. This appears to have some mechanical function during morphogenesis of the optic stalk. Cell death occurs in the ventral midline of the optic cup during formation of the choroidal fissure, which provides a passage for intraocular blood vessels and retinal axons (J. Silver and Hughes, 1973).

Morphogenetic cell death is a widespread phenomenon found, for example, during changes in shape in the formation of the otocyst and olfactory pit (Glücksmann, 1951). It also occurs during degeneration of the interdigital tissue in the vertebrate limb (Saunders, 1966, review; Saunders and Fallon, 1966; Whitten, 1969). Cell death during morphogenesis of the chick wing is the most fully investigated case of morphogenetic cell death (Saunders, 1966, review). Fallon and Saunders (1968) have shown that when the cells of the posterior necrotic zone (PNZ, a region of mesodermal cell death at the posterior junction of the wing bud and body wall) from chick embryos at Stages 17–23 are grafted to another embryo or are explanted to a culture medium, cell death occurs on schedule, when the PNZ cells reach Stage 24. Death of PNZ cells appears to be preprogrammed. However, the PNZ cells can be saved from death by grafting them before Stage 22 to the dorsal side of the wing bud or by placing them *in vitro* in association with dorsal wing bud mesoderm. Although the causes of survival of PNZ cells in those cases are not known, it can be concluded that death of cells in the PNZ need not be inevitable. Another instance of programmed death of cells occurs in the placenta, in which the trophoblastic giant cells die in tissue culture at an age that corresponds with their life span *in vivo* in the rat (Dorgan and Schultz, 1971). The conclusion to be drawn from these examples is that morphogenetic cell death involves the obsolescence of cells whose functions have been completed as part of a program of development of tissues and cells. By contrast, histogenetic cell death of nerve cells occurs before the cells have become functionally mature, and it appears to be a means of selection of cells whose functions are most effectively adapted to the final ensemble.

Histogenetic cell death is strongly contingent on conditions outside the cells that die, that is, on interactions with other cells, and on nutritional, hormonal, and "trophic" influences. Histogenetic death of neurons occurs if they are unable to form effective synaptic connections. This is most obviously seen when the neuron's synaptic targets are removed before its axon arrives at the target zone. For example, after removal of a limb in a vertebrate embryo, the spinal motoneurons and spinal sensory ganglion neurons die a short time after their axons have grown to the target region of the limb if they find no synaptic targets on muscles and sensory cells (Prestige, 1967*a*,*b*).

It should be noted that not only does removal of an eye produce changes in the visual centers that receive afferent nerve fibers from the eye, but also neurons are affected that send their axons to the eye, for example, the neurons of the isthmo-optic nucleus (ION) in birds which give rise to centrifugal axons to the retina. All the neurons of the ION originate as postmitotic cells over a period of less than 48 hours, from E5 to E7 in the chick embryo (Cowan and Wenger, 1968*a;* P. G. H. Clarke *et al.,* 1976; Cowan and Clarke, 1976). The cells assemble to form the nucleus in the usual way, in temporospatial order, from ventrolateral to dorsomedial. At 13 days of incubation the ION contains about 22,000 neurons, but 60 percent of the cells die in the following 5 days, leaving about 9500 cells in the nucleus at hatching (Fig. 7.7). Cell death occurs uniformly throughout the nucleus, showing that death of a cell is not determined by the time of its origin. In the duck ION there is a similar sequence of events: the number of neurons reaches a maximum of about 6000 cells on E15, but cell death on the following 3 days reduces the number of cells to about 3500 by 21 days of incubation (Sohal and Narayanan, 1974). After removal of the retina or optic cup on E3 in the chick embryo, the loss of cells in the contralateral ION is greatly increased so that no neurons remain in the nucleus at E18 (Cowan and Wenger, 1967; P. G. H. Clarke *et al.,* 1976). The proliferation, migration, and differentiation of ION neurons are not affected by removal of their targets, the amacrine and displaced ganglion cells in the retina. The neurons die only after they fail to connect with those targets.

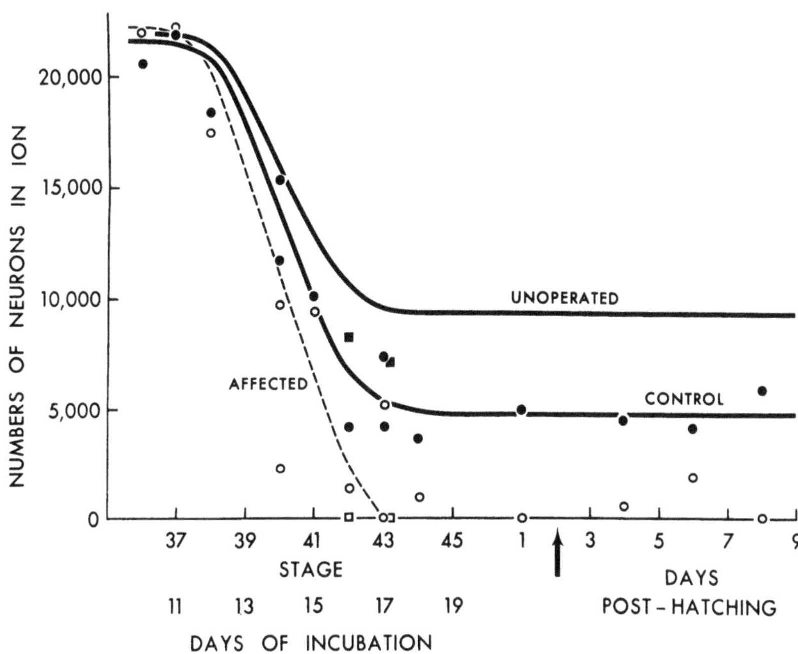

Figure 7.7. Cell death in the isthamo-optic nucleus (ION) of the chick embryo shown by the decline in numbers of ION cells in normal embryos ("unoperated" curve). After removal of one eye at 2–3 days of incubation, the number of cells declines to virtually zero in the ION contralateral (affected curve) and declines to about half normal numbers in the ION ipsilateral to the enucleated eye ("control" curve). Circles and squares denote removal of the eye and removal of the retina, respectively. From P. G. H. Clarke, L. A. Rogers, and W. M. Cowan, *J. Comp. Neurol. 167:* 125–142 (1976).

This result has exactly the same significance as the observation by Harkmark (1956) that after removal of the cerebullum of the chick embryo, the neurons of the inferior olivary nucleus originate, migrate, and differentiate normally, but degenerate when their outgrowing axons fail to find connections in the absent cerebellum.

Similarly, in the staggerer mutant mouse, the cerebellar granule cells die after their axons, the parallel fibers, fail to find their normal synaptic targets, the dendritic spines of the Purkinje cells, because the spines are defective in the mutant (see Section 3.4.5). These examples of the most exaggerated forms of cell death of neurons deprived of their synaptic targets suggest that the so-called histogenetic death of nerve cells during normal development may also occur because the cells fail to find synaptic targets. It seems that this may not be the only factor, as is shown by the fact that all the isthmo-optic (P. G. H. Clarke *et al.*, 1976) and probably all the spinal motoneuron axons (A. F. Hughes and Egar, 1972; Prestige and Wilson, 1974) reach the proximity of their targets, and the axons that arrive at the target zone last do not appear to have a lower probability of survival than those that arrive there first (P. G. H. Clarke *et al.*, 1976). The fact that preganglionic axons make functional synapses in the ciliary ganglion before dying (Landmesser and Pilar, 1974, 1976) shows that death is not merely due to failure of synapse formation. Death may, however, be due to failure of the neuron to make a sufficient number of synapses. Selection of the survivors does not seem to be on the basis of "first come, first served," but rather on a more subtle criterion of most effective matching between presynaptic and postsynaptic elements. There may also be interactions between the presynaptic terminals themselves as well as between presynaptic and postsynaptic elements (R. Levine and Jacobson, 1975). Finally, one cannot reject the possibility that the presynaptic terminals compete for a limited quantity of an agent, essential for their survival, which is produced by the target cells.

The evidence that cell death can be reduced in chick embryos by providing additional postsynaptic targets (Shieh, 1951; Hollyday and Hamburger, 1976) is important in showing that the cells that die are neither intrinsically defective nor preprogrammed to die. Shieh (1951) transplanted cervical spinal cord in chick embryos in place of thoracic spinal cord at a stage before the onset of death of the ventrolateral motoneurons and found that some motoneurons survive that would normally have died. Hollyday and Hamburger (1976) showed that an additional leg grafted near the normal hindlimb in chick embryos results in an increased number of motoneurons innervating the extra limb, and that those neurons, derived from thoracic and rostral lumbar spinal cord levels, are a different population from those that innervate the normal hindlimb (Fig. 7.8).

It has been suggested that histogenetic cell death is ubiquitous in all parts of the developing central nervous system (e.g., Hollyday and Hamburger, 1976). However, cell death has not been seen in most parts of the nervous system. In some regions, this may reflect the rapidity of degeneration and the efficiency of removal of cellular debris. However, there are good reasons for suspecting that cell death is not ubiquitous but is found in those neurons that form connections only with a single postsynaptic target and are unable to make connections elsewhere if that target is unavailable. The type of neuron that does not die during normal development is one that sends axonal branches to connect with more than

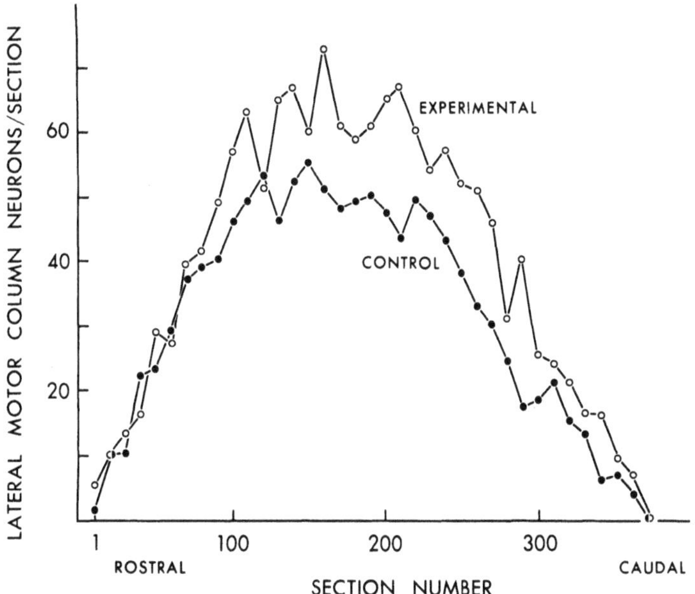

Figure 7.8. Cell counts of the lateral motor column neurons on the experimental (right) and control (left) sides of a 12-day chick embryo in which an extra right hindlimb had been grafted on the right side at 3½ days. The extra limb was innervated by spinal segments 22, 23, 24, and 25. There was a 25.5 percent increase in the number of lateral motoneurons on the right side, and these motoneurons were mainly in spinal segments not normally supplying the limbs. From M. Hollyday and V. Hamburger, *J. Comp. Neurol. 170:*311–320 (1976).

one neuronal set or whose axon connects with more than one type of postsynaptic cell. Such neurons die only when deprived of all their postsynaptic targets. This hypothesis of "sustaining collaterals" (Ramón y Cajal, 1928; Fry and Cowan 1972) applies also to the severity of chromatolysis after axotomy in fully developed neurons, showing that the neuron's dependence on the postsynaptic target cells persists throughout life. The type of neuron that has axonal branches arising relatively close to the cell body shows little chromatolysis and does not usually die after one of its axonal branches is cut, presumably because it is sustained by the synaptic connections of the intact axonal branches. By contrast, the type of neuron that has a single long axon that branches close to its targets is very vulnerable: section of the main axonal trunk results in marked chromatolysis and leads to neuronal death if axonal regeneration does not reconnect the cell to its postsynaptic targets.

7.7. Dependence of Motoneurons on Peripheral Connections

7.7.1. Cell Death in the Trochlear Nucleus of the Chick Embryo

Normal development of the trochlear nucleus in the chick embryo and the effects of removing its peripheral field, the superior oblique muscle, have been studied by Dunnebacke (1953) and by Cowan and Wenger (1967). This system has several advantages over many others: The trochlear nucleus is composed of a homogeneous population of neurons that are clearly separate from surrounding structures, and it is a small nucleus composed of about 1000 neurons, according to Dunnebacke (1953), and about 1400, according to Cowan and Wenger (1967). At 72 hours of incubation the trochlear nucleus can first be recognized lying immediately dorsolateral to the medial longitudinal bundle in the floor of the aqueduct of Sylvius. The trochlear nucleus innervates only a single muscle, the superior oblique, whose anlage can be almost totally excised at 1½ days of incubation, before the trochlear nerve fibers start sprouting at day 4 of incubation. The trochlear fibers decussate and emerge from the brain to innervate the superior oblique muscle on the opposite side. The fibers reach the muscle by the end of day 5 of incubation. There is no evidence of addition of neurons to the trochlear nucleus after day 4 or 5, and the nucleus attains its maximal complement of neurons at 5 days (Dunnebacke, 1953). Dendrites appear on the trochlear neurons on day 5, and the neurons continue growing until hatching.

Dunnebacke (1953) found no evidence of cell death and reduction in the number of trochlear neurons during normal development. However, Cowan and Wenger (1967) reported a progressive decrease in the number of trochlear neurons, resulting (at hatching) in the survival of only 50 percent of the original number of neurons. The largest loss of neurons occurs between days 9 and 17 of incubation (Fig. 7.9). No significant reduction occurs after hatching.

Extirpation of the optic vesicle and surrounding mesoderm, including the anlage of the superior oblique muscle, at 1½ days of incubation results in development of only 10–26 percent of the superior oblique muscle, and causes death of up to 83 percent of the trochlear neurons supplying the reduced muscle (Dunnebacke, 1953). Although the superior oblique muscle has been removed at 1½ days of incubation, there is no effect on proliferation, migration, and differentiation of

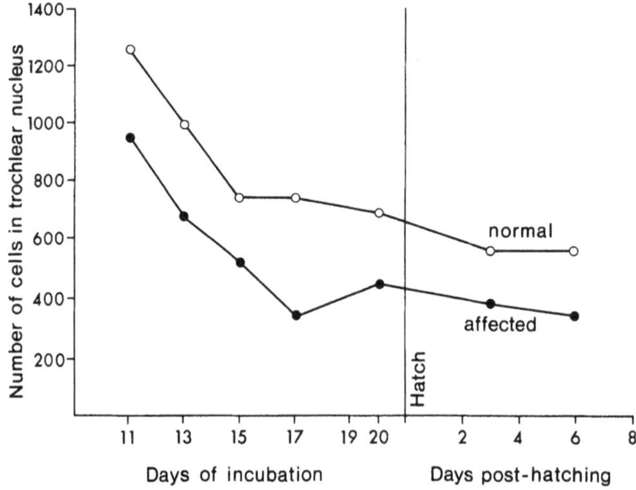

Figure 7.9. Number of cells in the trochlear nucleus of the chick at different intervals after removal of the optic vesicle on one side at embryonic Stages 11–13 of the Hamburger and Hamilton (1951) series (that is, between 34 and 50 hr of incubation), showing that the rate of cell loss in the trochlear nucleus was the same on the normal and affected sides and that there was a constant difference between the two sides. From W. M. Cowan and E. Wenger, *J. Exp. Zool. 164*:276–280 (1967).

trochlear neurons until after day 5, when they normally begin innervating the muscle. A less radical extirpation of the optic vesicle and superior oblique anlage results in loss of about 80 percent of trochlear neurons (Cowan and Wenger, 1967). The number of neurons is reduced from an estimated 1300 at 9 days, to 1000 at 11 days of incubation, to 300 at 6 days after hatching (Fig. 7.9). Degenerating cells are only rarely seen, even when the loss of cells is at a maximum (Dunnebacke, 1953; Cowan and Wenger, 1967), and there are no signs of glial proliferation or invasion by macrophages. However, the loss of neurons is slow in the trochlear nucleus compared with the rapid loss in those situations where cell debris accumulates and where macrophage activity is evident, for example, in the spinal visceromotor column of the chick embryo or in the spinal cord and spinal ganglia after amputation of a limb. The severity of neuronal death after limb amputation is probably increased by the combination of retrograde and transneuronal effects resulting from simultaneously depriving both the motor and sensory neurons of their peripheral fields.

7.7.2. Peripheral Influences on Development of Spinal Motoneurons

Motoneurons in the spinal cord are greatly influenced by the developing limb, and experiments to determine whether this effect is on the proliferation, migration, differentiation, or maintenance of the neurons have consisted of grafting additional limbs or of amputating a limb. The effect of these limb operations on the adjacent region of the spinal cord appears to be similar in all vertebrates. Amputation of the developing limb results in a reduction of the total number of motoneurons that survive to maturity, whereas an extra limb results in an increase in the number of motoneurons. These changes in the final number of neurons might eventuate from changes in cellular proliferation, migration, differentiation, and death, and there is some uncertainty about the relative changes in these four processes that result from amputating or grafting a limb. Although the problem has not been fully solved, some progress has been made recently as a result of attention given to differences in the immediate and late effects of amputating the limb at various stages of development. These studies show that proliferation and early differentiation of motoneurons are not affected by the limb, that outgrowth of motor axons occurs in the absence of the limb, and that the axons grow out to the vicinity of the peripheral targets, but that some neurons degenerate because their axons fail to make stable peripheral synaptic connections.

As I have pointed out before, the analysis of the influence of the periphery is complicated by the fact that normally there is a large overproduction of neurons, which is followed by degeneration of all the neurons that fail to make peripheral synaptic connections. That is, the number of neurons that survive seems to be the number required for saturation of the periphery. This comes about because the skeletal muscle fibers, with rare exceptions, will accept only a single motor axon terminal in mammals (see Section 8.1) or a limited number of terminals in the submammalian vertebrates (Tiegs, 1953). The reader's attention is directed to my comment in Section 7.11 about the significance of cell death during normal development.

The normal maturation and subsequent vitality of the motoneurons depend on their connections with muscle. Proliferation, migration, and initial differentiation of motoneurons, including outgrowth of their axons to contact muscles, occur autonomously and are not affected by removal of the muscles. The latter results in failure of maturation of the neuron—initially in atrophy of its dendrites and finally in degeneration of the whole neuron. For example, after removal of a developing limb, hypoplasia is found in the spinal motoneurons of anuran amphibians (R. M. May, 1930; Beaudoin, 1955; Hughes and Tschumi, 1958; Hughes, 1961; Prestige, 1967*b*, 1970), whereas hyperplasia of spinal motoneurons in frogs results from grafting of additional limbs (R. M. May, 1933; Hollyday and Mendell, 1976). Bueker (1945*b*) observed motoneuron hyperplasia of 22.7 percent in a frog with three functional right hindlimbs. Polydactyly in the chick (Baumann and Landauer, 1943) and the mouse (Tsang, 1939) is also associated with an increased number of motoneurons in the spinal cord segments supplying the extra digits.

The evidence obtained by Detwiler (1936, review) showing that the motoneurons in *Ambystoma* are unaffected by removal of a limb is in conflict with the results obtained in anuran amphibians, the chick embryo, and mammalian fetuses. In part, these differences may be due to the difficulty of distinguishing young motoneurons from other cells in the mantle layer of the spinal cord of *Ambystoma*,

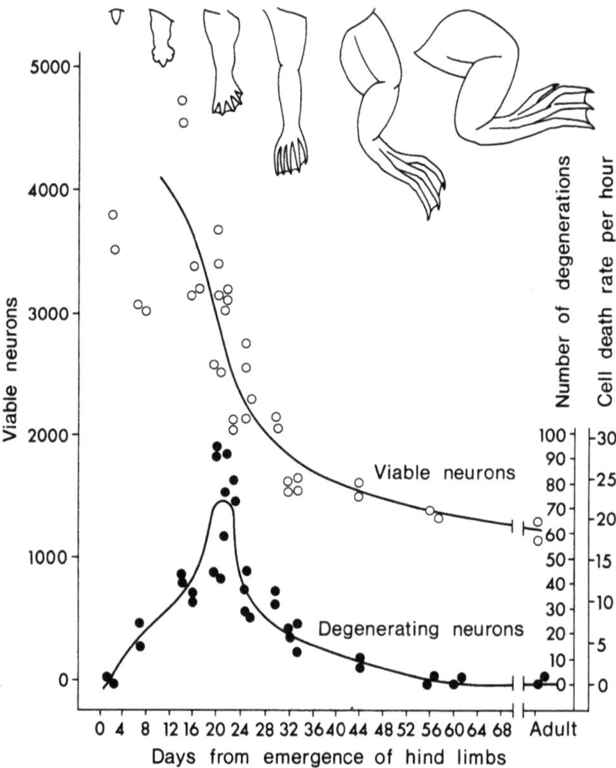

Figure 7.10. Numbers of viable and degenerating neurons in the ventral horn of the lumbar spinal cord of *Xenopus* at different stages of development of the hindlimbs. The number of degenerating neurons is based on a degeneration time of 3.2 hr. Modified from A. F. Hughes, *J. Embryol. Exp. Morphol.* 9:269–284 (1961).

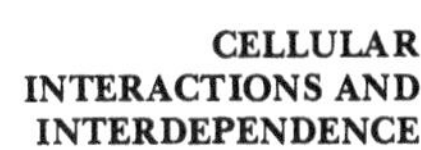

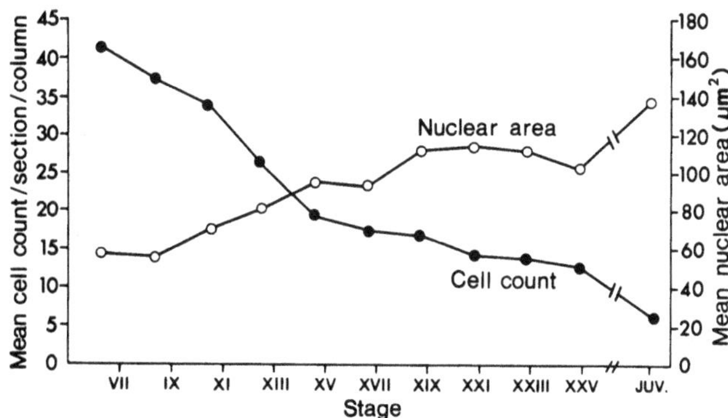

Figure 7.11. Changes in the number of lateral motor neurons and the mean area of their nucleus measured in sections of the brachial spinal cord of the frog at different stages of development. The abscissa shows the Taylor and Kollros (1946) stages in the normal development of *Rana pipiens.* From E. D. Pollack, *Anat. Rec. 163:*111–120 (1969).

and in part they may be due to the unique organization of the motor system in the urodele amphibians (Straus, 1946; Székely and Czéh, 1967). However, there has been a brief report of hypoplasia of spinal motoneurons in *Ambystoma* observed several months after limb bud amputation (Stultz, 1942).

The motoneurons in anurans form a column in the ventrolateral part of the spinal cord (M. L. Silver, 1942; D. W. Kennard, 1959; Cruce, 1974). The normal development of this lateral motor column has been described in *Rana* (Beaudoin, 1955; Race and Terry, 1965; Hughes, 1968*a,b,c;* Pollack, 1969), *Xenopus* (Hughes, 1961; Prestige, 1967*b*), and *Eleutherodactylus* (Hughes, 1966, 1968*a*). Newly formed motoneurons migrate from the ventricular germinal zone laterally into the mantle layer of the spinal cord. This migration occurs during the early development of the limb bud, and the motoneurons grow slowly until midlarval stages. Lateral motoneurons at lumbosacral levels develop earlier than those in the brachial cord (Pollack, 1969). There is no evidence of death of young motoneurons until midlarval stages, but thereafter, through metamorphosis, 60–80 percent of the lateral motor column neurons degenerate.

Hughes (1961) counted the motoneurons in the lumbar ventral horn of the spinal cord in the clawed frog *Xenopus* at different stages during development, and found that for every neuron that finally survives to metamorphosis about eight degenerate. At Stage 53 (of the normal series of Nieuwkoop and Faber, 1956) there are about 4000 neurons in the lumbar region of the spinal cord, whereas at metamorphosis there are only 1200 (Fig. 7.10). Microglial cells appear at Stage 53 and phagocytose degenerating neurons. The peak of degeneration at larval Stages 54–56 coincides with the onset of movements in the hindlimbs, and this can be correlated with the formation of neuromuscular junctions as determined by cholinesterase staining (Hughes, 1961). The surviving neurons are presumably those that have formed peripheral connections. Their nuclear size almost doubles from midlarval stages to the completion of metamorphosis (Beaudoin, 1955; Race and Terry, 1965). Pollack (1969) observed a further increase in nuclear size after metamorphosis in the brachial lateral motoneurons of *Rana* (Fig. 7.11).

The development of the motoneurons in amphibians is partly under the control of the thyroid gland (Hughes, 1974, review). Although the production and initial differentiation of the motoneurons can occur in the absence of thyroxine in hypophysectomized frogs (Race, 1961), their full growth depends on the presence of thyroxine. High doses of thyroxine given to metamorphosing *Rana pipiens* result in precocious cytodifferentiation and death of spinal motoneurons (Reynolds, 1963). The corollary to this experiment is that an antithyroid drug, thiourea, prevents the cell death that normally occurs in the spinal cord and spinal ganglia of *Xenopus* from larval Stage 53 to metamorphosis (Prestige, 1965).

Beaudoin (1955) found that removal of the hindlimb bud of the frog *Rana pipiens* at an early larval stage (I or III of the normal stages of A. C. Taylor and Kollros, 1946) does not affect normal development of the motoneurons until after midlarval stages (IX), when rapid disappearance of motoneurons occurs on the operated side of the spinal cord and results in 82 percent hypoplasia by Stage XVI. Production, migration, and the initial stages of differentiation of motoneurons in the frog spinal cord do not appear to be affected by amputation of the hindlimb.

The most satisfactory analysis of the factors that determine the final number of motoneurons in the ventral horn of the spinal cord of the clawed frog *Xenopus* has been made by Prestige (1967*b*, 1970). Removal of a hindlimb before larval Stage 53, when the limb is in the palette stage, has no effect on the production and early maturation of spinal motoneurons (Hughes and Tschumi, 1958; Prestige, 1967*b*). Axons can be seen in the limb bud as early as Stage 49 (Hughes and Tschumi, 1958), and these have been shown to be motoneuron axons which transport horseradish peroxidase from the site of its injection into the Stage 50 limb bud to the motoneurons in the ventral horn of the spinal cord (Lamb, 1974). At these stages, the ventral horn neurons have not established neuromuscular connections in the limb. Peripheral neuromuscular connections are made soon after Stage 53 and movements of the hindlimb start at larval Stage 54. At the same time, histogenetic degeneration of neurons is first seen in the ventral horn of the spinal cord as well as in the spinal sensory ganglia supplying the hindlimbs. Amputation of a hindlimb at Stage 54, when the leg has reflex movements and therefore has sensory and motor connections, results within 3–4 days in massive degeneration of neurons in the ventral horn of the spinal cord. Death of spinal motoneurons during normal development in *Xenopus* reaches a peak at larval Stages 54–56 and then declines gradually to metamorphosis (Hughes, 1961). According to Hughes's calculations, the number of degenerating cells is greater than the decline in cell numbers, and therefore he concluded that cell proliferation continues during the period of cell degeneration. More direct evidence of the duration of cell proliferation should be obtained by determining how much [^{3}H]thymidine is incorporated into the DNA of newly generated spinal motoneurons in *Xenopus* at different larval stages.

Prestige (1967*b*) has pointed out that the effects of amputation of the developing limb differ according to the stage of maturation of the neurons. Before larval Stage 53, the ventral horn consists entirely of recently formed neurons with scanty cytoplasm. Outgrowth of axons from some of these neurons has commenced and some axons have entered the limb bud by Stage 50 (Hughes and Tschumi, 1958; Lamb, 1974), but neuromuscular connections are not made until

Stage 54. Limb bud amputation before Stage 53 has no effect on the young neurons, which continue to develop until the stage when their axons normally form connections with the limb muscles. In the absence of these muscles the motoneurons die at Stages 54–56. This shows that injury to the axon as a result of amputation of the limb bud is not the primary cause of cell death, because when the limb is amputated after the motoneurons have grown into it but before they have made neuromuscular connections, their death is delayed until the stage when they normally would have formed connections.

Prestige (1967*b*) found that the earlier the limb is removed, the shorter the latent period before the motoneurons start to degenerate. If the limb is amputated at larval Stage 54, when the majority of ventral horn cells are in the process of forming neuromuscular junctions, the resulting degeneration occurs within 3–4 days of amputation. Limb amputation at still later stages, after Stage 56, when the motoneurons are in the final stages of maturation, results in a gradual onset of chromatolysis and cell death. The latent period between limb amputation and death of spinal motoneurons depends on the maturity of the neurons at the time of amputation. When this is performed at Stages 55–56, final loss takes place after about 3 weeks; after amputation at Stage 57, during the fourth week; after amputation at Stage 61, during the third and fourth months; and after amputation as juveniles, not until the fourth to seventh months. "Young neurons therefore die after amputation very quickly, while older ones take longer. Thus the times at which cells die after amputation plot out a maturity spectrum for the cells in the ventral horn at the time of the operation" (Prestige, 1967*b*).

It is worth noting that in no case has complete absence of either sensory or motor neurons resulted from amputation of a limb in amphibian larvae or in the chick embryo. Even the most radical peripheral extirpation, short of damaging the spinal cord, results in survival of 10–20 percent of the motor or sensory neurons, and when only the limb is amputated a greater percentage of neurons survive. Either the surviving neurons innervate sense organs or muscles proximal to the amputated limb or some neurons survive for a long time in the absence of peripheral connections, perhaps because they were sustained by intracentral connections or do not require sustenance from sense organs or muscles.

The effects of amputation of a limb bud in the chick are similar to those in frogs. Shorey (1909) first showed that removal of a limb in chick embryos results in cellular hypoplasia in the spinal motoneurons and spinal sensory ganglia. Hamburger (1934) also found that removal of the wing bud of the chick embryo at 2½–3 days of incubation results, after 5 or 6 days, in reduction of between 28 and 61 percent in the number of motoneurons in the ventrolateral column of the spinal cord. The loss of motoneurons is roughly proportional to the amount of muscle that is removed. However, even the most radical excision of the limb results in survival of about 10–20 percent of the somatic motoneurons (Bueker, 1945*a*). Removal of the hindlimb bud results in catastrophic death of motoneurons in the lumbosacral region of the spinal cord of the chick. Hamburger (1958) has estimated that 20,000 motoneurons die within a period of 3 days after removal of the hindlimb bud. An even more catastrophic death of virtually all visceromotor cells in the cervical spinal cord occurs between the fourth and fifth days of incubation in the chick embryo during normal development (Levi-Montalcini, 1949), as is shown in Fig. 7.12. Less dramatic loss of neurons, amounting to about 70 percent

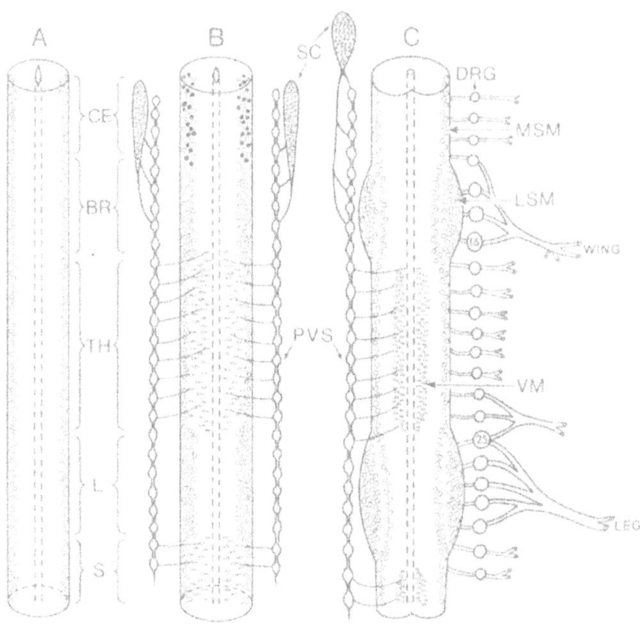

Figure 7.12. Origin and migration of motoneurons in the spinal cord of the chick embryo at 3 days (A), 4½ days (B), and 8 days (C) of incubation. The motoneurons originate uniformly at all levels from the germinal zone surrounding the central canal. Visceromotor neurons (spindle-shaped) migrate toward the central canal to form the visceromotor column (of Terni) at thoracic levels. Degenerating motoneurons at cervical levels are shown in black. The somatic motoneurons form into a medial column that supplies axial muscles and proximal limb muscles and into a lateral motor column that supplies distal limb muscles. In C, the spinal nerves and ganglia have been omitted on one side and the sympathetic ganglia on the other. BR, Brachial; CE, cervical; DRG, dorsal root ganglia; L, lumbar; LSM, lateral somatic motor column; MSM, medial somatic motor column; S, sacral; PVS, sympathetic ganglia; SC, superior cervical ganglion; TH, thoracic; VM, visceromotor. From R. Levi-Montalcini, *J. Morphol. 86:*253–283 (1950).

of the original number of visceromotor neurons, occurs during normal development of Hofmann's nucleus of the chick spinal cord during the last 10 days of incubation (Dubey *et al.,* 1968). A gradual loss of about 30 percent of the motoneurons in the ventral horn of the spinal cord occurs in normal mice between days 2 and 12 after birth (Romanes, 1946).

In summary: The case of the effects of limb amputation on spinal neurons provides a good example of the probabilistic nature of histogenetic cell death. The life of spinal motoneurons appears to be unaffected by the peripheral field during the early stages of neuronal differentiation. Only at the time when the motoneuron makes peripheral connections, and its functional adequacy is put to the test, do large numbers of motoneurons die. The number of neurons that die can be altered experimentally by removal or addition of peripheral organs. Such experiments have shown that the mechanism of this type of cell death involves a failure of neurons to achieve adequate connections with peripheral organs. However, the balance between life and death of the neuron may also be weighted by nutritive and hormonal factors.

The development of motoneurons does not occur synchronously throughout the spinal cord. Their development is most advanced in the hindbrain and there is a rostrocaudal gradient of maturity in the spinal cord. However, even at any given level of the spinal cord, there is asynchrony in the time of generation and the rate of development of different types of motoneurons. Some motoneurons arc already in an advanced stage of differentiation while production of motoneurons by division of ventricular germinal cells is still in progress. The peak of mitotic activity is seen in the basal plate of the chick spinal cord on day 3 and in the alar plate at day 6 of incubation (Hamburger, 1948). Mitosis declines rapidly from E6, and the great majority of neurons are formed in the spinal cord by E8. Thus tritiated thymidine injected after the eighth day of incubation does not label any spinal cord neurons, showing that DNA synthesis and mitosis in neuron precursors in the cord have ceased by E8 (S. Fujita, 1963, 1965*b*). From E8 to E21, glial cells increase steadily in the white matter of the spinal cord, as is shown in Fig. 2.6 (Bensted et al., 1957; H. Fujita and Fujita, 1964), and only the glial cells are labeled by tritiated thymidine injected into the chick embryo during this period of development (S. Fujita, 1963, 1965*b*).

The initial differentiation of motoneurons begins while they are still in the course of migration out of the ventricular germinal zone. At 40 hours of incubation, the first silver-impregnated neurofibrils can be seen in young motoneurons in the hindbrain near the otic invagination and in the cranial nerve nuclei (Cowdry, 1914). By 59 hours, silver impregnation can be seen in commissural fibers in the cord and in spinal ventral roots (Tello, 1922*a;* Hughes, 1955). Axons of the motoneurons continue to grow out into the ventral roots during E3, E4, and E5. The first motor axons make contact with anterior trunk muscles at 3½ days. The first motor axons arrive at the proximal muscles of the limb on day 5 of incubation. Barron (1946) named these the "primary motor neuroblasts"; those that sprouted axons on days 5 and 6 he named the "secondary" motoneurons, but there is no compelling evidence in favor of this conjecture. The axons of most of these late-differentiating neurons are commissural, but some do exit via dorsal and ventral roots (Windle and Orr, 1934). Barron (1943, 1946, 1948) observed that the development of dendrites of spinal motoneurons occurs shortly after their axons connect with the muscles, and postulated that the sprouting of dendrites is triggered by the contact of the axon with muscle fibers.

It is convenient, at this juncture, to summarize the development of the spinal reflex circuits in relationship to the onset of reflex behavior. Reflexes can first be elicited by stimulating the skin on day 6, and this can be correlated with the growth of the central processes of dorsal root ganglion cells into the spinal cord on days 5 and 6, and the first appearance of synapses in the spinal cord on day 5. The reflex arcs from the skin, which pass via the dorsal root ganglia and spinal interneurons to motoneurons ending in muscles, are completed on days 5–7 at different spinal levels. The onset of stretch reflexes is delayed until days 10 and 11, when the monosynaptic reflex circuit from the muscle spindles to motoneurons is completed (see Section 8.6).

In the chick spinal cord the motoneurons are arranged as follows: The lateral somatic motor column, which supplies the limbs, is present only in the brachial (segments 12–16) and the lumbar (segments 22–30) enlargements of the cord. The medial somatic motor column, which innervates the axial musculature, extends throughout the length of the cord (Fig. 7.12). The visceral preganglionic neurons lie in the ventrolateral column (of Terni) and send axons to the prevertebral autonomic ganglia. There are also segmental groups of neurons situated laterally in the spinal cord just beneath the pia mater, which have been called *marginal nuclei* or *Hofmann's nuclei*. They are probably preganglionic visceromotor neurons.

Levi-Montalcini (1950) has described the histogenesis of the ventrolateral motor column of the spinal cord of the chick embryo as follows: The ventrolateral motor column is formed by migration of neurons from the ventricular germinal zone of the basal plate starting on the second day of incubation. Migration starts at the cervical level and extends rapidly caudally so that mitotic figures are uniformly distributed in the basal plate throughout the cord. Neuron production reaches a maximum on the third day of incubation (Hamburger, 1948; Corliss and Robertson, 1963). Neurons develop uniformly throughout the spinal cord, apparently as a result of a uniform rate of motosis in the germinal zone of the basal plate (Hamburger, 1948). At that stage, all the young neurons in the ventrolateral motor column are morphologically identical when stained with hematoxylin or silver. However, Levi-Montalcini (1950) has shown that they are functionally heterogeneous: some young neurons differentiate further into somatic motoneurons whose axons grow into the ventral roots to the muscles, whereas others differentiate into visceral preganglionic neurons whose axons run in the rami communicantes to the prevertebral autonomic ganglia. The growth of the rami communicantes occurs at 3–4 days of incubation at all levels of the spinal cord except the brachial and lumbosacral, where they are absent. In the cervical region of the spinal cord, all the preganglionic visceral neurons degenerate and disappear in a short period of about 12 hours between 4½ and 5 days of incubation (Fig. 7.12). This occurs at the same time as the headward migration of the prevertebral cervical sympathetic ganglia to form the orthosympathetic cervical ganglia. Using the electron microscope, Wechsler (1966*a,b*) found evidence of cell degeneration, seen maximally in the anterior horn of the spinal cord of 4½-day chick embryos. At E4½, degenerating neuroepithelial germinal cells, young neurons, and glioblasts were identified, but there are reasons for skepticism about the accuracy with which these types of cells can be recognized and distinguished from each other on electron photomicrographs, particularly when they are in various stages of degeneration.

It is noteworthy that the initial growth of capillaries into the neural tube of the chick embryo at 4½–6 days of incubation occurs at the same time as the onset of cell degeneration (Ramón y Cajal, 1929*b;* Hughes, 1934; J. F. Feeney and Watterson, 1946). Capillarization of the spinal cord of *Xenopus* also occurs during the period of maximal cell death (Sims, 1961). This correlation of ingrowth of capillaries and the appearance of macrophages that remove the debris of dead cells is consistent with the concept of the hematogenous origin of brain macrophages (see Section 2.6).

Migration of young motoneurons in the spinal cord of the chick embryo starts at 4½ days as follows: At E4, all the young motoneurons of the chick spinal cord form a compact ventrolateral column of cells, uniform at all levels. The most medial neurons at thoracolumbar levels start migrating medially from the ventrolateral column at E4½ (Fig. 7.12). They form a column of preganglionic visceral neurons which become visibly differentiated after E5, and they can be distinguished from the somatic motoneurons by the much larger size of the latter. From E5, the young somatic motoneurons grow much more rapidly than the young visceral neurons, so that at hatching the visceral motoneurons are about one-tenth the size of the somatic motoneurons.

Beginning at E5, the ventrolateral motor column enlarges at the brachial and lumbosacral levels of the spinal cord, mainly as a result of growth of the somatic motoneurons. At the same time, the somatic motoneurons segregate into a small medial and a large lateral column. The medial column runs through all levels of the spinal cord. The lateral column is absent at the thoracolumbar and cervical regions, having degenerated in the cervical region and having migrated medially to form the visceromotor column in the thoracolumbar region of the cord, as is illustrated in Fig. 7.12 (Levi-Montalcini, 1950, 1964*a,b*).

The development of Hofmann's nucleus major of the chick spinal cord has been described by Dubey *et al.* (1968). The cells that form these nuclei arise by separation of the most lateral neurons of the marginal layer of the spinal cord at about 6 days of incubation. At E7–E10, there are 25–27 pairs of nuclei, arranged segmentally, one on each side of the spinal cord just beneath the pia mater. The eight pairs of nuclei in the lumbosacral region enlarge during E8–E14 and form bilateral prominent bulges on the ventrolateral aspect of the spinal cord. Between E10 and E14, the number of cells in Hofmann's nuclei is greatly reduced, but the surviving cells increase in size. Dubey *et al.* (1968) found that only 31 percent of the cells present in Hofmann's nuclei of the embryo survive in the adult. They also found that the number of cells is not affected by amputation of the limb buds or by grafting of an additional limb, and they concluded that neurons of Hofmann's nuclei do not supply the limbs, but are probably visceral preganglionic neurons.

Almost all the available evidence, which will be summarized below, shows that the proliferation and initial differentiation of motoneurons are not influenced from a distance by the peripheral organs. The analysis is complicated because of the errors inherent in methods of measuring cellular proliferation in the nervous system, which were discussed in Section 2.3. It is equally difficult to obtain a meaningful measure of the rate of cellular differentiation because development of neurons does not occur synchronously; therefore, in any region of the neural tube, cells can be seen in different phases of proliferation, migration, and differentiation. It has also proved impossible to remove the limb rudiment in the chick embryo before the stage at which some motoneurons have already reached a relatively advanced state of differentiation. For example, the brachial spinal cord of the 72-hour chick embryo has the following appearance, according to Hamburger (1934): "Large number of mitoses are found around the central canal. Neuroblasts in various stages of differentiation may be found in the wall. Small groups of motor neuroblasts are already assembled in the anterior horn region. Some of them have sent out their axons which form a tiny anterior root. The spinal ganglia are already formed; they have established their first connections with the spinal cord by forming the dorsal root and the first sensory fibers have joined the motor fibers." The earliest stage at which the wing bud has been amputated in order to test its effect on the development of the brachial spinal cord has been at 2½ days of incubation, and the ensuing reduction in the number of mitotic figures is barely significant and occurs only after days 5 and 6 of incubation (Hamburger and Keefe, 1944), by which stage the production of neurons in the brachial region has almost ceased. It thus seems that glial cell production rather than neuronal production is affected by limb bud amputation. Moreover, the mitotic activity in the basal plate of the spinal cord, which is the source of the motoneurons supplying the limbs, reaches a peak on day 3 of incubation and declines to a low level thereafter (Hamburger, 1948). After removing a limb bud on day 3 of incubation, Hamburger (1958) found no reduction in the number of lateral motoneurons until day 5, after which there was a rapid degeneration of well-differentiated motoneurons.

There is considerable evidence that proliferation of neuroepithelial germinal cells and the initial stages of neuron differentiation are independent of the periphery, and that the neurons become affected by the periphery only after the stage when their axons have grown into the peripheral organs. Connection between the axon and its postsynaptic target is essential only for the final maturation of the neuron and for the maintenance of the neuron. Thus amputation of a limb bud in anuran amphibians has no effect on the proliferation and early differentiation of cells in the spinal cord and spinal ganglia (Beaudoin, 1955; Perri, 1956; Hughes, 1961; Prestige, 1967*a,b,* 1974). In amphibians, amputation of a limb results in death of neurons at the stage of development when they would normally have formed peripheral connections. In the chick embryo the evidence, given below, leads to the same conclusion.

The brachial and lumbar enlargements of the chick embryo spinal cord, which innervate the limbs, do not have more mitoses than at other levels (Hamburger, 1948, Corliss and Robertson, 1963). The increase of neurons at limb levels of the spinal cord is due to a relative decrease of cell degeneration and reduction of the number of cells migrating out, rather than to an increase in cell proliferation (Levi-Montalcini, 1950). Yates (1961) found no differences of proliferation rate in spinal ganglia isolated on the chorioallantoic membrane in 5-day chick embryos, compared with the proliferation rates in the spinal ganglia of intact 3- to 12-day chick embryos. There are also no changes to be seen in the paravertebral autonomic ganglia examined 5 days after amputation of the wing bud of 3-day chick embryos, but at 19 days of incubation the brachial ganglia show hypoplasia of from 20 to 80 percent (Simmler, 1949). Therefore, it seems likely that cellular proliferation in the ganglia is unaffected but that immature neurons die in the absence of the limb they normally innervate.

The available evidence shows that removal of muscles in the chick embryo does not affect the proliferation and initial differentiation of the motoneurons. For example, after excision of the superior oblique muscle anlage in the chick embryo at 1½ days of incubation, the proliferation, migration, and differentiation of trochlear motoneurons proceed normally until the full complement of trochlear neurons is formed at 5 days. No difference is found at 5 days of incubation between the trochlear nucleus on the side that is in possession of its peripheral field and the nucleus on the side that lacks its peripheral field (Dunnebacke, 1953; Cowan and Wenger, 1967). After amputation of a leg of a 2½-day chick embryo, Hamburger (1958) found that the development of the lateral motor column continues normally up to 5 days, but the majority of lumbosacral lateral motoneurons die at 5–8 days, during the period that they would normally have made connections in the leg.

The evidence does not support the opinion that the periphery can influence the centers from a distance, before the outgrowing axons make peripheral contacts. The only way in which such an action at a distance could occur is by the release of humoral agents from the peripheral organs into the bloodstream or extracellular fluid, and it is difficult to imagine such an effect localized to a specific group of neurons. On the contrary, the evidence shows that proliferation of neuroepithelial germinal cells and the initial differentiation of neurons occur normally in the absence of the peripheral organs, and that degeneration of neurons occurs only after their axons have reached close to their targets in the peripheral organs or have actually formed connections with them. Contacts between terminals of the axons and the peripheral organs seem to be essential for the maturation of the neuron and for the maintenance of the neurons. If this is true, the possibility must be entertained that materials are transferred from the peripheral tissues to the tips of the axons, and a message is then transmitted up the axon to the neuron soma, resulting in growth and maturation of the neuron. Flow of materials from axonal endings toward the cell body was first seen by Hughes (1953) in isolated spinal dorsal root ganglia in culture, and reported by Nakai (1956) in isolated neurons from dorsal root ganglia. More recent studies of retrograde axonal flow are discussed in Section 4.9. The nature of the putative factor or factors is not known. Prestige (1967*a,b*) has suggested that there is a "maintenance factor" that is transported by retrograde axonal flow from the periphery to the developing cell body. The delay in degeneration after removal of the limb bud indicates that the "maintenance factor" is stored in the cell body and that the cell dies when its stores are exhausted. This idea is entirely consistent with the evidence and is essentially the same as that of the delayed onset of atrophy of muscle and cutaneous sense organs after their supply of trophic factors is cut off: the longer the peripheral stump of the axon, the larger the reservoir of trophic factor and the longer the delay before the onset of atrophy in the muscle and sensory cells (J. M. D. Olmsted, 1920*b;* Parker, 1932; Parker and Paine, 1934; J. V. Luco and Eyzaguirre, 1955). The notion that the motoneurons become "dependent" on the "maintenance factor" follows, according to Prestige (1970), from the observation that the motoneurons are not dependent on the limb before they have formed peripheral connections, but after forming connections they become dependent on the integrity of the axonal lifeline conveying the "maintenance factor" from the postsynaptic cells.

7.9. Peripheral Influences on the Development of Neurons in Spinal Sensory Ganglia

Amputation of a developing limb in amphibian larvae results in reduction in the number of cells in the spinal ganglia supplying the limb in urodeles and anurans (Shorey, 1909; Dürken, 1911; Detwiler, 1924; Wieman and Nussman, 1929; R. M. May 1930, 1933; Hughes and Tschumi, 1958; Prestige, 1967*a,* 1974, Hughes and Carr, 1978, review).

Although the neurons in the spinal ganglia of the amphibians all have the same histological appearance, there must be at least two functional types that have not been identified histologically. One type must supply the muscle spindles and tendon stretch receptors, and the other type must provide sensory nerves to the skin. Amputation of the limb bud would remove the peripheral field of both types.

Increase in the number of cells in the spinal sensory ganglia occurs as a result of peripheral overloading. For example, heteroplastic transplantation of a limb from the larva of a large species of salamander (*Ambystoma tigrinum*) in place of the limb of a smaller species (*Ambystoma punctatum*) results in cellular hyperplasia of the spinal ganglia supplying the limb (Detwiler, 1930*b;* Schwind, 1931). Heteroplastic transplantation of a limb from *Ambystoma tigrinum* to the head of *Ambystoma punctatum* results in hyperplasia of cranial ganglia (Detwiler, 1930*a*). Hyperplasia of spinal sensory ganglia occurs after grafting of additional limbs in amphibians (Detwiler, 1920*b*, 1933*a*, review; R. M. May, 1933). In a frog with three functional right legs, Bueker (1945*b*) found hyperplasia of more than 70 percent in spinal ganglia S8 and S9 connected with the extra limbs.

It should be noted that there are several authoritative reports of the absence of either sensory or motor hyperplasia in amphibians with additional limbs (Harrison, 1924*b;* Nicholas, 1924; Weiss, 1937*b*). The conditions of these experiments must have differed in some unknown way from those that resulted in hyperplasia in other experiments.

Very limited conclusions about the mechanism of control of cell numbers in the sensory ganglia can be drawn from all these experiments, mainly because the effects were observed at relatively long intervals following limb bud amputation or transplantation. A more satisfactory analysis has been made of the mechanisms controlling the number of cells in the spinal ganglia of the clawed frog, *Xenopus* (Hughes and Tschumi, 1958; Prestige, 1965, 1967*a*, 1974).

The number of neurons that finally mature in the spinal ganglia is determined by the number generated, as well as by the number that die before maturation. During normal development, cell death is first seen in the spinal ganglia S8, S9, and S10, which supply the hindlimbs of *Xenopus,* at larval Stage 53, just before movement of the limb begins (Prestige, 1965). Histogenetic degeneration in the ventral horn of the spinal cord starts at about the same time (Hughes, 1961; Prestige, 1967*b*).

Prestige (1965) counted the total number of cells and the number of degenerating cells during development in the spinal ganglia S8, S9, and S10, and found that two neurons degenerate for every one that survives to maturity. Degeneration starts at Stage 54, when the toes of the hindlimb are being formed. The hindlimbs have spontaneous movements at that stage, but they are insensitive until Stage 55, when reflex movements can be elicited by stimulating the skin of the legs (Hughes and Prestige, 1967). Degeneration of neurons in spinal ganglia supplying the hindlimb reaches a peak at Stages 55–56. In spinal ganglia S8, S9, and S10 on one side, 1500 neurons at Stage 50 increase to about 10,000 at Stage 55, which are later reduced to about 8000 at Stage 65. An estimated 20,000 neurons degenerate during this period of about 60 days. In the trunk ganglia S5, S6, and S7, which do not supply the limbs, the number of neurons increases from about 1500 at Stage 50 to over 3000 at Stages 55–57, and decreases to 2500 at Stage 65. An estimated 4000 neurons degenerate in these ganglia; that is, two die for every one that matures. These estimates should be regarded with caution because they are based on the unsupported assumption, initially made by Hughes (1961), that the degeneration time is about 3 hours.

7.10. Development of Spinal Sensory Ganglia in the Chick Embryo

A great deal of effort has been devoted to investigating the influence of the periphery on the development of the spinal ganglion neurons, especially in the chick embryo. Before giving an account of these studies, it is necessary to outline the chronology of normal development of spinal dorsal root ganglia.

The spinal ganglia are formed by migration of neural crest cells (see Section 1.4). This occurs during the first 2½ days of incubation in the chick embryo (Weston, 1963; Weston and Butler, 1966; Johnston, 1966). At 2½ days of incubation, the first signs of neuronal differentiation and growth are visible in the ventrolateral part of the spinal ganglia, and these ventrolateral neurons are then distinguishable from the smaller cells in the mediodorsal part of the ganglion, which do not start their growth spurt until 9 days of incubation (Table 7.1). At the end of the third day of incubation, the central processes of the ventrolateral cells reach, but do not yet enter, the spinal cord in the brachial region (Tello, 1922*a;* Levi-Montalcini and Levi, 1943). They enter the cord and form the dorsal roots on day 5, just before the spinal motor reflexes can be elicited by cutaneous stimulation on day 6, thus indicating that the peripheral processes of the ventrolateral cells in the spinal ganglia form connections in the skin (Visintini and Levi-Montalcini, 1939). The large ventrolateral cells grow in size and gradually assume their characteristic pseudo-unipolar form on days 8–10 of incubation. They do not develop an affinity for silver until 9–10 days, and neurofibrils can be seen in them from that time (Hamburger and Levi-Montalcini, 1949).

The small mediodorsal cells differentiate and grow in size from day 9. Neurofibrils are first seen in silver-impregnated mediodorsal cells at 10 days (Visintini and Levi-Montalcini, 1939), coincident with the arrival of the sensory

Table 7.1. Differences between Ventrolateral and Mediodorsal Cells in Spinal Ganglia of Chick Embryo[a]

	Ventrolateral cells	Mediodorsal cells
Position in ganglion	Ventrolateral	Mediodorsal
Size	Large	Small
Origin	Neural crest	Neural crest
Development	Differentiate early (2½–8 days incubation)	Differentiate late (9–15 days incubation)
Functions	Cutaneous sensation; connect with dermis at 7 days of incubation	Proprioceptive; connect with muscle stretch receptors at about 11 days of incubation
Effect of removing peripheral field (wing bud amputation)	Rapid degeneration	Slow atrophy
Effect of increasing peripheral field (grafting extra limb)	Increased cell number as a result of reduced cell death	No effect
Effect of nerve growth factor	No effect	Increased RNA and protein synthesis; increased growth; perhaps protection from cell death

[a]Adapted from Hamburger and Levi-Montalcini (1949).

nerves at the muscle spindles (Tello, 1922*b*). This also coincides with the time when stretch reflexes can first be elicited on flexing the hindlimbs. Therefore, Hamburger and Levi-Montalcini (1949) suggested that at least some of the mediodorsal cells of the spinal ganglia are connected with sensory terminals in muscle spindles. From day 9 the mediodorsal cells grow faster than the ventrolateral cells, so that from day 15 it is no longer possible to distinguish the two cell types histologically. By day 20 of incubation, cells of all sizes are distributed throughout the ganglion except at its ventrolateral margin, where a rim of ventrolateral cells persists.

Differentiation of spinal dorsal root ganglion cells of the chick embryo has been studied with the light and electron microscope (Pannese, 1968, 1969; Pannese *et al.,* 1971). The most interesting findings are that until day 5 of incubation the young neurons have scant cytoplasm, little rough endoplasmic reticulum, and few polyribosomes. After day 5, they show all the signs of mature neurons that are exporting materials into the axon: well-developed rough endoplasmic reticulum, a large number of free ribosomes, mitochondria, and an extensive system of Golgi cisternae. The neurons, which are in close apposition until day 5, become separated by ensheathing glial cells. Acetylcholinesterase (AChE), assayed histochemically with the electron microscope, is detectable in the chick embryo spinal dorsal ganglion cells at 3 days of incubation (Pannese *et al.,* 1971). In the rabbit embryo, AChE is present in the spinal ganglia at 10 days of gestation (Tennyson *et al.,* 1967). In these cases, as well as in *Ambystoma* embryos, AChE appears before the neurons form either peripheral or central connections.

Mitotic activity in the spinal ganglia reaches a peak on days 5–6, and is completed at day 9 (Levi-Montalcini and Levi, 1943; Hamburger and Levi-Montalcini, 1949). Proliferation of glial cells is said to start after day 9 and to continue through hatching (Bensted *et al.,* 1957), but the electron microscopic observations indicate that glial cells are present as early as day 5 and that they totally ensheath the neurons by day 10 (Pannese, 1969). The earlier studies of histogenesis in the spinal ganglia were made by counting cells and mitotic figures, and they have recently been supplemented by the more reliable technique of tritiated thymidine autoradiography (Carr, 1975, 1976). The latter studies show that production of neurons ceases by 6½ days in the ventrolateral region and by 7½ days in the mediodorsal region, and that only glial cells continue to be produced in the spinal ganglia after 7½ days of incubation.

The pattern of normal cell death in the spinal ganglia of the chick embryo is as follows: Few degenerating cells are seen before 4½ days, but cell death reaches a maximum at 5–6 days, then decreases rapidly, and is virtually completed at the end of day 7 (Hamburger and Levi-Montalcini, 1949). Little or no cell death occurs in the ganglia that supply the limbs, namely brachial ganglia 14–16 and lumbosacral ganglia 24–29. Cell death is maximal in the cervical and thoracic ganglia, which do not supply the limbs. Cell death is localized to the ventrolateral part of the ganglion, which is occupied by the large, early-differentiating neurons. Therefore, Hamburger and Levi-Montalcini (1949) postulated that only "differentiated neurons are affected by degeneration." In the following paragraphs, evidence will be given to show that the ventrolateral neurons in the check spinal ganglia are much more sensitive than the mediodorsal neurons to changes in the peripheral field produced by amputating or grafting limbs. It should be noted that the converse is true of the responses of these cells to nerve growth factor (see Section 6.7.3).

Increase or reduction in the size of the peripheral innervation zone has different effects on ventrolateral and mediodorsal cells of the chick spinal ganglia. According to Hamburger and Levi-Montalcini (1949), amputation of a limb of the chick embryo at 2½–3 days of incubation has the following effects on spinal ganglion cells: the majority of differentiated ventrolateral cells degenerate at 5–6 days of incubation, while the mediodorsal cells slowly atrophy. This shows that the neurons die in the absence of the limb in which they normally form connections.

Grafting an extra limb on the chick embryo at 2½–3 days of incubation results in an increase by as much as 80 percent in the number of neurons that differentiate to form ventrolateral cells in the spinal ganglia innervating the extra limb. The mediodorsal cells appear to be unaffected. Hamburger and Levi-Montalcini (1949) also observed an increase of about 20 percent in the number of mitoses in the spinal ganglia at the level of the grafted limb. From these observations they concluded that "two basically different mechanisms operate in the control of spinal ganglion development by peripheral factors: (a) the periphery controls the *proliferation* and *initial* differentiation of undifferentiated cells which have no connections of their own with the periphery; (b) the periphery provides the conditions necessary for *continued growth* and *maintenance* of neurons following the first outgrowth of neurites." The weight of available evidence is against these conclusions. The evidence shows that production of neurons and the outgrowth of their axons occur without regard to the presence or absence of the peripheral tissues. However, *contact* between the axons and peripheral tissues seems to be necessary for the maturation and maintenance of the neurons. The growth of the neurons appears to stimulate production of neuroglia so that one of the effects of amputation of a limb bud is to reduce glial cell proliferation. This has been shown by tritiated thymidine autoradiography of the brachial dorsal root ganglia after amputation of the wing bud of the chick embryo at 2½ days of incubation (Carr, 1976). Neuron production is unaffected by wing bud amputation until day 6½ of incubation, after which a considerable reduction of proliferation is observed in the ventrolateral region only. Carr (1975, 1976) showed that proliferation in the ventrolateral region after day 6½ is exclusively neuroglial; it is clear that amputation of the wing bud results in diminished production of glial cells but not of neurons. Carr (1976) found that grafting an additional wing bud does not increase proliferation, as shown by no increase in labeling with [^{3}H]thymidine, in the ganglia that innervate the graft as compared with the normal ganglia on the other side.

Another set of sensory neurons that has been shown to depend on the size of its peripheral field is the trigeminal mesencephalic nucleus, which supplies the sensory nerves to the muscle spindles in the jaw muscles. One of the advantages of this nucleus is that the neurons are large and easy to count, and are clearly distinguishable from glial cells. Excision of the mandible from salamander larvae results in marked reduction of the number of cells in the mesencephalic nucleus (Piatt, 1946). Conversely, heteroplastic grafting of the large mandible of *Ambystoma tigrinum* in place of the smaller mandible of *Ambystoma punctatum* during embryonic stages results in considerable increase in the number of neurons in the mesencephalic nucleus. In this case, the mechanism of the hyperplasia has not been studied. In the light of what is known, it is most likely to have resulted from survival of neurons that would have died in the absence of a large enough peripheral field to provide targets for all the mesencephalic neurons that are produced. This has been more definitely demonstrated for the trigeminal mesencephalic nucleus of the chick embryo (L. A. Rogers and Cowan, 1973). The neurons are produced in the neural folds or neural crest on days 3 and 4 of incubation, and by day 6 the total number, about 4500 neurons, has assembled in the mesencephalic nucleus. Cell death in the nucleus becomes appreciable during the next 4 days and reaches a maximum on days 11–12. From the 13th day of incubation, the number of cells remains stable at about 1000. Thus, of the neurons that are produced and migrate to form the trigeminal mesencephalic nucleus, about 75 percent die, almost certainly after their axons have reached the periphery.

The controversy about whether changes in the size of the peripheral field affect cellular proliferation in the nervous system can now be said to have been finally resolved. In summary, it can be said that the production of neurons occurs independently of the peripheral tissues that the neurons are destined to innervate. The neurons die or fail to grow if their axons do not make synaptic connections, and this may result in a reduced production of glial cells associated with the neurons deprived of their peripheral targets.

It follows from all these reports of hyperplasia of sets of neurons which have been given extra targets that the cells which normally die, but survive in such experiments, are not predestined to die. Such neurons are not defective, nor are they incapable of forming connections if provided with targets. Death of such neurons cannot be regarded as a form of "error correction," but is the consequence of saturating the targets with more neurons than they can support. In the event, the gross overproduction of neurons ensures that every target receives a nerve fiber. Matching a set of neurons with a set of targets which are produced independently may require a one-to-one correspondence between neurons and targets, or some less rigid many-to-many form of correspondence between neurons and targets. The evidence that additional targets can save neurons from death proves that the neurons are not matched one-to-one with targets. Evidence that sense organs and muscles can be cross-innervated by foreign nerves (see Chapter 8) shows that the specificity of sensory nerves for sense organs and of motoneurons for skeletal muscle is not absolute. The question of whether there is a range of specificities which are expressed only when nerves compete for targets cannot be answered in this case. If, as I have postulated (M. Jacobson, 1970*a,b,* 1973), the neurons within a set are not identical, they may compete for the available target cells, the survivors being selected according to one or other criterion of fitness. This is discussed further in the following section.

7.11. Variations, Anomalies, and Errors of Neuronal Ontogeny and Their Significance

Invariance of the structure of the nervous system is so striking that less attention has been given to the variations of brain structure between individuals or between different strains within a species. Variations are the essential prerequisites for evolution by natural selection, but they have an evolutionary effect only when they result in selective advantages or disadvantages. As I have pointed out (M. Jacobson, 1970*a,b,* 1974*b,* 1975*a*), variability is largely found in the structures that develop last: in the Type II neurons and in the dendrites of Type I neurons.

These structures may be affected by mutations which may have no selective advantage or disadvantage; that is, they may be neutral. It is postulated that such neutral mutations will accumulate because they are not eliminated by natural selection, and in time this accumulation will result in an increase in the polymorphism of the nervous system. As the polymorphism increases, certain structures may become advantageous or disadvantageous. The repository of neutral or nearly neutral mutations, which may provide the individual with negligible functional advantages under one set of environmental conditions, may become of significant advantage under a different set of conditions.

This hypothesis of a mechanism of neural evolution, like all hypotheses of mechanisms of evolution, is difficult or impossible to prove. It depends on several converging lines of evidence. First, it depends on the evidence of variability in the structure of the nervous system. Neuronal types and typical patterns of neuronal organization can be recognized because of their invariant features, but anyone who has had some experience of neuroanatomy and neurocytology is aware of the variability within cells of a given class and is struck by the frequency of anomalous patterns of neuronal organization in normal individuals in which such anomalies do not result in abnormal functions.

Distinction between true errors and variations is easily made in theory but is more difficult to make in practice. Variations are inherited differences between strains of the same species. Errors are unpredictable deviations from normal structure that are not determined genetically, except in the sense that everything in the organism is under some degree of genetic control. In practice, the distinction between variations and errors is made by showing that the former are inherited while the latter are not. The variability in what are generally considered to be extremely invariant neuronal structures appears to have been overlooked. Whenever a careful search has been made, variability has been found even in the invertebrate nervous system, which has generally been regarded as very stereotyped. In the locust nervous system, two types of variability have been seen. Individual variations have been seen in the structure of identified neurons which conform to their type but show variability in the fine patterns of axonal and dendritic branching (Bullock and Horridge, 1965; Macagno *et al.,* 1973). Major variations occur in the brain of the locust, including cases in which axons project to lobes of the brain in which they are not normally found (C. Goodman, 1974). Duplication of cells has been seen as a rare anomaly in the ocellar interneurons of the locust (C. Goodman, 1974) and in the Mauthner's neuron of amphibians (Stefanelli, 1951). Even in the projection of the retinula axons in the fly, which in most cases show great precision of their connections, some "erroneous" connections are occasionally found in "normal" animals (Meinertzhagen, 1972). In a leech that was found with more cells than usual in many of its ganglia, the supernumerary cells formed normal connections (D. P. Kuffler and Muller, 1974).

In newborn rats and newly hatched chicks, there is considerable individual variability in brain DNA content, which is an index of the total number of cells (neurons plus glial cells). For example, about 0.25 percent of chicks and 0.4 percent of rats have brain DNA content at birth or hatching that is well above the range of brain DNA content of individuals from the same litter or same batch of eggs (Zamenhof *et al.,* 1971*c*). It is not known whether these rare cases of high brain cell number result from increased cell proliferation or from diminished cell death, nor is it known whether neurons or glia are affected. It is also not known whether the increased brain cell number results from a superior nutrient supply or whether it is caused by conditions within the embryo. No studies have been undertaken to determine whether the variability in brain DNA content is inherited. However, genetically determined variability in the number of neurons of the hippocampal formation has been found in mice (Wimer *et al.*, 1976).

Differences in brain structure which depend on the genotype have been described in many species, but such "neurological mutants" (see Section 3.4.5 for mutations affecting the cerebellum and Section 9.10 for anomalous visual pathways in albinos) are usually at such a large selective disadvantage that they could not have survived in natural conditions. However, a striking variation in brain structure, which appears to have little or no selective value and may be neutral, occurs in mice of the strain BALB/cJ. In these mice, the hippocampal mossy fibers do not form the usual *infra*pyramidal synaptic field but form an *intra*pyramidal synaptic field instead (Barber *et al.*, 1974). This instance of genetically determined variability is particularly striking, first, because it is seen in a structure, the hippocampal formation, that is generally thought of as quite invariant. Second, the variation is found in the mossy fibers, which are the axonal terminals of the granule cells, typical Type II neurons. Such slight variations that are inherited in inbred strains of mice have no known functional effects, and have neither selective advantage nor disadvantage. However, accumulation of such mutations may ultimately become advantageous or disadvantageous. Such variations in structure should not be regarded as "errors" of development. Errors are chance deviations from the normal range, and any structure that occurs with a high probability in all individuals of the species cannot be called an error. Transient structures that appear only for a short period of development should not be termed "errors" if they occur predictably in all individuals. Such, for example, are the transient excesses of the number of neurons in many parts of the nervous system which arise and disappear predictably at specific stages of development (see Section 7.6).

Anyone who has handled many brains will have reached the conclusion that no two brains of individuals of the same species are exactly alike. There are always small individual variations. The range of such variability in the human brain is large enough to have to be taken into consideration by neurosurgeons who probe the human brain stereotaxically, for example, to make lesions in the basal ganglia (Van Buren and Maccubin, 1962). Individual variability is most easily seen in the gyri and sulci of the human cerebral hemispheres (Bailey and von Bonin, 1951). Variations in the dimensions of the cerebral convolutions were the main evidence used by Gall (1810) to support his hypothesis that such individual variations are correlated with individual personality traits (see Section 3.6). The functional significance of individual variations of human brain structure is not known, and neither are the genetic and developmental mechanisms that may give rise to individual variability in brain structure. There is, however, one case in which left–right asymmetry of cerebral cortical structures is known to be related to specific brain functions, namely to the lateralization of language functions in the cerebral hemispheres. This lateralization, which is probably genetically determined, is correlated with an increased size of the temporal planum and the frontal operculum, gyri related to cortical language functions, in the speech dominant hemisphere (Geschwind and Levitsky, 1968; Geschwind, 1970, 1972). This asymmetry becomes measurable as early as the 29th week of gestation, and is well developed at birth (Witelson and Pallie, 1973; Wada *et al.*, 1975).

Other asymmetries of brain structure also appear to be inherited, for example, the left–right asymmetry of the habenula nuclei in teleosts and amphibians

(Braitenberg and Kemali, 1970). An additional habenular nucleus starts developing on the left side at the beginning of metamorphosis in frogs, and attains full size about 2 months after metamorphosis (M. J. Morgan *et al.*, 1973). The same asymmetry—the presence of an accessory left habenular nucleus—is found in newts, but the asymmetry is reversed in newts with *situs inversus,* either produced by making lesions in the gastrula or present in natural populations in about 2 percent of individuals (von Woellwarth, 1950, 1969). Ludwig (1932) has reviewed the problem of the origins and functional effects of left–right asymmetry, but he was unable to adduce any general conclusions. The functional significance, developmental mechanisms, and evolutionary origins of left–right asymmetries in the nervous system remain largely unknown. They should not be thought of as "errors" of development.

Anomalous location of single neurons is fairly common, and even groups of ectopic neurons are found in a large percentage of adult human and primate brains when they are examined thoroughly (H. R. Schneider, 1968). This type of individual variability has been termed *heteromorphism* by Feremutsch (1952, 1960). Displaced and disoriented neurons are often found close to blood vessels which appear to have obstructed their migration. According to Ramón y Cajal (1929*a*), "In all neural organs one occasionally sees atypical and accidental arrangements with regard to the path and orientation of axons. . . . All these aberrations are produced during fetal development and can be explained by obstacles which the neurons must surmount during their migration."

Ectopic neurons are found in the human brain in a number of pathological conditions and are occasionally seen in individuals with no neurological disease (see reviews by Ostertag, 1956; Crome and Stern, 1972; Norman, 1966). That some of these ectopias are the result of arrested migration is shown by the fact that the displaced neurons are situated in one of the migratory paths (Wiest and Hallervorden, 1958; Rakic, 1975*a*). Thus ectopic olivary neurons, arrested in the medulla during migration from the rhombic lip via the pontobulbar body to the inferior olive, are seen in cases of pachygyria and of lissencephaly (A. E. Walker, 1942; Hanaway *et al.*, 1968). In almost all cases of trisomy 18, ectopic neurons are seen arrested in the course of their migration along the corpus geniculothalamicum to the thalamus (Norman, 1966; Sumi, 1970; Terplan *et al.*, 1970). In the cerebellum, ectopic granule cells are often seen in the molecular layer in normal rabbits (Špacek *et al.*, 1973) and in normal humans (Brustowicz and Kernohan, 1952) as well as in a number of diseases of various etiologies. Although the mechanism of production of the ectopias is not known, the common factor in all these cases appears to be defective migration of the granule cells. In the reeler and weaver mutant mice, where the failure of migration of granule cells has been established with certainty, the underlying cellular defect is not known (see Section 3.4.5). Possible causes of the migration defect may be failure of development of some component of the mechanism of cell locomotion or failure to acquire the cell surface properties that are necessary for neurons to interact with cells along their paths of migration.

There are several ways in which errors of positioning, of orientation, or of the number of neurons may be corrected at later stages. The first means of eliminating malpositioned or disoriented cells is by cell death, yet the malpositioned cells survive in all the cases that have been cited above. The possibility remains that many malpositioned cells die because their axons fail to find the correct synaptic targets. This form of "error correction" by elimination of redundant cells is what has been termed "natural selection" of nerve cells in the first edition of this book (M. Jacobson, 1970*b*, p. 161). This concept originated with Wilhelm Roux in his book *Der Kampf der Theile im Organismus* (1881), and of course I am in agreement with other authors who have followed me in accepting the concept of "natural selection" of neurons (Cowan, 1973; Prestige, 1974, Hollyday and Hamburger, 1976), but I must part company with them when they adopt the view that death of redundant neurons in the spinal sensory ganglia or death of spinal motoneurons represents a mode of "error correction." In my view, the excess production of neurons is in itself not an error. It is an invariant stage of development found in all individuals of the same species, and is part of the normal developmental program, determined genetically in the first instance and performing a constructive function during development. This is a normal means of matching one set of neurons to another set, and the misconception that it is a form of "error" correction directs attention away from its significance as a mechanism of achieving optimum matching between pre- and postsynaptic elements.

As Wilhelm Roux (1881) was the first to recognize, the nervous system of vertebrates consists of a very large number of types of cells, with each type showing a range of variations of structure and function. Many more cells of each type are produced during normal development than survive in the mature animal. Although the range of variability within each type of neuron in the large intitial set and in the reduced final set has not been measured, it seems unlikely that all the cells in the initial set are identical. As is well known (Mayr, 1970, p. 82 *et seq.*), a range of variation may enhance the adaptability of a population: the greater the variation, the greater the "efficiency of the exploration of the resources of the environment by the living matter" (Dobzhansky, 1951). Therefore, such polymorphism is adaptive. The selection of the survivors that form the final set must be determined on the basis of some type of benefit, functional effectiveness, or what I have termed "functional validation" (M. Jacobson, 1970*b*). There is a competition between neurons which results in elimination of some neurons and the survival of others contingent on their fitness to survive (M. Jacobson, 1970*b*, p. 161, 341, 1974*b*; Hirsch and Jacobson, 1975). That a larger number of cells may survive if they are provided with additional peripheral targets shows that the death of cells is not inherently predetermined within the dying cells but is determined by factors in the postsynaptic target cells (see Section 5.7). The present understanding is that there is a quantitative disparity between the presynaptic set of elements and the postsynaptic targets on which they form synapses. It may also be assumed that there are qualitative differences between the elements of the presynaptic set and also between the elements of the postsynaptic set such that an element in one set will associate with an element in the other set, with a probability that varies as the range of different properties in each set of elements. Very slight differences between individual elements in each set may be sufficient to result in a struggle between the presynaptic elements for space on the postsynaptic cell or for a limited supply of some vital material produced by the target cells. Competition is keenest between individuals that are most similar, and will finally result in one type completely displacing the other (Gause, 1932, 1934; Mayr, 1970; L. M. Cook, 1971).

Returning to the mechanisms of "error correction" in cases of malpositioning or misalignment of cells, there is considerable evidence that many such malpositioned neurons survive embryonic development and persist in the adult. An example of migration up to 700 neurons beyond their usual assembly zone occurs in the isthmooptic nucleus of the chick embryo (P. G. H. Clarke and Cowan, 1976; P. G. H. Clarke *et al.,* 1976). In this case, the majority of the misplaced neurons die, with the result that the anomaly is party but not entirely corrected. A few of the misplaced neurons of the chick embryo isthmo-optic nucleus survive beyond hatching (P. G. H. Clarke and Cowan, 1976), and in these cases one may regard such "errors" as a means of giving rise to a new form of neuronal organization, and one may conceive of this as one way in which evolution of neuronal systems can occur. In many such cases, it seems that the ectopic neurons have formed essentially normal connections. For example, in the reeler mouse, the neurons of the cerebral cortex are malpositioned, yet interhemispheric connections through the corpus callosum are normal, and it is probable that the correct connections are made within the cortex (Caviness, 1976; Caviness and Yorke, 1976). In the cerebellum of the reeler mutant mouse, the malpositioned Purkinje cells receive their normal synaptic connections (Rakic and Sidman, 1972; Bliss and Chung, 1974), and in the weaver mutant mouse, the mossy fibers usually synapse normally on the ectopic granule cells (Rakic and Sidman, 1973*b*). The significance of aberrant synaptic connections which are formed in the cerebellum of the weaver mouse is discussed in Section 3.4.5.

Displaced cells persist either because they are integrated into the existing circuitry, as appears to occur even in some extreme cases of neuronal malpositioning, for example, the reeler mouse, or because they form novel functional systems or extend the functional capabilities of preexisting systems. If variations arise because of mutations whose effects are neutral or are corrected at later stages of development, they will not be subject to natural selection but will tend to accumulate. Neuronal development need not be as invariant as is commonly supposed, provided that variants are either corrected or eliminated, or, if they persist, are neutral or advantageous.

8

Development of Peripheral Neural Connections with Muscles and Sensory Receptors

8.1. Development of Neuromuscular Connections

The nerve supply of skeletal muscles is very constant; except for rare anomalies, each muscle is innervated by a specific group of motoneurons. This has been demonstrated by cutting various peripheral nerves and then observing that chromatolysis is confined to a localized group of motoneurons whose axons have been cut (Romanes, 1946; Szentágothai, 1948, 1949). More recently, accurate mapping of relations between muscles and motoneurons has been done by tracing the retrograde flow of horseradish peroxidase injected into the vicinity of motor nerve terminals in the muscles (Kristensson and Olsson, 1971, 1973; Kristensson, 1975, review). Not only do the axons of motoneurons supply specific muscles, but also their dendrites form specific connections within the spinal cord with the neurons that are involved in postural and locomotor reflexes. It is not known how the motoneurons form the appropriate peripheral and central reflex associations. It is therefore still necessary to survey the alternatives.

The possibility that there is a high degree of affinity between a particular motor nerve and a particular muscle has been eliminated by the many experiments in which limbs grafted to abnormal positions have become functionally innervated by foreign nerves. Lack of neuromuscular specificity between different mammalian species is shown by the development of functional connections between rodent spinal cord and human skeletal muscle in tissue culture (S. M. Crain *et al.,* 1970). Experiments also show that heterotopic grafts of parts of the nervous system innervate muscles nonselectively (Braus, 1905; Detwiler, 1923,

1925, 1930*a;* Nicholas, 1930*a,* 1933 Piatt, 1940). The fact that muscle can be experimentally innervated by foreign motor nerves makes it unlikely that the nerve grows to the appropriate muscle as the result of either an attraction or an affinity between the two, but it does not exclude the possibility that the nerve is guided to the muscle by extrinsic factors. The stereotyped pattern of peripheral innervation is mainly due to the fact that the nerves are not free to grow at random, but tend to grow along tissue planes, particularly along blood vessels. Another important factor in determining the pattern of muscle innervation is the order in which the motoneurons sprout their axons. Romanes (1941, 1946) has shown that the motoneurons in the ventral horn of the spinal cord of the rabbit fetus mature and sprout their axons in a spatiotemporal order that is correlated with the order of innervation of muscles in proximodistal sequence in the limbs. The first axons to reach an uninnervated muscle will neurotize it, and at the same time will exclude other nerves and constrain them to terminate elsewhere. The muscles are thus innervated in an orderly sequence in the limb (A. C. Taylor, 1943, 1944; Roncalli, 1970). However, the evidence obtained by recording muscle activity in response to nerve stimulation shows that there is no clearly defined proximodistal order of innervation in the hindlimb of the chick embryo, most muscles apparently becoming innervated at the same time (Landmesser and Morris, 1975). It is very unlikely that the earliest innervation of muscles was detectable in those experiments. More plausibly, a stereotyped pattern of innervation—for example, of a limb—can be explained on the basis of a timed outgrowth of motor axons, mechanical guidance of the motor nerves, and the exclusion of motor nerves that arrive after the muscles have already been innervated (Braus, 1905; Harrison, 1907*a;* A. C. Taylor, 1943, 1944; Piatt, 1940, 1957*a,b,* 1958). "It is not necessary to imagine, as a number of writers do, that the growing nerve would have to wend its way through a labyrinth of differentiated tissues, extending from the hip to the toes, in order to reach its end organ, but merely that the nerve must grow independently as far as the base of the undifferentiated limb bud, the rest being provided by the development of the limb itself" (Harrison, 1907*a*).

Full neurotization is assured by the production of a large excess of motor axons and the degeneration of those that do not make peripheral connections. This is the teleological explanation for the overproduction of motoneurons followed by degeneration of the large percentage that fail to connect with muscles. That the maintenance and maturation of the motoneuron depend on the formation of peripheral connections with muscle is well supported by experimental evidence (Weiss *et al.,* 1945*a*; Cavanaugh, 1951; Aitken *et al.,* 1947; D. H. L. Evans and Vizoso, 1951; Prestige, 1967*b*). The muscle affects the neuron by an undiscovered mechanism which results in the maintenance and maturation of the neuron. This trophic action of the muscle on its motoneuron is an example of retrograde transsynaptic stimulation. We may posit that a message is transmitted from the muscle to its nerve. In order to produce an effect on the cell body, the message has to travel centripetally in the axon. It has been suggested that one of the effects of the muscle on the motoneuron is to stimulate the growth of its dendrites (D. H. Barron, 1943, 1946, 1948); another suggested effect is to direct the growth of its dendrites into the correct synaptic reflex associations (Weiss, 1936, 1952). The latter effect has been named "modulation" by Weiss, and will be considered at length in Section 9.4.

8.2. Development of Skeletal Muscle Innervation

In mammals, each muscle fiber is innervated by a single myelinated axon terminating in one end plate, usually located near the middle of the muscle fiber. The constancy of this pattern of innervation in mammals is in contrast to the presence in lower vertebrates of unmyelinated motor collaterals and *en grappe* motor terminals (Tiegs, 1953; Bone, 1964; R. C. L. Hudson, 1969). The morphology of the neuromuscular junction of vertebrates has been reviewed by Couteaux (1963) and Coërs (1967). Elimination of some neuromuscular junctions occurs as a normal event during development of innervation of skeletal muscle in newborn mammals. Although each skeletal muscle in adults is innervated by a single motor nerve ending, the initial innervation is polyneuronal, with an average of three to five synapses per muscle fiber in newborn rats (Redfern, 1970; M. R. Bennett and Pettigrew, 1974; M. C. Brown *et al.,* 1976) and newborn cats (Bagust *et al.,* 1973). In the soleus muscle of the rat, M. C. Brown *et al.* (1976) found that the percentage of muscle fibers that are innervated by more than one nerve ending decreases from 91 percent at 10 days after birth to 2.5 percent at 15 days of age (Fig. 8.1). The total number of motor units remains constant, but their size decreases during the period of elimination of polyneuronal innervation (M. C. Brown *et al.,* 1976). The elimination of polyneuronal innervation occurs, first, as the result of increase of the number of muscle fibers that continue to be formed after the initial polyneuronal innervation (Chiakulas and Pauly, 1965) and, second, by retraction and degeneration of axonal branches at the periphery, but not by degeneration of entire motoneurons. This results in a constant density of innervation, with neither overinnervation nor underinnervation of muscle fibers.

There appears to be no specificity or selectivity in the establishment of connections between motor nerves and muscles, either during normal development or following nerve regeneration. If such specificity plays any role in the normal development of neuromuscular connections, the specificity is overruled by other factors in experiments in which muscles are provided with foreign nerves.

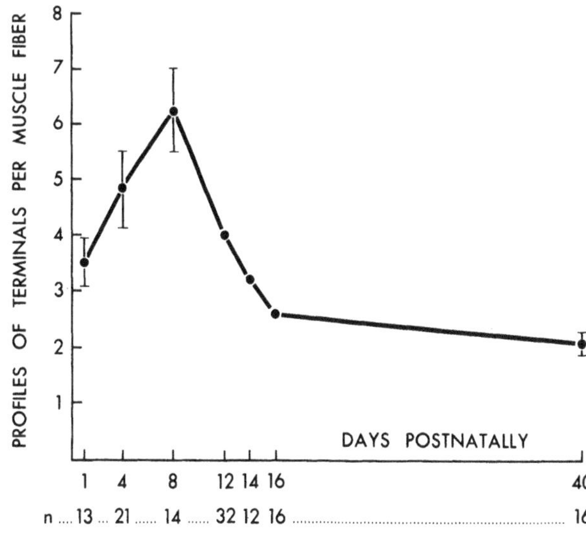

Figure 8.1. Reduction of polyneuronal innervation of skeletal muscle fibers in newborn rats from 1 to 4 days after birth ±1 standard error of the mean. *n,* Number of end plates examined at each age. From H. Korneliussen and J. K. S. Jansen, *J. Neurocytol.* 5:591–604 (1976).

Piatt (1940) showed that when segments of spinal cord of *Ambystoma* are grafted to new positions they can supply any muscle indiscriminately. He concluded that the developing motoneuron of *Ambystoma* possesses no functional specificity or inherent affinity for the muscles that they normally supply. "The fact that in normal ontogeny these neurons form constant and regular patterns of distribution must be the result of factors extrinsic to the nerve fibers themselves, but not referable to specific attraction exerted by different muscle groups" (Piatt, 1940). This is in agreement with the evidence that limb buds devoid of nerves ("aneurogenic limbs") which have been transplanted to the trunk of the frog tadpole become functionally innervated by the spinal nerves at the level of the grafts (Braus, 1905; Harrison, 1907*a*). In *Ambystoma,* limb buds transplanted to the head become functionally innervated by cranial nerves (Braus, 1905; Nicholas, 1933; Hibbard, 1965*b*). The muscles of a limb bud transplanted to the orbit of the newt become innervated by the nerves that normally supply the extraocular muscles (Nicholas, 1930, 1933). Tail muscle transplanted to the position of the limb becomes innervated by limb segments of the spinal cord in the frog tadpole (Letinsky, 1974). Another bit of evidence showing nonselectivity of neuromuscular associations is that sartorius muscle transplanted to the thorax of the adult frog may become innervated by the vagus nerve, and these preganglionic autonomic nerve fibers prevent the muscle fibers from atrophying but do not alter the functional characteristics of the muscle. Neither are the properties of the vagus nerve fibers altered by synapsing with skeletal muscle: the vagus nerve fibers retain their small diameters and high threshold for electrical stimulation (Landmesser, 1971).

If a mammalian skeletal muscle is denervated and then reinnervated by its own and a foreign motor nerve, the two nerves neurotize the muscle fibers at random (Steindler, 1916; Elsberg, 1917; Weiss and Hoag, 1946; Bernstein and Guth, 1961; Miledi and Stefani, 1969). By contrast with these observations, there are many others that show selective association between motoneurons and the appropriate muscle. For example, Mark and his associates have reported that functional synapses will form between motor axons mismatched with skeletal muscles as a result of nerve crosses, but that such synapses become "functionless," although morphologically intact, when the muscle is innervated by the matching nerve (reviewed by Mark, 1974*a*) (Fig. 8.2). The upshot of Mark's work is that matching of nerve and muscle is not absolute in salamanders but that the correct match is more stable and, moreover, suppresses the function of incorrectly matched neuromuscular junctions. This conclusion has not gone unchallenged (S. A. Scott, 1975). However, even if the recognition between nerve and mammalian skeletal muscle is relatively weak, the mere existence of such selectivity poses the problem of its mechanism. The same problem is posed more clearly in the case of selective reconnection of muscle with regenerated motoneurons in the cockroach (Bodenstein, 1957; Guthrie, 1962, 1967; Jacklet and Cohen, 1967*a,b*; D. Young, 1972; K. G. Pearson and Bradley, 1972; Denburg *et al.,* 1976).

Specificity of reinnervation in the invertebrate nervous system has been studied most fully in the leech *Hirudo medicinalis.* In this organism, each segment contains a ganglion composed of a few recognizable motor and sensory neurons (Nicholls and Baylor, 1968; Kuffler and Nicholls, 1976, pp. 354–371, review). In this organism, the nerves can re-form connections either by regeneration or by reconnection. After a lesion to the connectives between sequential ganglia, the axons re-form the appropriate connections (Baylor and Nicholls, 1971; Jansen

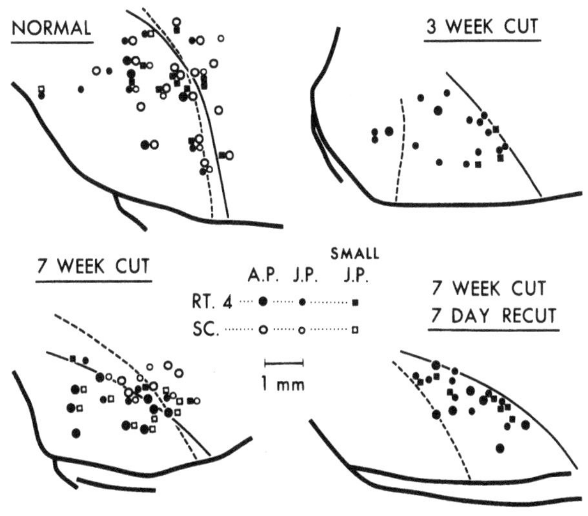

Figure 8.2. Dynamics of functional innervation of the supracoracoideus muscle of the shoulder of the axolotl. The muscle is normally innervated by the main nerve (SC.) and by a branch of root 4 (RT. 4). Three weeks after SC. has been cut, expansion of the territory of RT. 4 occurs. Seven weeks after SC. has been cut, the latter regenerates to restore its territory of functional innervation and repress the junctions of RT. 4. Rapid recovery of repressed neuromuscular junctions of RT. 4 occurs within 7 days of recutting the main nerve (SC.) The solid line shows the boundary of root 4 innervation, while the dotted line shows the corresponding boundary on the opposite side. Symbols show the types of electrical responses recorded with an electrode in muscle fibers. A.P., Action potentials; J.P, junction potentials; small J.P., small, ineffective junction potentials; RT. 4, root 4 nerve; SC., supracoracoideus nerve. From R. K. Mark, Ciba Foundation Symposium No 29, new series, pp. 289–307 (1975).

and Nicholls, 1972). Peripheral nerve lesions are also followed by recovery of the appropriate connections with muscles and skin in the proper positons in the body wall. Sensory nerves regain their formed stimulus modality (touch, pressure, or noxious stimuli) and motor neurons reinnervate either circular or longitudinal muscles selectively (Van Essen and Jansen, 1977). We do not know whether such highly specific intercellular association is the result of chemotaxis, guidance of regenerating axons along their route to their targets, specific recognition between motor nerve terminals and muscles, or a combination of several of these mechanisms.

Sensory nerve fibers cannot innervate muscle. Although the axons of sensory nerves grow in close apposition to the sarcolemma, no neuromuscular junctions are formed (Langley and Anderson, 1904*b*; Gutmann, 1945; Weiss and Edds, 1945; Zalewski, 1970*b*). The different capacities of sensory and motorneurons to form neuromuscular junctions are already determined in the neural plate. When pieces of neural plate, jacketed in ectoderm and mesoderm, are cultured *in vitro*, only the presumptive motor regions and not the presumptive sensory regions are able to form functional neuromuscular junctions in the explant (Corner, 1964).

The ability of a neuron to innervate a skeletal muscle is apparently limited only by its transmitter: as Dale (1935) first suggested, only cholinergic nerves can reinnervate denervated skeletal muscle. Thus autonomic preganglionic neurons can innervate denervated skeletal muscle (Langley and Anderson, 1940*a,b*; Landmesser, 1971), but postganglionic sympathetic nerves cannot (Hinsey, 1934; Bowman and Nott, 1969; L. Olson and Malmfors, 1970; C. F. Luco and Luco, 1971).

Muscle with its nerves intact will not accept any new innervation (for example, when foreign motor nerves are implanted in the muscle), but will accept such implants after denervation (Aitken, 1950; H. Hoffman, 1951*b*; J. Koenig, 1971). No neuromuscular junctions are formed by the peroneal nerve implanted into the gastrocnemius muscle when its normal innervation (the tibial nerve) is intact, although the implanted nerve fibers grow freely into the muscle. Preimplantation of the peroneal nerve into the gastrocnemius muscle 30 days before cutting of the tibial nerve is followed by the formation of neuromuscular junctions by the peroneal nerve within 2 days after the tibial nerve has been cut (Fex and Thesleff, 1967). After reinnervation or after cross-innervation, the neuromuscular junctions are formed at original sites on many muscle fibers, which shows that the position of the original junction has special properties (M. R. Bennett *et al.*, 1973*a,b*). Hyperinnervation of muscle has been produced by partially denervating it and allowing regeneration of the severed motor axons. As a result, many end plates become dually innervated by the collateral sprouts of residual motor axons as well as by regenerated axons (H. Hoffman, 1950, 1951*a*; Guth, 1962).

Morphogenesis of the neuromuscular junctions in the intercostal muscles of the rat fetus commences at 16 days, as seen with the electron microscope (Teräväinen, 1968; A. M. Kelly and Zacks, 1969). Junctions are first seen when the muscle is at the myotube stage of development. All the junctions are not formed simultaneously, but muscle cells and neuromuscular junctions at various stages of development are seen in the same muscle throughout the fetal and early postnatal period. During the first stage of development of the neuromuscular junction, a primary synaptic cleft is not present, and there is merely an irregular gap between the axon terminal and muscle fiber. The motor nerve terminal contains mitochondria and synaptic vesicles 500 Å in diameter. The postsynaptic region of the muscle plasma membrane thickens and an amorphous basement membrane forms. At 18 days of gestation the junction is composed of several axon terminals enveloped in a Schwann cell, separated by a 500 Å primary cleft from the thickened but unfolded muscle plasma membrane. Secondary synaptic clefts form as invaginations of the postsynaptic membrane during prenatal day 20 to postnatal day 4. As the maturing motor nerve axons increase in diameter, the size of the motor end plate increases in proportion to the diameter of its axon (Flamm, 1968).

Several different criteria have been used to indicate the time of development of neuromuscular junctions, namely observations of the time of arrival of the motor nerves in the muscle, or of the time at which cholinesterase can be shown histochemically, or of the onset of muscle movements. Neuromuscular contacts have been seen, using silver-impregnation techniques, in the neck muscles of the chick at 2½ days of incubation, just before the onset of spontaneous motility in the neck muscles on day 3 (Visintini and Levi-Montalcini, 1939; De Anda *et al.*, 1963; Filogamo and Gabella, 1967). In the forelimb of the rat fetus, muscular contractions can first be elicited by electrical stimulation at 16 days of gestation, which corresponds with the time at which neuromuscular contacts are first visible histologically (Straus and Weddell, 1940). The neuromuscular junctions form later in the hindlimbs than in the forelimbs, and are first seen in the muscles of the hindlimbs of the chick embryo only at 7–13 days of incubation and continue to form for several days later (H. Hirano, 1967*a,b*; Landmesser and Morris, 1975).

The development of the neuromuscular junctions has been studied electrophysiologically in frog tadpoles (Letinsky, 1974; Letinsky *et al.*, 1976), and with the electron microscope in newborn rats (A. M. Kelly and Zacks, 1969; Juntunen, 1973*a,b*; J. Koenig, 1973) and in the chick embryo (H. Hirano, 1967*a*; A. M. Kelly and Zacks, 1969; Daneo and Filogamo, 1974). The development of neuromuscular junctions in the sartorius muscle of the chick embryo has been studied with the electron microscope (H. Hirano, 1967*a*; A. M. Kelly and Zacks, 1969). Neuromuscular junctions develop in the sartorius muscle at 13–20 days of incubation. At 13 days, the muscle cells are at various stages of differentiation. Myoblasts and immature muscle fibers are seen in the same muscle bundle. The nerves that grow into the muscle are unmyelinated axons, 0.2–2 μm in diameter, enveloped in Schwann cells. The first visible sign of the formation of the junction is an increase in the thickness of the muscle plasma membrane in the region opposite an approaching nerve terminal. This occurs when the approaching nerve fiber is separated from the muscle by a gap of between 2000 and 3000 Å. The nerve terminal contains vesicles similar in appearance to synaptic vesicles in the mature motor nerve terminals. The changes in the postsynaptic membrane are thought to be caused by the release of acetylcholine or other "trophic" substances from the motor nerve terminals. The development of the neuromuscular junction in the chick continues for several days after contact between the nerve terminal and muscle fiber. The neuromuscular junctions in the sartorius muscle have a mature appearance (as illustrated by Couteaux, 1963) by 20 days of incubation, but additional folding and branching of the postsynaptic membrane occur after hatching.

Three stages are described in the development of skeletal muscle: myoblast, myotube, and myofiber (Boyd, 1960, review). The elongated myoblasts differentiate from mesodermal cells. Proliferation of myoblasts is followed by fusion of myoblasts to form myotubes. Myofibrils appear at the periphery of the myotubes. The myofiber develops as the membranes of the T-system develop, the cell becomes filled with myofibrils, and the nuclei are displaced to the periphery of the mature muscle fiber. In developing muscles of higher vertebrates, some myocytes differentiate into the intrafusal muscle fibers of the muscle spindles. This requires the presence of sensory nerves. The development of muscle spindles in relation to their innervation is considered in some detail in Section 8.8.

In all species studied, the muscle differentiates to the myotube stage before it becomes innervated during normal development (Teräväinen, 1968; A. M. Kelly and Zacks, 1969). In amphibians the muscles can develop normally to maturity in the absence of nerves (Harrison, 1904; Hooker, 1911; Hamburger, 1928). Development of muscle occurs normally during limb regeneration in axolotl larvae continuously immobilized under general anesthesia (Carlson, 1973). However, in birds and mammals, only the initial phases of development (to the myotube stage) can occur in denervated muscle and in regenerating muscle (Allbrook and Aitken, 1951; Jirmanová and Thesleff, 1972), and full maturation of the muscle is dependent on a motor nerve supply (Anders, 1921; E. A. Hunt, 1932; Hamburger and Waugh, 1940; Eastlick, 1943; Eastlick and Wortham, 1947). Apparently there is a phylogenetic increase in the dependence of muscle on nerve supply.

The influence of nerves on regeneration of skeletal muscle has recently been reviewed by Carlson (1973). Regeneration of muscle in many respects recapitulates its ontogeny. So-called satellite cells, which lie between the sarcolemma and basement membrane of the muscle fibers, persist in adult muscle and are the stem cells which proliferate after muscle injuries to provide myoblasts (Mauro, 1961; Church, 1969, 1970; Shafiq, 1970). Not only large injuries can be repaired, as was known in the last century (Waldeyer, 1865; Volkmann, 1893), but also an entire muscle such as the gastrocnemius can regenerate from minced fragments to about one-third of its former mass (Carlson, 1973). Regeneration can proceed to the myotube stage in the absence of nerves, but the muscle then degenerates if nerves are lacking. The muscle spindles also contain satellite cells which can give rise to intrafusal muscle fibers (Elliott and Harriman, 1974). The failure of muscle spindles to develop in regenerated muscles (Zelená and Sobotková, 1971) is apparently due to absence of Ia sensory nerves, which are an absolute requirement for the differentiation of muscle spindles (See Section 8.8).

Neuromuscular junctions develop in tissue culture of nerve and muscle of amphibians (Harrison, 1907*b*; Corner and Crain, 1964; M. W. Cohen, 1972), chicks (Szepsenwol, 1947; James and Tresman, 1969; Fischbach, 1972), and rats and mice (S. M. Crain, 1966; Bornstein *et al.*, 1968; Robbins and Yonezawa, 1971). Functional neuromuscular junctions develop between separate pieces of spinal cord and muscle of the chick embryo (Veneroni, 1968; Veneroni and Murray, 1969; Nakai, 1969) and mammalian fetus (S. M. Crain, 1964, 1966, 1968; E. R. Peterson and Crain, 1968), cultured in close proximity (S. M. Crain, 1974, 1976, reviews). That sensitivity of muscle to acetylcholine is not required for the development of neuromuscular junctions is shown by the fact that neuromuscular connections develop in skeletal muscle and nervous tissue cultured in the presence of curare in concentrations which greatly reduce the sensitivity of the muscle to acetylcholine (S. M. Crain and Peterson, 1967, 1974; M. W. Cohen, 1972; Steinbach *et al.*, 1973). Neuromuscular junctions form in the chick embryo injected with an agent that blocks neuromuscular transmission—curare, botulinum toxin, hemicholinium, or α-bungarotoxin—although severe muscular atrophy occurs (Giacobini *et al.*, 1973; S. S. Freeman *et al.*, 1976). Neuromuscular connections also develop in rat skeletal muscle that is immobilized (Juntunen, 1973*a*). However, immobilized skeletal muscle later undergoes atrophy (Jirmanová and Zelená, 1970; Riley and Allin, 1973; Tomanek and Lund, 1974).

In the rat fetus, the first muscular contractions are seen in the neck at 16 days of gestation and in the muscles of the trunk and limbs at 19 days (Angulo y Gonzalez, 1932; Straus and Weddell, 1940). This is correlated with the stages at which electrical stimulation of the motor nerves results in muscle contractions (Windle *et al.*, 1935; Straus, 1939). The first developing neuromuscular junctions have been seen in the rat at 16 days of gestation (Straus and Weddell, 1940).

8.3. Neural Control of the Differentiation of Skeletal Muscle

In adult mammals, the skeletal muscles contain fibers of two major types, slow- and fast-twitch fibers, which have different structures, contract at different speeds, and contain different amounts of myoglobin and enzymes. Some differences between slow and fast muscle fibers are summarized in Table 8.1. Some skeletal muscles (for example, soleus) are composed mainly of slow fibers. Other muscles such as flexor hallucis longus, flexor digitorum longus, and gastrocnemius are composed mainly of fast fibers, whereas others contain different proportions of slow and fast fibers.

Three types of mammalian skeletal muscle fibers have been identified. According to differences in the content of the enzyme succinic dehydrogenase, they have been classified as A, B, and C fibers by J. M. Stein and Padykula (1962).

Table 8.1. Differences between Slow and Fast Mammalian Skeletal Muscle Fibers and Effects of Cross-Innervation

Characteristic	Slow muscle	Fast muscle	References	Effects of cross-innervation	References
Structure	Myofilaments are not arranged into separate bundles (Felderstruktur) Sparse sarcoplasmic reticulum; Z bands irregular	Myofilaments arranged in discrete myofibrils (Fibrillenstruktur) Extensive sarcoplasmic reticulum; Z bands straight	Krüger and Günther (1955), Shear and Goldspink (1971)		
Speed of contraction	58–193 msec	18–70 msec	Denny-Brown (1929), McPhedran *et al.* (1965), Wuerker *et al.* (1965)	Reversal of speed of contraction	Buller *et al.* (1960*b*), Close (1965, 1967)
Nerve supply	Tonic α-motoneurons; axons with slow conduction velocity	Phasic α-motoneurons; axons with fast conduction velocity	Eccles *et al.* (1958*a*)		
Color and myoglobin content	Deep red; high myoglobin content	Pale red; low myoglobin content		Reversal of myoglobin content	McPherson and Tokanuga (1967)
Enzymes	High in enzymes of oxidative metabolism; low in glycolytic enzymes	High in glycolytic enzymes; low in enzymes of oxidative metabolism	Dubowitz and Pearse (1960), Romanul (1964), Dawson and Romanul (1964)	Reversal of enzyme profile	Romanul and Van der Meulen (1967), Yellin (1967*b*), Karpati and Engel (1967)
Sensitivity to acetylcholine	Over entire fiber	Restricted to endplate region	Miledi and Zelena (1966), Miledi *et al.*, (1968)		
Capillary supply	Rich	Poor	Romanul (1965)		

The histochemical reaction for actomyosin adenosine triphosphatase (ATPase) also reveals three types of skeletal muscle fibers designated α, β, and $\alpha\beta$ (Guth *et al.*, 1970; Samaha *et al.*, 1970).

The functional characteristics of the muscle fibers are closely matched with the size and type of the α-motoneurons that innervate them. Mammalian fast muscles are innervated by large motoneurons (phasic α-motoneurons) and slow muscles are innervated by small motoneurons (tonic α-motoneurons) (Granit *et al.*, 1956; Eccles *et al.*, 1958*a*; Wuerker *et al.*, 1965; Henneman *et al.*, 1965; Henneman and Olson, 1965). The phasic α-motoneurons have rapidly conducting axons and respond reflexly with a brief high-frequency burst of action potentials. The tonic α-motoneurons have axons with lower conduction velocities, and they have a prolonged low-frequency discharge in response to sustained reflex stimulation. The frequency of repetitive discharge from α-motoneurons is thus matched by the speed of contraction of their muscles so that maximum efficiency is achieved. This is the teleological explanation for why the motor nerve induces matching functional characteristics in its muscle (Eccles *et al.*, 1958*a,b*). One of the consequences of the different functional properties of motoneurons that innervate the two types of muscle is that fast muscles are excited infrequently and for short durations while slow muscles are excited for much longer periods. This difference in the total time of usage has important implications because there is considerable evidence that the properties of the muscle are determined by the total amount and probably also the pattern of contractile activity.

Miledi (1962) demonstrated that if frog skeletal muscle is divided into an innervated and an uninnervated portion, the latter will accept new innervation and the former will not. The presence of an intact neuromuscular junction prevents the muscle fiber from forming new motor end plates. The formation of new motor end plates is not due to injury, since a foreign nerve simply laid on a denervated muscle and not implanted into an incision can neurotize the muscle (Gwyn and Aitken, 1964). Nor is the acceptance of new innervation merely the result of muscular inactivity, because implanted nerves cannot form end plates in tenotomized muscle that has atrophied from disuse but has a normal nerve supply (Aitken, 1950).

Muscle poisoned with botulinum toxin forms functional neuromuscular junctions with an implanted nerve, even when its own innervation is intact (Fex *et al.*, 1966). The only known effect of botulinum toxin is to prevent the release of acetylcholine from the nerve terminals. However, it is conceivable that the release of some other unidentified substances from the nerve terminal may also be prevented by botulinum toxin. After botulinum poisoning, the ingrowing foreign nerve fibers form new end plates quite separate from the old ones, which remain intact (Fex *et al.*, 1966). Therefore, there does not seem to be any attraction of reinnervating nerve fibers by the old end plates such as M. R. Bennett *et al.* (1973*a,b,c*) observed after reinnervation of mammalian and avian skeletal muscle.

8.3.1. Neural Control of Muscle Acetylcholine Sensitivity

After denervation, or after botulinum poisoning, the whole muscle fiber becomes sensitive to acetylcholine applied iontophoretically through a micropipette (Axelsson and Thesleff, 1959; Thesleff, 1960; Miledi, 1960*a*). In normally innervated muscle fibers the end plate region is most sensitive to acetylcholine applied through a micropipette, and there is a steep gradient of diminishing sensitivity extending for about 500 μm along the length of the muscle fiber (Miledi, 1960*b*). Miledi concluded that the highest density of acetylcholine receptors is found on the muscle membrane in the region of the end plate, which is 20–30 μm in diameter, and there is a gradientwise decline in the density of receptors in the extrajunctional region. There are differences between the fast- and slow-twitch fibers in mammalian skeletal muscle as regards the spatial distribution of their acetylcholine sensitivity. In fast muscle fibers, the sensitivity to acetylcholine is confined to the neuromuscular junction, while the slow fibers, in addition to a region of high sensitivity at the junction, have a low sensitivity to acetylcholine throughout their length (Miledi and Zelená, 1966; Albuquerque and Thesleff, 1968).

J. Diamond and Miledi (1962) studied the development of sensitivity to acetylcholine in muscle fibers of the diaphragm in rats from 17 days of gestation to maturity. The presence of miniature endplate potentials shows that neuromuscular junctions are present as early as day 17 of gestation. The frequency of miniature endplate potentials, recorded intracellularly from the muscle fiber, increases about a hundredfold from day 17 of gestation to maturity (Fig. 8.3). This large increase shows that a change has occurred, during development, in the spatial distribution of sensitivity of the muscle fiber to acetylcholine. Before birth, application of acetylcholine to any part of the muscle fiber produces a depolarization. Although the whole fetal muscle fiber is sensitive to acetylcholine, the sensitivity is greatest near the middle of the fiber and lowest at its ends. Toward the end of the fetal period and during the first 3 postnatal days, the acetylcholine sensitivity diminishes at the ends of the muscle fiber, and the sensitivity continues to diminish in the extrajunctional regions of the muscle fiber during the following days. The muscle fibers attain their adult sensitivity at 2 weeks after birth, with acetycholine sensitivity restricted to the end plate and surrounding region.

The changes in spatial distribution of receptors for acetylcholine in the muscle membrane are reversed by denervating the muscle or by blocking the release of acetylcholine from the motor nerve terminal by means of botulinum

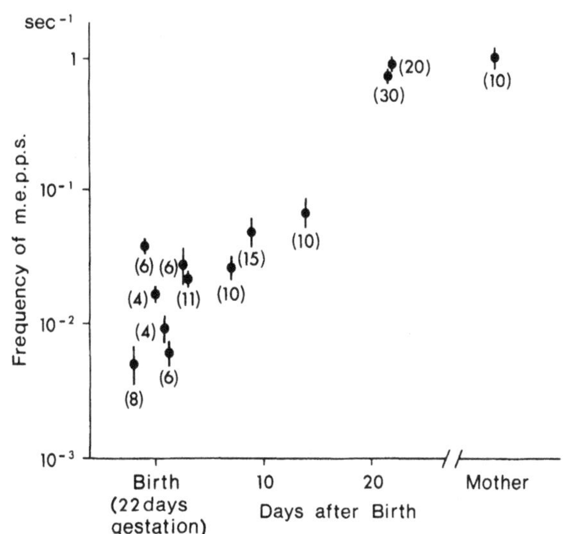

Figure 8.3. Frequency of miniature end plate potentials (m.e.p.p.s) in muscle fibers of the diaphragm of the rat at different ages. The number of fibers examined is given in parentheses. From J. Diamond and R. Miledi, *J. Physiol. (London) 162:*393–408 (1962).

toxin. Figure 8.4 illustrates the gradual increase in sensitivity of the rat diaphragm after denervation (Fambrough, 1970) and shows that the sensitivity to acetylcholine increases uniformly over the whole denervated muscle fiber.

The observed redistribution of acetylcholine sensitivity may be due to (1) redistribution of preexisting acetylcholine receptors, (2) activation of latent receptors, or (3) synthesis of new receptors. The first has been ruled out by the experiments showing that acetylcholine sensitivity increases in a fragment of muscle lacking an end plate (Katz and Miledi, 1964), by the fact that sensitivity increases simultaneously over the entire muscle (Fambrough, 1970), and by the fact that the total number of acetylcholine receptors is greatly increased after denervation (Berg *et al.*, 1972; Hartzell and Fambrough, 1972; Fambrough, 1974*a*). That protein and RNA synthesis are required for the increase in acetylcholine receptors after denervation indicates, but does not prove, that new receptors are synthesized (Fambrough, 1970; Grampp *et al.*, 1971). Proof that new receptors are synthesized following denervation was obtained by Brockes and Hall (1975), who showed that ^{38}S-labeled methionine is incorporated into extrajunctional receptors after denervation of rat diaphragm.

Measurement of the number of acetylcholine receptors on the muscle membrane can be made by measuring the specific binding of iodinated α-bungarotoxin or of cobra α-toxin. These toxins bind specifically and irreversibly to the nicotinic acetylcholine receptors on muscle membrane. The density of acetylcholine receptors at the neuromuscular junction is $1.4–4.7 \times 10^7/\mu m^2$ in various vertebrate skeletal muscles, and the receptor has a molecular weight of about 250,000 (Karlin, 1974), so the receptors must constitute about 90 percent of the protein of the junctional membrane. By contrast, the extrajunctional receptor density is less than $5/\mu m^2$ (Hartzell and Fambrough, 1972; Barnard *et al.*, 1974). The number of

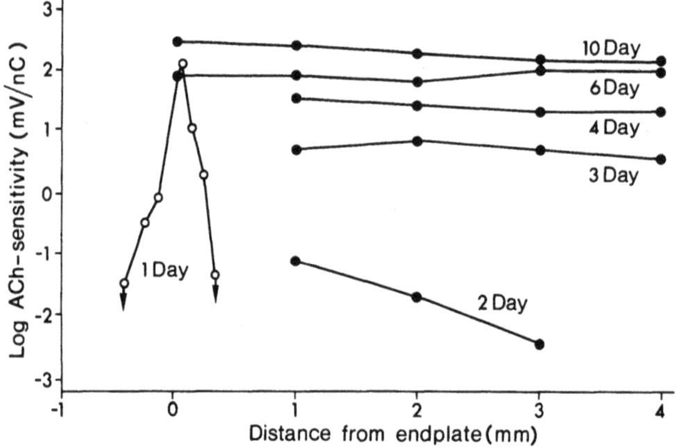

Figure 8.4. Development of hypersensitivity to acetylcholine (ACh) by muscle fibers of the rat diaphragm after denervation. The left hemidiaphragms of adult rats were denervated by cutting the left phrenic nerve about 1 cm from the surface of the muscle. The ACh sensitivity 1–10 days later was measured by iontophoretically applying ACh to the surface of the muscle fiber while recording the transmembrane potential with an intracellular microelectrode. Sensitivity was calculated as millivolt depolarization per nanocoulomb of iontophoretic current. Each point (•) shows the average log sensitivity of four to eight muscle fibers. Open circles (○) indicate single measurements for individual end plates. By courtesy of Dr. D. M. Fambrough.

junctional acetylcholine receptors is greatly decreased in myasthenia gravis and in rats treated with neostigmine (Fambrough *et al.*, 1973).

Changes in the density of acetylcholine receptors after denervation have been measured by the use of radioactively labeled α-bungarotoxin. After denervation of rat diaphragm, the extrajunctional receptor density begins to increase after about 2 days and increases approximately linearly from a normal level of $5/\mu m^2$ to $635/\mu m^2$ at 14 days, subsequently decreasing to $529/\mu m^2$ as the muscle atrophies (Fambrough, 1974*a,b*). This increase in extrajunctional receptor density is accompanied by a large increase in the total number of receptors (Hartzell and Fambrough, 1972). The turnover time of extrajunctional receptors is rapid, with a half-time of about 20 hours in chick muscle in culture (Devreotes and Fambrough, 1976*a,b*), as well as in rat diaphragm *in vivo* (Chang and Huang, 1975). The junctional receptors turn over much more slowly, with a half-time of about 7.5 days (Chang and Huang, 1975). The cell deals differently with the junctional and with extrajunctional receptors, not only as regards their rates of degradation and replenishment but also as regards their density and localization. It is not known to what degree these differences are due to regional differences in the membrane or to biochemical differences between junctional and extrajunctional receptors.

The distribution of acetylcholinesterase on the muscle membrane is correlated with the distribution of acetylcholine receptors. Use of a histochemical technique for staining acetylcholinesterase (AChE) in the chick embryo shows that AChE is diffusely distributed throughout the myoblasts at 3–6 days of incubation, and recedes toward the endplate region and myotendinous junction on subsequent days (Begliomini and Moriconi, 1960; Mumenthaler and Engel, 1961). This occurs during the myotube stage in all vertebrates that have been examined (Mumenthaler and Engel, 1961; Wake, 1964; Filogamo and Gabella, 1967; H. Hirano, 1967*b*; H.-C. Liu and Maneely, 1968). The local concentration of AChE at the end plate occurs only after the nerve has made contact with the muscle fiber and appears to be caused by neuromuscular contact (Mumenthaler and Engel, 1961; Filogamo and Gabella, 1967). Localization of AChE to the motor end plates is first seen on day 10 in the paraspinal muscles and on days 12–13 in the distal leg muscles of the chick embryo (Drachman, 1965). In the absence of innervation, as in muscle fibers in tissue culture, a weak AChE activity is found throughout the muscle, and the localization of cholinesterase to the end plate does not occur (Engel, 1961). However, direct electrical stimulation of cultured chick embryo skeletal muscle results in a decrease of the AChE (C. R. Walker and Wilson, 1975).

8.3.2. Neural Control of the Speed of Skeletal Muscle Contraction

In newborn mammals all the limb muscles are slow, and differentiation into fast and slow muscles occurs only postnatally; for example, during postnatal weeks 3–6 in the kitten (Denny-Brown, 1929; Koshtoyantz and Ryabinovskaya, 1935; Buller *et al.*, 1960*a*; Buller and Lewis, 1964; Buller, 1966) and during the first 5 postnatal weeks in the rat (Close, 1964; Yellin, 1967*a,b*). After birth all muscles show an increase in the speed of their contractions, but after a few weeks those destined to become tonic muscles stop increasing their rate of contraction while the phasic muscles continue to increase their speed of contraction. Shortening of the contraction time of the muscles is not related to changes in their motor nerves. The conduction velocity of all the motor nerves increases tenfold from birth to maturity, owing to increase in fiber diameter and to the distance between nodes of the myelin sheath, but the ratio of conduction velocities of motor nerves that supply fast and slow muscles remains constant (Ridge, 1967).

Denervation of slow or fast muscles results in alterations in the speed of contraction, myoglobin content and enzyme content to levels intermediate between those of normally slow and fast muscle fibers (Romanul and Hogan, 1965; Hogan *et al.*, 1965; McPherson and Tokunaga, 1967; Yellin, 1967*a,b*). Reinnervation by the same nerve results in a return of the characteristics of the muscles to their normal levels (Buller *et al.*, 1960*b*; Close, 1965). Like denervation, treatment with botulinum toxin results in a change of the histochemical profile of muscle to a level intermediate between that of fast and slow muscle (Drachman and Romanul, 1970).

Cross-innervation of slow muscle by a nerve that normally supplies fast muscle, and *vice versa,* results in reversal of the characteristics of the muscle: speed of contraction (Close, 1965), myoglobin content (McPherson and Tokunaga, 1967), total soluble proteins (Guth and Watson, 1967), and levels of oxidative and anaerobic enzymes (Romanul and van der Meulen, 1967; Yellin, 1967*b*; Karpati and Engel, 1967). Cross-innervated muscle has mechanical properties intermediate between those of fast and slow muscles. The conversion of the mechanical properties of fast to slow muscle is much more complete than conversion of the mechanical properties of slow to fast muscle after cross-innervation (Buller *et al.*, 1960*b*; Buller and Lewis, 1965). Muscles that are partially reinnervated by their own nerve and partially cross-innervated contain areas of fast and areas of slow fibers. They contract rapidly or slowly depending on the nerve that is stimulated (Romanul and van der Meulen, 1967). The effects of cross-innervation apparently occur only where both slow and fast types of muscle fibers have focal *en plaque* innervation (Tiegs, 1953; Bone, 1964), and they have been observed in mammals and frogs (Miledi and Orkand, 1966). In birds, the fast and slow muscles differ in their innervation pattern as well as in their ultrastructure, enzymes, myoglobin, and speed of contraction. Fast muscles (for example, posterior latissimus dorsi) have focal *en plaque* innervation, while slow muscles (for example, anterior lastissimus dorsi) have multiple *en grappe* innervation with motor end plates occurring every 600–1000 μm along the entire muscle fiber. Cross-innervation of anterior and posterior latissimus dorsi in the chick does not alter the speed of contraction or the ultrastructure of these muscles (Hník *et al.*, 1967). The pattern of innervation is dependent on the muscle rather than on the nerve that supplies it: thus anterior latissimus dorsi muscle of the chicken retains its multiple *en grappe* pattern of innervation when cross-innervated with the nerve to posterior latissimus dorsi (M. R. Bennett *et al.*, 1973*c*). In cats, Guth *et al.* (1970) showed that cross-innervation of the soleus muscle (which contains mainly β fibers) with the nerve from flexor hallucis longus muscle (which contains α, β, and $\alpha\beta$ fibers) results in the appearance of many α fibers in the soleus muscle. They concluded that qualitative changes in the type of actomyosin ATPase that occur as a result of cross-innervation indicate that the nerve regulates synthesis of the enzyme by altering gene expression.

The conversion of many major components of slow into fast muscle, and *vice versa,* after cross-union of their motor nerves shows that the nature of the muscle is determined by the nerve that supplies it. The biochemical differences between slow and fast skeletal muscle are specified by the nerve, and the interconversion from one type of muscle to another can occur at any age. The mechanism by which the motoneuron regulates the function of its muscle is unknown, but several possibilities have to be considered: (1) the amount of contractile activity, regardless of how it is produced; (2) the number, frequency, or pattern of nerve impulses in the motor nerves; and (3) the influence of trophic substances produced by the motor nerves.

8.4. Mechanism of Trophic Action of Motoneurons on Muscles

The possibility that trophic agents released by the motor nerve induce the changes in the muscle that have been observed during innervation and denervation was never more than a hypothesis. It persisted as long as the evidence for the other alternatives was slight. The trophic factor hypothesis has diminished in plausibility as the evidence has increased showing that virtually all the effects of denervation can be produced by pharmacological blockade of cholinergic transmission at the neuromuscular junction. The evidence that the differentiation of muscle depends on the amount of muscle contraction, regardless of whether it is produced by stimulation via the neuromuscular junction or by direct electrical stimulation of the muscle, has, in the absence of equally strong direct evidence of a trophic agent, reduced the need to invoke such an agent. The putative trophic agent, appropriately termed "mysterine" by Drachman (1976), cannot be entirely dismissed, for several reasons. First, most but not all the effects of denervation are reproduced by blocking cholinergic neuromuscular transmission (Drachman, 1976, review). The residual functions of muscle that persist after treatment with botulinum toxin could be ascribed to the spontaneous release of acetylcholine. Furthermore, the end plate persists after botulinum treatment but degenerates after nerve section, so that the two are not entirely equivalent in their effect on the muscle. Second, although most of the effects originally attributed to the hypothetical trophic agent have been shown to be mediated by neuromuscular transmission and the subsequent events that lead to muscle contraction, some evidence of a different kind indicates that there may be some aspects of muscle differentiation that are controlled by a trophic factor. It should be noted, however, that valid interpretations of these experimental results can also be made without invoking a trophic agent. For example, the demonstration that radioactively labeled amino acids are transferred from the motor nerve to the muscle (Kerkut *et al.,* 1967; I. M. Korr *et al.,* 1967; I. M. Korr and Appeltauer, 1974) falls far short of showing that the transferred material has any trophic effect. Another type of experimental result suggests but does not directly demonstrate that the motor axon has a store of trophic agent which, after cutting of the motor nerve, is gradually depleted in the peripheral nerve stump. Thus there is a latent period between cutting of the nerve and the onset of fibrillation in the denervated muscle which is proportional to the length of the peripheral stump (Gutmann *et al.,* 1955). This might mean that the proximodistal flow of the trophic agent is about 2–5 mm per hour (J. V. Luco and Eyzaguirre, 1955; J. B. Harris and Thesleff, 1972). This is within the range of rapid axonal transport (see Section 4.8), and might only indicate that the length of the peripheral stump is related to a reservoir of materials transported distally in the axon for maintenance of the nerve terminal (Droz, 1973) and for release of acetylcholine rather than release of a trophic agent. In fact, Miledi and Slater (1970) have shown that the latent period before onset of fibrillation is the period during which spontaneous release of acetylcholine persists after nerve section. Another type of evidence, purportedly showing that a trophic agent is transported in the axon to the nerve terminal, is that inhibition of axonal transport produces some of the effects of denervation in the muscle but does not prevent traffic of nerve impulses or release of acetylcholine at the neuromuscular junction (Albuquerque *et al.,* 1972; W. W. Hoffman and Peacock, 1973; Juntunen, 1973*b*; Max and Albuquerque, 1975). The same method, involving application of a cuff containing a local anesthetic, colchicine, or vinblastine, has been used to block flow of a presumed trophic agent in sensory nerve fibers (Aguilar *et al.,* 1973; J. Diamond *et al.,* 1976). The difficulty of interpretation of this type of experiment stems from the direct effects of the colchicine or other agents on the muscle. However, regardless of their mechanism of action, these experiments show that denervationlike effects on muscle can be produced without blocking cholinergic transmission and apparently without reducing muscle contractile activity.

The evidence that muscle contraction is an important if not the sole factor that determines the functional properties of muscle is of three kinds. First, there is the evidence that muscles that are used frequently during normal activity tend to have slow speeds of contraction. Second, there is evidence that resting a muscle, which can be achieved by several methods mentioned below, results in denervationlike changes in the functional characteristics of skeletal muscle. Third, there is evidence that direct electrical stimulation of denervated muscle is able to retard or prevent the effects of denervation.

The total amount of contraction and probably the temporal pattern of contraction are important in determining the functional properties of muscle. Guth and Yellin (1971) conclude that "muscle cells undergo continual alterations throughout life in adaptation to changing functional demands and that the histochemically demonstrable 'fiber types' merely reflect each muscle fiber's constitution at a given moment in time." In normal development and during normal life, the activity is determined by the type of motoneurons. Attention has already been directed to the relationship between the functional characteristics of the muscle and those of the motoneuron that innervates it. The pattern and frequency of nerve impulses may determine the nature of the muscle (Eccles *et al.,* 1958*a,b*; Vrbová, 1963*a,b*; Henneman and Olson, 1965; Wuerker *et al.,* 1965; C. B. Olson and Swett, 1966, 1969; Salmons and Vrbová, 1969). Muscles that are innervated by large motoneurons contract rapidly and develop large amounts of tension but are used phasically at irregular intervals. Muscles that are innervated by small motoneurons contract slowly and develop small amounts of tension, but they are used frequently or tonically.

Frequent use of a muscle, regardless of its type of motoneuron, apparently results in slowing of the muscle contraction time (Gutmann *et al.,* 1969; Guth, 1971). By contrast, a slow muscle such as the soleus muscle increases its speed of contraction when it is rested, as occurs after cutting of the achilles tendon (Vrbová, 1963*a,b*). This increase in the speed of contraction can be prevented by long-term electrical stimulation of the soleus muscle at frequencies of 5 or 10 per second, but not by stimulation at frequencies of 20 or 40 per second (Salmons and Vrbová,

1969). Tenotomy in 4-day-old rats prolongs the period of polyneuronal innervation in the tenotomized soleus muscle (Benoit and Changeux, 1975). Reduction in the amount of contractile activity of muscles has also been attempted by splinting, casting, or pinning a limb. These procedures result in an increase in the extrajunctional acetylcholine sensitivity (Solandt *et al.,* 1943; Fischbach and Robbins, 1969) and a decrease in the contraction time of slow muscles (Fischbach and Robbins, 1969; Mann and Salafsky, 1970). Another method of reducing the impulse traffic in motor nerves is by isolating the spinal cord connected to the hindlimb of the dog, dividing the cord above and below the lumbosacral segments, and cutting the dorsal roots supplying the hindlimb (Tower, 1937*a,b*). This results in slow atrophy of the muscle and in an increase in extrajunctional acetylcholine sensitivity which is not as great as that after denervation (Johns and Thesleff, 1961). Other methods of reducing or totally preventing muscle contraction have been to block nerve conduction by injection of tetrodotoxin into the sciatic nerve of rats (Pestronk *et al.,* 1976*b*) and to maintain cats under deep nembutal anesthesia (Davis, 1970; Montgomery, 1972). These procedures result in denervationlike changes including increase of speed of contraction after barbiturate anesthesia, and increase in extrajunctional acetylcholine receptors after nerve conduction block.

Finally, the evidence that electrical stimulation of muscle is sufficient to prevent most of the atrophic effects of denervation is inconsistent with the hypothesis that a trophic agent is transmitted from nerve to muscle. The appearance of extrajunctional acetylcholine sensitivity can be completely prevented by repetitive stimulation of denervated muscle (Drachman and Witzke, 1972; Lömo and Rosenthal, 1972; R. C. Kauffman *et al.,* 1974; Frank *et al.,* 1975). Reinnervation of denervated rat soleus muscle by foreign nerves is diminished by electrical stimulation of the muscle (Jansen *et al.,* 1973).

The present evidence cannot entirely exclude the possibility of one or more specific trophic factors that are released from the motor nerve terminal and control the various properties of skeletal muscle. Moreover, the evidence that no single experimental case of cholinergic block or of muscle disuse completely reproduces the effects of total denervation leaves open the possibility that the residual muscle functions are mediated by one or more trophic agents. If the effects of denervation could be completely reproduced by total block of cholinergic neuromuscular transmission (using both botulinum toxin and α-bungarotoxin), the trophic factor hypothesis would be rendered untenable, at least as regards skeletal muscle. For the present, while the trophic factor cannot be entirely excluded, it is nevertheless easy to conceive of a mechanism of trophic action on skeletal muscle in which acetylcholine is the sole mediator between nerve and muscle. According to this hypothesis, each muscle phenotype is regulated independently by an intracellular control circuit that includes a different part of the excitation–contraction mechanism. For example, the mechanisms controlling the number of extrajunctional acetylcholine receptors would include membrane depolarization but would not include muscle contraction and would not be directly sensitive to the amount of muscle contractile activity. By contrast, the control of muscle twitch duration would include part of the contractile mechanism and would be sensitive to the amount of muscle contractile activity. According to this hypothesis, the functions that remained after any experimental procedure, such as treatment with botulinum toxin or immobilization, as compared with the total loss of functions after denervation, would reflect the residual functions of the muscle that had been spared by the experimental procedure. The less parsimonious alternative is that each experimental procedure, short of axotomy, leaves some muscle functions intact because it produces only partial block of a single trophic agent or blocks some but not all of several trophic agents.

Economy of means gives us a particular pleasure in nature as in art. Who fails to respond to the sepia washes of Claude or to the evocation of color by a seemingly infinite variety of black ink tones and textures? To have found another example of parsimony in nature is always pleasing, but we should not allow such instances to narrow our perspective of the equally pleasing diversity of means by which particular ends have been reached during evolution.

8.5. Formation of Connections between Sensory Nerves and Sensory Receptors

Sensory nerves always arrive before sensory receptor cells start differentiating in the skin, taste buds, lateral line organs, muscle spindles, tendon organs, and other chemoreceptors, thermoreceptors, and mechanoreceptors in the viscera and blood vessels. This leads one to suspect that the presence of sensory nerve may be required for the differentiation of sensory receptor cells. The evidence that sensory nerves "induce" the development of sensory receptors is discussed in the following pages.

It is well known that each type of sense organ can respond only to a specific stimulus modality and to a limited range of intensities. An attempt will be made to answer the question of whether the sensory nerve determines the modality specificity of the sense organ, or *vice versa,* or whether a reciprocal interaction between nerve terminal and sense organ determines their functional specificity. At present, no direct evidence has been obtained by recording from developing sense organs, and we have to rely mainly on the evidence from studies of denervation and reinnervation of sense organs.

All types of sensory cells degenerate after denervation and may regenerate or differentiate anew after reinnervation. If the denervated sense organelles survive, the effects of denervation may be completely reversed after reinnervation. Whether regenerating sensory nerves reconnect with the sense organs with which they were originally connected or whether reinnervation is totally nonselective is a problem that has not been fully resolved. Some evidence of selective reinnervation is given below.

Some observations show that regenerating sensory nerves may be attracted or guided to the positions occupied by degenerating sensory cells. R. M. May (1925) observed that regenerated nerve terminals return to the positions previously occupied by taste buds in catfish. After cutting the dorsal lateral line nerve and cutaneous nerves in frog tadpoles, Speidel (1964) observed a marked preference for reinnervation of lateral line organs by lateral line nerves rather than by cutaneous nerve fibers. A similar preferential reinnervation is seen after regeneration of cutaneous nerves to the hairy skin of the cat: the nerves show a distinct tendency to regenerate to their original terminal positions in relationship to specialized epithelial (Merkel) cells (Burgess *et al.,* 1974). Two problems are raised by such observations: First, how do the regenerating axons find their way to their original locations? Are they guided there by the Schwann cells that mark their original paths, or are they attracted by alluring substances emanating from the degenerating receptors? Second, what is the source of the cells that differentiate as new receptors? It is known that the original cells can participate in the formation of receptors after nerve regeneration, but that is impossible in cases where the original receptors have completely degenerated before the nerves return. In that case, the nerves induce differentiation in the epithelial cells, and we wish to know whether all epithelial cells have this capability or whether there are special precursor cells that remain undifferentiated until they are contacted by a sensory nerve fiber. Partial solutions to these problems will be given in the following sections.

8.6. Development of Nerve Connections with Muscle Spindles

Muscle spindles are stretch receptors found in vertebrate skeletal muscle (Reviews by Barker, 1974; C. C. Hunt, 1974). They consist of specialized intrafusal muscle fibers innervated by the γ-motoneurons and by sensory nerve terminals of the Type Ia axons from the spinal dorsal root ganglia. These neurons develop from the small mediodorsal cells of the spinal ganglia (see Section 7.10). There are two main types of intrafusal muscle fibers in mammalian muscle spindles: the large nuclear bag fibers and the smaller nuclear chain fibers, so called because of the arrangement of their nuclei. The neuromuscular junctions are confined to the poles of the intrafusal muscle fibers, whereas the sensory axons are confined to the equatorial zone of the spindle where they form the annulospinal and flower-spray nerve endings. The normal development of muscle spindles has been described in many papers which should be consulted for details of the structural changes that occur during development (Sutton, 1915; Tello, 1922*b*; Cuajunco, 1927*a,b*; Kalugina, 1956; Barker and Milburn, 1972; Landon, 1972*a,b*; Milburn, 1973*a,b*).

In the hindlimb of the chick embryo, the muscle spindles can first be seen on day 9 of incubation, and no additional spindles develop after day 13 (Tello, 1922*b*). Because stretch reflexes can be elicited from days 10–11, sensory nerves must have connected with the spindles before then (Visintini and Levi-Montalcini, 1939; Hamburger and Levi-Montalcini, 1949). The innervation of muscle spindles in the jaw muscles of the chick embryo probably occurs between days 9 and 13 of incubation, as indicated by the death of neurons in the trigeminal mesencephalic nucleus which fail to connect with spindles (L. A. Rogers and Cowan, 1973).

The muscle spindles develop under the influence of their nerves, but here the problem is complicated by their dual innervation. The initial development of the intrafusal muscle fibers, to the myotube stage, occurs in the absence of innervation. However, the differentiation of mature intrafusal muscle fibers requires both sensory and motor innervation. In the rat, the muscle spindles begin to appear in the limbs on day 18 of gestation. Initially, the intrafusal muscle fibers are innervated only by sensory nerve terminals. In the hindlimb of the rat, sensory innervation of the muscle spindles develops on day 18 of gestation while the neuromuscular junctions develop at the polar regions of intrafusal muscle fibers only at birth and on the subsequent days. At birth, the muscle spindles are immature, containing two myotubes with nuclear bags and one satellite myotube. Postnatally, intrafusal myotubes fuse to form another satellite myotube. The two myotubes that are formed last develop nuclear chains, and this completes the full complement of intrafusal fibers in the rat by 4 days after birth. However, the polar zones of the spindles do not become fully differentiated until 12 days after birth.

The differentiation of muscle spindles beyond the myotube stage of the intrafusal muscle fibers is under control of the sensory nerves and remains so throughout life. Elimination of the sensory nerve supply by cutting the dorsal roots in adult cats and dogs, leaving the motor supply intact, results in degeneration of the muscle spindles (Tower, 1932). Denervation of rat muscle spindles on day 19 or 20 of gestation (60–72 hours before birth) results in rapid degeneration (Zelená, 1957). Since the only innervation present at the time of the operation before birth is the sensory nerves, they must be required for differentiation of the muscle spindles. On the other hand, if the sensory nerves remain intact, spindle development is little affected, but the intrafusal muscle fibers slowly degenerate following selective motor denervation (Zelená, 1964, 1965; Zelená and Soukup, 1973, 1974*a,b*).

With increasing age, muscle spindles in the rat hindlimb have a progressively decreasing dependence on their nerve supply (Zelená, 1957, 1964). In newborn rats, denervation results in atrophy and degeneration of the muscle spindles within 10 days. Denervation in rats 20 days after birth, when the muscle spindles are fully differentiated, merely results in slight atrophy of the intrafusal muscle fibers 10 days later. There is a critical period during which muscle spindles will degenerate if deprived of their innervation, but the spindles will survive if they are denervated after that period. In the gastrocnemius muscle of the rat, the spindles require innervation until 6–8 days postnatally, after which they survive if denervated (J. K. Werner, 1973).

Although the intrafusal muscle fibers are highly specialized, they resemble the extrafusal muscle fibers in having neuromuscular junctions which apparently are cholinergic. The question thus arises why the intrafusal fibers degenerate after removal of their sensory nerve supply even when their motor nerve supply is intact. This case is apparently in conflict with the hypothesis that cholinergic stimulation, or at least muscle contraction, is the trophic stimulus (see Section 8.6). Although the evidence is inadequate to permit a conclusive explanation, some sense can be made of the existing data. First, it might be thought that cutting the dorsal roots opens the γ loop and virtually eliminates impulse traffic in the γ-motoneurons to the intrafusal muscle fibers, thus causing disuse atrophy. However, that explanation is not convincing because cutting the γ nerve fibers does not result in the rapid degeneration that follows cutting the sensory nerve supply. Therefore, the sensory nerve itself must exert the trophic effect. The observation that there are specialized junctions, resembling synapses, between the sensory nerve and the intrafusal muscle suggests that the sensory nerves may release a trophic agent that stimulates the muscle, and the presence of light- and dense-cored vesicles in the sensory nerve ending and of coated invaginations in both the muscle and axonal membrane is consistent with this hypothesis (Zelená and Soukup, 1973). The synapselike structure may also mediate transmission from the muscle to the sensory nerve.

8.7. Development of Cutaneous Sensory Innervation

The density of cutaneous innervation and the number of sensory corpuscles in each region are remarkably invariant. These appear to be regional characteristics of the epithelium and are probably determined during early development, before entry of the nerves, by interactions between the epithelium and underlying mesenchyme (McLoughlin, 1968). The distribution of hairs and feathers is also determined by interactions between epithelium and mesenchyme (Wessells, 1965; Wessells and Roessner, 1965). Virtually nothing is known about the early stages of development of the epithelium when the local properties of the epithelium are determined which control the density of innervation and of sensory corpuscles.

The nerves growing into the skin appear to be confronted with a large number of potential targets from which each nerve has to select one. The situation creates the impression of a very difficult multiple-choice problem which is further complicated by the fact that the density of cutaneous innervation and the number of sensory corpuscles are quite constant in each region of the skin. These aspects of the problem were first fully grasped by Ramón y Cajal, who, in a remarkable paper published in 1919, established the concepts into which all subsequent contributions to the problem have ineluctably had to be fitted. If anyone has seen further into this problem than Ramón y Cajal, it is only by standing on his shoulders. He believed that both selective growth (that is, chemotropism) and selective terminal connection (that is, chemoaffinity) probably play a part in regulating the pattern of cutaneous innervation. He pointed out that the density of innervation of each region of the skin is precisely determined and that "each fiber is destined for an epithelial territory devoid of nerves, and there are no vast aneuritic spaces in some regions nor excessive collections of fibrils in others" (Ramón y Cajal, 1919). He suggested that the nerve fibers are attracted by chemicals in the epidermis, which are either used up or neutralized by the nerves as they grow into the skin, so that "after invasion of the epithelium a state of chemical equilibrium is created, by virtue of which the innervated territories are incapable of attracting new sprouts."

In addition to the general attractive effect of the epithelium, Ramón y Cajal proposed a more specific neurotropic effect to account for the specific innervation of different types of sensory organelles and muscles. He pointed out that this specificity is unlikely to be the result of mechanical guidance, because then "it becomes difficult to understand how, of the large nervous contingent arriving at the mammalian snout, some fibers travel without error to the cutaneous muscle fibers, others toward the hair follicles, others to the epidermis and finally some to the tactile apparatus of the dermis. A similar multiple specificity is found in the tongue, where hypoglossal fibers invade the muscle, trigeminal fibers innervate the ordinary papillae, and facial (geniculate ganglion) and glossopharyngeal fibers go to the gustatory papillae" (Ramón y Cajal, 1919).

Neurotropic substances have not been identified in the skin, but a number of observations indicate that there may be some kind of biochemical control of the density of cutaneous innervation. For example, denervation of a region of skin results in collateral sprouting of adjacent nerve fibers, which grow into the denervated region (Weddell *et al.,* 1941; Livingston, 1947). This kind of growth adjustment of nerve endings was studied in the tail fin of the frog tadpole by

Speidel (1941), who concluded that "in some manner the denervated zone constitutes a local stimulus with sufficient influence to evoke new sprouts from nearby fibers which otherwise would not have given rise to them." Collateral nerve sprouting is the normal method of innervation during development and growth of the skin. Regulation of the density of cutaneous innervation continues throughout life. Nerve endings and sense organelles in the skin and mucous membranes are continually destroyed as a result of normal wear and tear. The innervation of these tissues remains in a steady state because replacement of epidermal cells, nerve endings, and sense organelles exactly compensates for their loss (Tello, 1932; Cowdry, 1932, Vol. 1, p. 24; Fitzgerald, 1962; Beidler, 1963; Beidler and Smallman, 1965). The observation by Fitzgerald (1961, 1962) that during development of the pig snout the number of axonal branches increases in proportion to the number of epidermal ridges is consistent with Ramón y Cajal's concepts of the control of cutaneous innervation density.

Direct observation of the process of growth adjustment of peripheral nerves can be made in the tail fin of the living tadpole. Speidel (1933, 1935*a,b,* 1941, 1942) observed the growth of nerves in the dermis of the tail fin of the living tadpole almost continuously over a period of several weeks (Figs. 4.5 and 4.6). Collateral branches occur at any position in unmyelinated axons and at the nodes of Ranvier in myelinated axons. The branches may extend, retract, or degenerate, and as a result the pattern of innervation is constantly changing. Speidel (1942, p. 63) concluded: "It seems very probable to me that the endings of terminal arborizations within the central nervous system undergo adjustments quite like those of terminal arborizations of the skin." This has proved to be true, and evidence is given in Sections 5.7 and 5.8 of sprouting of presynaptic terminals which occupy synaptic sites on partially denervated neurons in the central nervous system.

Denervation of a region of skin results in collateral sprouting from neighboring nerves (Fig. 8.5). The collateral branches grow into the denervated region of skin, which then regains its sensitivity (Speidel, 1941; Weddell *et al.,* 1941; Livingston, 1947). This type of regeneration is clearly adaptive, and one is struck by the correlation between the degree of degeneration and the number of extra axonal branches that restore the original density of cutaneous innervation. There seem to be homeostatic mechanisms which regulate the density of innervation of skin or muscles so that after the peripheral organs become saturated with nerves, no more axon collaterals are produced and the excess collaterals degenerate.

Ramón y Cajal's concept that the epithelium regulates axonal sprouting by producing a neurotropic factor that is neutralized by the nerve has recently been amplified by evidence that an antisprouting factor is transported in the axon to the nerve terminal. This is considered at greater length in Sections 5.7 and 5.8 in relation to sprouting and plasticity of axonal endings. Aguilar *et al.* (1973) and J. Diamond *et al.* (1976) blocked axonal transport by means of colchicine applied to one of the three cutaneous nerves to the leg of the salamander and observed collateral sprouting of neighboring nerves into the peripheral field of the colchicine-treated nerve. They concluded that a substance is transported to the nerve endings which neutralizes the sprouting factor produced by the epithelium. The story has now come full circle back to Ramón y Cajal's original hypothesis. Diamond *et al.* (1976) propose an additional hypothesis, that cutaneous nerves are allotted domains of body space, and that their axons are hindered from responding to the sprouting stimulus emanating from denervated skin in a different domain. However, within a domain there is no apparent constraint on axonal sprouting in response to partial denervation of skin (Fig. 8.6).

The alternative mechanisms of innervation of the skin and formation of cutaneous sensory corpuscles are the following: First, there may be a coincidence between the time of arrival of nerves and the time at which their targets originate or are mature enough to accept innervation. The evidence does not show any regular pattern of temporal coincidence of the sort that would be consistent with such a hypothesis. Second, guidance or attraction to the appropriate endings may account for the specificity of innervation, and there is evidence of such targeting of nerve fibers on Merkel cells in the skin of the salamander. In this species the Merkel cells can be seen with the electron microscope before they become innervated, thus raising the possibility that they may differentiate prior to their connecting with nerves (E. Cooper and Diamond, 1977; E. Cooper *et al.,* 1977).

There is evidence, discussed below, that regenerating cutaneous nerve fibers might use the Schwann cell strands as guides to the positions that they originally occupied in the skin (Burgess *et al.,* 1974). If there are cytological markers along the route of the axon's growth, it is unlikely that Schwann cells carry the markers or provide mechanical guidance, because the Schwann cells do not precede the

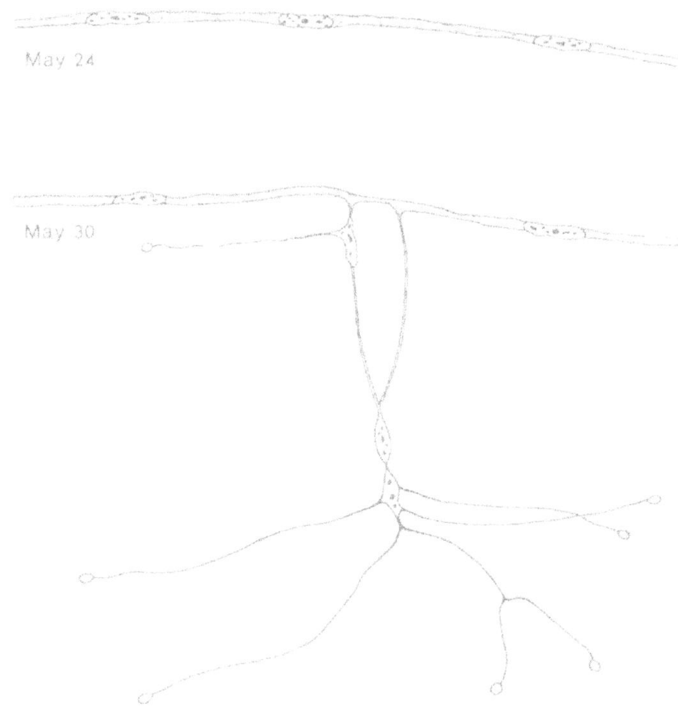

Figure 8.5. Origin of collateral sprouts from an axon following experimental denervation of an adjacent zone of the skin on the tail fin of a frog tadpole. On May 24 a zone of the tail fin was deprived of its nerve supply. The nerve illustrated was at the edge of the denervated region. Two new sprouts arose, one on May 27 and one on May 28. These grew, and by May 30 had given rise to seven endings which supplied a part of the denervated zone. From C. C. Speidel, *Harvey Lect. 36:*126–158 (1941), copyright Academic Press, Inc.

nerves but the growing nerves bring their Schwann cells with them into the peripheral tissues. Speidel (1933, 1935*a,b*, 1941, 1942) observed the growth of nerves in the tail fin of the living frog tadpole and noted that peripheral nerve fibers enter the skin before the Schwann cells migrate out over the nerves to their terminals. The crucial experiment showing that Schwann cells are not essential for development of nerves was performed by Harrison (1924*a*). He showed that a normal pattern of peripheral nerves functionally innervating sense organs and muscles develops in the absence of Schwann cells after removal of the neural crest in amphibian embryos. The corneal nerves of mammals develop and regenerate in the complete absence of Schwann cells (Rexed and Rexed, 1951; Zander and Weddell, 1951).

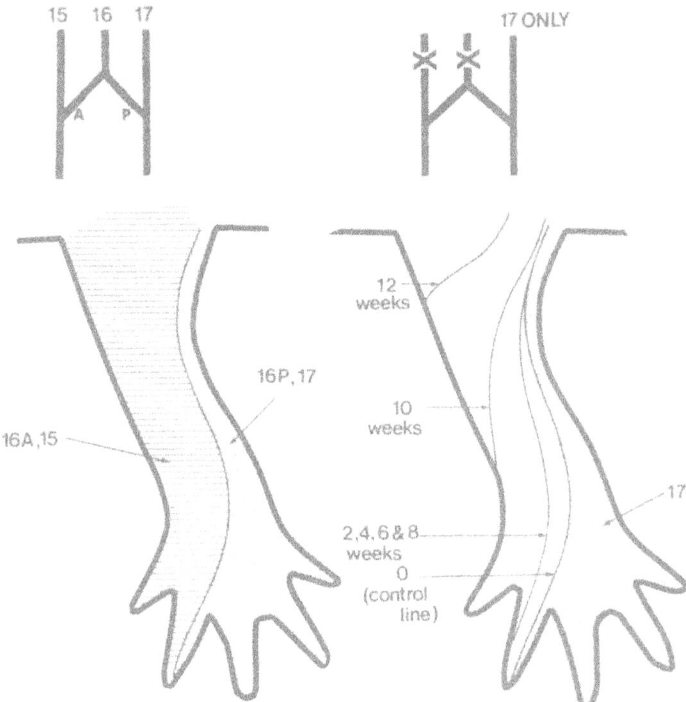

Figure 8.6. Nerve sprouting in the skin on the dorsum of the hindlimb of the salamander (narrowest region approximately 6 mm). Cutaneous sensory fields of spinal nerves 15, 16, and 17 were mapped by recording action potentials in the nerve trunks evoked by mechanical stimulation of the skin with a fine bristle. Normal cutaneous fields are shown on the left: fields of nerves 15 and 17 meet on a common boundary which is also that separating the fields of the anterior and posterior divisions of nerve 16. Changes in the cutaneous field of nerve 17 after cutting of nerves 15 and 16 are shown in the diagram of the limb on the right. In all such animals, sprouting stops for 8 weeks after a small initial extension of the 17th field. Thereafter, the 17th field expands rapidly until it covers the entire dorsal surface of the limb by 12 weeks postoperatively. Other nerves behave similarly when sprouting into a foreign domain. Although the capacity of the nerve to sprout into a foreign field is delayed, it sprouts into its own field immediately after partial deafferentation. Only intact nerves are so constrained: regenerating nerves sprout without delay into foreign fields so that a single regenerating nerve can enlarge its field continuously to innervate the entire dorsum of the limb. Unpublished results of J. Diamond and L. Macintyre.

It seems essential to invoke some sort of specific affinity between nerve endings and their target organs to account for the specific association of different kinds of nerve fibers with the appropriate kinds of cells in the skin and subcutaneous tissues. However, it is not necessary to invoke chemotaxis to account for selective terminal connections. Correct connections would form with a high degree of probability as a result of chemoaffinity between nerve terminals and their appropriate target cells plus extensive preterminal branching and random contacts between nerve terminals and their target cells.

The studies of Saxod (1978, review) on the development of innervation of Herbst and Grandry corpuscles in the duck beak are the most complete of their kind, and they show that those cutaneous receptors, which normally form at the endings of the ophthalmic branch of the trigeminal nerve, can be made to form *de novo* in relation to spinal sensory nerves. This makes it unlikely that there is an all-or-none affinity between the nerve ending and its target cells in the skin. Of course, all such cross-innervation experiments, in which only one kind of nerve fiber innervates the target cells, cannot rule out the possibility that nerve terminals of one kind have a greater affinity than those of another kind for the target cells but that if both kinds innervate the targets those with the greater affinity will displace those with less affinity.

In general, receptors have the same functional characteristics after regeneration as before, regardless of the source of their sensory innervation. This has been most thoroughly studied in the cutaneous sensory nerves of the cat (A. G. Brown and Iggo, 1962; Burgess and Horch, 1973; Burgess *et al.,* 1974). Type I sensory fibers in the cat's hairy skin innervate sensory structures called domes or Merkel tactile discs, containing 20–50 specialized Merkel cells. Each dome is supplied by a single axon which branches to supply the Merkel cells. Section of the Type I cutaneous nerve results in degeneration of the domes supplied by the nerves. Domes reappear after regeneration of the nerve and recover their normal response properties. Not all domes reappear, but the positions of those that reappear after nerve regeneration are closely coincident with the preoperative positions of domes (Fig. 8.7). Coincidence is as good with foreign invading nerves as with the normally reinnervating nerves. After excision, the domes can reappear in regenerated skin. This eliminates the possibility that there are a limited number of dome sites ("intrinsic target specificity" of Burgess *et al.,* 1974), but it does not show whether there are specific types of cells which can be induced to differentiate as Merkel cells or whether all types of skin cells have this potentiality. Burgess *et al.* (1974), in discussing their results, considered the other alternative hypotheses, which they call "extrinsic terminal specificity" and "specific conduit guidance," meaning, respectively, that domes are potentially able to form anywhere but their actual position is determined by sensory nerve terminals and that regenerating sensory axons are guided, perhaps by Schwann cells, to the positions of the domes they had originally innervated. Either or both these mechanisms could have resulted in the observed pattern of receptors.

Another experiment to determine whether there is any specificity in the formation of connections between sense organelles and sensory nerves was performed by Kadanoff (1925). He exchanged hairy skin of the snout and hairless skin of the soles of the feet in mice and guinea pigs. Reinnervation of both types of grafts occurs. In some cases, the innervation pattern of the graft resembles what was normal for the grafted skin and not for the skin that the nerves originally supplied. This is most clearly seen in the case of hair follicles that are innervated normally in snout skin transplanted to the soles of the feet.

In birds, sensory nerves arrive in the skin long before the development of the feather follicles and the sensory corpuscles which they innervate. The first sensory nerves arrive in the skin of the back as early as day 4 of incubation in the chick embryo (Saxod, 1978). From days 4–10 of incubation the nerves form a dense plexus which surrounds and innervates the developing feather follicles. The cutaneous sensory corpuscles begin to appear synchronously in different regions at 17 days of incubation in the chick and at 20 days in the duck embryo.

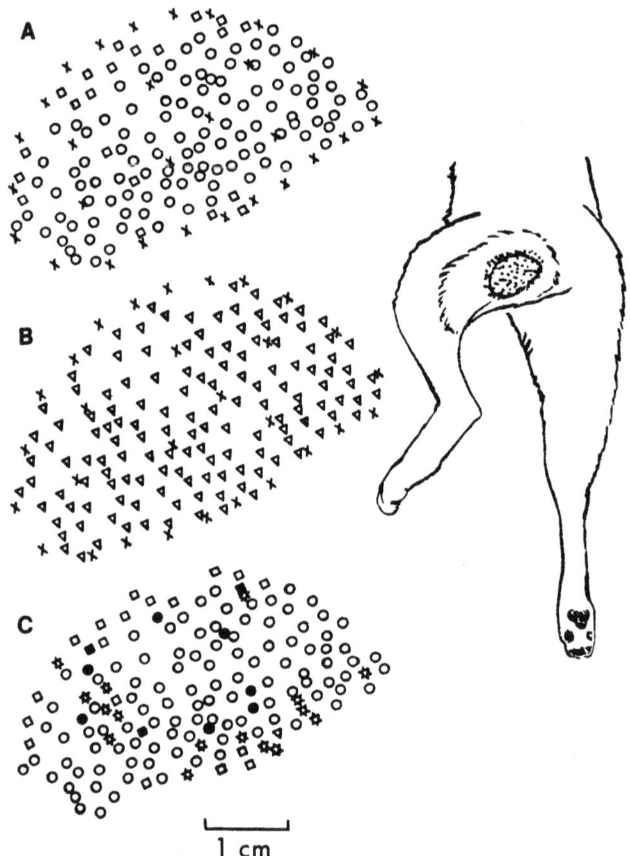

Figure 8.7. A: Distribution of domes on the cat thigh at the time of the original recording. Domes producing a discharge in the femoral cutaneous nerve are circled, those that did not are enclosed by squares, and x's indicate reference tattoo marks. Recordings were made from the femoral cutaneous nerve in this experiment, after which the nerve was crushed or cut. B: Tracing of one of the photographs of the dome distribution in the same animal made 113 days after the distribution in A was mapped. The nerve was not recorded from at this time and the domes were located by visual inspection at 25×. Hence femoral cutaneous and nonfemoral cutaneous domes are not distinguished, and each location is indicated with a triangle. C: Tracing in A amended to show the changes in dome distribution that occurred during the 113-day experimental period. No tattoo marks are shown. The symbols have been filled in where domes were lost; new domes are indicated by stars. From R. P. Burgess, K. B. English, K. W. Horch, and L. J. Stensaas, *J. Physiol. (London) 236:*57–82 (1974).

Herbst and Grandry corpuscles are specialized, encapsulated sensory corpuscles in the dermis which function as rapidly adapting mechanoreceptors. There are several thousand corpuscles situated on the beak and tongue of the duck, where they are supplied by the ophthalmic branch of the trigeminal nerve. Similar corpuscles are found on the skin of other parts of the body in many birds. Studies of their morphogenesis with the light microscope (Heringa, 1918; Tello, 1932) have been greatly extended by Saxod (1967, 1970*a,b*) using the electron microscope. The subject of their development has been reviewed in all its aspects by Saxod (1978). Saxod (1973*a*) used autoradiography to study the formation of Herbst and Grandry corpuscles in the duck beak. Injection of [^{3}H]thymidine as a pulse any time before day 16 of incubation results in equal probability of labeling any of the types of cells in the corpuscles as well as other cells of the dermal mesenchyme. From days 18 to 20 the sensory cells associated with the nerve endings undergo their final mitosis (inner bulb cells of Herbst corpuscles and Grandry cells of Grandry corpuscles). The inner space cells and capsular cells of the Herbst corpuscle and the satellite cells of the Grandry corpuscle are generated as postmitotic cells on days 20–24 of incubation.

Herbst and Grandry corpuscles thus start developing at 20 days of incubation on the duck beak, and they are fully developed by the final 3 days of embryonic development (days 26–28). The constituent cells are assembled progressively from the center to the periphery around the nerve fiber, and they also differentiate in an inside-out order (Fig. 8.8). This seems to be the rule for other encapsulated sensory corpuscles, for example, Pacinian and Meissner corpuscles.

The origins of the various types of cells that compose the sensory corpuscles, such as the Herbst corpuscle and the Pacinian corpuscle, remained the subject of surmise and speculation until new techniques made it possible to analyze this question. There are three cell types in Herbst corpuscles, which are arranged concentrically. The nerve ending, in the center of the corpuscle, is surrounded by inner bulb cells, the latter are surrounded by inner space cells, and those are surrounded by capsular cells (Saxod, 1970*b*, 1971, 1978). Grandry corpuscles are composed of a nerve ending, flattened in the shape of a disc, on either side of which is a large Grandry cell. These are surrounded by satellite cells which are enclosed by a capsule. The various hypotheses of the origins of these cells are thoroughly reviewed by Saxod (1978), and it is necessary only to point out that until the cells could be identified by radioactive or cellular markers their origins remained a matter of surmise. Thus Shantha and Bourne (1968) suggested that the corpuscles are modifications of the sheaths of the peripheral nerves; Pease and Quilliam (1957) thought that the inner bulb and inner space cells are modified fibrocytes of mesodermal origin; while others, correctly as it now seems, believed the inner bulb cells to be modified Schwann cells and thus derived from the neural crest (Rhodin, 1963; Polacek, 1966; Chouchkov, 1971). The capsular cells were generally thought by these authors to be modified fibrocytes. The origins of these cells in the Herbst corpuscle have been finally determined by Saxod (1973*a,b*). He combined the frontal bud (which gives rise to the beak) from the quail with Gasserian ganglion from the duck or frontal bud from the quail with sensory ganglion from the chick. Chimeric Herbst corpuscles are formed in which the quail cells can be identified by a large chromatin granule made visible by Feulgen staining (see Section 1.4 for the same technique used to identify cells derived from the neural crest). Saxod (1973*a,b*) showed that all or almost all the inner bulb cells and some inner space cells accompany the nerve during its outgrowth from the Gasserian ganglion, and are thus of neural crest origin, while all the other cells are derived from dermal mesenchyme. The origins of the cells of the two other types of corpuscles in birds, the Grandry and Merkel corpuscles, have not yet been resolved.

The influence of the nerve on development of Herbst and Grandry corpuscles has been studied in a number of ways: by determining whether the corpuscles will develop in the absence of nerves; by observing the effects of denervation on the developing and mature corpuscles; by determining whether the corpuscles can be innervated by foreign nerves. Saxod and Sengel (1968) transplanted skin before the development of innervation from the duck beak to the chorioallantoic membrane, where the skin grows but no corpuscles develop in the absence of nerves. Moreover, removal of the innervation of the corpuscles during their development results in their degeneration. Likewise, in the adult duck, crushing the ophthalmic branch of the trigeminal nerve results in atrophy of the sensory corpuscles to about one-third their normal size in 14 days. The corpuscles become reinnervated at about 14 days after the nerve crushing, and the sensory corpuscles double in size during the following 14 days and attain parity with normal corpuscles at the end of a month (Quilliam, 1962).

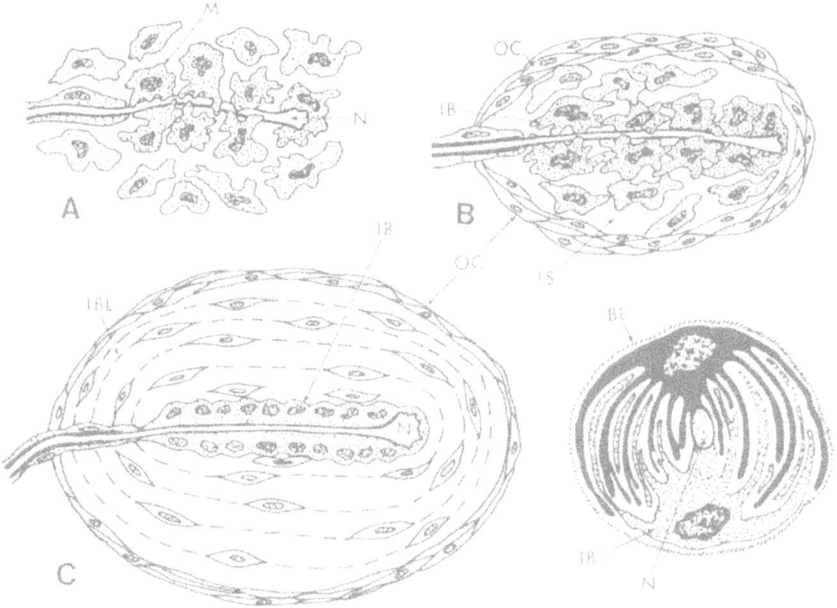

Figure 8.8. Histogenesis of the Herbst corpuscle of the duck beak occurs in an inside-out sequence. A (day 20 of incubation): Large multipolar cells are grouped around the sensory nerve terminal. B (23–26 days of incubation): These cells form two rows of lamellar cells of the inner bulb. Flat cells form an outer bulb. The inner space is narrow. C (at hatching, day 28): The inner bulb consists of about 20 lamellar cells, shown in transverse section on the lower right. The inner space contains concentric perforated lamellae. BL, Basal lamina; IB, inner bulb; IBL, perforated lamellae of inner bulb; M, multipolar cells; N, nerve ending; OC, outer capsule. By courtesy of Dr. R. Saxod.

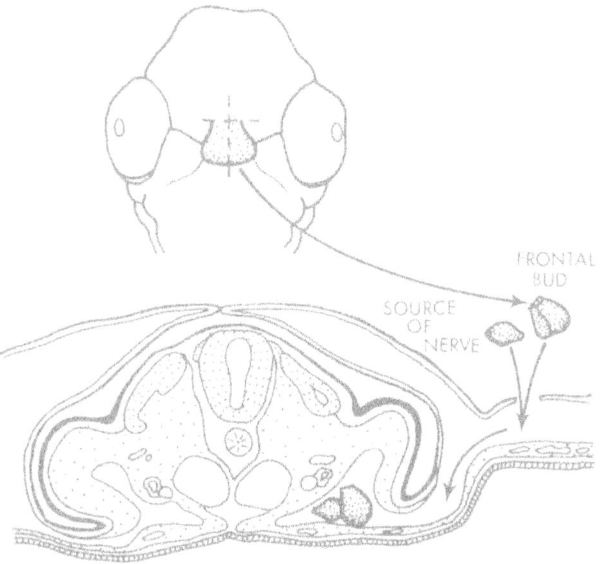

Figure 8.9. Grafts of frontal bud (donated from a 2-day duck embryo, shown above) combined with nervous tissue (e.g., spinal ganglion) develop in the extraembryonic coelom (shown in transverse section of a 35-somite host embryo at the level of the 20th somite). Courtesy of Dr. R. Saxod.

The reinnervation of corpuscles by foreign nerves was first clearly demonstrated by Dijkstra (1933), who transferred skin containing Herbst and Grandry corpuscles from the duck's beak to its foot, which normally lacks these corpuscles. Many of the corpuscles degenerate after transplantation but re-form when the graft is reinnervated by sensory nerves of the foot. This suggests that the foot sensory nerves can exert the same trophic effect as the trigeminal nerve in maintaining the corpuscles. Because these experiments were done on adult ducks, they do not show whether cutaneous nerves of the foot can induce the formation of Herbst and Grandry corpuscles *de novo.* This question was answered by Saxod and Sengel (1968) by showing that Herbst and Grandry corpuscles develop *ab initio* in beak skin grafted to other parts of the body and innervated by spinal nerves. The question of which nerve fibers (sensory, motor, sympathetic) innervate the corpuscles was dealt with by Saxod (1972*a*) by associating frontal buds with various sources of innervation in grafts grown in the extraembryonic coelom (Fig. 8.9). Coelomic grafts of frontal bud alone or frontal bud and sympathetic ganglia develop no corpuscles. Similarly, no corpuscles develop when frontal bud is innervated by motoneurons growing from ventral half of the neural tube. By contrast, corpuscles develop in all frontal buds that are innervated by Gasserian or spinal ganglia (Saxod, 1972*a*). The same results are obtained when xenoplastic combinations of frontal buds and sensory ganglia are made between chicken, duck, and quail but not between duck and mouse or lizard embryos.

These experiments show that the presence of sensory nerves is an absolute requirement for the initial formation, maturation, and subsequent maintenance of corpuscles. Although the grafts are innervated by foreign sensory nerves, the type of corpuscles, the number of corpuscles, and their spatial distribution are determined by the origin of the skin graft. Other experiments also indicate that the corpuscles have an inherent capacity to differentiate in a special way and that the nerves provide only the stimulus and do not determine the mode of differentiation of the corpuscles that they innervate. Thus Pacinian corpuscles develop in the cat mesoderm innervated by the saphenous nerve (Ilyinsky *et al.*, 1973) or by the hypogastric nerve (Schiff and Loewenstein, 1972). The maintenance of taste buds after cross-innervation, discussed below, is also consonant with the other evidence showing the nonspecific inductive or trophic influence of sensory nerves on sensory end organs.

Saxod (1972*b*) made heterochronic associations of pieces of duck beak at various embryonic ages with nerves at a fixed age (4.5 days). In other experiments, the frontal bud was allowed to develop in the coelom in the absence of innervation for 7–20 days before grafting the frontal bud to the wing of a 4.5-day embryo, where it becomes innervated. The results of those experiments show that the stage at which corpuscles begin to develop depends on the absolute age of the skin and not on the time of innervation. The nerves must be more than 14 days of embryonic age in order to respond to the action of the cutaneous mesenchyme that controls the proliferation and differentiation of the inner bulb cells, which are modified Schwann cells. The corpuscles can develop under the influence of the nerve ending only after the skin reaches the age of 19–20 days of embryonic development. These morphogenetic interactions, leading to differentiation of Herbst corpuscles, thus seem to occur some days before the time of origin of the inner bulb cells on E18–E20 and of the inner space cells on E20–E24, according to Saxod (1973*a*). Knowing the time of the cellular interactions should make it easier to discover the mechanisms by which the nerve induces development of the corpuscle. The regional specificity of the dermal mesenchyme, which determines the types and numbers of corpuscles, is acquired at a much earlier age—it is present in the frontal bud at E4½—and the origins of that specificity remain completely unknown.

8.8. Development of Taste Buds

There are three types of gustatory papillae that bear taste buds in mammals, namely fungiform, foliate, and circumvallate papillae on the tongue, and there are numerous fungiformlike papillae on the soft palate and epiglottis. The fungiform papilla has two or three taste buds on its oral surface. The circumvallate papilla has a circular moat, the walls of which can contain up to 279 taste buds in man and 375 taste buds in the rat. The taste bud consists of flask-shaped cells of epithelial origin grouped like staves of a barrel. The apices of the taste cells bear the taste receptors, which communicate with the oral cavity by a taste pore. Each taste cell has a synaptic connection with an ending of one of the taste nerves. In addition to differentiated taste cells, the taste buds contain supporting cells whose functions are unknown and basal cells which divide to form new taste cells. The latter have a life expectancy of 10–12 days and have to be continually replaced (Beidler and Smallman, 1965; Conger and Wells, 1969). The morphological development of the gustatory papillae is well reviewed by R. M. Bradley (1972) and Mistretta (1972).

The sensory nerve supply to the epithelium always develops before the taste buds appear. The gustatory nerve supply to the anterior two-thirds of the tongue epithelium is the chorda tympani branch of the lingual, while the glossopharyngeal nerve supplies the epithelium of the posterior third of the tongue. There is also a nongustatory sensory nerve supply by the trigeminal nerve to the anterior two-thirds of the tongue, by the vagus nerve to the posterior third, and by sympathetic fibers which enter the papillae (Gabella, 1969).

The time of development of the taste papillae which bear the taste buds, their number, and their distribution are remarkably invariant in all individuals of the same species. This has been studied most thoroughly in the rat (Farbman, 1965, 1971; Mistretta, 1972), and essentially the same developmental sequence, on a longer time scale, is seen in the human taste papillae and taste buds (Bradley and Stern, 1967; Bradley, 1972). In the rat, the fungiform papillae all appear on the same day at 14–15 days of gestation. Initially, they are small eminences on the surface of the front of the tongue, formed by a cluster of epithelial cells in which taste buds have not yet differentiated. There is a single circumvallate papilla in the rat, on the posterior surface of the tongue, which also appears on day 15 of gestation. Papillae can be seen in the 6- to 7-week human fetus as thickenings of the epithelium, which acquire a connective tissue core and become raised in the next few weeks. The distribution and number of taste papillae in the embryo are the same as those of the adult, show great invariance, and are probably determined by interaction between epithelium and mesenchyme during early development. At that stage, they are uninnervated. The gustatory nerves grow into the papillae and innervate the epithelium at the same time as taste buds appear. This first occurs on day 20 of gestation in the rat (Farbman, 1965, 1971), and taste buds can be seen on the fungiform papillae of the human fetus at 7 weeks and have been seen on circumvallate papillae at 11 weeks *in utero* (Bradley and Mistretta, 1975; review). All the taste buds do not appear simultaneously. Their numbers increase in relation to branching of the gustatory nerves into the epithelium. Maturation of the taste buds and development of a taste pore, by which each bud communicates with the oral cavity, occur during the third month of gestation in the human fetus but do not occur until the first 2 weeks after birth in the rat. Maturation of the taste buds in the rat correlates with their ability to discriminate between differently flavored solutions. Newborn rats show no preference between water and solutions of saccharin or quinine until 9 days of age, when they begin to prefer the sweet solution, but they reject the bitter solution only after 14 days of age (H. L. Jacobs and Sharma, 1969).

There is a continual turnover of all the epithelial cells of the tongue, including those of the taste buds. The average life span of a taste bud in the tongue of the rat and mouse is about 10 days (B. E. Walker, 1960; Beidler, 1963; Beidler and Smallman, 1965; Conger and Wells, 1969). The cells in the taste bud are displaced from the periphery of the bud, where mitosis occurs, to the center of the bud, where they degenerate. This has been observed in the taste buds of the catfish (R. M. May, 1925), frog (N. Robbins, 1967*a*), and rat (Beidler, 1963; Beidler and Smallman, 1965). Presumably the nervous connections do not change as the cell moves, but it is not known how the nerve endings make connections with new taste cells and disconnect from those that die.

The olfactory receptor cells pose a similar problem (Graziadei, 1973, 1974; Graziadei and Monti Graziadei, 1978, review): they undergo continual replacement in all vertebrates (Fig. 8.10). The receptor cells in the olfactory mucosa are neurons whose axons form the olfactory nerve. Newly formed olfactory cells have to send their axons in the olfactory nerve to the olfactory bulb to make synaptic connections with the second-order neurons. It is not known whether olfactory receptors with different response properties reconnect selectively with matching second-order neurons, but that seems to be necessary if this continual disconnection and reconnection of synapses in the glomeruli of the olfactory bulb occur without any change in the overall functions of the olfactory system.

It is not known whether the gustatory nerves have an effect on cellular proliferation in the taste buds. Guth (1963) proposed that epithelial cell proliferation is independent of nerves and that nerves stimulate only differentation of taste cells. N. Robbins (1967*a*) found that DNA synthesis in the taste buds of the frog is almost totally abolished by cutting the lingual nerve. However, as the rate of mitosis is very slow in the frog's taste buds, the difference between the normal rate and that after denervation is barely significant.

Treatment of castrated male rats with testosterone for 30–60 days results in the development of taste buds on abnormal locations—on the upper surface of the vallate papillae of the tongue (Allara, 1952; Zalewski, 1969*b*). This phenomenon was investigated by Zalewski (1969*b,c*), in order to determine whether testos-

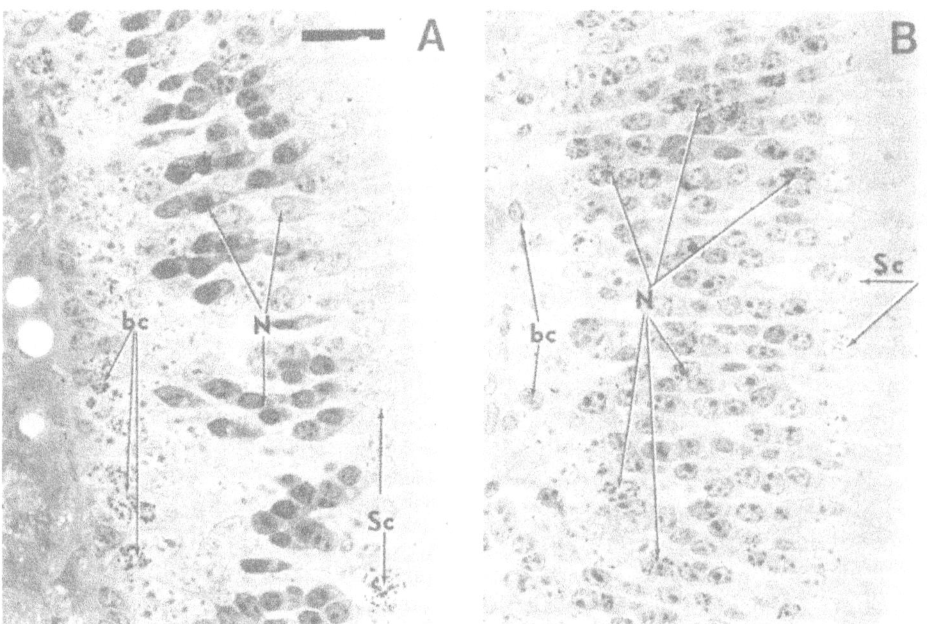

Figure 8.10. Turnover of neurons in the olfactory epithelium of the adult mouse shown autoradiographically after injections of [^{3}H]thymidine, in A at 12, 18, and 24 hours before death, and in B after injections twice daily for 5 days and survival for 14 days after the final injection. In A, many basal cells (bc) and one supporting cell (Sc) are labeled but neurons (N) are unlabeled. In B, many neurons are labeled but no basal cells remain labeled because they have either differentiated into neurons or diluted their label by repeated mitoses. Labeled neurons disappear from the olfactory epithelium 30–35 days after incorporation of the label. Bar equals 10 μm. Courtesy of P. P. C. Graziadei and A. Monti Graziadei.

terone might be the trophic agent for taste buds. He found no obvious change in the number of taste buds after castration. Testosterone does not maintain old taste buds or stimulate the formation of new ones in the absence of gustatory nerves. The action of testosterone on taste buds depends, in some unknown way, on the presence of normal innervation.

8.9. Trophic Actions of Nerves on Taste Buds

Dependence of taste buds on their sensory nerves was first demonstrated almost a century ago by showing that the taste buds degenerate after denervation (Von Vintschgau and Hönigschmied, 1876; Von Vintschgau, 1880). Since then, there have been numerous reports of the degeneration of denervated taste buds and their regeneration after reinnervation (J. M. D. Olmsted, 1920*a;* R. M. May, 1925; Torrey, 1934; Zalewski, 1968, 1969*a,b,c,* 1970*a;* Guth, 1958, 1971, review). Degeneration occurs only if the gustatory nerve itself degenerates (Torrey, 1936); if the nerve is cut proximal to the ganglion, degeneration does not occur (Kamrin and Singer, 1953; Donegani and Gabella, 1967). The rate of degeneration of taste buds after denervation depends on the species. In the rat and rabbit, reduction in size of taste buds on the tongue is evident 8 hours after denervation, and the taste buds disappear completely in 4–7 days (Beidler, 1963). The taste buds on the barrels of the catfish show atrophic changes within a few days of denervation and disappear in 11–19 days (J. M. D. Olmsted, 1920*a,b;* R. M. May, 1925). Complete degeneration of the frog taste buds is delayed for up to a year after denervation (N. Robbins, 1967*a*).

The evidence given above does not show whether the trophic effect is specific or unspecific, that is, whether a particular type of gustatory nerve can exert a trophic effect on only one or on all types of taste buds and whether the effect can also be produced by nongustatory nerves. This has been investigated in mammals by reinnervation of taste buds by other gustatory nerves or by nongustatory nerves, and in submammals by heterotopic grafting of the tongue to regions where it is reinnervated by foreign nerves.

In the rat, the taste buds normally supplied by the glossopharyngeal nerve degenerate after denervation and regenerate after innervation by another gustatory nerve, namely the vagus (which is a gustatory nerve of the pharynx and larynx) or the chorda tympani nerve (Guth, 1958; Zalewski, 1969*c*). However, the taste buds do not regenerate after reinnervation by the hypoglossal, which is a pure motor nerve (Guth, 1958; Zalewski, 1969*c*). Another nongustatory sensory nerve, the auriculotemporal, is not able to maintain old taste buds or induce the development of new ones in the rat tongue (Zalewski, 1969*c;* Oakley, 1974*a,b*). Therefore, the trophic action required for the induction and maintenance of taste buds seems to be restricted to gustatory nerves and to be absent in motor nerves or nerves of general sensation. The specificity of trophic action of gustatory nerves on taste buds seems to be absent in urodele amphibians. In newts and salamanders, taste buds, innervated by foreign nerves, develop in tongue transplanted to the side of the body (L. S. Stone, 1933, 1940) or the orbit (Mintz and Stone, 1934, Poritsky and Singer, 1963). Taste buds also develop in tongue transplanted to the liver of the newt, apparently in the absence of innervation (Wright, 1964).

There are several types of taste receptor cells, and the nerve fibers from each type (sweet, salt, bitter, etc.) are largely segregated in their central projections via the chorda tympani and glossopharyngeal nerves (H. Burton and Benjamin, 1971). The way in which the appropriate connections are formed between receptor cells and nerves is not known. In theory, there are three ways in which the receptors of different types may form connections with matching taste nerve fibers. The first alternative is that specific types of nerve fibers impose their functional specificity on the taste cells with which they connect. This is not entirely ruled out by the evidence given below that cross-innervated taste buds in adult rats retain their original specificity, because the initial specification that occurs *in utero* may be imposed by the nerves but may not be modifiable thereafter. The second alternative is that the receptors have inherent functional specificities which they impose on the unspecified nerves. If the receptor cell has an inherent transducer action and imposes this action upon its nerves, how is the information dealt with centrally? This is the question asked by nineteenth-century psychologists: If the optic and auditory nerves were crossed, would the thunder be seen and the lightning be heard? Or would there be a compensatory change in the central nervous system? That question is considered further in Sections 9.4 and 9.5. There may be no need for central reassociation of gustatory nerves during normal development because from the onset of their growth into the tongue the chorda tympani and glossopharyngeal nerves segregate to supply different regions of the epithelium, with little overlap. This peripheral segregation of nerves occurs independently of the taste buds, which develop only after the nerves reach the epithelium. This eliminates the need for large adjustments of central connections but does not account for the formation of nervous connections with different functional types of receptors within the area supplied by one nerve. The evidence that different branches of the same nerve fiber innervate receptors of the same type is evidence against the hypothesis that receptors impose their functions on the nerve (Oakley, 1974*a,b*). The third alternative is that both receptors and nerve fibers are specified independently, in parallel, and that nerve fibers of each type recognize the appropriate type of receptor cells and selectively connect with them. Oakley's (1967, 1970) observations on the responses of cross-innervated taste buds in the rat tongue do not greatly help to distinguish between these alternatives: the fact that the responses of the receptors are not altered after cross-union of the glossopharyngeal and chorda tympani nerves might be interpreted as evidence that the receptors can accept any gustatory nerve indiscriminately, or it could mean that, because fibers with the same functional specificity are present in both nerves, connections are formed only between matching nerve fibers and receptors. The same problem of interpretation arises in connection with the cross-innervation experiments on the frog, performed by N. Robbins (1967*b*). He showed that taste buds on the tongue can be prevented from degenerating after denervation when they are reinnervated by a cutaneous branch of the trigeminal nerve. This may signify either that the trophic action of sensory nerves on taste buds is less specific in frogs than in mammals or that the trigeminal nerve, which innervates chemoreceptors on the skin of the frog head, contains gustatory nerve fibers.

In theory, the most attractive feature of the hypothesis of independent parallel specification of nerves and receptors is that it can account for the way in which nerves form connections with a continually changing population of receptor cells. Provided that all types of receptors are continually produced, each nerve ending has only to select a receptor of a type that matches its own.

The possibility of growing tongue epithelium with different sources of innervation in organ culture or in the anterior chamber of the eye might allow a more rigorous analysis of the interactions between nerve and receptor. Farbman (1972) has succeeded in growing taste buds on circumvallate papillae innervated by various cranial ganglia of the rat *in vitro.* Zalewski (1972, 1974*a,b*) has been able to obtain regeneration of taste buds on circumvallate papillae in combined grafts of the tongue epithelium and vagal nodose ganglion of the rat in the anterior chamber of the eye. Lumbar spinal sensory ganglia also innervate the taste buds and stimulate their regeneration in the grafts to the eye (Zalewski, 1973). Either the spinal ganglia contain gustatory nerves, which is unlikely, or the taste buds modulate the nerves that innervate them from the spinal ganglia.

The question that remains to be answered is how the nerve exerts its trophic effect on the taste receptor cells. In lieu of direct evidence, only very tentative conclusions based on indirect evidence are possible. The hypothesis that the trophic effect is mediated by an agent transmitted from the nerve to the taste cells originated with J. M. D. Olmsted (1920*a,b,* 1925), who proposed that some substance "of the nature of a hormone" is released by the gustatory nerve endings. This hypothesis was elaborated by R. M. May (1925), who postulated the "flow of a hormone-like substance from the cell body of the neuron to its terminations," and by Parker (1932).

These were the first suggestions in modern times of a flow of materials in nerve fibers. For 30 or more years the hypothesis was not widely accepted because of its resemblance to the ancient belief in the flow of animal spirits in the nerves and because of a preoccupation at that time with the mechanisms of transmission of action potentials that drew attention away from other functions of the neuron. Now it seems, since the transport of many substances in both directions in the axon has become so familiar, that the concept of transmission of trophic substances has become accepted too uncritically. As the master of Epicurean wisdom put it: "There is nothing so easy that it does not at first seem harder to credit than it later is; and nothing that is so great or so wonderful that mankind, little by little, abandon their surprise" (Lucretius, *On the Nature of Things,* Book II).

Parker (1932) and Torrey (1934) discovered that the latent period between cutting of the nerve and the onset of atrophic changes in denervated sense organs is proportional to the length of the distal stump of nerve. After the lateral line nerve of the catfish has been cut, degeneration of the lateral line organs spreads proximodistally from the cut at a rate of about 2 cm per day (Parker, 1932; Parker and Paine, 1934). A similar correlation has been found between the length of the peripheral stump of a severed motor nerve and the time of onset of atrophic changes in the muscle (J. V. Luco and Eyzaguirre, 1955; Emmelin and Malmfors, 1965). These results suggest that the latent period might be due to the gradual depletion of a reservoir of "trophic substance" in the peripheral stump of the nerve, which is released at the nerve terminals. J. V. Luco and Eyzaguirre (1955), after cutting the motor nerve to the tenuissimus muscle of the cat, showed an apparent proximodistal flow of "trophic substance" at the rate of 2 mm per hour for the first 73 hours, and from 1.4 mm per hour to 0.5 mm per hour thereafter. It seems that a "trophic substance" may flow proximodistally in sensory and motor nerves at about the same rate, that is, on the order of 2–4 cm per day.

In the opening section of Chapter 7, I wrote that the neurotrophic factor hypothesis has survived for lack of crucial evidence against it rather than because there is any direct evidence in favor of it. Although a scientific hypothesis may be important regardless of its eventual proof or disproof, reading papers by the proponents of the neurotropic factor hypothesis often makes one wish that Newton's maxim *hypotheses non fingo* had found more adherents.*

It cannot be denied that the trophic factor hypothesis has stimulated the research that has provided most of the evidence that makes the original hypothesis more dubious. This positive effect is balanced by the negative effect that the hypothesis directs attention away from alternative mechanisms by which the nerve may regulate muscle or receptor cell phenotypes. The implication of the trophic factor hypothesis is that each type of motor or sensory nerve releases a different trophic factor which has an instructive action on the genome of the target cell. Other alternatives are that the nerve has a permissive effect only and that a single factor may mediate different effects on target cells with different inherent responses. In the case of the muscle, acetylcholine mediates almost all the trophic effects, and its effects depend on the amount and pattern of stimulation. There is also some evidence that acetylcholine may have a role in the trophic action on sense organs. The synapse between the taste receptor cell and nerve has all the characteristics of a chemical transmitting synapse. For example, in the frog's taste bud, DeHan and Graziadei (1973) showed that the sensory nerve endings are filled with clear vesicles. These endings are probably cholinergic since they contain cholinesterase, while the receptor cell contains dense-cored vesicles that show fluorescence, which is typical of catecholamines. The catecholamine is most likely the chemical synaptic transmitter from the taste receptor cell to the nerve ending, while it is likely the acetylcholine mediates the trophic action of the nerve on the receptor cell.

Other evidence also implicates acetylcholine in the trophic action on taste cells. The drug hemicholinium-3, which blocks uptake of choline into nerve endings, administered to larval salamanders (*Ambystoma tigrinum*) in subparalytic doses, results in atrophy of the taste buds and lateral line organs in 2–5 weeks and total degeneration of taste buds in 15–20 weeks without damaging the nerves (Hui and Smith, 1972). The possibility that acetylcholine may play a role in the trophic effect of nerve on taste buds is also suggested by the fact that people with the hereditary disease familial dysautonomia lack taste buds and have a high taste threshold (A. A. Smith *et al.*, 1965*a*). Their taste threshold is reduced to normal within 10 minutes after administration of methacholine (Henkin and Kopin, 1964; A. A. Smith *et al.*, 1965*b*; A. A. Smith and Hui, 1971).

It is not known how muscle cell differentiation is regulated by cholinergic stimulation, and it is even more difficult to conceive of a neurotropic effect on sensory receptors involving acetylcholine. The hypothesis of specific trophic factors transmitted by sensory nerves to their receptor cells persists, not because of direct evidence to support it, but only because of insufficient understanding of the mechanisms of transmission between the sensory receptor cell and the nerve ending.

*This famous remark in the General Scholium of the second edition of Newton's *Principia* (1713) is appropriately applied to hypotheses about mysterious factors. It did not refer to hypotheses in general but only to the cause of gravity, about which Newton considered there were insufficient data to put forward any hypothesis, in anticipation of Leibniz's charge that gravity is either an occult agent or a perpetual miracle. For a discussion of Newton's dictum, see Koyré (1956).

9

Neuronal Specificity and Development of Neuronal Circuits

9.1. The Concept of Neuronal Specificity in Historical Perspective

History shows that the most advanced concepts and theories in biology are only gradually assimilated by neurobiology, and the concept of neuronal specificity is no exception. Concepts and theories such as those of adaptive evolution; of the matching of features of the outer world with functions of the organism; of the relations between structural and functional organization, which include the concepts of levels of organization and of localization of function; of homeostasis as a means of ensuring the integrity of structures and stability of functions—these were all appropriated by neurobiology from general biology in the nineteenth century. The present purpose is to show how the concept of neuronal specificity is related to and derived from the neuron theory and earlier concepts.

The neuron theory was an inevitable deduction from the cell theory.* These theories arose at the same time as the techniques were invented for demonstrating individual differences between nerve cells, developments that made it possible, for the first time, to interpret the structural differences in terms of cellular functions

*The neuron theory, as finally enunciated by H. W. G. Waldeyer in 1891, drew from Ramón y Cajal the quip that "all Waldeyer did was to publish in a weekly newspaper a résumé of my research and to invent the term 'neuron.'" This is a common accusation down the ages; Galileo complained similarly, "This assertion of mine, passing by word of mouth, found loving fathers who adopted it as a child of their own ingenuity." In fact, the neuron theory, like the theory of neuronal specificity, has more venerable ancestors than those who may lay claim to the immediate parentage. If one regard Ramón y Cajal, His, and Forel as the fathers of the neuron theory, then Purkinje and Remak are its grandfathers. Thus the origins of the neuron theory can be traced to the period before 1839 when Schwann's masterwork was published in which the cell theory was worked out. However, the neuron theory was a mere bud when the cell theory was a fully blown flower, albeit on the same branch.

(see Chapter 4). The concept of cellular specificity grew out of these advances in knowledge of cell structure and function.

The concept of cellular specificity has a venerable history, supported by classical observations such as those on the specificity of chemotaxis, first reported by Pfeffer in 1884, and the specificity of serological reactions (Landsteiner, 1899, 1936). Such observations and the general idea of cellular specificity were in the minds of those who tried to explain the selectivity with which neurons connect with one another and with muscle and epithelial cells (*cf.* Ramón y Cajal, 1909, p. 658, 1928, p. 392). The concept of functional specificity in the nervous system, that is, that specific functions are subserved by specific types of neurons, can be said to have originated between 1833 and 1840 with Johannes Müller, in whose laboratory Schwann spent the 4 critical years (1834–1838) which led to the final synthesis of the cell theory in 1839.

Cells show their specificity by their particulars and peculiarities in the mature organism, and also by their behavior during normal development and in experimental situations *in vivo* or *in vitro.* One of these peculiarities by which cell specificity can be assayed is the preference shown by any type of cell for associating with other cell types. Thus the observation that reaggregating cells tend to sort out to regain their former intercellular relations in the tissue (H. V. Wilson, 1907; Holtfreter, 1939; Townes and Holtfreter, 1955) made it obvious that nerve cells may exercise a similar selectivity in choosing a pathway along which to migrate or to extend axonal or dendritic processes and in selecting other neurons with which to form synaptic connections. It was a small step from Holtfreter's demonstration of "Gewebeaffinität" to the notion that the self-assembly of nerve cells results from intercellular recognition, which is, in turn, based on distinctive cytochemical properties of nerve cells. That, in essence, is the chemoaffinity hypothesis of neuronal specificity.

The chemoaffinity theory of neuronal specificity as proposed by Sperry (1950*a,* 1951*a,b,* 1963, 1965) holds that neuronal circuits are assembled as a result of selective biochemical affinities and disaffinities between nerve cells. Its origins from concepts of cell biology have been outlined, but historically the significance of the chemoaffinity theory is that it was a reaction to the extreme empiricist view, widely held in the 1930s, that use and experience organize neuronal circuits out of initially equipotential networks. In emphasizing the predominant role of nature in the nature–nurture controversy, Sperry (1963) suggested that "the patterning of synaptic connections in the nerve centers, including those refined details of network organization heretofore ascribed mainly to functional molding in various forms, must be handled instead by the growth mechanism directly, independently of function, and with very strict selectivity governing synaptic formation from the beginning. The establishment and maintenance of synaptic association were conceived to be regulated by highly specific cytochemical affinities that arise systematically among the different types of neurons involved via self-differentiation, induction through terminal contact, and embryonic gradient effects."

Although it is now apparent that use and experience have a larger role in development of the nervous system than Sperry's formulation allowed, his principal thesis has been upheld. The main processes of neuron production, differentiation, and growth, including the formation of functional nerve circuits, are controlled by intrinsic developmental processes, unaffected by sensory stimulation and use.

The principal criterion of neuronal specificity, according to the chemoaffinity hypothesis, is the selective formation of synaptic connections. This specificity is shown with respect to the *types* of neurons that form connections, with respect to their *positions* in the cell population, and, on a finer level of resolution, with respect to the *positioning of the postsynaptic sites* on the neuron. The selective association between different types of neurons is an expression of *neuronal phenotypic specificity*. In addition, a neuron may have an affinity or disaffinity for other neurons depending on its position in the multicellular context, and thus express its *locus specificity*. Finally, the formation of synapses at specific places on the cell is an expression of *synaptic site specificity*. That some readers may find these terms rather high-sounding ways of asserting the obvious shows how thoroughly the concept of neuronal specificity has permeated our thinking about the nervous system. The reader can easily think of many examples to illustrate the different levels of neuronal specificity. Phenotypic specificity is manifested, for example, by the invariant association between the different types of neurons in the cerebellar cortex (see Section 3.4). Locus specificity is expressed in systems in which the topographical order of the presynaptic set of neurons is mirrored by the spatial order of their connections with the postsynaptic set of neurons, for example, the retinal ganglion cell projection to the visual centers (see Section 9.6). It seems as if each element (one or more neurons at the same locus) has a local address, defined by coordinates on the anteroposterior, dorsoventral, and mediolateral axes. However, when several cells share the same address (form an element of the cell population), it may be misleading to speak of the specificity as the unique property of a single cell. It should be clear that because an individual neuron has a specific property it does not necessarily mean that the property is held exclusively by one neuron or that it is independent of the presence of other neurons. Synaptic site specificity can be illustrated by the localized distribution of inputs to the dendrites of hippocampal pyramidal cells (see Section 5.5) and by very many other instances of localization of specific types of presynaptic endings to restricted regions of the postsynaptic membrane of the nerve cell.

Several experimental methods have been used to assay the specificity of neurons. The first method consists of transplating neurons or deflecting their axons to form connections with aberrant targets, either in competition with or in the absence of the normal inputs to those targets. The aberrant targets can differ from the normal targets in their locus specificity only (which is the usual case in which synaptic connections form in such experiments), or they may also differ in their phenotypic specificity. However, in the latter case, synaptic connections rarely develop.

In the second method, neurons are destroyed in order to determine whether their connections and functions can be taken over by other neurons. Third, mutations that produce derangements in the positions of neurons and that produce aberrant nerve fiber pathways have been studied in attempts to discover the genetic control of assembly of neuronal circuits. This has been discussed in Section 3.4.5. The strong tendency for correct connections to be made by malpositioned neurons can give an indication of their specificity. Finally, developmental anomalies of neuronal positioning and alignment (see Sections 4.6 and 7.11) may eventually reveal the mechanisms by which neurons become correctly positioned and how they change when they are malpositioned. One advantage of the mutations and developmental anomalies is that they produce changes in the pattern of cell position with a delicacy that is impossible to achieve by surgery. Mutations may selectively alter one or more types of cell without directly affecting others, although indirect effects invariably result. Finally, the limits of genetic control may be assayed by comparing the structure and connectivity of homonymous neurons in different individuals that are identical genetically (Macagno *et al.,* 1973).

How specific is the specificity that we are talking about? That is rarely defined, and the word is often used with the implication that specificity is all-or-nothing. Posing the problem as such a sharp antithesis between specificity and nonspecificity distorts the concept of biological specificity: few of us think that the specificity of any biological process is absolute, but rather that there are degrees of specificity, and we use the term in that sense (M. Jacobson, 1966, 1969). For example, the distribution of locus specificities in a population of retinal ganglion cells is not thought to be tessellated, discontinuous from cell to cell, but rather to be a continuously distributed function of the positions of the cells in the population (Sperry, 1950*a;* M. Jacobson, 1966, p. 360). Historically, the concept of relative rather than absolute specificity has precedence. Even the most characteristic type of biological specificity, the specificity of reactions between antibodies and antigens, was defined by Landsteiner (1936), the founder of immunochemistry, merely as "the disproportional action of a number of agents on a variety of related substrata." It is well known that although antibody A will react best with antigen B, cross-reactions with antibody C and antibody D are always found (F. F. Richards *et al.,* 1975). The specificity of lectins is also only relative (W. C. Boyd, 1974). Why should the specificity of presynaptic structure A for postsynaptic structure B not be of the same kind, in which "cross-reactions" with C and D also occur and will predominate in the absence of B? In other words, **specificity means that there is a preferential but not an obligatory association between neurons, and that the strength of the preference will vary according to the type of neuron and the conditions in which the specificity is expressed.** That is, the specificity is a contextual function, and the sensitivity to the context will be different for different sets of neurons.

Context-sensitive systems of the kinds which respond to an experimental perturbation by changing the relationships between pre- and postsynaptic elements exhibit a well-known form of neuronal plasticity (see Sections 5.7 and 9.9). For example, the system can be altered by removal of some neurons or addition of some neurons, so that a disparity is created between presynaptic and postsynaptic sets. In a context-sensitive system, the usual response is expansion or compression of the residual part of the set that was reduced or enlarged, so bringing the presynaptic elements into new associations with the postsynaptic elements. It is a general rule that, when such contextual changes occur in a system that normally has an orderly and continuous projection of the presynaptic set on the postsynaptic set, the order and continuity of the projection are preserved although one or both sets have changed in size (Fig. 9.1). Some examples of this form of plasticity or elasticity are given in Section 9.9.3.

In such cases, there are at least four cellular attributes that may be context sensitive, and there is no way of predicting *a priori* which of those cellular attributes will be sensitive to a given perturbation in a given system (R. K. Hunt and Jacobson, 1974*c*; M. Jacobson, 1974*b,c,* 1976*b*). Thus *cell deployment* (proliferation, migration, assembly, and death) can be context sensitive in systems in which the experimental intervention occurs while cell deployment is under way. An example of this kind is removal of an eye from an embryo or fetus during the period of cell deployment in the eye and visual centers (see Section 7.3). *Cellular properties* such as position-dependent properties can be context sensitive: removal of some cells, addition of some cells, or relocation of some cells in the population may result in a change in cellular properties in the entire set. Contextuality may be shown by *cellular operations* such as the selection of an axonal pathway; and, finally, the *selection of a synaptic site* may be context sensitive so that perturbations of a part of the system affect the system as a whole, resulting in formation of synapses between neurons that would not have formed connections normally.

While specificity implies a certain element of selectivity in the association between neurons, it does not mean that in all cases the association is one-to-one. Unique one-to-one associations are rarely found. For example, because the Mauthner's neuron is a unique cell, it is obliged to have some such associations. However, one-to-many and many-to-many associations between neurons are far more commonly seen. To the extent that the association between any presynaptic and any postsynaptic element may be influenced by other elements, the association is context sensitive and the specificity is contextual (R. K. Hunt and Jacobson, 1974*c*). Within any given context, the association between presynaptic and postsynaptic elements is invariant. Variability within such systems may be attributed to random perturbations in the genetic and developmental processes, that is, to noise in the system. The amount of such variability will depend on the level of resolution at which the system is observed. Thus the Mauthner's neuron, which is a neuronal class consisting of one cell, at the cellular level of resolution exhibits microprecision and invariance of connectivity. However, one does not require a computer to determine that the Mauthner's neurons on the two sides are not identical in all subcellular details. Similarly, microvariability is seen when comparing homonymous neurons in genetically identical organisms. For example, in the small

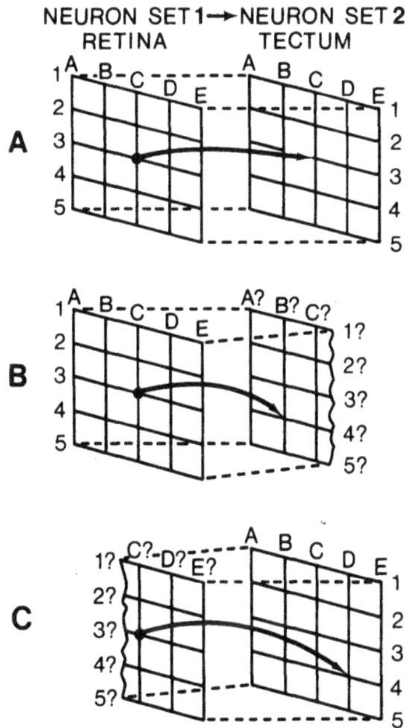

Figure 9.1. Relations between complete and partial neuronal sets. A: Mapping of neuronal set 1 (retina) onto set 2 (tectum), with elements linked at position C3 in both sets. B,C: What might be found some time after removal of part of the retina or tectum. The relations appear to have changed, but one cannot know what changes have occurred because the identities of elements at various positions cannot be determined from the map. From M. Jacobson, Neuronal recognition in the retinotectal system, pp. 3–23, in *Neuronal Recognition,* S. Barondes (ed.), Plenum, New York (1976).

crustacean *Daphnia* (Macagno *et al.*, 1973), there are great similarities between individuals and between corresponding cells on the two sides in the same animal when the position of cell bodies and the branching and synaptic pattern of nerve fibers are recorded to a resolution of a few micrometers. However, when the resolution is increased five- to tenfold, variations are recorded which are as large between the two sides of the same animal as between different animals of the same clone. Such microheterogeneity may be regarded as an indication of "the noise level of the genetic control of structure." Microheterogeneity may be seen in every system, and apparently is functionally neutral. In some systems, there may be less requirement for functional precision, and therefore less constraint is put on precise connectivity (M. Jacobson, 1969, 1970*a*) so that what may be termed "macroheterogeneity" can be tolerated without resulting in malfunction.

Finally, the degree of specificity may depend on the developmental stage of the system in question: early in development, the postsynaptic elements may have a lower average specific affinity for the presynaptic elements than later in development. Such systems attain their final state of specificity only after all growth has ceased, that is, in the adult. To take the retinotectal system as an example, I have written that "It would seem that, during embryonic development, the mapping of the retina on the tectum is independent of the size or shape of either the retina or the tectum, and that the topographical order of the retinotectal map would develop regardless of the relative sizes of retina and tectum. . . . Only the relative positions of the connections are determined, and only the topographical order of the retinotectal projection is invariant. The absolute position of each connection apparently becomes fixed at a later stage, as the experiments on adults show" (M. Jacobson, 1969). This refers to the frog, but it applies as well to all vertebrates if by an "adult" we mean an individual in which growth of the nervous system has been completed.

Any theory of neuronal specificity must account for the progressive loss of modifiability that occurs during development of the nervous system. There is a reduction, with advancing age, of recovery of structure and function of neurons after surgical ablation, transplantation of parts of the brain, or disruption of neuronal connections. Moreover, for reasons that are not understood, gradual removal of parts of the mammalian brain, in several operations over a period of weeks, results in less functional deficit than removal of the same volume of brain in one operation, even in adult mammals (Chow and Randall, 1964; D. G. Stein *et al.*, 1969; J. Rosen *et al.*, 1971). In general, in all species, repairs of structure and function are always greater in the earlier than in the later stages of development, and they virtually cease after development of the central nervous system has been completed.

No single method for assaying neuronal specificity has yet been devised that can deal with all its different levels. This is especially true under experimental conditions that alter the context in which the specificities originate and are expressed during normal development. Some of these difficulties have been reviewed by R. K. Hunt and Jacobson (1974*c*). The nihilistic attitude that one is forced to adopt with regard to behavioral or electrophysiological methods of assaying neuronal specificity is somewhat mitigated when different methods of assay yield the same result. However, the problems of behavioral or microelectrode mapping assays arise because of their indirectness. They cannot provide direct assays of the cellular properties or functions in which the specificity resides, but merely give some indication of the effective exhibition of neuronal specificity in the organized multicellular system. No doubt, this problem will persist until direct assays of the cytochemical basis of neuronal specificity have been devised. Some steps in that direction are reviewed in the following section.

9.2. Cellular Mechanisms of Neuronal Specificity

Selective associations of nerve cells, as of other types of cells, involve many cellular activities. *Morphogenetic movements* (Townes and Holtfreter, 1955; Trinkaus, 1966) of cells or of cellular outgrowths such as neuronal axons and dendrites provide the opportunities for *selective cell affinities* or *cell recognition* to come into play. To stabilize the association between cells, *contact inhibition of cell movements* may occur (Abercrombie, 1970) and stable intercellular adhesions or junctions may be formed.

The evidence that cell recognition plays an important role in morphogenesis comes largely from studies of reaggregation of sponge cells (H. V. Wilson, 1907; Humphreys, 1967; Burger, 1974, Burger *et al.,* 1975) and reaggregation *in vitro* of cells from amphibian, avian, and mammalian embryos (Holtfreter, 1939; 1944; Townes and Holtfreter, 1955; Moscona 1962, 1968; Steinberg, 1962*a,b,* 1963, 1970). Johannes Holtfreter was the first to show how differential cellular affinities and migrations could account for many aspects of morphogenesis of vertebrate embryos (Holtfreter, 1939, 1944; Townes and Holtfreter, 1955). He found that different types of cells sort themselves out when dissociated cells are mixed and allowed to reaggregate. In experiments in which fragments from different tissues are fused or in which isolated cells of different types are mixed under conditions that allow them to reassemble, the cells of different tissues tend to regain the relative positions in the aggregate that they normally occupy in the embryo. By using mixtures of cells with different appearances, Holtfreter was able to demonstrate that sorting out is due to cell migration. Selective cellular reaggregation is also shown by chick cells segregating from mouse cells (Moscona, 1962) and by sorting out of chick embryo cells labeled with tritiated thymidine from unlabeled chick cells of a different type when the two dissociated cells types are mixed and then allowed to reaggregate (Trinkaus and Gross, 1960).

Holtfreter regarded the sorting out of cells as a manifestation of "tissue affinities" or of "cell specific differences in surface tension" (Holtfreter, 1939, 1944), while Weiss (1941*a*) referred to "selective adhesiveness" as an important factor in morphogenesis. Townes and Holtfreter (1955) concluded that sorting out of embryonic cells is due to selective cell adhesion and to chemotactic migration of cells along a radial concentration gradient. Steinberg (1962*a,b*) ruled out the latter and showed that sorting out can be due entirely to differential cell adhesion. He found that when two types of cells are sorting out they do not move directly, by radial pathways, to their correct positions but rather form small clusters which gradually fuse to form a single aggregate of one cell type which becomes enveloped by cells of the other type. Steinberg (1963) tested all 15 pairs that can be formed among six different types of chick embryo cells in sorting-out experiments, and demonstrated a hierarchical order of affinity in which cells of higher rank in the hierarchy always envelop those of lower order.

According to the "differential adhesion hypothesis" (Steinberg, 1963, 1964, 1970), sorting-out and morphogenetic movements of embryonic cells occur because (1) cells adhere to one another with adhesive strengths which are specific for the cell type, and (2) the cells within a tissue assume an equilibrium arrangement, determined by their intercellular adhesive strengths, such that the interfacial or adhesive free energy of the system is at a minimum. The "differential adhesion hypothesis" predicts that a mixture of two types of cells will eventually form an aggregate in which cells of the less cohesive type envelop the cells with greater cohesion.

From the results of these studies, the hypothesis has evolved that cell recognition is mediated by macromolecular components on the cell surface that function as cell recognition sites and as ligands between cells. The specificity with which cellular associations are formed leads to the hypothesis that the cell recognition sites and intercellular ligands are specific properties of cell types which differ from one type of cell to another. In support of these hypotheses is the finding that cell aggregation factors are given off by cultured cells into the culture medium. Addition of these factors to a fresh suspension of cells enhances their reaggregation. This effect is cell type specific but not species specific. Thus the reaggregation factors obtained from chick neural retina enhance the aggregation of neural retinal cells but not of other types of neurons or other types of cells (Lilien, 1968; Garber and Moscona, 1972*a,b;* Moscona, 1974, review). The retina-specific cell aggregation factor released into the medium by cultured cells from the neural retina of the 10-day chick embryo is a glycoprotein of molecular weight about 50,000 (Hausman and Moscona, 1975). A similar factor can be isolated from the cell membranes of neural retina cells from chick embryos up to 13 days of age, and its aggregating effect is restricted to chick retinal cells from embryos younger than 13 days (Hausman and Moscona, 1976). One of the serious limitations of these experiments is that they do not show which types of retinal cells are involved in the aggregation. A factor that merely results in aggregation of neural retinal cells, without any greater specificity, could not be the basis of selective associations that develop between different types of retinal neurons. These limitations are found in all the other types of assays for specific cellular recognition and adhesion.

The specificity of attachment of retinal to tectal cells can be assayed fairly directly by measuring the adherence of cells from dorsal or ventral retinal halves to halves of the tectum of chick embryos (Barbera *et al.,* 1973; Marchase *et al.,* 1975; Barbera, 1975). A suspension of single cells from 7- to 12-day chick embryos (Stages 31–38) is labeled with ^{32}P, and about 5×10^6 labeled cells are incubated *in vitro* with tectal halves excised from 12- to 14-day chick embryos (Stages 38–40). After 1 hour, the tectal halves are washed and counted in a scintillation counter to determine the numbers of cells that have adhered. Cells from the ventral half-retina adhere selectively to dorsal half-tectum, and cells from the dorsal half-retina adhere preferentially to the ventral half-tectum. No selectivity is shown in adhesion of nonretinal nerve cells to tectum. Thus the adhesive selectivity of retinal cells to tectum in these experiments mimics the selectivity of retinal axons for tectal neurons. If the mechanisms of selectivity in this experiment are similar to those in real life, the results show that the molecules responsible for neuronal adhesive selectivity are present on the cell bodies as well as on the tips of axons. Because cells of the retinal pigment epithelium derived from dorsal or ventral retinal halves also show adhesive selectivity for dorsal or ventral tectal halves (Barbera *et al.,* 1973), the specificity appears to depend on retinal position, not on cell type.

The main limitations of these assays are that they do not show which cells of the neural retina adhere to the tectum and that they do not show to which tectal structures they attach. It would be premature to conclude that the adhesion shown in these experiments occurs at the same sites as those that determine retinotectal synaptic specificity, or even that the retinal and tectal cells that interact during normal development are the same cells that interact in these experiments.

The biochemical basis of the selective adhesion between cells of the neural retina and tectum of the chick embryo has been investigated by Marchase (1976). The cell adhesion is reduced by low temperature and by inhibition of general metabolism. Treatment of retinal cells with proteases reduces the adhesion of ventral retina to dorsal tectum, but does not affect adhesion of dorsal retina to ventral tectum. However, the latter is affected by treating the tectum with proteases, which suggests that adhesion of dorsal retina to ventral tectum depends on protein located on the ventral half of the tectum.

Another assay of retinotectal selective adhesion has been invented by D. I. Gottlieb *et al.* (1976). They assayed the adhesion of individual ventral or dorsal retinal cells to monolayers of ventral or dorsal tectal cells and report that dorsal retinal cells adhere selectively to ventral tectal cells and ventral retinal cells adhere to dorsal tectal cells.

One of the attractive features of the differential affinity hypothesis is that it demands little genetic information to specify cellular adhesiveness or affinity, and thus the genetic control of morphogenesis may be substantially simplified. It is much simpler for the egg to contain instructions for a program of development than to contain all the information to specify the structure of the fully developed organism. The amount of information required to specify the structure of the fully developed brain in every minute detail cannot be contained in the genome (Bremmermann, 1963; M. Jacobson, 1966, 1969). A more parsimonious use of genetic information to specify a program of histogenesis, cell migration, and cellular interactions, including a sequence of changes in affinities and disaffinities between cells, could result in self-assembly of neural circuits without requiring genetic control of the cell movements and interactions or genetic specification of all the details of the fully developed structure.

There is little point in debating whether 1 percent or 95 percent of the genome is devoted to specifying the structure of the nervous system. In fact, attempts to assay the proportion of the genome that is expressed in the brain are hampered by the complexity of the repeated sequence of nucleotides in the DNA of vertebrates. The fact that RNA from mouse brain hybridizes with about 10 percent of nonrepeated mouse DNA, while the comparable figure for mouse liver or kidney is 3 percent, indicates that a greater proportion of the genome is expressed in the brain than in the other organs (Hahn and Laird, 1971; Grouse *et al.,* 1972; Brown and Church, 1972; Soga and Takahashi, 1975, 1976).

It would be trite to say that "heredity" plays a role in all biological processes and structures: the problem is to trace the causal chain from genes to final structures and functions. This is difficult because there is no single correspondence (isomorphism) between genetic information and the neuronal structures that it generates. This is because the neuronal structures are not specified in detail in the genome. The latter contains only instructions for a developmental program leading to the formation of the nervous system. The relationship between the genes and the nervous system is not isomorphic but homeomorphic; one-to-one correspondences are found between genes and proteins but genes and higher levels of cellular organization are connected by many-to-many relationships. The path of migration of the neuron, the direction of growth of its axon and dendrites, the orientation of the dendritic branches, and the precise location of synapses have not been traced back to the genes. Mutations have been found that affect a large variety of structures and functions in the developing nervous system, but in no case has the causal nexus from mutant gene to mutant phenotype been unraveled.

9.3. Development of Neuronal Specificity in Spinal Cord Segments Controlling Limb Movements

How coordinated motor activity develops and how the patterns of movements are related to neuronal circuits remain largely unsolved. Yet this is one of the simplest cases of how structure and function are related during development of the nervous system. Integrated movements, such as those during walking, depend on the development of central generators of patterned motor output. Sensory input, while it can modify motor activity, is not necessary for coordinated motor behavior (Weiss, 1937*c;* Székely *et al.,* 1969; Harcombe Smith and Wyman, 1970; Grillner and Zangger, 1974). In principle, there are two ways in which the central programming of coordinated motor activity could be organized during development. Either the central circuits develop their organization independently of the muscles and sense organs, or the central programs are organized as a result of connections with the peripheral tissues. We may call the first way central specification of motor activity while the second may be called peripheral specification of motor activity. The first alternative presupposes that the central circuits controlling coordinated limb movements develop in parallel with the peripheral targets, but there is no presumption regarding the selection of those targets by motorneurons or sensory neurons. We have to discover whether the peripheral connections are formed at random or whether the central neurons form connections selectively with muscles and sense organs. The second alternative does imply that the peripheral tissues are specified and that their specificity is somehow responsible for organizing the activities of the central neurons.

The evidence to be adduced in this section shows that species-specific patterns of motor coordination develop according to an intrinsic program within the central nervous system. Patterns of movement that develop in transplanted limbs or in transplanted muscles or after cross-union of nerves to antagonistic muscles are in accordance with the inherent specificity of the motoneurons regardless of their peripheral connections and regardless of the functional utility of the movements.

Studies of the motility of grafted limbs have played an important part in research on the development of locomotion in tetrapods. Braus (1905) and Harrison (1907*a*) observed movements in limbs transplanted in amphibian embryos and showed that nerves that are not normally destined for the limb can innervate limb muscles. Coordinated movements in transplanted limbs were first studied and carefully analyzed by Detwiler (1920*a*, 1925) and later by Weiss (1922, 1924, 1937*a,b,c,d*). They found that when a limb bud from donor urodele amphibian embryo is grafted caudal to the normal limb bud of another embryo of the same species, it often develops movements that are coordinated with those of the limbs of the host.

This phenomenon was later called "homologous response" or "myotypic response" by Weiss (1937*a,b,c,d*). The movements of the grafted limb are coordinated with those of the host regardless of the orientation of the limb or its functional efficiency. For example, limbs transplanted with their axes reversed develop a coordinated sequence of movements that tend to propel the animal backwards (Weiss, 1937*d*). These maladaptive movements are unaffected by experience and are not corrected by learning. Sensory input does not play an essential part in the development of the coordinated movements of grafted limbs, as they are unaffected by deafferenting the limb (Weiss, 1937*c*). The coordinated movements occur even when the grafted limb is supplied by a single nerve that branches to supply all the muscles at random (Weiss, 1928*b*), provided that the nerve is one that normally supplies the limb (Detwiler, 1920*a*).

Detwiler (1920*a*) observed a gradual loss of function of the grafted limb as it is transplanted farther away from its normal position. Normally, the forelimbs of salamanders or newts are supplied by the third, fourth, and fifth nerves arising from the brachial segments of the spinal cord. Detwiler showed that some coordinated movements of the grafted limb develop even when it receives a single limb nerve. In cases where the limb grafted to the trunk is supplied by the trunk nerves as well as the fifth spinal nerve, section of the latter abolishes the coordinated movements of the grafted limb (Detwiler and Carpenter, 1929). Limbs grafted to the trunk and innervated exclusively by trunk nerves display feeble and incoordinated movements (Detwiler, 1930*b*). Limbs grafted to the head and innervated by cranial nerves do not develop movements that are coordinated with those of the normal limbs, but display mass contractions associated with movements of the eyes, jaw, or gills, depending on the source of innervation of the limb (Nicholas, 1933; Detwiler, 1930*a,b;* Székely, 1959*b;* Hibbard, 1965*b*).

The foregoing experiments show that although limb muscles can be innervated functionally by motoneurons at any level of the spinal cord, the mechanisms for coordinated limb movements are restricted to the brachial and lumbosacral regions of the spinal cord; thoracic segments of the spinal cord or cranial motor nuclei are unable to participate in the control of limb movements. Additional evidence showing that the limitation is in the spinal cord and not in the limb is given below. For example, W. M. Rogers (1934) found that limbs may be innervated by a supernumerary segment of the spinal cord grafted between the normal cord and the limb bud in salamander embryos. Normally integrated limb movements occur when the graft consists of the third, fourth, and fifth segments of the cord, which normally innervate the forelimbs, but feeble and uncoordinated movements occur when the limb is innervated by a graft of the seventh, eighth, and ninth spinal cord segments.

Other experiments, showing that the character of limb movements is determined by the region of spinal cord from which it is innervated, were performed by Székely (1963) on newts and by Straznicky (1963) on the chick embryo. Székely showed that an extra limb grafted on the trunk of a newt embryo develops coordinated movements if innervated by a segment of brachial cord transplanted in place of thoracic spinal cord. An extra hindlimb grafted on the trunk and innervated by lumbosacral segments of the spinal cord transplanted in place of thoracic cord moves synchronously with the normal hindlimbs. Straznicky (1963) showed that after brachial segments of the spinal cord have been transplated in place of lumbosacral segments in the chick embryo, the leg moves synchronously with the wing on the same side. If a leg is grafted in place of a wing, the leg, innervated by brachial spinal nerves, makes winglike movements.

In all the experiments that have been described, the difference between limbs with integrated locomotor movements and those with uncoordinated movements is not in the adequacy of neuromuscular connections, because the limb muscles appear to receive an adequate supply of nerves. The differences have been shown to reside in the functional organization of the spinal cord supplying the limb.

Other experiments have established that early in development the spinal cord segments at limb levels develop functional specificity for fore- or hindlimbs. There is evidence that the motor functions of the spinal neurons are specified in the late neurula and that specification increases progressively during development. This evidence has been obtained by transposing segments of the spinal cord in a series of amphibian and chick embryos at different stages of development. Székely (1963) showed that interchanging the brachial and lumbosacral regions of the spinal cord of newt embryos after the time of closure of the neural tube (Stage 20) results in reduced and uncoordinated movements of the limbs. Normal limb movements develop if the interchange of presumptive fore-and hindlimb regions of the spinal cord is made at earlier stages of development. Specification of spinal cord segments controlling limb movements also occurs in the early neural tube of the chick embryo. Straznicky (1967) has shown that interchanging brachial and lumbosacral segments of the spinal cord in chick embryos on day 3 of incubation results in development of limb movements corresponding to the origin of the spinal segments innervating the limb. In the chick embryo it is not certain whether the control of limb movements by spinal cord segments is already irreversibly specified before the motoneurons have made contact with muscles. According to Levi-Montalcini (1950), the axons of motoneurons can be seen in the ventral roots at 50 hours of incubation, and they reach proximal muscles at 2½ days and distal muscles on days 3 and 4. Spontaneous, uncoordinated movements of the trunk start on day 3½, before spinal reflex circuits have been established. The movements of the limbs commence on day 6. They are spontaneous, are not coordinated, and are due to random discharges in the spinal motoneurons. Reflex movements of the hindlimbs can be elicited only after day 7–7½, when the reflex circuits are completed in the brachial and lumbar segments of the spinal cord. The motility of chick embryos is considered fully in the masterful review by Hamburger (1973).

Landmesser and Morris (1975) have shown, by electrophysiological recording from individual muscles and motor nerves in the chick embryo, that the nerves always connect with the appropriate muscles from the beginning, that the innervation is quite invariant for each muscle, and that there is no proximodistal sequence of innervation. The specific pattern of innervation is seen from the time movement can first be elicited on day 6 (Stages 27–28). These observations tend to rule out random innervation of limb muscles followed by death of motoneurons that make connections with inappropriate muscles.

In the newt, too, the specification of limb-moving segments of the spinal cord occurs either shortly before or during the period of innervation of limb muscles. From the evidence now available, it is not possible to decide whether contact of the motor axon with the muscle precedes specification of the motoneuron and thereby causes motoneuron specification, as Weiss (1928*b*, 1941*b*, 1947) has proposed. In newts and salamanders there is a relatively long period during which the spinal cord is not specified as regards limb movements, and transposition of segments of the cord does not affect the subsequent development of limb movements. Detwiler (1923) showed that thoracic segments of the spinal cord are able to regulate when transplanted in place of brachial cord in tailbud stages of *Ambystoma* so that normally integrated limb movements result. Straznicky and Székely (1967) have shown that this capacity of thoracic segments of the cord to sustain coordinated limb movements is gradually lost at later stages of development. They showed that grafting thoracic segments in place of brachial segments of spinal cord in newt embryos at Stage 22 results in the development of normal forelimb movements. Progressively poorer limb movements develop when the limbs are innervated by thoracic segments of spinal cord grafted at Stages 23–27. Incoordinated movements develop when the spinal cord grafts are made after Stage 27. No forelimb movements develop when thoracic cord from an embryo at Stage 28 is grafted in place of brachial spinal cord of a Stage 22 embryo (Straznicky and Székely, 1967). These experiments establish that spinal cord segments at limb levels are at first unspecified as regards limb movement, but later develop functional specificity for fore- or hindlimb movements.

Homologous response develops in the transplanted limb only if it is grafted before a critical stage, which in *Xenopus* is at Stage 54 (Hollyday and Mendell, 1976). This is when the death of motoneurons in the lateral motor column has reached a peak (see Section 7.7.2), so that one of the limitations may be an inadequate motoneuron pool in the regions of spinal cord not normally connected to limbs. Stage 54 is also when neuromuscular connections develop, hindlimb movements commence, and limb reflexes can first be elicited. Hollyday and Mendell (1975) have suggested that it becomes impossible to form new spinal reflex connections once normal reflex connections are established in the spinal cord. The problem of whether these specificities develop before the spinal nerves form connections in the limbs has not been resolved. Therefore, we still have to consider the hypothesis that the primary specificities are in the muscles, which impart their specificities to the motor nerves that innervate them (Weiss, 1924, 1928*a,b,* 1931, 1941*b,* 1947, 1952).

9.4. Theories of Motoneuron Specification

To explain the phenomenon of myotypic response, that is, the movement of muscles in a normal limb in apparent synchrony with homologous muscles in a nearby grafted limb, Weiss at first suggested that "the nervous system does not form connections with muscles by means of special pathways, but by specific forms of excitation" (Weiss, 1928*a*). This theory of selective signaling he called the "resonance theory" (Weiss, 1928*b*, 1931). The nerves were believed to connect indiscriminately with muscles, but the muscles were supposed to be "tuned" to receive only a specific pattern of impulses. This theory had to be abandoned when Wiersma (1931) showed that impulse traffic is present only in motor nerves to muscles involved in reflex contraction, whereas nerves to inactive muscles are quiescent. Weiss then shifted the selective role from the muscle or neuromuscular junction to the axon or the motoneuron as a whole. He proposed that "each muscle gradually transforms ('modulates') its motor neurons into what from then on will be selective receivers admitting only the one type of impulse proper for that particular muscle. Such a modification affecting the neuron in a centripetal direction might gradually extend beyond the motor neurons and spread to other central neurons" (Weiss, 1935). The idea of the motoneuron as a selective filter of nerve impulses eventually gave way to the concept of myotypic modulation or specification (the terms are synonymous) of the synaptic connections between motoneurons and premotor neurons in the central nervous system. The return of normal limb movements even when the pattern of peripheral innervation appears grossly abnormal was taken by Weiss as evidence that rearrangement of synaptic association must occur. As no such rearrangement was evident at the neuromuscular junctions, Weiss assumed that synaptic plasticity must occur centrally in response to modulation by the muscle. This notion was developed further by Sperry, who agreed that contact of the nerve with the muscle might result in the formation of central synaptic associations that are appropriate to the actions of the muscle (Sperry, 1950*a,b,* 1951*a,b*). He introduced the idea that matching specificities develop independently in the muscles and premotor neurons; the muscles then confer their specificities on the motoneurons, causing them to synapse with the premotor neurons that have matching or homologous specificities.

Temporal and spatial restrictions to the process of myotypic specification have been considered above. There also appear to be important phylogenetic restrictions. In salamanders and newts, myotypic specification seems to occur after grafting of limbs at any stage of development, even in the adult, provided that the grafted limb is supplied by some nerves from lumbosacral or brachial segments of the spinal cord. In anurans and the higher vertebrates, myotypic specification appears to be restricted to early stages of development and to become irreversibly lost during maturation—earlier in the higher vertebrates than in the lower. If this is indeed correct, switching peripheral connections later in life would not be expected to result in any compensatory adjustments of central synapses. For example, cross-innervated muscles would be expected to contract in accordance with the original connectivity of the motoneuron, with resulting incoordination of movement.

Cross-innervation of muscle fibers inevitably occurs after nerve regeneration in the higher vertebrates. Even if the cut ends of the nerve are carefully sutured together, the nerve fibers are disarranged during regeneration and they innervate muscle fibers at random. After nerve regeneration in mammals, at any age after birth, recovery of voluntary or reflex movements is always incomplete; muscle power is diminished, and the timing and sequence of muscle contractions are permanently disordered. The incoordination is most marked in muscles involved in fine and complex movements. Reeducation may lead to compensatory use of muscles that are not affected by the injury, but careful studies have shown that, in man, incoordinated movements of the affected muscles are not improved by practice, even after many years. For detailed documentation of this conclusion, the reader should refer to the masterly review by Sperry (1945*a*).

Sperry's experiments on the effects of cross-uniting nerves to antagonistic muscles have shown the lack of plasticity in the neuronal circuits mediating coordinated movements of skeletal muscles in mammals. After crossing nerves to antagonistic muscles in the limbs of rats and monkeys, Sperry (1941, 1942, 1947) observed that reversal of movements and malfunction of the limb persist permanently. Reorganization of reflex movements is never observed, even when the operations are performed on young animals. However, it remains to be seen whether any functional adaptation may occur in the mammalian fetus after rearrangement of connections between motor nerves and muscles.

The greater functional recovery that occurs in lower vertebrates after rearrangements of muscle innervation indicates that there may be important differences in the recovery process between lower and higher vertebrates. So much of the evidence of myotypic specification has been obtained from salamanders and newts that it is important to emphasize that "urodeles so differ from other tetrapod vertebrates respecting nerve–muscle relationships that they form a group unto themselves" (Straus, 1946). In all vertebrates except urodeles the motoneurons of the ventral horn of the spinal cord are arranged in a ventromedial longitudinal column supplying trunk muscles and muscles in the proximal part of the limb, and in a lateral longitudinal column supplying distal limb muscles. There is no distinct columnar arrangement or even a distinct ventral horn in urodeles. This should be compared with the motor system of the frog, in which the columnar arrangement of spinal motoneurons is similar to that in tetrapod reptiles, birds, and mammals (M. L. Silver, 1942; Stussi, 1960; Cruce, 1974). In addition to these differences, the motoneurons are not so well arranged in somatotopic order (according to the relative positions of their muscles) in urodeles as they are in mammals. The significance of this in the analysis of homologous limb movements will be discussed below.

Székely and Czéh (1967) have provided additional evidence that questions the validity of the phenomenon of homologous response and that calls for a reappraisal of the theory of myotypic specification. They determined the arrangement of the brachial spinal motorneurons innervating the forelimb of the axolotl, *Ambystoma mexicanum,* by observing muscle contractions elicited by microelectrode stimulation in the spinal cord. The motoneurons in rostrocaudal sequence in the cord project to muscles in anteroposterior sequence in the shoulder girdle and proximodistal sequence in the forelimb. However, within this sequence there is considerable overlap of the central representation of different muscles, which blurs the precision of the somatotopic arrangement of motoneurons (Fig. 9.2). The overlap is such as to bring together the motoneurons of functionally related muscles. Székely and Czéh concluded: "In the light of our results it seems that an extra limb, being innervated by the 4th or 5th spinal nerve, has a good chance to receive the complete set of nerves which are necessary for the control of walking movements without assuming any kind of specification. Some probable shift in the phase of muscle action will be too small to be detected, and the movement of the grafted limb will appear to be synchronized with that of the normal limb."

Their final point is important because it raises grave doubts about the adequacy of naked-eye observations of the movements of grafted limbs. Czéh and Székely (1971), recording muscle activity from freely moving normal and supernumerary limbs, report that the electromyograms show asynchrony of contraction of homologous muscles when the movements appear to be synchronous. Electro-

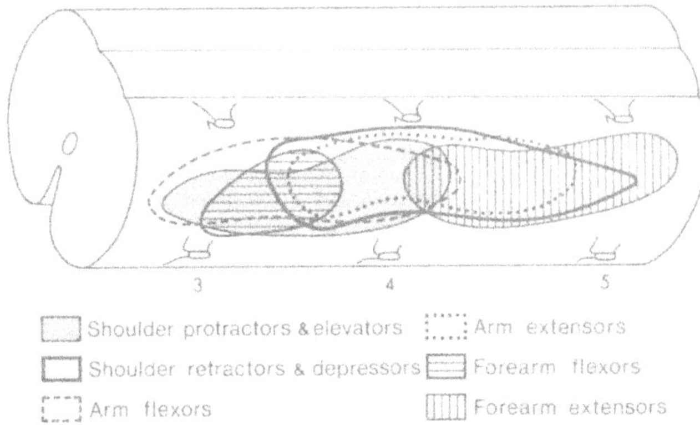

Figure 9.2. Projection to the lateral surface of the salamander spinal cord of the positions of motoneurons supplying muscles of the forelimbs via spinal roots 3, 4, and 5. The positions of motoneurons were determined by electrical stimulation with a microelectrode in the cord, and by observing the resulting contractions of individual muscles. From data in G. Székely and G. Czéh (1967) and G. Székely (1968).

myography reveals incoordination of contraction of extensor muscles innervated by flexor nerves in the cat hindlimb, even though no abnormality is apparent to the naked eye (McIntyre and Robinson, 1958). Electromyography also shows the complexity of timing of contraction, including co-contraction, of agonists and antagonists in the limb during locomotion (Paillard, 1960; Engberg and Lundberg, 1962; Székely *et al.*, 1969), as is shown in Fig. 9.3. These studies show that slight differences in the timing of contractions of individual muscles in the normal and grafted limb, which can be revealed by electromyography, might escape detection by naked-eye observation or even by the slow-motion cinematography used by Weiss (1941*b*).

At variance with the conclusions drawn from electromyographic recordings from freely moving salamanders are observations of Hollyday and Mendell (1976) of homologous reflex movements evoked by mechanical stimulation of the skin. These authors report synchronous electrical activity in nerves to homologous muscles as well as in the muscles themselves. A full range of reflex movements occur despite a limited sequential innervation of the grafted limb. This, and the finding that homologous reflex movements occur only if the limbs are grafted before Stage 54, is evidence in favor of myotypic specification of motoneurons connected to the transplanted limb. However, the possibility has not been excluded that the grafted limb receives a nerve supply from collateral branches from spinal nerves normally supplying the limb. The capacity of nerve fibers to find their proper muscle targets, even after deflection of the nerve, has to be considered in all such cases (Grimm, 1971).

Finally, there are considerable variations in the pattern of innervation of specific muscles of the limbs in urodeles (Piatt, 1939, 1942), as well as multiple innervation of muscle fibers by *en grappe* motor nerve terminals (Bone, 1964; Mark *et al.*, 1966). Mark *et al.* (1966) have suggested that selective connections between motor nerves and muscle fibers might be possible in muscles with multiple *en grappe* innervation, but are not possible in muscles with focal *en plaque* innervation. Each mammalian muscle fiber has a single motor end plate, and as a rule will accept no more. Therefore, the first motor nerve terminal to arrive at the muscle fiber will innervate it, regardless of whether or not it is functionally suitable. In fish and urodeles, on the contrary, multiple innervation of muscle fibers occurs normally in the adult as well as after nerve regeneration. In these animals, each muscle fiber is supplied by several nerve terminals, either branches of one axon or branches of different axons belonging to the same motor nerve. The hypothesis is that if motor nerve fibers of different central origin grow into the urodele or fish muscle, the nerve terminals with the greatest selective affinity for the muscle will compete with fibers having less affinity and will displace the latter from the muscle. A similar competitive growth process has been postulated by Guth and Bernstein (1961) to explain the selective reestablishment of synapses in the superior cervical ganglion of the cat after regeneration of the preganglionic nerve fibers.

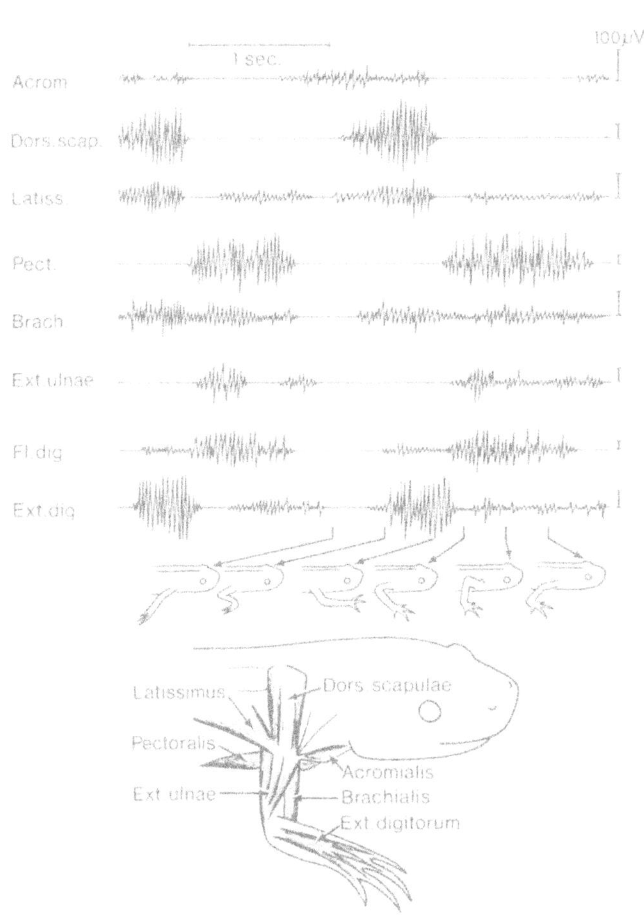

Figure 9.3. Activity pattern of eight forelimb muscles recorded electromyographically in the freely moving newt. The position of the limb is shown in different phases of the step, corresponding with the electrical records from muscles. The anatomical positions of the muscles used for recording (with the exception of flexor digitorum) are shown below. From G. Székely, G. Czéh, and G. Vörös, The activity pattern of limb muscles in freely moving normal and deafferented newts, *Exp. Brain Res.* 9:53–62 (1969).

The nerve–muscle specificity in fish and urodeles is not "all or none," but appears to be graded. This is indicated by the observation that motor nerves will connect with any muscle if constrained to do so by surgical cross-union of nerves or by implantation of motor nerves into foreign muscles, but selective connections tend to be made if the nerve fibers regenerate at random and are permitted to compete for the correct muscle fibers. For example, selective reconnection with extraocular muscles occurs after regeneration of the oculomotor nerve in a fish (Sperry and Arora, 1965). Regeneration of the nerves supplying the fin muscles of a fish results in recovery of coordinated fin movements, but incoordinated movements occur after cross-union of the nerves to the pectoral and pelvic fins (Sperry and Deupree, 1956). Mark (1965) confirmed that simply cutting the nerves of the brachial plexus in a teleost fish results in regeneration of the motor nerves and recovery of normal movements. However, reversed fin movements result when the nerve to the retractor muscle is implanted into the protractor muscle, and *vice versa*. The reversed fin movements persist for at least 18 months, but normal movements are restored by cutting the brachial plexus and allowing the nerves to regenerate at random into the fin muscles. These experiments indicate that recovery of coordinated movements of fin muscles in teleosts is due to selective reconnection between motor nerves and muscles rather than to myotypic specification of the central connections of the motoneurons. The suggestion has been made by Mark (1969) that the homologous response in urodeles might occur because of selective peripheral connections.

Studies of the reinnervation of muscles that move the eyes of fish also show that there is a specific selection process involved in the formation of neuromuscular junctions. The initial observations are quite conventional and in accord with the notion of functional specificity of motor nerves, namely that when the superior oblique eye muscle is reinnervated by its own nerve, the normal rotation of the eye is restored, but reversed eye rotation ensues after the superior oblique muscle is denervated and cross-innervated by the oculomotor nerve (Marotte and Mark, 1970*a*). Unexpectedly, however, Marotte and Mark found that when the superior oblique muscle is first innervated by the incorrect nerve, and later hyperinnervated by the correct one, the incorrect eye movements are converted to normal movements. This conversion of ocular movements occurs rapidly and completely on the first day of reinnervation by the correct nerve as if the incorrect nerve has lost its functional connections with the muscle. However, Marotte and Mark (1970*a,b*) could see no abnormalities in the neuromuscular junctions of the doubly innervated muscle, examined with the electron microscope. Therefore, they concluded that the correct motor nerve terminals take command of the muscle previously innervated by an incorrect nerve by suppressing the function of the incorrect neuromuscular junctions without altering their morphology. After random regeneration of motor axons from the IIIrd and IVth cranial nerves to the inferior oblique muscle, the normal action of the muscle is restored. Although incorrect or foreign axons enter the muscle, and their electrical impulses can be recorded there, the foreign nerves have no detectable effect on the muscle, which contracts only in response to impulses in the correct nerve. From this evidence, Mark *et al.* (1970) concluded that "a subtle but strong selectivity must operate to block transmission of excitation from foreign nerves as long as the correctly matched nerves are present." These findings are in conflict with other evidence that foreign motor nerves remain functionally effective after a muscle is reinnervated by its normal motor nerves. This has been reported in goldfish extraocular muscles (S. A. Scott, 1975), perch gill muscles (Frank and Jansen, 1976), frog skeletal muscle (Miledi, 1963), and mammalian skeletal muscle (Tonge, 1974*a,b,c;* Frank *et al.,* 1974). The very phenomenon of functional inactivation or repression at the synapse and the theoretical edifice of modifiable neuronal networks that has been raised upon it (Mark, 1974*b*) are no longer a *chose jugée;* they are now an open question.

9.5. Can Peripheral Organs Specify the Central Connections of Their Nerves?

Having questioned the validity of the theory of specification of motoneurons by muscles, it is now necessary to critically reevaluate the theory of specification of sensory neurons by sense organs. The evidence given in Chapter 8 shows that interaction between sensory nerve terminals and cutaneous cells is necessary for the differentiation of cutaneous sensory organelles. The question now being considered is whether the interaction between the skin and nerve also affects the differentiation of the neuron so that the central connections of the sensory neuron are specified according to the function and position of the receptor. The problem was posed by Weiss (1942) as follows: "Is the biochemical diversification of the nerve fibers of central or peripheral origin? Logically, both possibilities exist: Either each nerve fiber receives its biochemical characteristics from its center, and then makes selective connections with a peripheral receptor of the appropriate type, or the fibers become specialized only after connecting with the receptors, each fiber assuming the distinctive character of its terminal organ." An experimental strategy for distinguishing between these two alternatives has been to graft an eye (Weiss, 1942) or skin (Miner, 1956; M. Jacobson and Baker, 1969; Sklar and Hunt, 1973; E. M. Bloom and Tompkins, 1976) to a different position, cutting the sensory nerves during the operation, and then to determine the central connections of the sensory nerves that reinnervate the grafts. As we shall see, all these studies merely show changes in reflexes that result from the operations; they fall far short of demonstrating whether the reflex changes are due to changes in the pattern of central connections or whether they are due to changes in the sensory nerves supplying the grafts.

Weiss (1942) and Kollros (1943*b*) transplanted an additional eye of the larval newt to other parts of the head and then observed the reflexes elicited by stimulating the cornea of the grafted eye. In normal newts, retraction of the eye (lid closure reflex) can be elicited by stimulating the cornea, but only after metamorphosis. The reflexogenic zone for this reflex is restricted to the cornea and the skin close to the eye, and is mediated by branches of the trigeminal nerve. Stimulation of the rest of the head, also innervated by the trigeminal nerve, does not elicit a lid closure reflex but stimulates only reflex withdrawal of the head. Weiss (1942) showed that gentle tactile stimulation of the cornea of an extra eye grafted to the nose or ear region results in a lid closure reflex of the normal eye on the same side (Fig. 9.4). Weiss interpreted this observation in terms of his "modulation" theory, namely that the cornea of the grafted eye transfers its local specificity to the branches of the trigeminal nerve in the nose or ear region, causing them to connect selectively with the motoneurons to the retractor muscle of the eye. The same result is obtained when an additional eye grafted to the gill region is innervated by the vagus nerve; stimulating the cornea of the grafted eye results in reflex retraction of the normal eye on the same side (Kollros, 1943*b*). The experiment was repeated and the result was confirmed by Székely (1959*a*). He observed that before metamorphosis, tactile stimulation of an eye grafted to the gill region results in gill movements, but the response changes after metamorphosis, when the corneal reflex normally develops in the newt; stimulation of the cornea of the grafted eye results in retraction of the normal eye.

The difficulties of interpreting these experiments on grafted eyes are increased by other experiments of Székely (1959*a*) in which he grafted a limb to the gill region in larval newts and salamanders. Neither corneal reflexes nor gill reflexes can be elicited by stimulating the grafted limb. However, after amputation of the terminal part of the grafted limb, a regeneration blastema is formed, and when this is stimulated a reflex retraction of the normal eye on the same side occurs. Székely inferred that the patterns of nerve impulses originating in the naked nerve endings of the regeneration blastema and of the cornea are so similar that the central nervous system responds to them in the same way. This is a version of the theory of impulse selectivity, according to which the origin and modality of a sensation are encoded in a pattern of nerve impulses. Székely (1966, 1968) has invented a formal model for this theory, which is implausible because there is no evidence from electrophysiological experiments to support it.

A general criticism of all the experiments that have been described above is that they merely show changes in reflexes and infer the anatomical pathways and patterns of connectivity. There may be several alternative explanations of the changes in reflexes in terms of patterns of connections, as the discussion of myotypic specification has shown. One of the alternative explanations—that the cutaneous nerves grow selectively to the correct places in the graft—was examined more carefully in some experiments on the effects of translocating skin between the back and belly of frog tadpoles (Miner, 1956; M. Jacobson and Baker, 1968, 1969; R. E. Baker and Jacobson, 1970).

Miner (1956) removed a piece of skin on one side of the body of a frog tadpole and replaced the skin with its dorsoventral and anteroposterior axes inverted. The skin undergoes self-differentiation so that, after metamorphosis, dark dorsal skin develops on the belly and light ventral skin on the back (Fig. 9.5).

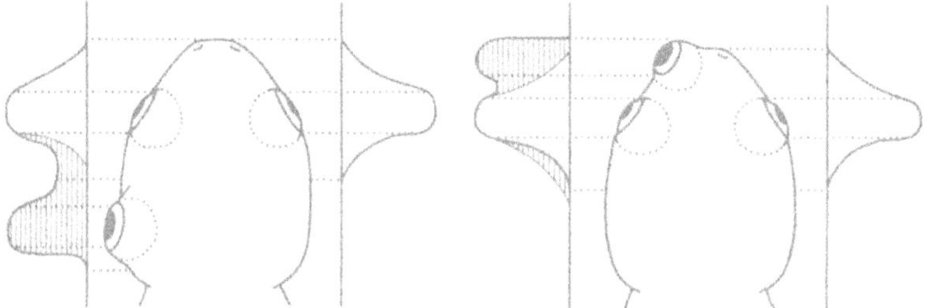

Figure 9.4. Sensitivity profiles for lid closure reflex in newts with eye-to-ear grafts and eye-to-nose grafts. The ordinates of the profiles represent sensitivity; shaded areas under the curves indicate the increase of sensitivity due to the presence of the grafts. From P. Weiss, *J. Comp. Neurol.* *77:*131–169 (1942).

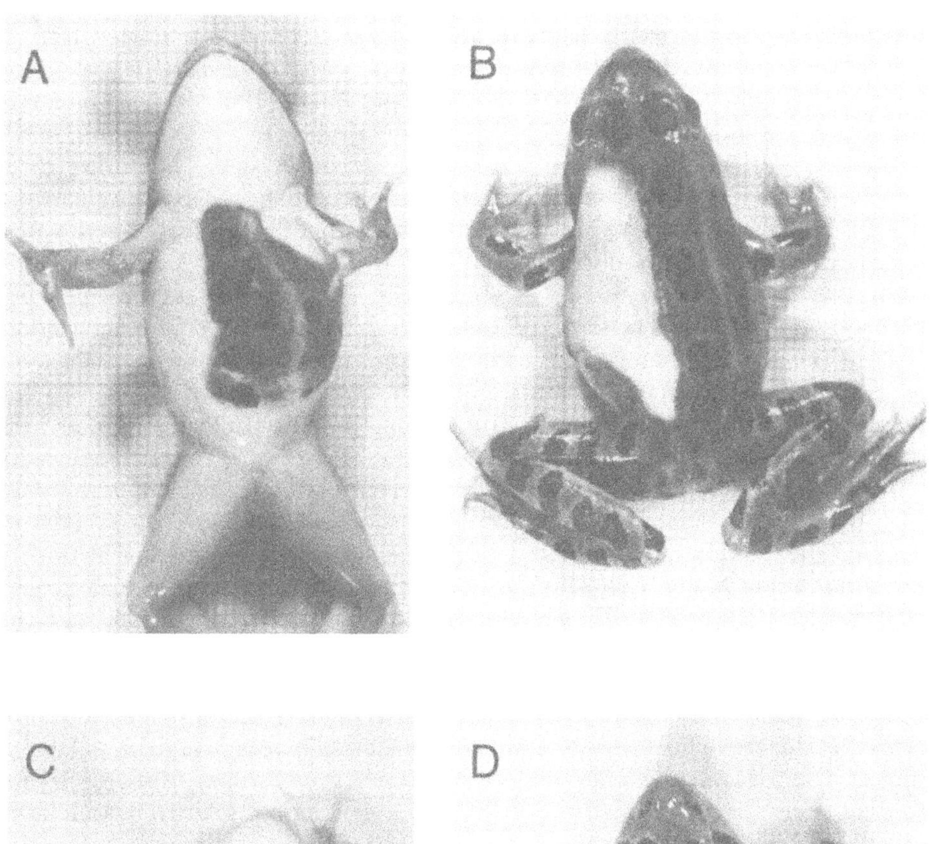

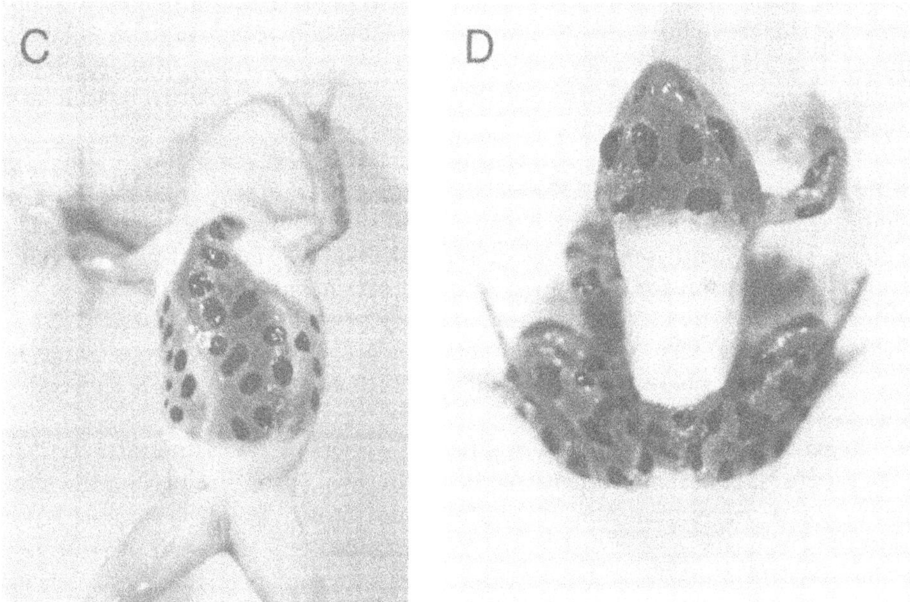

Figure 9.5. Frogs *(Rana pipiens)* with back-to-belly inverted skin grafts made at midlarval stages. A,B: Ventral and dorsal views of the same frog. C,D: Views of another frog in which the development of the reflexogenic zone giving rise to misdirected reflexes is shown in Fig. 9.6. From M. Jacobson and R. E. Baker, *J. Comp. Neurol.* *137:*121–142 (1969).

Tactile stimulation of the skin graft elicits a reflex movement of the leg aimed at the original position of the skin and not at the point of stimulation: when the back is tickled, the frog scratches its belly, and *vice versa.* These misdirected reflexes persist permanently and are not modified as a result of experience. These observations were confirmed by M. Jacobson and Baker (1968, 1969). The misdirected reflexes indicate that the skin, after being grafted to a new position, is able to signal its original position to the central nervous system. There are three possible explanations of the mechanisms of this phenomenon. First, the cutaneous nerves might grow back to their original places in the skin as the result of a selective attraction of the nerves by the skin; or, merely as a result of trial and error, the nerves might selectively reconnect with a place in the skin for which they have a specific affinity. The second possibility is that the nerves connect at random with the skin and are then respecified by the skin. As a result of the respecification, the central connections of the skin might undergo compensatory changes so that the central and peripheral sensory connections become congruent. Finally, the localization of the stimulus on the skin might be due to different patterns of impulses in sensory nerves connected to different places in the skin.

In order to distinguish among these possibilities in a more direct way, we mapped the peripheral connections of cutaneous nerves originating in normal and grafted skin of the frog. This was done by recording action potentials evoked in cutaneous nerve fibers by stimulating the skin gently with a fine hair (M. Jacobson and Baker, 1968, 1969). This experiment revealed no differences in the pattern of nerve impulses in nerve fibers originating from different places in the skin. Each nerve fiber connects with a small area of skin; action potentials can be evoked in the nerve fiber only by stimulating within this receptive field, as Fig. 9.6 shows. There is no evidence that nerve fibers grow a long distance in the subcutaneous tissues or in the skin in order to connect selectively with their original places in the skin graft.

These experiments also show that reversal of reflexes occurs only when skin grafts are inverted before larval Stage XV in *Rana pipiens* (M. Jacobson and Baker, 1969). Baker (personal communication) found that only normal reflexes develop in *Rana clamitans* and *Rana catesbiana,* regardless of the stage at which the skin is inverted. The reason for these species differences is not known. In *Rana pipiens,* normal and correctly localized reflexes develop when the inverted skin grafts are made after larval Stage XV, during metamorphosis, or in adult frogs. Stage XV occurs several days before metamorphosis, which starts at Stage XX and ends at Stage XXV (A. C. Taylor and Kollros, 1946).

Regardless of the stage of development at which inverted skin grafts are made in larval frogs, reflex movements of the limbs, evoked by stimulating the graft, commence at the normal time during metamorphosis (M. Jacobson and Baker, 1969). The reflexes are normal at first, either from the whole graft or from most of the graft. In some cases, misdirected reflex movements of the leg are elicited from a small area of the graft; in others, normally localized reflexes are evoked from the entire graft (Fig. 9.7). In the cases that show only normal reflexes, the origin of the grafted skin does not affect the reflex connections of its sensory nerves. The peripheral receptive fields of cutaneous nerves, mapped electrophysiologically, are normal in size, shape, and distribution.

These results show that the cutaneous nerves, which are cut close to the skin, initially regenerate nonselectively into the nearest skin regardless of their origin, with the result that normal cutaneous sensory localization is restored. After a period of normal behavior lasting several days or weeks, misdirected reflexes first appear on stimulation of a small region of the graft, shown in black in Fig. 9.7, while normal reflexes are elicited from the rest of the graft. In the majority of cases, the region of each graft giving rise to misdirected reflexes gradually increases in diameter at a rate of about 1 mm per day, until misdirected reflexes can be elicited from almost the entire graft. These misdirected reflexes persist indefinitely. The change from normal to maladaptive behavior is the reverse of that expected to result from learning. Whatever the mechanism of the change of behavior, it is not influenced by the animal's experience.

Because we could not detect any changes in the receptive fields of cutaneous sensory nerves during the period when reflexes changed from normal to misdirected, we inferred that the changes must have occurred in the central nervous

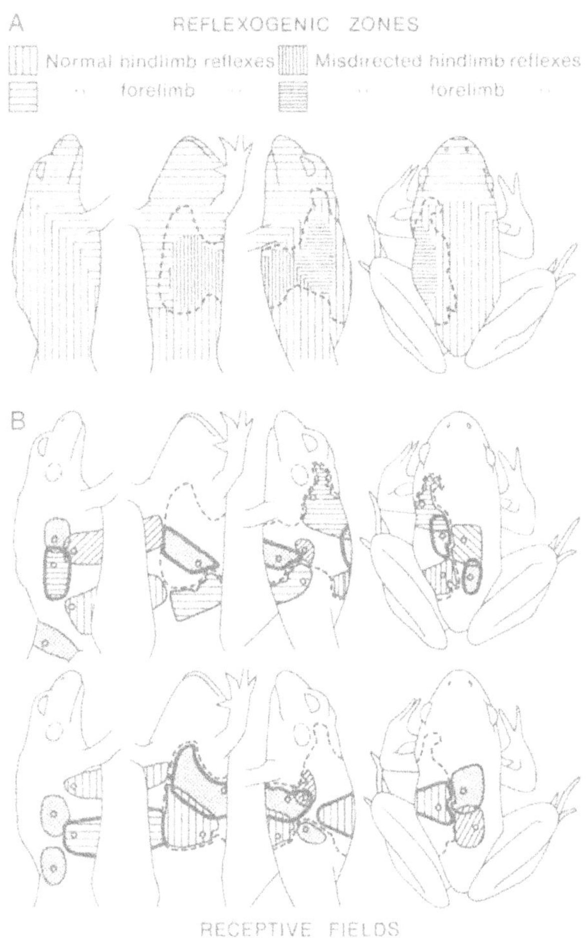

Figure 9.6. A: Reflexogenic zones of the skin shown in four views of a frog with a back-to-belly inverted skin graft (dashed outline) made at larval Stage XIV. The reflexogenic zones remained as shown during frequent tests from 31 to 280 days after the grafting operation. The frog aimed accurately at the position of a stimulus on a normal reflexogenic zone, but stimulation of a zone for misdirected reflexes on the back evoked movement of a limb to the belly, and *vice versa.* B: Receptive fields of cutaneous sensory nerves of the frog shown in A, mapped electrophysiologically 280 days after skin grafting. Each nerve entered the skin at the position shown by the small circle in its receptive field. From M. Jacobson and R. E. Baker, *J. Comp. Neurol. 137:*121–142 (1969).

system. We did not assert that this mechanism had been demonstrated, merely that it is considered probable pending further verification. Such rearrangements of connections in the spinal cord are conceivably possible in frogs because of extensive rostrocaudal spread of motoneuron dendrites for up to 2 mm (Stensaas and Stensaas, 1971), as well as rostral and caudal extension of dorsal root axons for several spinal cord segments (C. N. Liu and Chambers, 1958; B. Joseph and Whitlock, 1968).

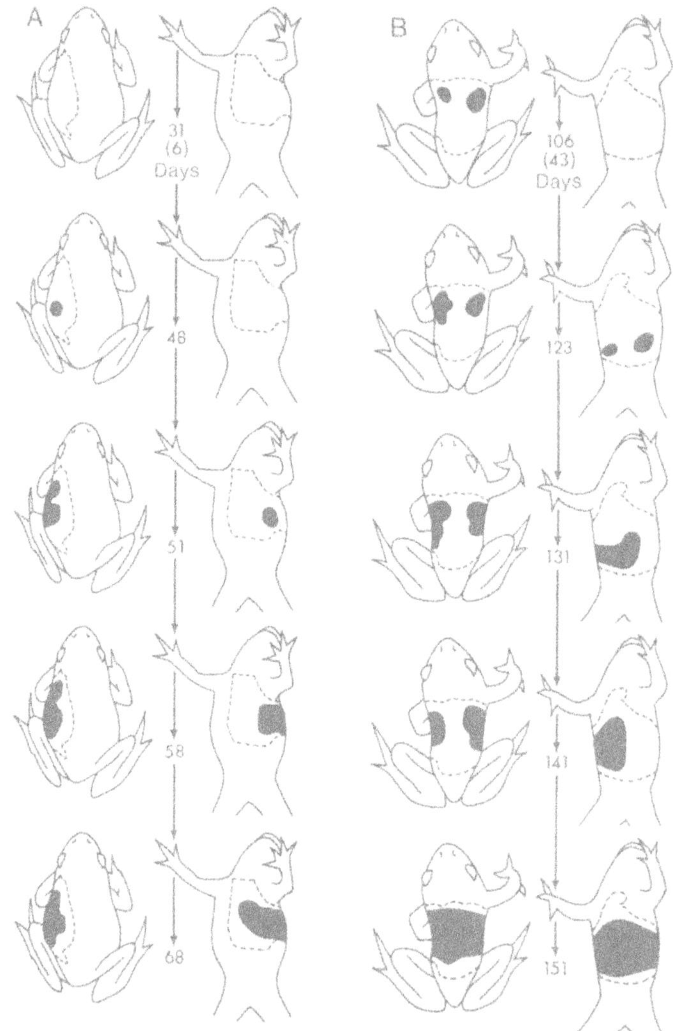

Figure 9.7. Tickling the frog in the area shown in black resulted in a reflex movement of a leg aimed at the original position of the skin graft. The back-to-belly inverted skin graft is outlined by dashed lines. Normal reflex movements, aimed at the point of stimulation, were evoked from the area of skin left white. Skin grafts were made in midlarval stages. Reflex movements of the limbs, evoked by tickling the skin, appeared only after metamorphosis and were at first normal. Misdirected reflexes appeared later from a small area of the graft, shown in black, which gradually enlarged. This is shown in frog A when tested 31 days postoperatively (6 days after metamorphosis), and 48, 51, 58, and 68 days postoperatively, and in frog B when tested 106 days postoperatively (43 days after metamorphosis), and 123, 131, 141, and 151 days after the operation. From M. Jacobson and R. E. Baker, *J. Comp. Neurol. 137:* 121–142 (1969).

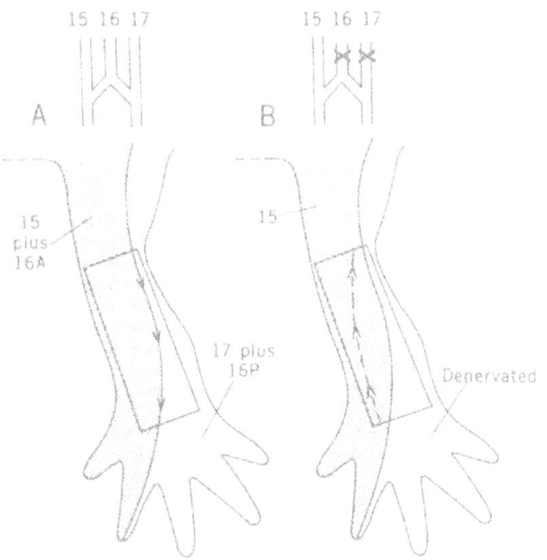

Figure 9.8. Effects of rotating skin areas on mechanosensory nerve fields in the salamander hindlimb. The rectangle of skin (approximately 6 mm wide) shown in limb A was rotated 180° in limb B. In the control limb A, the common field supplied by nerves 16 (posterior branch) and 17 is unshaded, while the field of nerve 15 and the anterior branch of 16 are shaded. In limb B, the 16th and 17th nerves had been cut at the time of skin rotation; the unshaded area shows the denervated region of skin. The dashed line in the skin rectangle of limb B shows the original boundary between the 15th and 17th fields in the skin before its rotation. This was also the boundary between the 16A and 16P fields. The nerves that invade the rotated skin patch pay no heed to the original position of the patch but form a boundary in the identical position in body space to that in the control limb. In some experiments of this kind, the original boundary is not reformed, but there is an unusually large extension of the remaining field into the denervated skin, both within the patch and outside it, without respect to the orientation of the patch. It is likely that the patch is innervated by regenerating nerve fibers in the latter cases, while in the former cases the graft is innervated by collaterals from intact fibers adjacent to the border of the grafted patch. Regenerating fibers ignore the spatial constraints which operate so effectively on sprouting fibers of intact nerves. From J. Diamond, E. Cooper, C. Turner, and L. Macintyre, *Science 193*:371–377 (1976).

Another explanation of the results is that the skin graft is initially reconnected with the nearest nerves, for example, back nerves to belly skin on the back, but later an entirely new contingent of nerves grows from the spinal sensory ganglia to target on their appropriate type of skin. This might not be detected by gross dissection if the belly nerves take the back nerve route and *vice versa.* Methods of tracing the peripheral nerves to their cell bodies, by filling them with cobalt or by retrograde transport of horseradish peroxidase, might reveal the identity of the axons by the positions of their cell bodies in the spinal ganglia.

The possibility of peripheral selection of connections has not been conclusively eliminated, and some evidence, also not conclusive, has recently been adduced in favor of selective reconnection of nerves with translocated skin grafts (Sklar and Hunt, 1973; E. M. Bloom and Tompkins, 1976). By contrast, J. Diamond *et al.* (1976) rotated large pieces of skin (up to 100 mm^2 rotated 180°) on the hindlimb of the salamander and found that ingrowing nerves show no preference for the skin to which they originally were connected. The nerves pay no regard to the axes of the skin but occupy a peripheral field that is the same, in relation to the entire limb, as they had previously occupied (Fig. 9.8).

Other attempts to find solutions to the problems of the development of reflex circuits, and to resolve the antithesis between central and peripheral selectivity, have also been inconclusive. An extremely favorable situation in which to study the development of specific connections is the circuit from muscle spindles to their homonymous motoneurons. Group la afferent nerve fibers from muscle spindles make monosynaptic connections only with α-motoneurons of the same muscle and its synergists. Each spindle-afferent nerve fiber branches to terminate on a large percentage of the motoneurons of its muscle, and, conversely, a single motoneuron receives branches of afferent fibers from almost all the spindles in its muscle (Mendell and Henneman, 1968, 1971). How these specific connections develop in the embryo is an unsolved problem. Because of the high degree of specificity with which spindle-afferents connect with motoneurons, any aberrant connections can be detected by microelectrode recording from single motoneurons while stimulating the Group 1a afferents from individual muscles.

To study the specificity of the connections between muscle spindle-afferent nerves and their homonymous motoneurons, Eccles *et al.* (1960, 1962*a,b*) cross-united the nerves to antagonistic muscles of the hindlimb of the newborn kitten (medial gastrocnemius and peroneus muscles, or lateral gastrocnemius and plantaris). Some months after such nerve crosses, the Group 1a monosynaptic input from muscle spindles was recorded intracellularly from α-motoneurons. As a result of the nerve crosses, the peroneal motoneurons acquire a statistically significant increase in Group 1a input from the synergic muscles, lateral gastrocnemius, and plantaris. There is also a significant decrease in the Group 1a inputs which have become functionally inappropriate as a result of crossing the nerves. No such rearrangements are found after cutting and self-union of the nerves to medial gastrocnemius and peroneal muscles (Eccles *et al.*, 1962*a*). The results indicate that new monosynaptic reflex pathways form, to a limited extent, and tend to reverse the effects of cross-union of nerves to antagonistic muscles. Such slight changes cannot be detected by testing the reflex activity of the whole limb or by naked-eye studies of limb movements. Cross-union of nerves involves axotomy and results in degeneration of up to two-thirds of the spinal ganglion cells. It is likely that the surviving Group 1a afferent neurons sprout new terminal branches to occupy the synaptic sites left vacant by the degenerating Group 1a afferents. Under such conditions, it is conceivable that only those synapses that are functionally effective are selected and that inappropriate synaptic connections are eliminated. Eccles *et al.* (1960, 1962*a,b*) were cautious in their interpretation of the results and were unwilling to distinguish between the latter hypothesis and that of myotypic specification.

Experiments similar to those described above, but involving cross-union of nerves to agonistic muscles, were done by Mendell and Scott (1975). They cross-united the nerves to synergistic muscles (ankle extensors) in the kitten 5–8 days after birth, and studied the effects on the connections of 1a fibers to the cross-united motoneurons. Under those conditions, they observed no rearrangement of synaptic connections. This evidence, showing lack of myotypic specification following nerve regeneration in newborn kittens, does not exclude the possibility that myotypic specification may occur during development. There clearly is some retrograde transsynaptic effect of muscle on motoneurons shown by the changes that occur in the motoneuron after it is disconnected from the muscle (see Section 7.4). In addition, reconnection of the motoneuron with the muscle can result in a recovery but not in a change in the functional properties of the motoneurons, which retain their original properties regardless of the type of muscle with which they reconnect (Kuno *et al.*, 1974*a,b*).

There are some other experiments (so far inconclusive) on invertebrates that may help to explain how neuronal circuits develop. Jacklet and Cohen (1967*a*) found that a metathoracic ganglion from one cockroach implanted into the coxa of the leg of another cockroach supplies only those muscles of the leg that were previously denervated. The neurons that reinnervate particular muscles were not identified, and Jacklet and Cohen did not obtain any evidence that muscles are selectively reinnervated or that respecification of motoneurons occurs. Such evidence might be obtained by denervating a single muscle of the host, which would then become selectively reinnervated by the grafted ganglion. Then the central origin of the reinnervating nerve fibers might be determined by microelectrode recording, or nerve cell bodies undergoing chromatolysis might be identified after cutting of their axons.

Sahota and Edwards (1969) have shown that an extra leg grafted to the mesothorax of the fifth instar of the house cricket develops muscles and nerves. However, there is no evidence of myotypic specification; the grafted limb either develops incoordinated movements or remains immobile.

Although these experiments have yielded inconclusive results, they show what might be done with insects and other arthropods. The arthropods seem ideal material with which to build model nervous systems consisting of small populations of neurons that can be manipulated experimentally. They combine some of the advantages of tissue culture with those of maintaining the cells *in vivo.* In such relatively simple systems it should be possible to map all the connections of a designated neuron under various conditions—for example, when connected with different peripheral organs. We shall then, perhaps, have found a system that will provide unambiguous answers to some of the problems raised but not solved in this chapter.

9.6. Expression of Neuronal Specificity in the Development of Neuronal Projection Maps

A neuronal projection map develops when one set of neurons projects its axons to form connections with one or more neuronal sets so that the spatial order of the elements of one set is preserved in the spatial order of the connections to the other set or sets. Such orderly and continuous neuronal projection maps are found ubiquitously (Werner, 1970), for example, in the projection from the sensory receptors from lower to higher levels of the neuraxis. The topographical representation of the distribution of sensory neurons is preserved in such maps, but neurons with different functional properties at different levels introduce qualitative changes in the functional operations that are performed at successive levels of the projection. These anamorphic changes are best illustrated by the vertebrate visual system (Fig. 9.9) but also occur in all other sensory systems. The spatial order of the visual image is preserved, although processing of visual information occurs as the information passes from the receptors, through retinal interneurons, to retinal ganglion cells, and then to the optic tectum, lateral geniculate nucleus, and cerebral cortex. Although the retinotopic organization of the visual projection is preserved at ali levels in the brain, new kinds of functional organization, of increasing complexity, are created at higher levels of the projection by convergence and synthesis of inputs from the lower levels.

It is obvious that a rank order of complexity exists in the nervous system—the higher orders corresponding with higher levels in the sense introduced by Hughlings Jackson and Charles Sherrington. The possibilities exist for combining inputs from one level to the next, and for introducing entirely new functional classes of neurons at each level. Hierarchical structures of this kind can be analyzed, according to Weyl (1949), in three steps of increasing resolution: (1)

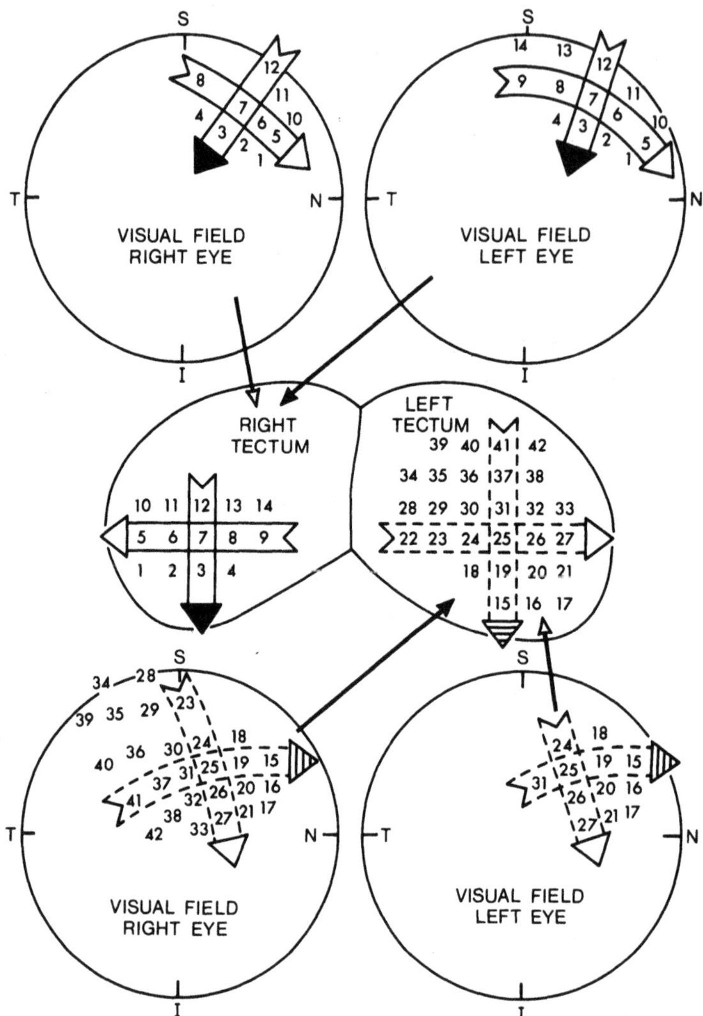

Figure 9.9. Map of the visuotectal projection in the frog, *Rana pipiens*. Each number in the visual field shows the position at which the visual stimulus optimally evoked electrical potentials recorded by a microelectrode at the position indicated by the same number in the tectum. Tectal electrode positions were spaced 250 μm apart. The projections from both eyes were mapped with the right eye centered on the visual field. In this position a large part of the left tectum and the rostral half of the right tectum can be mapped. Much of the ventral half of the visual field cannot be mapped because it projects to the lateroventral aspect of the tectum (not shown) which cannot be reached by a microelectrode. Four representations of the visual field are shown for convenience but all four are actually superimposed in the same visual space (see Fig. 9.30). The visual field extends 100° from the center and its poles are designated I (inferior or ventral), N (nasal or anterior), S (superior or dorsal), T (temporal or posterior).

morphology, which describes the form as a whole; (2) *topology,* which deals with the combinatorial relationships of the elements; and (3) *geometry,* which deals with the metrics of the system. This structural analysis has to be associated with a functional analysis, and both have to be integrated into the analysis of the changes that occur during development. It is obvious that such an analysis is far from being achieved.

Development of projection maps requires at least four steps: (1) Differentiation of the types of neurons that are proper to each set, that is, expression of their phenotypic specificity. (2) Development of locus specificities in each neuronal set. These are defined as the position-dependent properties acquired by each element in the neuronal set which predispose it to connect selectively with an element at the corresponding position in other sets. (3) Expression of the specificities in the selection of the pathway along which axons from one set grow to another. (4) Expression of the locus specificity of each element of one set in selecting, as a synaptic target, an element at a corresponding position in another set.

Neuronal sets develop in different places in the neural tube, and the question arises how each set develops the appropriate phenotypic specificities and how all the necessary locus specificities become deployed throughout the neuronal population of each set so that the polarity of each set is aligned with other neuronal sets and with the polarity of the embryo as a whole (Fig. 9.10).

Both the polarity and the position-dependent properties in neuronal sets are, at present, occult entities. Search for a variable parameter extending gradientwise across the cell population, that might be a sign of polarity, has not been successful, although there are some promising results on the chick retinotectal system that have been discussed in Section 9.2. In the absence of objective criteria, therefore, the polarity of a neuronal population is conventionally defined with respect to the anteroposterior, dorsoventral, and mediolateral axes of the embryo as a whole. Any gradients of physiological parameters in a population of nerve cells such as the retina or tectum have to be shown to be related to formation of connections between the two populations, and neither in the case of the chick embryo retina and tectum discussed in Section 9.2 nor in any other case has such a relationship been shown. It has also to be shown that the polarity or gradient is the cause of such connectivity between neuronal populations and not its effect.

Number, order, and position are the threefold attributes of all things arranged in spatial patterns. One should beware of attaching special significance to the purely formal resemblance between patterns in different structures that have developed by different mechanisms. Richard Feynman, in discussing the

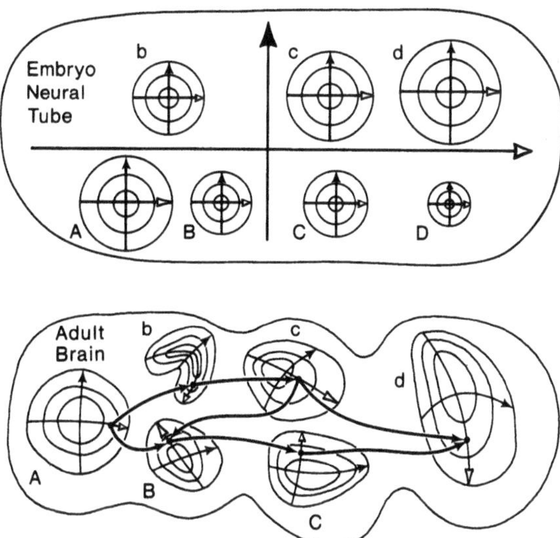

Figure 9.10. Development of neuronal sets. In the upper diagram, seven neuronal sets are shown in various places in the embryonic neural tube. They are aligned with one another and with the neural tube as a whole because they derive their AP and DV axes from an external source of axial cues or positional information. Within each set, the cells acquire position-dependent properties, termed *locus specificities,* with reference to the axes laid down in the neuronal set. The lower diagram shows that the sets change their size and shape, and may even disappear completely (set D), but connections between the sets are formed by linking neurons that have the same locus specificity in different sets. From M. Jacobson, Neuronal recognition in the retinotectal system, pp. 3–23, in *Neuronal Recognition,* S. Barondes (ed.), Plenum, New York (1976).

"underlying unity" of nature, observes that " . . . the thing which is common to all the phenomena is the *space*. . . . As long as things are reasonably smooth in space, then the important things that will be involved will be the rates of change of quantities with position in space. That is why we always get an equation with a gradient. . . ." (Feynman *et al.,* 1964).

It has been postulated that the locus specificities in neuronal populations are stable cytochemical properties of nerve cells that develop as a result of the cells' interpretation of *positional information* (Wolpert, 1969). The nature of the positional information is not known: it could be a gradient of a morphogenetic agent arising from a restricted source and distributed through the cell population by diffusion (Crick, 1970, 1971); it might be a gradient of a substance that is actively transported through the cell population; it might be information provided by the time delay between the arrival of two signals propagated at different velocities through the cell population (Goodwin and Cohen, 1969); or it might be a metabolic gradient based on many complex physiological processes rather than a gradient of a single agent (Child, 1941; Needham, 1942). For example, the positional information might be provided by a higher metabolic activity at one end of the cell population, or entire embryo, than at the other end. In fact, the dorsoventral polarity of the entire embryo of *Xenopus* is associated with a gradient of oxygen consumption with a maximum at the dorsal pole, and the embryo's polarity can be reversed by an imposed gradient of oxygen supply (U. Landström and Lövtrup, 1975). Polarity of the embryo as a whole, determined initially by the point at which the sperm enters the oocyte (Ancel and Vintemberger, 1948), may be a source of polarity of all cell populations, including those in the nervous system. If so, there would not be a time before which the cell population does not have polarity. Evidence to support this notion is that polarity is present in the retina of *Xenopus* at the earliest stage at which the retinal anlage can be recognized as an outgrowth of the brain, at Stage 22 when the retinal anlage contains about 100 cells. We isolated the retinal anlage of *Xenopus* embryos at Stages 22–24 *in vitro,* and when the cultured eye reached Stage 32 we implanted it into the eye socket of a Stage 32 embryo, and showed that the retinotectal projection formed by such an eye expresses the polarity of the eye in the original donor (R. K. Hunt and Jacobson, 1973*a*).

Another experiment indicates that the retinal cell population derives its polarity from a polarizing influence that is present outside the eye socket and may extend throughout the embryo. R. K. Hunt and Jacobson (1973*a*) showed that an eye of *Xenopus* at embryonic Stages 24–26 can reverse its polarity when implanted on the flank of an embryo at the same stage (Fig. 9.15). This observation suggests that other neuronal sets may also derive polarity from a common polarizing influence which is available throughout the embryo. This would result in alignment of the polarities of all neuronal populations with the polarities (DV, AP, and ML) of the embryo as a whole.

It is important to note that these experiements do not show when the locus specificities develop in the retinal ganglion cell population which are expressed in the development of the retinotectal map. The earliest time that such a map can be demonstrated in *Xenopus* is at Stage 47 (Gaze *et al.,* 1974) when the retina contains about 2000 ganglion cells (M. Jacobson, (1976*a*) and when about 2000 optic nerve fibers are present (Gaze and Peters, 1961; M. A. Wilson, 1971). It is assumed that the cellular processes resulting in the development of stable locus specificities in the retina occur continuously as more retinal ganglion cells originate, but that the presence of at least several hundred ganglion cells is required for the development of the few elements required to produce a retinotectal map organized in two axes (see Fig. 9.13).

In all theories of the origin of position-dependent cellular properties, regardless of the nature of the developmental signal or its mode of propagation in the cell population, the cellular response to the signal depends on its amplitude, and this varies according to the positions of the cells in the population. According to Wolpert (1969, 1971, 1974), the cells "interpret" the positional information. This may mean that a developmental program is triggered or initiated that results in development of stable cellular position-dependent properties. In all discussions of this topic it is assumed that the propagated signal is free of noise and that a significant difference in the amplitude of the signal or level of the gradient across a single cell can be detected and interpreted as a difference in positional information at those cells' positions, thus giving each cell a unique cellular address.

The hypothesis that cells are able to use positional information in the differentiation of position-dependent properties has proved of considerable heuristic value in our studies of the origins and expression of locus specificity in the retinotectal system (M. Jacobson and Hunt, 1973, review). However, in those experiments, as well as in other studies of neuronal connectivity, it is clear that neurons rarely form one-to-one connections, as might be expected if they are able to express unique cellular position-dependent properties. On the contrary, locus specificity is usually expressed by groups of cells in one neuronal set connecting with groups of cells in other neuronal sets. These cell groups have already been defined as an element of a neuronal set. Further evidence showing that such elements are composed of hundreds of cells in many neuronal systems will follow later. The immediate purpose is to consider how such a multineuronal element may develop.

Turing (1952) has proposed a "chemical theory of morphogenesis" which can account for the development of patterns consisting of stripes or discrete patches or spots. He showed how cells that are coupled through permeable junctions or are able to interact by diffusion, starting with uniform chemical conditions in all cells, can develop marked nonuniform conditions that are initiated by small fluctuations that are always present in the system. Turing coined the term "morphogen" to describe a molecule produced in the embryo, whose concentration at various loci in the field is interpreted by the cells to develop in a particular way. The spatial pattern generated by a morphogen may be a monotonic gradient, with a maximum at one side and a minimum at the opposite side over a tissue no larger than about 60 cells or 1 mm wide (Wolpert, 1969; Crick, 1970). However, Turing's model and other similar models in which more than one morphogen interact or in which there are inhibitory as well as excitatory interactions between cells (Gmitro and Scriven, 1966; Gierer and Meinhardt, 1972; Meinhardt and Gierer, 1974) can result in the formation of repeating patterns such as bands (e.g., cerebral cortical ocular dominance columns) or peaks and valleys (e.g., cerebral cortical barrels or columns). Turing's model, unlike that of Crick (1970), is not limited to a small number of cells, but is size invariant and can form a pattern over an unlimited area within a few hours (Bard and Lauder, 1974). Although the maximum wavelength that can be generated by Turing systems is about 1 mm, or about 60 cells 15 μm in diameter, the wave can be repeated, so that the size of the system is unlimited.

According to Bard and Lauder (1974), Turing systems generate periodic patterns that are "characterized by a general regularity rather than absolute precision," like the zebra's stripes and the hair follicles on the skin. Turing systems might well be responsible for generating the patterns of neuronal projection from the sensory receptors to the central nervous system, for example, the ocular dominance columns, the thalamocortical somatosensory projections, and the retinotectal projection. The element of such a system would be the group of cells that forms a discrete band or patch.

Although neuronal sets become different from one another in size and shape and in the number of neurons that compose a single element of the set, sets that connect together develop the same reference axes with respect to the polarity and axes of the embryo, and corresponding locus specificities develop along those axes in each set. An element carrying a particular locus specificity in one set—for example, the retina—will be able to connect with an element carrying the corresponding locus specificity in other sets—for example, the tectum, pretectal nuclei, and lateral geniculate nucleus. It is assumed that the terminal branches of the presynaptic axons from an element in set A recognize the synaptic sites on the neurons composing the corresponding element in set B. The molecular basis of this recognition is unknown.

For readers who are not familiar with the anatomical details, it is only fair to point out that anatomical data are usually insufficient to determine the size of an element as a morphological entity in most neuronal sets. In principle, the size of an element can be determined from its connections. For instance, the size of the subset of neurons in the retina that collectively connect with a subset of tectal neurons may give an indication of the developmental element since the locus specificity of the element is finally expressed in the development of those retinotectal connections.

It is also to be expected, although again there are few data, that the number of neurons composing an element may differ in different neuronal sets and may vary in the same set at different stages of development and under differing experimental conditions. An approximation to the size of an element of a map may be achieved anatomically in a few systems. To give the extremes in the mammalian brain, there is a one-to-one or, at most, few-to-few relationship between the climbing fibers arising from inferior olivary neurons and their targets, the cerebellar Purkinje cells (Brodal, 1940*b*; Palkovits *et al.*, 1971). At the other extreme, a single Type Ia afferent axon from the muscle spindle branches to make connections with almost the entire set of homonymous spinal motoneurons (Mendell and Henneman, 1968, 1971). In the first case, the element may consist of a single cell and certainly consists of no more than a few cells, while in the second case almost the entire homonymous motoneuron population, consisting of hundreds of cells, compose a single element. In these cases, there is some indication, but no firm evidence, that the elementary functional and structural unit is also the elementary developmental unit of the system. However, in no system has the relationship between a developmental element and an elementary unit of the fully developed system yet been finally established.

The concept of developmental elements of a neuronal set can be related to the concept that the mammalian cerebral cortex is organized as "elementary functional units" in the form of columns of neurons extending vertically from the surface through all layers of the somatosensory cortex (Mountcastle, 1957, 1974;

Powell and Mountcastle, 1959; E. G. Jones *et al.,* 1975), auditory cortex (Abeles and Goldstein, 1970), visual cortex ocular dominance columns (Hubel and Wiesel, 1963*a,b,* 1972; LeVay *et al.,* 1975), and orientation columns (Hubel and Wiesel, 1974*a,b*). Similar bands are found in the ipsilateral retinal projection to the superior colliculus of the cat (Graybiel, 1976). The hypothesis of columnar organization follows from the results of making sequential microelectrode penetrations perpendicular to the cortical surface. All the neurons encountered in a single penetration perfectly normal to the cortical surface respond to the same modality of sensation and have identical, or nearly identical, peripheral receptive fields, while neighboring penetrations, spaced 0.5–1 mm apart, encounter neurons in different columns. It has proved very difficult to relate the columns in the somatosensory cortex as defined by electrophysiological recording to anatomical columns, probably because the column diameter (upper limit 0.4–0.5 mm) is at the limits of resolution of the physiological recording technique. However, the structure–function relationship has been demonstrated in the ocular dominance columns in layer IV of the striate cortex (LeVay *et al.,* 1975; Wiesel *et al.,* 1974) and in the layer IV barrel field (Woolsey and Van der Loos, 1970), which will be discussed below.

Towe (1975) has calculated that if the columns are 0.4 mm in diameter, then 360 columns could be packed into the posterior sigmoid gyrus of somatosensory area I of the cat, while if the column diameter is 0.3 mm, the number of columns would be 640. Towe (1975) shows that there are about 170 nonoverlapping excitatory cutaneous receptive fields on one side of the cat's body, making it possible to represent four different modalities in 640 cortical columns. While these numbers are not precise, they show that the number of elementary functional units is not large, and suggest that these functional units may develop from a similar number of elementary developmental units. This is best illustrated by the barrels in layer IV of the somatosensory cortex, each of which is a multicellular unit that receives its sensory input from a single mystacial hair in rodents (Woolsey and Van der Loos, 1970). Similar cortical barrels are also found in the cat, macaque, and man (Feldman and Peters, 1973). The barrel is dependent for its development on the presence of its mystacial hair (Fig. 9.11). Removal of a row of vibrissae and cauterization of their follicles in the newborn rat result in failure of development of the corresponding row of barrels (Van der Loos and Woolsey, 1973; Welker and Johnson, 1975; Killackey *et al.,* 1976; Woolsey and Wann, 1976). The peripheral cutaneous element and the cortical element forming the barrel develop at the same time in the embryo (Rice and Van der Loos, 1977). Not only the barrel field, representing the vibrissae in the cerebral cortex, but also the representation of the sinus hairs on the lower jaw, the somatosensory projection from the feet (Welker, 1976), and probably the entire primary somatosensory thalamocortical projection (Killackey *et al.,* 1976) appear to be organized in the form of barrels (Fig. 9.12). Figure 2 of Killackey *et al.* (1976) shows that there are about 160 barrels forming the primary somatosensory thalamocortical projection from one side of the body of the rat.

In most instances, the resolution of both physiological and anatomical mapping methods falls just short of being able to resolve a single functional element in the cerebral cortex, and therefore falls short of being able to determine the extent of overlap of functional elements. However, some functional elements in the cerebral cortex do not overlap, for example, the cortical barrels representing whiskers (mystacial hairs) and the representation of toe pads (Fig. 3.16). In such cases, there is a clear anatomical separation between elements, which corresponds precisely with the functional separation between them. These separations between the functional elements in the adult cerebral cortex must arise from a large measure of developmental autonomy between the elements. In such cases, the functional elements may correspond with developmental elements.

A direct but rough estimate of the minimal sizes of developmental elements in the retinotectal system can be obtained from the sizes of the terminal arborizations of the optic axons as seen in histological preparations (Scalia *et al.,* 1968; Lázár and Székely, 1969; H. D. Potter, 1969, 1972) or as determined electrophysiologically (George and Marks, 1974). Such observations show that a single optic axon

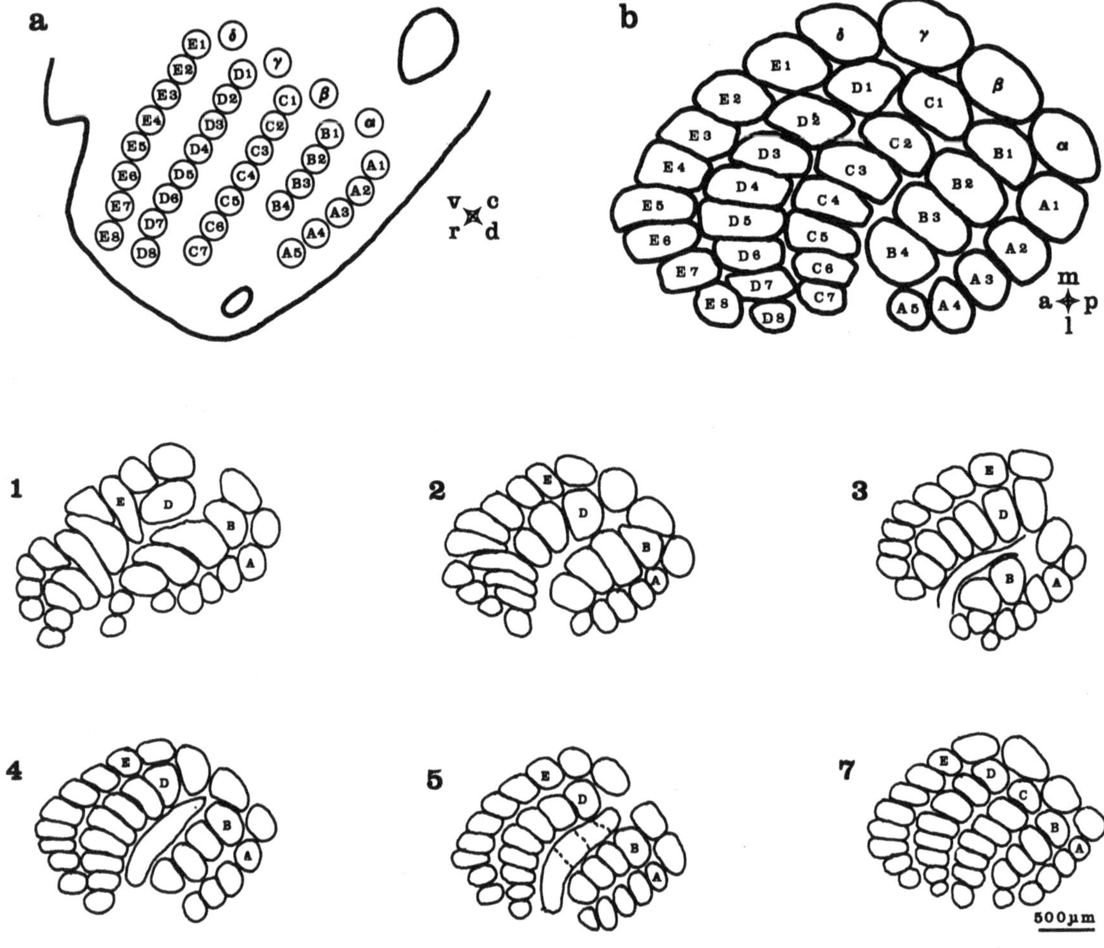

Figure 9.11. Mystacial vibrissae of the mouse on the right side of the face (a) project to the posteromedial barrel subfield (b) of the left cerebral cortex. Barrels, like the vibrissae, are arranged in five rows labeled A to E. Barrels are numbered within each row. Posteromedially, four barrels, designated α–δ, straddle the rows. The effect of cauterizing vibrissae of row C on the right side on different days after birth is shown in the lower set of diagrams. There is progressively less disruption of the pattern of barrels after lesions made on postnatal days 1, 2, 3, 4, 5, and 7. From T. A. Woolsey and J. R. Wann, *J. Comp. Neurol. 170:*53–66 (1976).

connects with many tectal cells and that an individual tectal cell receives synaptic inputs from many optic axons. However, the sizes of retinal and tectal elements cannot be deduced from those observations. An additional complication arises from the fact that there are four separate retinotectal maps superimposed in different laminae of the frog tectum (Maturana *et al.*, 1960; Witpaard and ter Keurs, 1975) and from the fact that each of the four classes of retinal ganglion

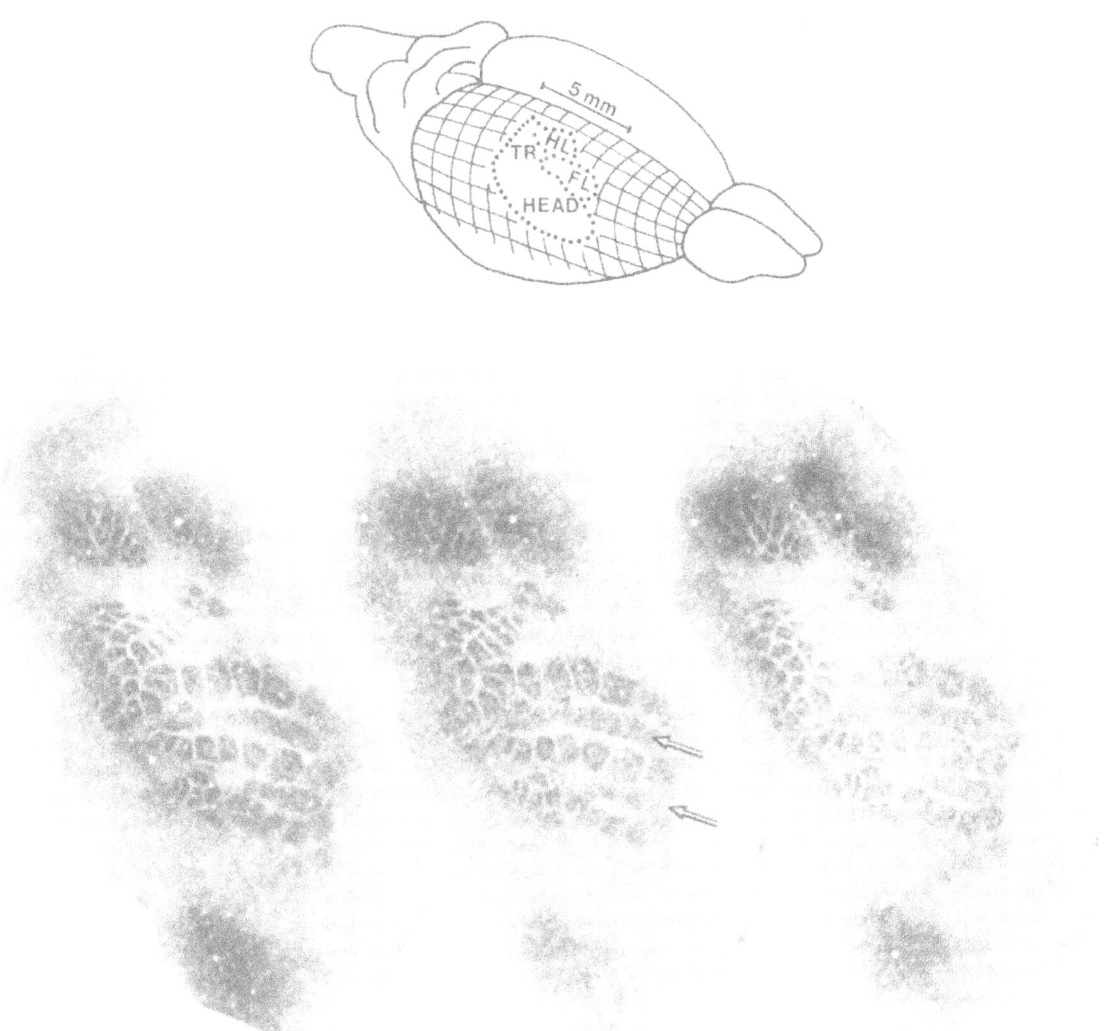

Figure 9.12. Mapping the thalamocortical somatosensory projection in the rat by means of the histochemical stain for succinic dehydrogenase, which is mainly localized in mitochondria which are concentrated in nerve endings, shows the barrellike organization of the projection extending beyond the projection from the face to the projection from the trunk and limbs. The histological sections, from left to right, are at progressively deeper levels of the cerebral cortex. In this case, the vibrissae of rows B and D (*cf.* Fig. 9.11) were removed at birth and the corresponding cortical barrels are disrupted (arrows: distance apart approximately 1 mm). The brain shows the sensory projection mapped electrophysiologically, superimposed on a 1 mm grid drawn on the surface of the cerebral hemisphere. The cortical projection zones are shown of the head, trunk (TR), hindlimb (HL), and forelimb (FL). Histological sections courtesy of G. Belford and H. P. Killackey.

cells differentiates at a different time extending over several weeks (Pomeranz, 1972). There are four different functional types of retinal ganglion cells, each of which expresses its phenotypic specificity by projecting to a different level in the tectum, and each type evidently synapses selectively with a different type of neuron at a different level in the tectum, as shown in Fig. 7.3. This shows that every retinal element contains all four types of ganglion cells. Ganglion cells of different types in the same element all express the same locus specificity, but express different phenotypic specificities in projecting to different levels in a single vertical column in the tectum. Independent expression of phenotypic and locus specificity is seen in other systems organized as vertical columns and horizontal layers, *par excellence* in the cerebral cortex, as discussed above.

How a discontinuous map of multineuronal elements may become converted into a continuous map, by means of tangential linkages, will now be considered. The hypothesis of specified nonoverlapping multineuronal elements requires that neurons in a retinal element connect exclusively with neurons in a corresponding tectal element and that there is little if any overlap between neighboring elements. However, it is well known that there is considerable overlap of peripheral receptive fields, and that receptive fields can rapidly change their functional states, including their sizes. It is obvious that a retinal receptive field does not correspond with a retinal element. By contrast, changes in the structure of multicellular developmental elements can occur only as a result of relatively slow developmental and growth processes. However, it is evident that rapid lateral interactions between elements must occur, first to convert the discontinuous, tessellated organization of the close-packed elements into a continuous topographical representation of the peripheral field (Werner, 1970) and second to achieve the combinations and permutations of receptive field characteristics that have been observed in different functional states. The lateral interactions are effected by systems of neurons, not included in the elements, that form tangential connections between elements. These neurons apparently do not share the locus specificities of the neurons composing the elements but are free to express their phenotypic specificity by connecting neighboring elements or even by connecting widely separated elements. It seems that such neurons originate and differentiate late in development, as a general rule. In the retina, the amacrine cells are of this type, and analogous types of tangentially arranged neurons are seen in the tectum.

Until precise counts can be made of the number of retinal axons of each class that synapse on each type of tectal cell and the number of tectal cells that serve as targets for the branches of a single retinal axon, resort has to be made to indirect methods. The sizes of retinal and tectal elements may be estimated from the minimal number of neurons that must be removed or transplanted in order to create a detectable discontinuity in the retinotectal map. Such assays are subject to the limitations of the retinotectal mapping methods which are discussed later. Nevertheless, deficits and discontinuities in the map can be detected: for example, if the optic nerve of a frog is cut and a small retinal lesion is made at the same time, the regenerating optic axons respect the gap in the retinotectal map that would have been occupied by the ablated cells. This scotoma in the retinotectal map can be shown by behavioral perimetry (Sperry, 1944) or by mapping of the retinotectal projection electrophysiologically in the frog (M. Jacobson, unpublished) or in the goldfish (M. Jacobson and Gaze, 1965). The smallest lesion that can be detected by these methods produces a scotoma which subtends an angle of about 5–10° in the visual field. This is equivalent to a line of about 10–20 ganglion cells in the central retina of the frog or about 100 μm on the tectum (M. Jacobson, 1962). This sort of observation gives a rough indication of the size of an element in the retinotectal system of the frog, namely a group of about 100–400 ganglion cells which projects to a region of tectum with a surface area of about 0.01 mm^2.

The number of tectal elements can be estimated from the experiment of rotating or translocating a small patch of tectum (area of 0.05–0.08 mm^2) which is shown to act as a target for the retinal axons with which it was originally connected (R. Levine and Jacobson, 1974; M. Jacobson and Levine, 1975*b*). Such patches, with an area considerably larger than expected for a single tectal element, nevertheless allow an estimate of the discrimination shown by a retinal axon that approaches the margin of the patch and chooses a target element either on the patch or outside the patch, but never on both sides of the margin. This can be mapped electrophysiologically with a resolution of 50–100 μm. A closer approximation to the size of a tectal element is obtained from the observation (M. Jacobson, unplublished) that the smallest tectal patch that acts as an independent target for retinal axons has an area of about 0.01 mm^2 in young adult *Xenopus,* in which the total surface area of the tectum is about 1 mm^2. This sets an upper limit to the size of the tectal element, but in such experiments that limit is determined by surgical limitations in translocating small tectal patches and by the limit of resolution of the mapping method. Assuming that the tectal elements are closely packed but not overlapping hexagonal prisms extending from the surface through all four layers of the tectal neuropil, the tectum of the young frog, shortly after metamorphosis, could contain 2000 elements if the diameter of an element is 25 μm, 500 elements if the diameter is 50 μm, or 125 elements if the diameter is 100 μm. Considering the packing density of tectal neurons and the spread of their dendrites into the superficial tectal neuropil where the optic axons terminate, it is very unlikely that the diameter of a tectal element is as small as 25 μm or even 50 μm, and a diameter of 100 μm is consistent with the evidence given above as well as with the observed spread of dendritic fields of tectal neurons (Lázár and Székely, 1967; Székely *et al.,* 1973). It then follows that, in *Xenopus,* there are about 125 nonoverlapping tectal elements and the same number of nonoverlapping retinal elements, each containing about 280 retinal ganglion cells. A retinal element would thus have a diameter of about 20 ganglion cells. It must again be emphasized that the developmental elements need not be directly equivalent to functional units.

These estimates of the number of retinal and tectal elements that compose the retinotectal map in the young adult frog, if they are correct, have implications for the mode of development of the retinotectal map. They dispose of the problems that would be raised if individual retinal neurons were uniquely matched with individual tectal neurons, or even if there were large numbers of retinal and tectal elements that were matched one-to-one. The sizes of retinal and tectal elements are consistent with the evidence that a few hundred ganglion cells originate at Stages 29–31 in *Xenopus,* and send the first contingent of a few hundred optic axons which arrive in the tectum at about Stage 40 (M. Jacobson, 1968*b*). These axons may compose a single element, which connects with the first and only tectal element to have developed before Stage 45 (M. Jacobson, 1976*b,* 1977). That no order is seen in the retinotectal map at Stage 46 (Gaze *et al.,* 1974) is consistent with the hypothesis that the map consists of a single retinal and tectal element at that stage (Fig. 9.13). At least three elements must be appropriately arranged to give a map ordered in two axes. Such a map can first be recorded at Stage 47 (Gaze *et al.,* 1974), when there are about six retinal elements and a similar number of tectal elements as judged from the number of optic nerve fibers and the size of the tectum. A daily increment of one or two retinal and one or two tectal elements occurs throughout development of the tadpole until the end of metamorphosis in *Xenopus,* and then the rate of increment slows considerably (M. Jacobson, 1976*b,* 1977).

The next sections will deal with the genesis of polarity and position-dependent properties in retinal and tectal cell populations, and the assembly of the retinotectal map in submammalian vertebrates. While it is unlikely that all the rules for assembly of that system apply to other sensory systems (there are indications that there are several modes of assembly of the retinotectal system itself (see M. Jacobson, 1977), it seems that all such systems are composed of a relatively small number of elementary developmental units, probably no more than several hundred in any system, and that the position-dependent properties deployed in each set of such elements may be derived from Cartesian reference axes in the entire embryo.

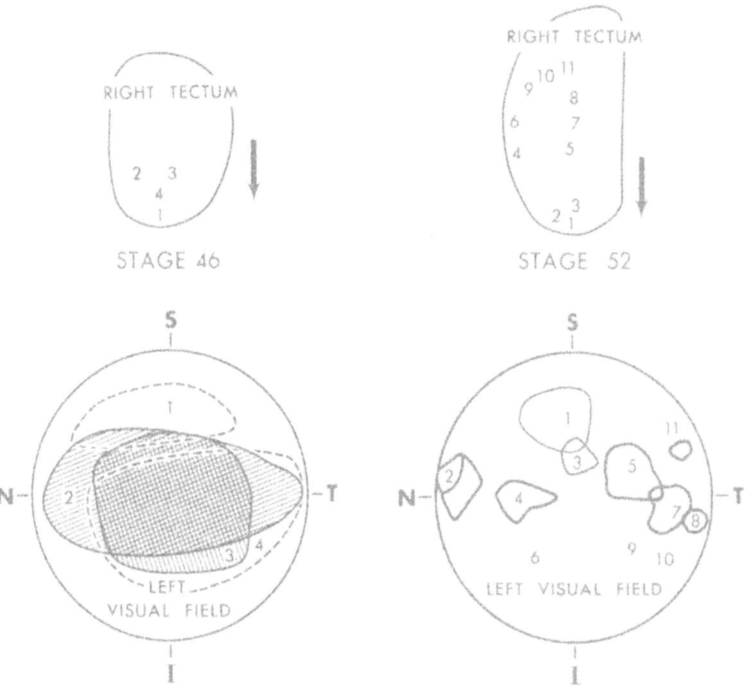

Figure 9.13. Development of the visuotectal map in *Xenopus* tadpoles. Numbers on the right tectum show positions of a microelectrode at which multiunit responses could be elicited from receptive fields numbered correspondingly in the left visual field of a Stage 46 tadpole soon after visuotectal responses first appear, and about 16 days later, in a Stage 52 tadpole. From R. M. Gaze, M. J. Keating and S. H. Chung, *Proc. Roy. Soc. (London) B Ser. 185:*301–330 (1974).

9.7. Development of Polarity and Position-Dependent Properties in the Retina

The term "neuronal specificity" has many connotations, and to avoid confusion it is essential to define the meaning of the term in particular cases. Does it refer to properties of an individual cell, of a group of cells, or of the entire cell population? Does it refer to the program of development, the intermediate states, or the final products of the program in which the specificities can be recognized? Are the program of development, the intermediate states, and the specific properties of the fully developed system invariant under all conditions or only under certain limited conditions? What are the various conditions under which the developmental program, the specific cellular properties, or the cellular mechanisms of expression of those properties may be altered? These are some questions that arise when attempting to understand the results of the experiments that are described and discussed below.

In our experiments over the past few years, we have adopted the strategy of surgically altering the position of the embryonic eye rudiment in relation to the tectum, or of explanting the eye rudiment to tissue culture, before challenging the retinal ganglion cells to complete their developmental program by projecting their optic nerve fibers to the tectum. From the relative order of the optic nerve fibers in the retinotectal map and from the conditions under which the eye develops (such as its orientation in the embryo or embryos into which the eye is grafted, or the conditions under which it develops *in vitro*), we can draw inferences about the transitions through which the retinal ganglion cells have passed in the development of their final set of locus specificities.

The experimental strategy is to reposition one eye of the embryo of the clawed frog, *Xenopus laevis,* at various stages of development before the eye starts forming nervous connections with the brain. The eye is either inverted *in situ* within the ocular orbit, transplanted to another position on the body, or explanted into tissue culture for some time. In all cases, the eye is reimplanted in the orbit in order to map the resulting retinotectal projection.

In the first type of experiment the eye rudiment is excised at various embryonic stages and then simply reimplanted in different orientations in its own ocular orbit (M. Jacobson, 1967, 1968*a*) or transplanted from a donor to a carrier at the same stage of development, as shown in Fig. 9.14 (M. Jacobson, 1967, 1968*a*). In control experiments a normal retinotectal projection always results after reimplantation or transplantation of the eye rudiment in its normal orientation at all stages of development. When the eye is rotated at embryonic Stage 28, it gives rise to a normal retinotectal projection. However, when an eye rotation occurs a few hours later at embryonic Stage 30, a retinotectal projection develops that is inverted in the anteroposterior axis of the retina, but normal in its dorsoventral axis. Slightly later, at Stage 31, eye rotation results in complete inversion of the retinotectal map. These experiments show that there is a change in the embryo, in a 5- to 10-hour critical period between Stages 28 and 31, during which there is a change in response of the retinotectal system to 180° rotation of the eye. These experiments permit three main conclusions:

First, the set of locus specificities that ultimately develop in an eye rotated before the critical period is spatially organized in accordance with the postopera-

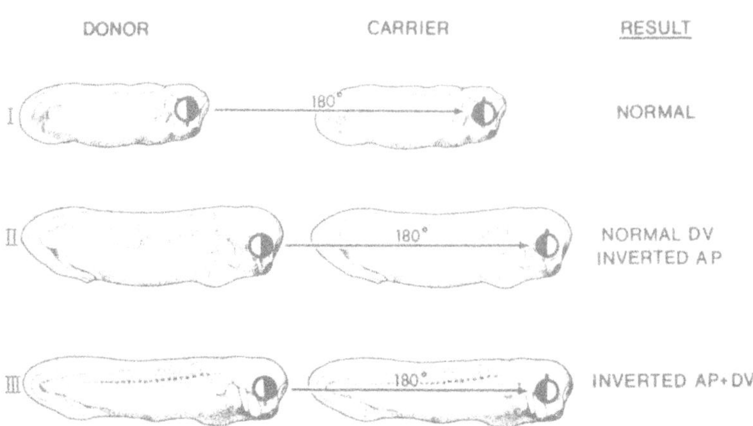

Figure 9.14. Inversion of the eye of *Xenopus* embryos at various stages of embryonic development has different effects on the retinotectal projection when mapped later in the adult frog. Inversion of the eye at or before Stage 28 results in a normal retinotectal projection (I). If the eye is inverted at Stage 30, the map is inverted in one axis (II). If the eye is inverted at Stage 31 or later, the map is completely inverted.

tive positions of the retinal cells and does not depend on the cells' preoperative positions. Second, on the other hand, in an eye rotated after the critical period, the set of locus specificities that ultimately develops is determined by the preoperative positions of the retinal cells and does not pay heed to their postoperative positions. Third, by rotation of an eye in the middle of the critical period, at about Stage 30, the set of position-dependent properties that develops in the retina has an anteroposterior component which is appropriate to the eye's preoperative position, but the dorsoventral component is appropriate to its postoperative position. Thus the position dependence of locus specificity has two axial components, one related to the ganglion cell's position in the anteroposterior axis of the retina and the other to the cell's position in the dorsoventral axis of the retina.

These experiments merely show a *terminus ad quem,* and the results should not, strictly, be used to infer antecedent mechanisms or the *terminus a quo.* That is, they show the stage of development at which the axes of the entire retinal cell population become irreversibly fixed, but they do not show when the specificity is first acquired, what the initial conditions are for specification, or whether the specification applies to individual cells or to groups of cells or only to the entire retina. Nevertheless, for convenience, the change of state that occurs in the *Xenopus* retina at Stages 29–31, and presumably at analogous stages in the retinae of other vertebrates, is termed "axial specification" or merely "specification," and the system is said to be prespecified before that time and to be specified thereafter. Apparently a similar process leading to specification, first in the anteroposterior axis and later in the dorsoventral axis, occurs in the limbs and ears in amphibian and chick embryos (Harrison, 1921, 1945; Swett, 1937; Hall, 1939; Chaube, 1959; Saunders and Gasseling, 1968).

Returning again to the strategies that we have used for studying the development of position-dependent properties in the retinal ganglion cell population, first we have to show that the position-dependent properties are truly dependent on position in the retinal cell population and are not merely an expression of some temporal order in development, such as the order of origin of retinal ganglion cells, the order of their differentiation, and the timing of the arrival of the retinal axons in the tectum. That the last is not the case is shown in experiments in which eyes are either grafted from Stage 32 embryos to the body wall for 30 days or explanted into tissue culture for several days before being reimplanted in the orbit and allowed to form connections with the brain. These eyes form normal, retinotopically organized projections with orientations which are appropriate to the positions of the eyes in the original donors (R. K. Hunt and Jacobson, 1972*a,b*).

These experiments show that the expression of locus specificities does not depend on the sequential order of arrival of nerve fibers from the eye into the tectum. It is then necessary to discover whether the position dependence is derived from the position of the ganglion cell within the retinal field or is derived from the position of the eye on the body surface. For this purpose we transplant a Stage 28 eye rudiment onto the body wall of a Stage 28 intermediate host in various orientations as is shown in Fig. 9.15 (R. K. Hunt and Jacobson, 1972*a*). After the eye has developed to mid-Stage 31, it is reintroduced to the orbit of a Stage 32 carrier embryo and allowed to form connections with the brain. The resulting retinotectal projections are normally organized and their orientation is appropriate to the orientation of the eye on the body wall. The retinotectal projection formed by the experimental eye, which has spent its critical period on the body wall, is indistinguishable from the retinotectal map of the normal eye which serves as a control. Therefore, the position dependence of locus specificity is derived not from some absolute position of the eye on the body surface but from the relative positions of the ganglion cells within the retinal field (R. K. Hunt and Jacobson, 1972*a*). Apparently, then, the eye is not directly instructed by the embryo about its absolute position on the body, but merely uses the body as a source of "positional cues" or "axial cues" for establishing properly aligned axes of its own. These "axial cues" are not unique to the tissues surrounding the eye but are also available to an eye on the side of the body. This raises the possibility that the same cues may be used to align the axes of other organ rudiments such as the limb or the ears. Like the eye, those organ rudiments may also receive "axial cues" from the surrounding tissues which then participate in aligning the axes of the organ rudiment with the axes of the embryo (Harrison, 1921, 1945; Swett, 1937; Hall, 1939).

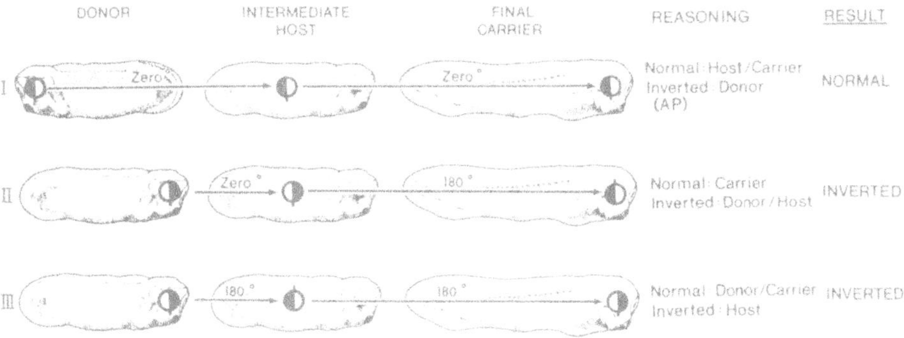

Figure 9.15. An eye that spends the critical period (Stages 29–31 in *Xenopus* embryos) while implanted on the body of a host embryo, and is later returned to the eye socket, forms a retinotectal map whose axes are derived from the eye's orientation on the body of the host. From R. K. Hunt and M. Jacobson, *Proc. Natl. Acad. Sci. U.S.A.* *69:*780–783 (1972).

The next question that arises is whether the transition from the prespecified to the specified state involves stable and irreversible changes in the retinal cells or whether, in contrast, the change in the state of the system reflects changes in the extraocular conditions in the embryo. An example of the latter change might be the disappearance of axial cues required to reorganize retinal axes after eye rotation or transplantation of the eye. To test whether the transition which occurs at Stages 19–31 involves irreversible changes in the eye or in the embryo, we back-grafted Stage 31–32 right eyes into the enucleated right orbits of Stage 28 embryos as shown in Fig. 9.16 (R. K. Hunt and Jacobson, 1972*b*). When the eye is back-grafted in an inverted position, the pattern of retinotectal projections which develops is retinotopically organized but inverted in both axes of the tectum. When the Stage 31–32 eye is implanted into a Stage 28 orbit in normal orientation, a normally oriented retinotectal projection invariably develops. These results show that the back-grafting procedures themselves do not alter the pattern of retinotectal connectivity and that a back-grafted Stage 31–32 eye develops locus specificities from positional information obtained in the original donor orbit and is not influenced by the host. The Stage 31–32 eye is thus refractory to the same conditions which are capable of providing positional information to a prespecified eye in a Stage 28 animal. These experiments provide strong evidence that the transition from the prespecified to the specified state involves stable and irreversible changes in the eyes between Stages 29 and 32, but whether irreversible changes also occur in the embryo remains unknown. That the axial cues persist until Stage 39 and are available to a Stage 28 eye implanted into a Stage 39 embryo is shown by the following experiment (Fig. 9.17). A Stage 23 eye is transplanted in rotated position into a Stage 28 host, allowed to traverse the critical period of that host, and then reimplanted into a Stage 39 carrier (R. K. Hunt and Jacobson, 1973*a*). The reimplantation is done before the eye itself has reached its critical period. Such eyes always develop normal retinotectal projections regardless of their orientation in the final carrier embryo. These experiments show that the trigger mechanism for the transition from prespecified to specified state is not the sudden disappearance at Stage 28 of the extraocular axial cues, which presumably participate in organizing the retinal axes and aligning them with the major axes of the body. Rather, the trigger mechanisms are within the eye itself. That the transition during the critical period is not due to extraocular agents which transiently arise between Stages 28 and 32 is shown in the following experiment (M. Jacobson, unpublished). Prespecified eyes before Stage 28 are transferred

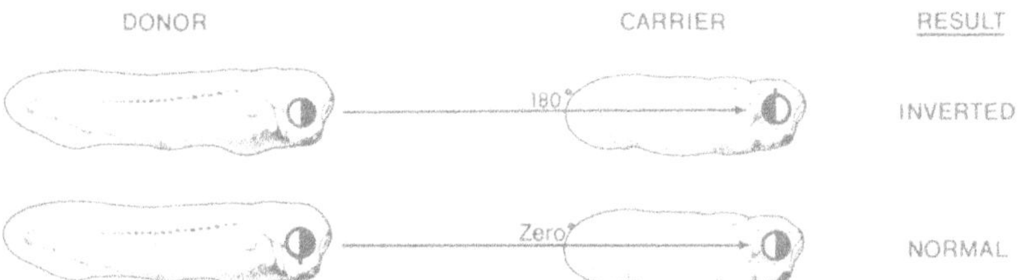

Figure 9.16. An eye "back-grafted" from a Stage 31 to a Stage 28 *Xenopus* embryo fails to realign its axes. When the eye is grafted in an inverted position, an inverted visuotectal map develops; when the eye is grafted in normal orientation, a normal map develops. From R. K. Hunt and M. Jacobson, *Proc. Natl. Acad. Sci. U.S.A. 69:*2860–2864 (1972).

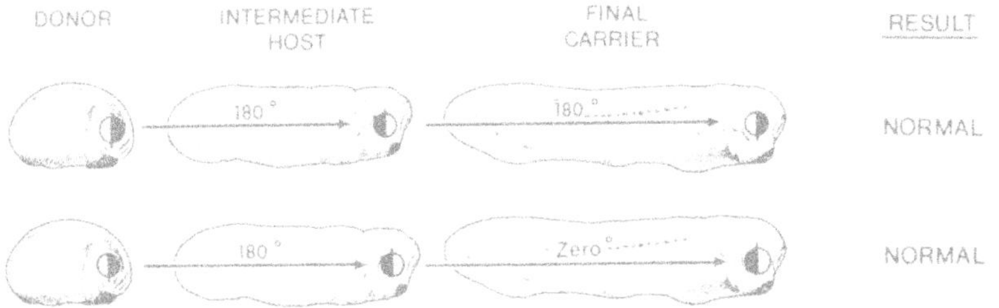

Figure 9.17. The change of state that occurs in the eye of the *Xenopus* embryo at Stages 29–31 is triggered from within the eye and is not altered by the stage of the extraocular tissues. From R. K. Hunt and M. Jacobson, *Proc. Natl. Acad. Sci. U.S.A. 71*:3616–3620 (1974).

directly to carrier embryos between Stages 32 and 39. In all cases in which a retinotectal projection develops (about 20 percent of animals) regardless of the orientation of the eye in the final carrier, a normally oriented retinotectal projection develops. Thus a normal pattern of retinotectal projections develops from an eye which has never been in contact with an embryo at the critical Stages 28–32. This experiment eliminates a classical induction model of specification in which extraocular agents arise transiently during the critical period and instruct or specify an unspecified retinal cell population.

That the specification process does not involve instructive action on the part of the embryo but merely a transition from a reversible to an irreversible state is shown by the experiment illustrated in Fig. 9.18 (M. Jacobson and Hunt, 1973; R. K. Hunt and Jacobson, 1973*a,* 1974*b*). Eye rudiments from Stage 22–25 embryos are cultured *in vitro* for periods of 2 to 10 days during which the explants develop the features of Stage 38 or 39 normal eyes. These mature explants are then reimplanted into Stage 39 carrier embryos (R. K. Hunt and Jacobson, 1973*a*). In these cases, the resulting retinotectal maps are normal when the eye is in its normal orientation in the final carrier, but when the eye is rotated the map is rotated to the same extent. This shows that the locus specificities in the retinal ganglion cell population are derived from the original donor and are not altered in the final carrier. Specification thus occurs in tissue culture in total isolation from the embryo and the eye as early as Stage 22 contains a set of reference axes properly aligned with the axes of the Stage 22 embryo. These axes can be reversed within 6 hours of surgical inversion of a prespecified eye (R. K. Hunt and Jacobson, 1974*b*). The embryonic eye in the prespecified state before Stage 28 possesses a stable but reversible set of axes. Whether these axes are physically the

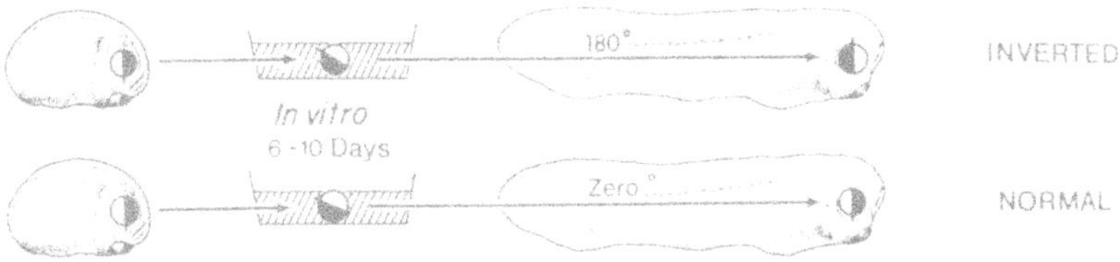

Figure 9.18. Specification consists of a transition from a reversible set of axes in the eye before embryonic Stage 28 to an irreversible state of ocular axes after Stage 28. This transition can occur in an eye isolated *in vitro.* From R. K. Hunt and M. Jacobson, *Proc. Natl. Acad. Sci. U.S.A. 70*:507–511 (1973).

same as those that are present after Stage 31 remains to be determined. However, it is certain that **the specification process merely consists of a transition from a reversible but stable set of axes in the prespecified retina to a stable but irreversible set of retinal axes in the specified retina.**

The foregoing discussion has defined the changes of state through which the retinal cell population goes in the development of definitive locus specificities, but it has left open the question of cellular mechanisms of (1) deployment of position-dependent properties in the retinal cell population, (2) substitution of new retinal axes after eye inversion, and (3) expression of the properties as locus specificities during the morphogenesis of the retinotectal projection. These questions are considered below.

The eye at Stage 31 contains only a few hundred retinal ganglion cells and retinal axons have not yet grown out of the eye, yet rotation of the eye at Stage 31 results in corresponding rotation of the entire retinotectal map of the adult eye, which contains about 50,000 retinal ganglion cells (M. Jacobson, 1968*a,b,* 1976*a*). Apparently a developmental program has been established in the embryo that affects the entire set of specificities that will arise in the adult retina, and the unsolved problem is how the retinal ganglion cells that originate after Stage 31 acquire their locus specificities. The retina grows by addition of new cells at its margin (Glücksmann, 1940; Hollyfield, 1971; Strazincky and Gaze, 1971; M. Jacobson, 1976*a,* 1977) where a population of retinal stem cells persists throughout embryonic and larval development. The retinal cells that are produced after Stage 31 at the circumference of the retina must obtain their positional information from other cells in the eye and not from extraocular cues, because rotation of the eye after Stage 31 always results in a completely rotated retinotectal map (M. Jacobson, 1967, 1968*a*). The newly produced retinal ganglion cells may derive their locus specificities by cell lineage, by cellular communication, or by a combination of both mechanisms.

In the cellular interaction mechanism the stem cells (M) at the retinal circumference do not possess locus specificities themselves and do not participate in the specification of their daughter cells, but serve merely to produce cells of the correct cellular phenotype; the daughter cell (x) is initially without locus specificity, but then interacts with the nearest specified neuron (n) and so acquires the locus specificity appropriate to its position in the array ($n+1$). This process is then repeated as follows:

$$\begin{array}{ll} 1.2.3 \ldots\ldots n.\,(M) & \\ \quad\quad\quad\quad\downarrow & \text{mitosis} \\ 1.2.3 \ldots\ldots n.\,(x)\,. & (M) \\ \quad\quad\quad\quad\downarrow & \text{interaction } (x \xrightarrow{n} n+1) \\ 1.2.3 \ldots\ldots n.n+1.\,(M) & \end{array}$$

In this cellular interaction model, all the stem cells that produce ganglion cells at the retinal circumference are qualitatively identical in space and time, as are the newly produced neurons (x) that lack locus specificity initially. Random destruction of some stem cells and (x) cells or inhibiton of DNA synthesis or mitosis in some stem cells would not alter the normal pattern of deployment of locus specificities, although the total number of cells would be reduced. However, inhibiton of cell communication, for example, with lithium ions, would be expected to alter the spatial pattern of locus specificities.

In a cell lineage mechanism locus specificities are inherited directly by retinal ganglion cells from the stem cells:

$$\begin{array}{l} 1.2.3 \ldots\ldots n. \, (M^{n}) \\ \qquad\qquad \downarrow \text{ mitosis} \\ 1.2.3 \ldots\ldots n.n + 1. \, (M^{n-1}) \\ \qquad\qquad \downarrow \text{ mitosis} \\ 1.2.3 \ldots\ldots n.n + 1.n + 2. \, (M^{n-2}) \end{array}$$

The stem cell line changes its specificity with each cell division, and the positional information is not communicated from cell to cell except at mitosis, from stem cell to daughter cell. If this is the case, destruction of stem cells will result in a deficit in the set of locus specificities. Such deficits can not be detected by the conventional retinotectal mapping methods (for reasons given in Section 9.1), but the completeness of the set of locus specificities in the experimental eye may be assayed by the double-eye comparison strategy (see Fig. 9.27).

According to the cell lineage model, alterations of the orderly schedule of cell proliferation in the retina would result in a derangement of the normal pattern of deployment of locus specificities. Finally, translocation of stem cells (such as are produced by combining parts of the eye rudiment in abnormal locations) would, according to the cell lineage model, give rise to predictable changes in the pattern of retinal locus specificities. Evidence that development of retinal locus specificity need not depend on cell lineage comes from experiments on recombination of retinal halves to form "compound eyes" (Gaze *et al.*, 1963, 1965; R. K. Hunt and Jacobson, 1973*b*) in which the final set of locus specificities in the surgically altered eye is different from the set that would have developed if each half of the eye had produced the half-set of specificities that it was destined to develop in the intact eye.

One of the problems raised by these experiments is that although the deployment of position-dependent properties is permanently stable and unmodifiable in an *intact* eye after Stage 31, disruption of the eye can result in redeployment of the locus specificities in the retinal ganglion cells at later stages of development. For example, mere vertical transection of a Stage 32 retina results in redeployment of the locus specificities so that each half of the eye appears to contain a complete set of locus specificities rather than the partial set that would be expected to develop in part of the intact eye (R. K. Hunt and Jacobson, 1974*a*).

At present, the only clues to a solution of those problems are certain correlations between retinal histogenesis and the genesis of locus specificities in the retinal ganglion cell population. First, the retinal ganglion cells that are born in the central region of the retina cease DNA synthesis at Stages 29–31 in *Xenopus* (M. Jacobson, 1967, 1968*b*), as shown in Figs. 9.19 and 9.20, and it seems likely that changes in their developmental programs accompanying their withdrawal from DNA synthesis and from the mitotic cycle initiate the transition from reversible to irreversible retinal axes, which is called "specification." This change of state, according to one hypothesis, occurs in many different neuronal populations as nerve cells become postmitotic (M. Jacobson, 1968*b*, 1969, 1970*b*). A similar close correlation between cessation of DNA synthesis at Stages 12½–13, withdrawal from the cell cycle, and histogenetic determination is seen in Mauthner's neuron of *Xenopus* (Vargas-Lizardi and Lyser, 1974). Similarily, in the retina of the chick embryo, ganglion cell specification occurs at about the same time as the first ganglion cells withdraw from the cell cycle. Cessation of DNA synthesis in chick retinal ganglion cells is seen at Stages 12–13, at 45–52 hours of development (Kahn, 1973, 1974), and some of these ganglion cells can be seen to have sprouted an axon by Stage 15, at 50–55 hours of development (K. T. Rogers, 1957; Goldberg and Coulombre, 1972). Crossland *et al.* (1974*a*) have showed that these retinal events are correlated with a change in the response of the chick retinotectal system to removal of part of the retina. They observed that removal of 15–75 percent of the retina before Stage 11 (40–45 hours of development) results in development of retinal connections to all parts of the tectum, whereas removal of part of the retina after Stages 12–13 leaves the corresponding part of the tectum free of retinal connections. This change in the capacity of the reduced retina to send axons to occupy the entire tectum is correlated with the time of origin of the first retinal ganglion cells at Stage 11. This seems to be analogous to the change of state that occurs in the retina of *Xenopus* at Stages 29–31. However, in *Xenopus*, the capacity of a part of the retina to fill the entire tectum with its axons persists for a few stages after Stage 31 (R. K. Hunt and Jacobson, 1974*a;* R. K. Hunt and Frank, 1975). In the adult frog, this capacity is considerably slowed (Udin, 1975, 1976) or lost (Meyer and Sperry, 1973). By contrast, in the adult goldfish, the retinotectal map can form between a piece of retina and the entire tectum (Yoon, 1972*a*) or between an entire retina and a residual fragment of the tectum (Yoon, 1971). This is discussed more amply in Section 9.9.

The change of state of the retina in its response to inversion of the eye or to partial removal of the retina may involve a change in the intercellular communication between retinal cells themselves, and between the cells of the eye and the cells of the surrounding tissues. According to this hypothesis, developing nerve cells, when grafted to another position, can acquire new position-dependent properties only if they can communicate with neighboring cells. The locus specificities of the grafted cells then develop in accord with their new positions. However, it seems that if the graft itself cannot communicate with neighboring cells, its locus specific-

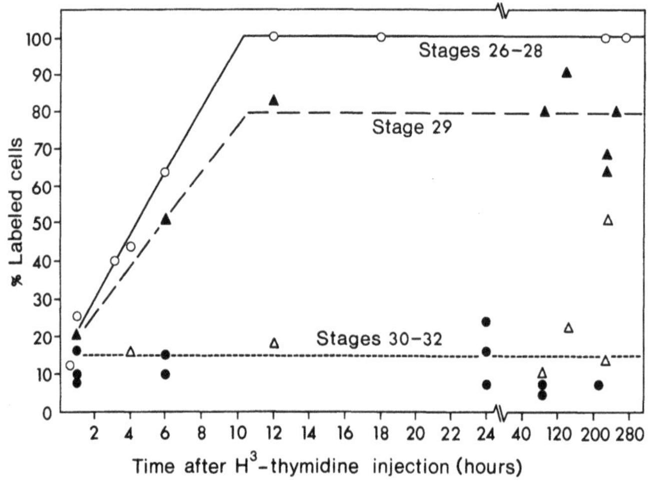

Figure 9.19. Percentages of labeled cell nuclei in the retina of *Xenopus* embryos after either one or several injections of tritiated thymidine. The stage at which the initial injection was given is indicated by the following symbols: ○, Stages 26–28; ▲, Stage 29; Δ, Stage 30; ●, Stages 31 and 32. From M. Jacobson, *Dev. Biol. 17:*219–232 (1968), copyright Academic Press, Inc.

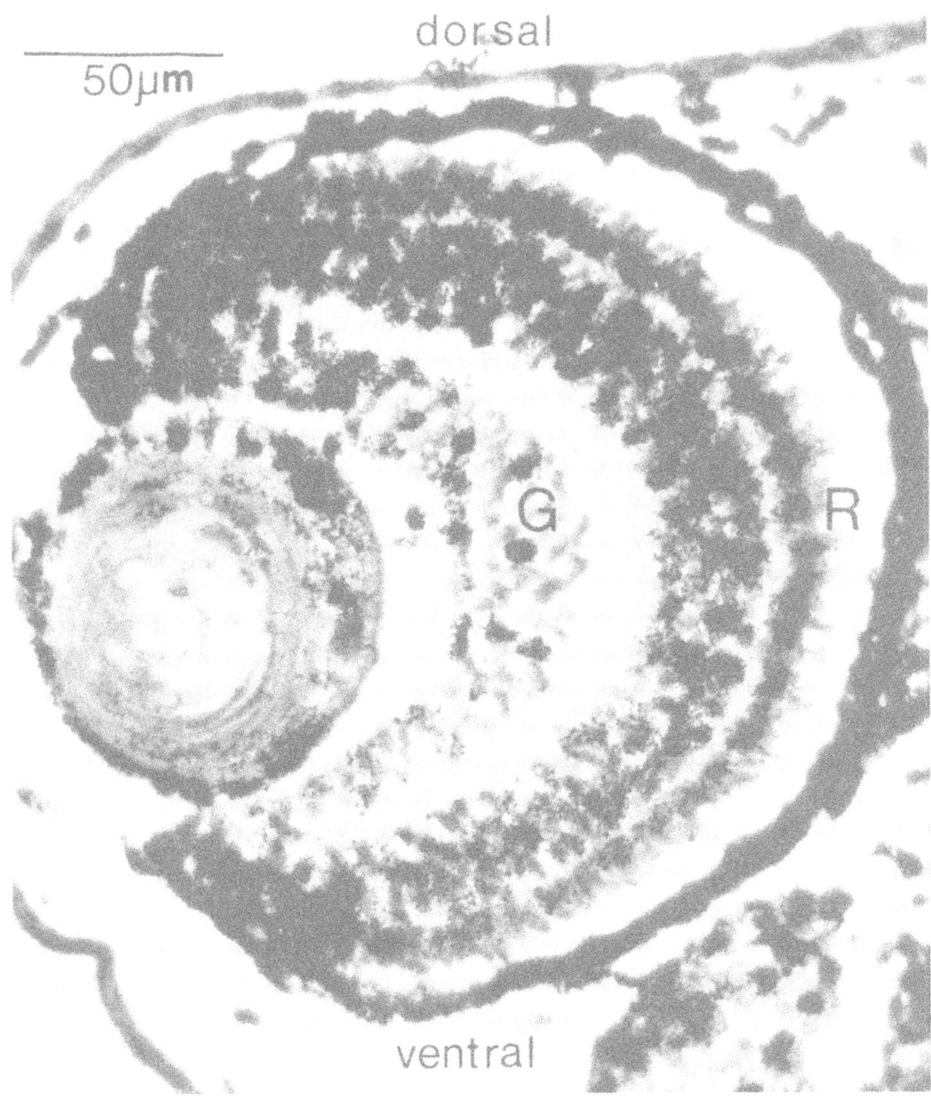

Figure 9.20. Autoradiograph of a vertical (coronal) section through the eye of Stage 43 *Xenopus* larva labeled cumulatively with tritiated thymidine, first injected at embryonic Stage 29. Note the gradients of labeling from receptor cells, R, to ganglion cells, G, and from dorsal to ventral in each layer of the retina. From M. Jacobson, *Dev. Biol. 17*:219–232 (1968), copyright Academic Press, Inc.

ities are derived from the preoperative position. Similarly, after surgical reduction in the size of the retina, the residual cells may be able to develop a complete range of position-dependent properties only as a result of cellular interactions. Such interactions probably require cell contact and may involve intercellular communication through specialized intercellular junctions (Loewenstein, 1968*a,b,* 1970, 1973, 1975) that provide intercellular pathways for ions and small molecules (Loewenstein, 1968,*a,b,* 1973; Warner, 1970; I. Simpson *et al.,* 1977). Evidence in support of this hypothesis is the observation that gap junctions have been found ubiquitously between the cells of the embryonic retina of *Xenopus* before Stage 29 (while the retina is composed of mitotically active stem cells), but disappear from the retinal cells in the center of the retina during the critical Stages 29–31 (as the first retinal nerve cells, destined to become ganglion cells, withdraw from the mitotic cycle), and at later stages persist only between the cells at the retinal margins, which remain mitotically active (Dixon and Cronly-Dillon, 1972; Hayes, 1976). Our experiments (Loewenstein, Rose, and Jacobson, unpublished) have demonstrated the passage of fluorescent-labeled molecules between cells of the embryonic retina before Stage 30, but have shown that such intercellular communication is impeded or absent at later stages of development of the retina. Because of their technical flaws, these results are little more than suggestive.

It seems that the change of state at the critical period involves withdrawal of retinal cells from the mitotic cycle and concomitant uncoupling of the postmitotic nerve cells from the rest of the retinal cell population. After uncoupling from the retinal population the nerve cell is characterized by a stable and irreversible program leading to development of a locus specificity. Development of this position-dependent specificity enables the young nerve cell to extend its outgrowing axon on the proper pathway and predisposes that axon to terminate at a specific position in the brain and to form synaptic connections selectively with particular nerve cells. It must be emphasized that the arguments associating specification with the terminal cell cycle are based on no more than circumstantial evidence, and the association with cellular uncoupling rests on a mere shred of evidence. We have yet to devise an experiment aimed at showing the neuron *in flagrante delicto* of specification.

9.8. Development of Polarity and Position-Dependent Properties in the Optic Tectum

The tectum must play an essential role in the formation of an orderly, continuous, and properly aligned retinotectal map, but whether the tectum merely aligns the map or whether it controls or directly influences the positions of individual elements of the map cannot be decided *a priori*. The problem can be generalized to include other orderly neuronal projections: either the entire presynaptic population may be deployed with reference to the polarity of the postsynaptic population as a whole, or individual presynaptic elements may position themselves with reference to the corresponding individual postsynaptic elements.

Polarity of the tectum as a whole, or at least two reference points giving the tectal axes, is the minimal condition for setting up a map of the retinal axon population properly aligned with the tectal axes or reference points, which are themselves aligned with the axes of the embryo as a whole. In that case, positions of individual retinal axons in the map would require interactions between the axons themselves in which they would express their retinal position-dependent properties (locus specificities) in selecting a place in the retinotectal map. Alternatively, or in addition to the expression of tectal polarity, individual tectal elements may have properties that depend on their positions in tectal space, and these positional markers may serve as targets for corresponding retinal elements.

Rotation of the tectum (rostrocaudal inversion), in part or whole, and then assay of the retinotectal map, behaviorally or electrophysiologically, has shown that the tectal polarity becomes irreversible (i.e., refractory to tectal rotation) only after the retinal axons enter the tectum. The experiments do not indicate whether tectal polarity is present before that stage, but they show that polarity is stable thereafter. In the first experiments of this sort, Crelin (1952) excised the tectum in *Ambystoma* embryos at various stages and replaced it back-to-front. When the operation is done before the stage at which the tectum is invaded by retinal axons, the animals develop normal vision. However, inversion of the tectum at later stages, while retinal axons are invading it, results in the development of confused visually guided behavior. These results are not easy to interpret because it cannot be shown how the altered behavior is related to the retinotectal map, and it is not demonstrated that the inverted tectum receives retinal inputs.

The possibility that the rotated tectum retains its original polarity if a "polarizing zone" is included in the rotated graft, but not if it is excluded, was suggested by R. Levine and Jacobson (1974). Evidence that the polarity of the tectum is determined by the diencephalon has been put forward by Chung and Cooke (1975). They showed that rotation of the mesencephalic anlage without including the diencephalon in *Xenopus* embryos at Stages 21–24 or at Stage 37 results in development of a retinotectal map that is normally aligned with the embryonic axes. This demonstrates that tectal polarity either is absent or can be reversed up to Stage 37. However, if the anlage of the diencephalon is included with the rotated mesencephalon, even at Stages 21–24, the resulting retinotectal map is inverted. In some cases, two retinotectal projections with opposed polarities develop in the same tissue, apparently showing that there are two sets of intermingled tectal cells which express their polarity independently (Fig. 9.21). These important experiments raise in an acute form the problem posed by rotation of the embryonic eye, namely how the information about polarity (or possibly about position) is transmitted from the few stem cells present at Stage 21 to the hundreds of thousands of tectal cells that do not come into existence until later stages. The first cells of the tectum originate as postmitotic neurons at Stages 39–40, and by Stage 46 the tectum contains less than 5 percent of the neurons that are present at Stage 66. The population of tectal cells in the frog is built up over a period of more than 2 months (Straznicky and Gaze, 1972; Currie and Cowan, 1974*b*, 1975; M. Jacobson, 1977).

The earliest time at which the tectal polarity becomes refractory to tectal inversion can be correlated with the production of the first postmitotic tectal neurons at Stages 39–40 and with the time at which optic axons invade the tectum, at about the same stage. However, these correlations are not as neat as they are in the eye (M. Jacobson, 1968*b*), as the tectum may "repolarize" after back-to-front inversion, even in the adult. In an unpublished series of experiments, I have reimplanted the entire midbrain, back to front (180° rotation and left–right inversion), in *Xenopus* embryos at different stages. In all the operated animals that recover vision, the optomotor reflexes as well as the ability to locate and pursue a visual lure are apparently unimpaired. Electrophysiological mapping of the retinotectal projection shows that 180° rotation of the tectum at Stage 45 results in development of a normally aligned retinotectal map. The same result has been reported by Chung and Cooke (1975) after rotation of the entire midbrain anlage at Stages 21–24 or at Stage 37, but they were unable to do the operations at later stages. In my experiments, operations done at progressively later stages, from Stage 45 to Stage 66, resulted in progressively more cases of inverted retinotectal

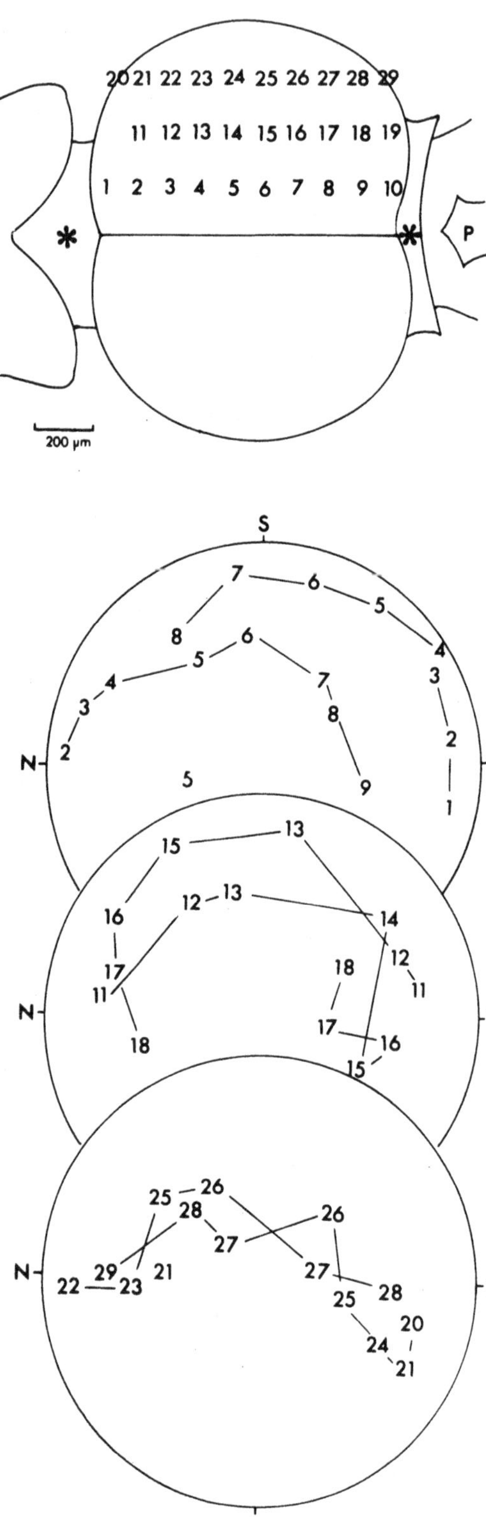

Figure 9.21. Visuotectal projection from the left eye to the right tectum of young adult *Xenopus* in which the midbrain anlage had been excised and reimplanted back-to-front at embryonic Stage 22. Asterisks show the positions of the duplicated diencephalon. With permission, from S. H. Chung and J. Cooke.

maps, but some normally aligned maps were found even after tectal rotation in the adult *Xenopus* (R. Levine and Jacobson, 1974).

The normal visually guided behavior of animals with demonstrable inversion of the retinotectal map may be due either to the fact that the behavior is not subserved by the tectum or to the fact that tectal rotation does not change intratectal circuits or alter the relationship between retinal afferents and tectal cell efferents. These results indicate that before Stage 46 the tectum either has no polarity or has a polarity that can be realigned or reversed when the tectum is rotated. Control experiments to determine whether a normally aligned map in an ostensibly rotated tectum might be due to derotation of the tectum or to tectal regeneration have not been successful.

The cases in which tectal rotation results in the expected rotation of the retinotectal map show unambiguously that tectal polarity is irreversibly established at the stage of the operation. There is no sudden change of the response of the tectum to rotation, such as occurs in the eye at Stages 29–31. Rather, the frequency of cases of rotated retinotectal maps increases as the operation is done at later stages of development.

Whether individual tectal elements have acquired position-dependent properties cannot be adduced from the results that have been discussed above. Therefore, we performed the additional experiment of rotating or translocating a small patch of tectum in larval and adult frogs (*Xenopus* and *Rana catesbeiana*) to see whether the patch expresses its original position-dependent properties independently or whether it expresses properties appropriate to its new location (R. Levine and Jacobson, 1974; M. Jacobson and Levine, 1975*a,b*). Rotation of a patch alters both the polarity and position of the patch relative to the surrouding tectum, whereas translocation without rotation changes the position but not the polarity of the piece of tissue. Both operations result in discontinuities in the retinotectal map, which show that the position-dependent entities in the tectum serve as targets for retinal elements (Fig. 9.22). That these tectal entities (positional markers, R. Levine and Jacobson, 1974) are expressed independently of the tectal polarity is shown by the discontinuity of the retinotectal map produced by moving a patch from anterior tectum to posterior tectum without rotation (M. Jacobson and Levine, 1975*b*). This shows that positional information used in setting up an orderly map in the tectum is vectorial and not merely scalar. Rotation of patches of tectum in the goldfish (Sharma and Gaze, 1971; Yoon, 1975*a,b,* 1977) has also shown that the tectal patch behaves autonomously in serving as a target for retinal axons.

Additional evidence of the active role of the tectum in establishing the polarity of the map is provided by experiments in which surgical removal of the caudal half of the tectum, which results in rostrocaudal compression of the entire retinal projection to the residual half of the tectum, also results in compression of the projection to a rotated patch in the residual half-tectum (Yoon, 1977). In such cases, the patch and the surrounding tectum each express their polarity independently in aligning the retinotectal projection to the patch and to the surrounding tectum, respectively (Fig. 9.23). In all cases, regardless of the orientation of the patch, including turning the grafted patch upside down, thus producing inversion in only one axis (Yoon, 1975*b*), the reestablished projection respects the original polarity of the patch, and a sharp discontinuity of the retinotectal projection

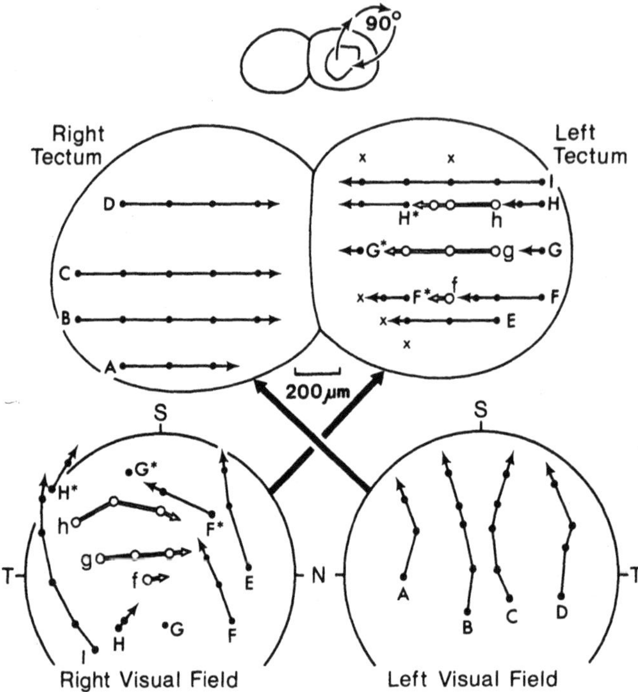

Figure 9.22. Expression of tectal positional markers in a rotated patch of tectum of adult *Xenopus* occurs independently of the expression of tectal positional markers in the surrounding tectum. Visuotectal map made 195 days after rotation of the patch shows that optic axons recognize the original positional markers in the patch, as well as those in the surrounding tectum. The conventions are the same as in Fig. 9.9. From R. Levine and M. Jacobson, *Exp. Neurol.* *43*:527–538 (1974).

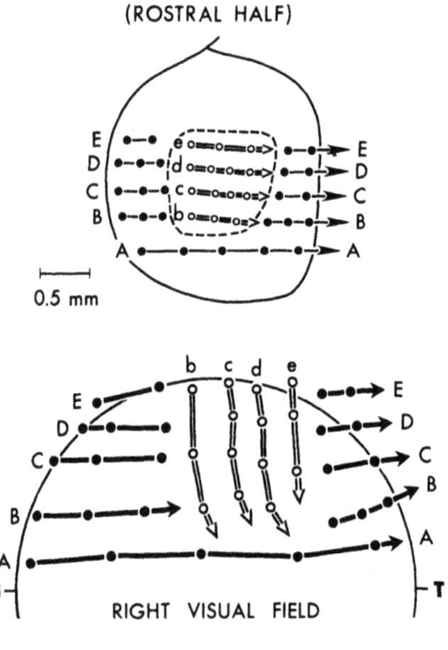

Figure 9.23. Compression of the visuotectal projection to a 90° rotated tectal patch in the goldfish with retention of the original polarity of the projection to the patch. The map was made 184 days after rotation of the tectal patch in the rostral half-tectum immediately after removal of the caudal half-tectum. The arrows on the tectum point to the caudal part of the tectum that had been removed. N, Nasal visual field; T, temporal visual field. From M. G. Yoon, *J. Physiol. (London)* *264*:379–410 (1977).

occurs at the patch margins. Such evidence in both the goldfish and the frog shows that the tectum as a whole, as well as a small tectal patch, has a sovereign effect in determining the polarity of the retinotectal projection, and that this effect is stronger than the tendency of optic axons, interacting only with one another, to assemble themselves in a continuous map.

9.9. Expression of Locus Specificity in the Assembly of the Retinotectal Map

Several methods have been used for studying the expression of neuronal locus specificity during development of the retinotectal map. First, the normal appearances of the map during normal development can be observed; second, the map can be studied during and after regeneration of the optic nerve in fish and amphibians; third, the response of the map to removal of neurons in the retina and/or tectum can be determined; and, fourth, the effects of drugs can be determined that destroy retinal and tectal cells or inhibit their proliferation or differentiation. As the destructive effects of these methods increase from first to fourth, their results become increasingly more difficult to interpret in terms of normal development. In each case, the retinotectal map that develops after experimental perturbation must be assayed and compared with the normal map, and the normal maps obtained at various stages of assembly must be compared with one another and with the adult map. Several methods of assaying the map are available: (1) tests of visually guided behavior, (2) histological methods of tracing the optic axons from the retina to the tectum and other visual centers, and (3) electrophysiological mapping. Each of these techniques has its advantages and its limitations. Thus the tests of visually guided behavior show whether there are functional connections between the retina and visual centers but do not localize the function to any particular visual centers or to any synapses in those centers. The anatomical methods do not show whether the demonstrated structures are functional. Electrophysiological mapping can show whether the pattern of the map is normal and orderly, and functional synapses can be demonstrated by recording postsynaptically.

Normally, a ganglion cell at a particular retinal position always projects its axon to a particular position in the map of axon endings in the tectum. Thus the axon terminals originating in the retina are deployed in the tectum in a spatial pattern or map which reduplicates the pattern of deployment of the ganglion cells in the retina. To demonstrate this electrophysiologically, a microelectrode is lowered into the tectum at a succession of positions farther and farther back on the tectum, and nerve action potentials are recorded at each of these successive positions only by providing the animal with a visual stimulus at appropriate and successively temporal positions in the visual field. In this manner, we can map the visuotectal projection (M. Jacobson, 1962; M. Jacobson and Gaze, 1964). This procedure has become the standard method of assaying the effects of experimental surgery to the retina or tectum (references on this topic include Gaze *et al.*, 1963, 1965; M. Jacobson and Gaze, 1965; Sharma, 1972*a,b,c,d;* Yoon, 1971,

1972*a,b,* 1976). In normal adult animals the visuotectal projection and the retinotectal projection can be regarded as equivalent, but they cannot be assumed to be equivalent in experimental animals with retinal lesions or during development when the intraretinal circuits and visual optics are changing. Because the map is obtained extracellularly from presynaptic terminals of retinal axons in the tectum, it does not show whether those terminals have formed functional synaptic connections in the tectum, and it should not be misused to make inferences about such connections. The retinotectal projection provides a convenient assay of the locus specificities of the retinal ganglion cells, but does not provide an assay of functional connectivity between them and tectal neurons. Such as assay can be obtained only by recording beyond the synapse, that is, by assaying the postsynaptic potentials arising in tectal neurons when retinal neurons are stimulated appropriately. This can be done by recording intracellularly from single tectal neurons (Witpaard, 1976), by recording extracellularly from individual tectal neurons (Lettvin *et al.,* 1961; Grüsser and Grüsser-Cornehls, 1968, 1973; Fite, 1969; Skarf, 1973; Skarf and Jacobson, 1974), or by recording extracellular field potentials in the tectum (J. A. Freeman and Stone, 1969; Chung *et al.,* 1974*a,b*).

The map is also limited with respect to the information that can be obtained from it. It provides no more than relative information about the disposition of the position-dependent properties across the retinal cell population. The map does not show which locus specificities are present; it only shows that the order of their spatial deployment in a retinal population occurs in a particular direction and across a population of cells within defined spatial boundaries. Thus it is extremely risky to try to correlate discontinuities or continuities in the retinal fiber projection to the tectum with a history of surgical manipulation of the retinotectal system. The main limitation of the mapping technique is that after experimental surgery to either the eye or the tectum, it cannot assay the range of the position-dependent properties in the retinal cell population or tell whether the set of properties that is finally expressed is complete, reduced, or augmented.

Exponents of retinotectal mapping with microelectrodes have a tendency to confuse the retinotectal map with the developmental mechanisms that produce it. There is some danger in this kind of confusion of levels because each level has unique concepts and research methods that are not applicable to other levels. Thus, on an abstract level, the expression of the developmental program of retinal ganglion cells can be represented as a series of retinotectal maps, but the latter do not indicate morphogenetic or biochemical mechanisms. The physicochemical level, which cannot be adduced from the maps, includes the program of synthesis and assembly of molecules in the retinal ganglion cells, which results in the acquisition of position-dependent cellular properties. The morphogenesis of the connection between retina and tectum is on yet another level, which cannot at present be adduced from either the maps or the biochemical assays.

Morphogenesis of the system can be assayed in terms of elongation and branching of axons, selection of axonal pathways, tentative or permanent contacts between optic axons and tectal cells, selection of synaptic sites, and formation of functional synapses. In this example, it is fair to believe that the mapping phenomena will eventually be explained in terms of morphogenesis and that the latter will be explicable in biochemical terms. Because we are so far from reducing one level to another and because different concepts and methods are used at the different levels, we have to respect the independence of the three levels of description of development of the retinotectal system. In order to avoid confusion we have to be very cautious in transferring data from one level to the others. Rarely, in developmental neurobiology has it become possible to grasp all the levels of description in a coherent synthesis.

9.9.1. Assembly of the Retinotectal Map during Normal Development

There are several ways in which the population of retinal ganglion cells can form connections with the tectal cell population during development. First, both retina and tectum may develop independently without forming connections until the development of both neuronal populations is complete. This seems to occur in the chick retinotectal system, in which retinal axons enter the tectum during the period of tectal histogenesis, but synapse formation is delayed until both retinal and tectal sets have been completed (LaVail and Cowan, 1971*a,b;* J. P. Kelly and Cowan, 1972; Crossland *et al.,* 1974*a,b;* Rager, 1976*b*). Second, synaptic connections between retinal axons and tectal cells may commence before the entire populations of retinal and tectal neurons have been produced. This occurs in the frog (Gaze *et al.,* 1974; T. M. Scott, 1974; T. M. Scott and Lázár, 1976; M. Jacobson, 1977), and probably in other amphibians and in fish in which the number of retinal and tectal neurons increases throughout life. In both the first and second cases, an individual retinal axon may form a connection only once with the "correct" tectal neurons, or it may initially form connections with the "correct" neurons and also with "incorrect" neurons from which it later retracts its connections; or, alternatively, the retinal axon may initially connect only with the "incorrect" tectal neurons, and may form a succession of temporary "incorrect" connections before finally making connections with the "correct" neurons. We do not know what really happens to individual retinal axons as they selectively connect with tectal neurons, but several hypotheses have been proposed.

In 1974, Gaze *et al.* put forward their hypothesis of "shifting retinotectal connections" which has captured the popular imagination. They proposed that each retinal axon in *Xenopus* forms a succession of temporary synaptic connections with different tectal cells as the axon adjusts its position in the retinotectal map to accommodate newly produced retinal axons and tectal neurons. This adjustment is required, they argued, because the patterns of growth of retinal and tectal cell populations appear to be grossly mismatched—circumferential rings of cells are apparently added to the retina (Straznicky and Gaze, 1971), while lines of cells are added at the caudomedial margin of the tectum (Straznicky and Gaze, 1972)—and because synaptic connections develop during this period of retinal and tectal growth starting at tadpole Stage 46 and continuing through metamorphosis (T. M. Scott, 1974; Chung *et al.,* 1974*b*). In postulating a shift of the retinal projection to the tectum on these grounds, they assumed that all retinal ganglion cells project to the tectum, in spite of evidence that the retina projects to several other visual centers (Scalia and Fite, 1974). Even if retinal growth does not match tectal growth, it may match growth of the visual centers as a whole.

While the tectal pattern of histogenesis has been confirmed (Currie and Cowan, 1974*b;* M. Jacobson, 1977), the original observations of Straznicky and

Gaze (1971) showing that retinal histogenesis in *Xenopus* is radially symmetrical have been refuted. The pattern of retinal histogenesis in *Xenopus* is markedly asymmetrical from tadpole Stage 53 through metamorphosis, with about 10 times as many cells added at the ventral as at the dorsal margin of the retina (M. Jacobson, 1976*a;* D. H. Beach and Jacobson, 1978). Thus the patterns of retinal histogenesis and tectal histogenesis are not grossly mismatched in *Xenopus* and thus the principal premise is refuted on which the "shifting connection" hypothesis was founded. I do not know of an example from the recent history of developmental neurobiology that more aptly illustrates the thesis that science advances by a series of conjectures and refutations (Popper, 1962). It is ironical, however, that although the hypothesis of "shifting connections" has been refuted in *Xenopus,* the species which gave rise to the initial conjecture, temporary connections are not thereby excluded in other species or in other systems. However, no method has yet been devised that can decisively demonstrate that an identified presynaptic ending has moved its connections from one postsynaptic element to another. There are many instances in which movement of synapses occurs over considerable distances because of displacement of the synapses by growth of the neuron, and especially of the dendrites, but there need be no break in the functional and structural stability of the synapse in such cases. Even in the case of the apparently transient connections between climbing fibers and somatic thorns of Purkinje cells, there is little evidence that the synapses are disrupted when they move from the cell body to the outgrowing dendrites of the Purkinje cells. Direct demonstration of the movement of an individual retinal axon terminal from one tectal cell to a succession of others is especially difficult because the movement is presumed to occur at the same time as the dendrites of tectal neurons extend into the superficial neuropil, and their synapses formed at one stage may be passively moved by hundreds of micrometers from their initial positions while maintaining the original pre- to postsynaptic relationships. Demonstration of the mere presence of synapses between retinal axons and tectal cells (T. M. Scott, 1974; Chung *et al.,* 1974*b*) is thus of little relevance to the problem of whether those synapses are permanent or labile or whether they are sessile or mobile.

Mapping the visuotectal projection in *Xenopus* tadpoles at different stages of development (Gaze *et al.,* 1974) is a singularly ineffective method of showing whether synapses are sessile or mobile—the map is made from presynaptic terminals and does not show whether they have formed functional connections. Even if such connections were to be demonstrated, the visuotectal map is not a retinotectal map, and it merely shows a changing relationship between visual space and tectal space during development without taking changes in visual optics or intraretinal circuits into account. For those reasons, the conclusions reached by Gaze *et al.* (1974) about movements of retinotectal connects are hardly worth taking seriously in the form in which they are presented, as a series of visuotectal maps. Such maps show that the retinal locus specificities are expressed in the assembly of an orderly retinotectal map from shortly after the time of arrival of the retinal axons in the tectum, and the observation that the alignment and order of the map do not change shows that the locus specificities continue to be expressed throughout development. The maps do not show whether the order is due entirely to interactions between retinal axons themselves or whether interactions between axons and tectal cells also occur. The tectum must, however, be involved in aligning the map even if the deployment of the axons is determined by interactions among themselves. That this role is not exerted by a single polarizing focus in the tectum but rather is distributed in small patches of the tectum is shown by the fact that retinal axons respect the polarity of a translocated and rotated patch of tectum in forming a map on the patch (R. Levine and Jacobson, 1974). Expression of the locus specificities of tectal patches independently of the locus specificities in the surrounding tectum shows only that in such experiments the affinities between retinal axons and tectal cells are greater than the affinities between retinal axons themselves; it does not exclude the possibility that axons interact with one another during normal development. A simple rule, that the affinity between axons is an inverse function of the distance between their ganglion cells in the retina, could result in assembly of the axons in retinotopic order. Affinities and disaffinities between axons have been observed *in vivo* (Speidel, 1942, 1964) as well as *in vitro* (Dunn, 1971) and are discussed in Section 4.5. However, the suggestion that interactions between retinal axons may play a role in assembly of the retinotectal map (M. Jacobson, 1960*a*, 1967, 1969, 1970*b*; R. Levine and Jacobson, 1974; J. E. Cooke and Horder, 1974) rests, at present, entirely on indirect evidence of the sort given above. Theoretical models of self-assembly of optic axons in the tectum (Prestige and Willshaw, 1975; Willshaw and von der Malsburg, 1976) ignore the evidence given above and in Section 9.8 that patches of tectum can exert an effect on the pattern of optic axons which clearly dominates any tendency that the axons may have to assemble themselves.

The relationship between retinal axons growing into the tectum and the timetable of tectal histogenesis has been studied in *Xenopus* by labeling the retinal axons with [^{3}H]proline injected into one eye, and at the same time injecting [^{3}H]thymidine to label the retinal and tectal cells originating at that time (T. M. Scott and Lázár, 1976; M. Jacobson, 1977). Using that technique, T. M. Scott and Lázár (1976) reported that when both labels were injected at Stage 50 in *Xenopus* and the animals were killed 3 days later, the labeled retinal axons and tectal cells were congruent. However, if the animals were killed 2 or 4 weeks after the injections, the proline-labeled axons extended about 150 μm caudal to the rostral limit of the band of labeled tectal cells. It should be noted that they measured the disparity between the two labels in the way which gives the maximum dispartiy, namely from the most rostral boundary of thymidine-labeled tectal cells to the most caudal boundary of the proline-labeled axons. As their Fig. 9 shows, the thymidine-labeled cells form a band about 200 μm wide rostrocaudally. In fact, the proline-labeled axons extend into, but not across, the band of thymidine-labeled cells. Therefore, their conclusions that the results show "that a shift *does* occur and that the amount of shift observed is consistent with the previous electrophysiological evidence of Gaze *et al.* (1974)" do not really follow from their results. I have measured the area of proline-labeled axons as shown in T. M. Scott and Lázár (1976) and find that the area increases in the 2 weeks after the injection, when the animal develops from Stage 50 to 54, but that no further increase occurs in the following 2 weeks during which the animal develops to Stage 55, although the tectum triples its surface area during that time.

Using the same technique of intraocular injection of [^{3}H]proline and intraperitoneal injection of [^{3}H]thymidine, but in a larger series of animals injected at various stages from 46 to 66, I have shown that proline-labeled axons remain juxtaposed with tectal cells that were present before the time of the operation and do not move later across the zone of labeled cells into the zone of cells added to the tectum in the survival period after the injection (M. Jacobson, 1977). Measurements of the surface area of the tectum containing labeled retinal axons at various times up to 37 days after the injection of the label show no increase in the proline-labeled area, although the total surface area of the tectum increases continuously, as shown in Fig. 9.24. In a control experiment, I crushed the optic nerve in frogs at Stages 53–56 after about 15,000 retinal axons had already entered the tectum, and those axons, labeled with [^{3}H]proline before the optic nerve crush, were later found to have regenerated to the area in the rostrolateral part of the tectum that they had previously occupied. During this regeneration, an additional 15,000 retinal ganglion cells had been born and their axons, unlabeled, had invaded the tectum concurrently with the labeled, regenerated axons. The unlabeled axons were also found to have taken their correct places in the tectum, and autoradiographs showed the unlabeled axons clearly segregated from the labeled axons in the tectum and in the correct juxtaposition to the band of tectal cells labeled

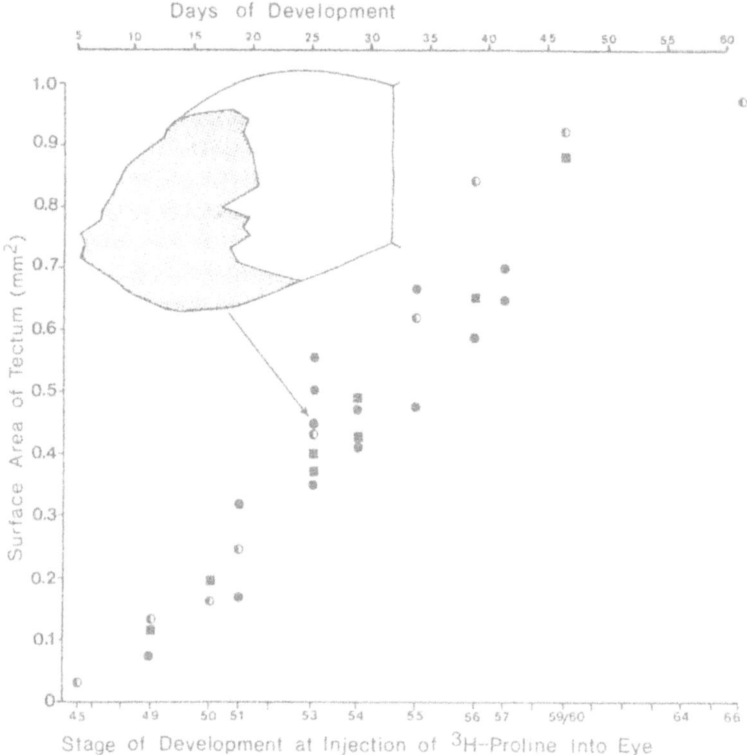

Figure 9.24. Surface area of the tectum to one side of midline (as shown at upper left of figure) in 21 tadpoles that each received a single injection of [^{3}H]proline at various stages of development. The tectal surface area over the labeled retinal axons in the superficial layers of tectum (stippled) was measured in autoradiographic serial sections in animals killed 1–2 days (■) or 16–37 days (•) after the injection, compared with the tectal surface area of uninjected normal controls (◐, each point the mean of four tecta). Regardless of the period of development after the injection, the labeled retinal axons occupy an area of tectum that correlates with the total tectal area of normal controls at the same stage of injection. The surface of the tectum shown at the upper left is from an animal that had received intraocular [^{3}H]proline at Stage 53, and was killed 33 days later, at Stage 66. The stippled area is the part of the tectum labeled with [^{3}H]proline. From M. Jacobson, *Brain Res. 127*:55–67 (1977).

immediately before the optic nerve was crushed. These results, of course, do not give any indication of the connectivity of individual elements of the map, but they show that the populations of labeled and unlabeled retinal axons and tectal cells retain constant spatial relationships during normal development as well as after regeneration of the optic nerve. Because label incorporated into optic axons before regeneration can easily be detected in the axons after they have regenerated to the tectum, and because the label is confined to axons in their correct positions, it can be concluded that extensive branching of axons into incorrect regions of the tectum does not occur. Thus the evidence shows that large movements of optic axons in relation to their associated tectal cells do not occur.

9.9.2. Assembly of the Retinotectal Map during Regeneration of the Optic Nerve

Adult fish and amphibians can regain vision as a result of optic nerve regeneration, and this phenomenon has provided a means of studying the mechanisms of regeneration of optic nerve fibers and of the formation of connections between optic axons and their targets in the visual centers. With the reservation that regeneration does not exactly recapitulate ontogeny, regeneration of the optic nerve may be used as a model of development of the retinotectal projection. Yet, in spite of much effort, studies of optic nerve regeneration have been of limited value in disclosing the mechanisms of nerve growth, pathway selection, target selection, and formation of synaptic connections. The salient result that emerges from all the investigations is that optic axons have a strong tendency to regain their positions in the retinotectal map, and that functional connections are formed after regeneration on the basis of the inherent specificities of the optic axons (Gaze, 1960, 1970, reviews).

A series of studies by Sperry (1943, 1944, 1945*b*, 1948; reviewed in 1951*a,b*) show that visuomotor coordination recovers completely after regeneration of the optic nerve in adult amphibians. These observations of behavior led him to infer that the optic nerve fibers regenerate to the correct positions in the visual centers, especially in the optic tectum. This has been confirmed more directly by recording the electrical activity in the optic tectum when stimulating the retina with a small spot of light or other suitable visual stimulus (Gaze, 1959; M. Jacobson, 1960*b*, 1961*a,b;* Gaze and M. Jacobson, 1963*a;* M. Jacobson and Gaze, 1965). Not only is an orderly, continuous, and properly aligned retinotectal map restored in many cases, but also the different functional classes of optic nerve fibers end at approximately normal depths in the tectum after regeneration of the optic nerve in adult frogs (Maturana *et al.,* 1959; Gaze and Keating, 1969).

Recovery of vision has been reported following a variety of surgical rearrangements of connections between the eye and brain in adult amphibians. Optic nerve section has been combined with inversion of the eye (Sperry, 1944, 1951*a;* L. S. Stone, 1944, 1948, 1953, 1960); an eye has been transplanted to the opposite orbit (L. S. Stone, 1930, 1941; L. S. Stone and Cole, 1943); the left and right eyes have been transposed (Sperry, 1945*b*); and the optic chiasm has been excised and each optic nerve deflected into the ipsilateral optic tract (Sperry, 1945*b*). Visual recovery also occurs in urodeles after transplantation of an eye to the orbit of another salamander of the same species (L. S. Stone, 1930; L. S. Stone and Cole,

1943) and after exchanges of eyes between different species of salamanders (Harrison, 1929; L. S. Stone, 1930: Twitty, 1932; L. S. Stone and Ellison, 1940). These observations on the formation of connections of optic axons in the wrong side of the brain show that optic nerve fibers treat the left and right sides of the brain as mirror-image replicas (this does not relate to the left–right asymmetry discussed in Section 7.11), and the capacity of an eye from one species of urodele to form a retinotectal map in the brain of another species shows that the same mechanisms operate in different species of urodeles and might thus be of greater universality.

In all cases, when the operation results in inversion of one or both axes of the retina, visuomotor reflexes are correspondingly inverted. For example, after 180° rotation of the eye, the animal's attempts to capture a fly in the nasosuperior quadrant of the visual field are misdirected toward the temporoinferior visual field. Optokinetic reflexes are also inverted: after 180° rotation of the eye, the frog or salamander follows vertical bars moving in a nasotemporal direction across the visual field, whereas normal amphibians respond only to temporanasal movement of the stimulus. The surgical operations result in inversion of spatial localization and movement detection, both of which depend for their realization on orderly connections of the eye with the brain, although not necessarily with the tectum. Some visuomotor behavior is mediated by the diencephalon (Muntz, 1962*a,b*). Optokinetic responses are mediated by pretectal nuclei and are unaffected by removal of the tectum (Székely, 1971; R. J. Mark and Feldman, 1972).

The inverted visuomotor reflexes are permanent and are not corrected by experience or learning (Sperry, 1944, 1951*a,b;* L. S. Stone, 1944, 1953). In one newt, inverted visuomotor reflexes were observed for 4½ years after inversion of the eye, but recovery of normal optokinetic reflexes and accurate localization of a lure occurred immediately after the eye was returned to its normal orientation (L. S. Stone, 1953). All these experiments show that the optic nerve fibers in adult amphibians regenerate to form a continuous map properly aligned in the optic tectum irrespective of the alignment of the eye from which they originate or the side of the brain with which they connect, and regardless of the functional effect. The observations that optic nerve fibers show a very strong tendency to regenerate to the tectum and to re-form a functional retinotectal map pose a number of questions, none of which can yet be answered fully.

First, there are several questions relating to the routes taken by optic axons to the visual centers. How do the fibers select the correct pathway? Does pathway selection require interactions between axons and cells along the pathway? Do regenerated axons make use of vestiges of the degenerated axons? Are the mechanisms of selective regeneration the same as those of selection of a pathway in the embryo? How do the fibers select the proper side of the brain to enter at the optic chiasm, and how do fibers diverge from the main visual tract to enter branches to various visual centers?

Second, there are several questions about interactions between fibers during their growth. If interactions between axons occur, do they take place all along their length or only close to or at their growing tips? Do the interactions occur only during outgrowth of the axon, or are they maintained after the system has reached a steady state in the adult? Are interactions only positive (i.e., affinities resulting in fasciculation), or are there inhibitory interactions or disaffinities between axons? What are the mechanisms of such interactions; what are their strengths and the ranges of their actions?

Third, there are several questions relating to the control of axonal elongation and axonal branching. It is known that axons growing from eyes transplanted to the nose, ear, or flank will continue growing indefinitely unless they arrive at one of the visual centers of the brain (R. M. May and Detwiler, 1925; R. M. May, 1927*a,b;* Van Campenhout, 1935; Rensch and Nolte, 1949*a,b;* Constantine-Paton and Capranica, 1975, 1976*a,b*). So the question arises, what determines that the axon stops elongating when it arrives at a target? Does the axon approach the target by random branching, or is it attracted by a neurotropic stimulus released from the target?

The direct trajectory of the optic axons from the retina to their targets in the various visual centers in the adult might lead us to think that they grow directly to their terminations without widespread branching and without deviating from the correct track. However, it is risky to make inferences about the development of any system without some knowledge of the intermediate stages leading to the final product. At present, it is safe to say only that there must be a sorting-out process to ensure that optic nerve fibers arising from different places in the retina will terminate in the correct places in the brain. Some sorting out must occur even before the optic axons enter the tectum, since the optic axons enter the correct branches of the optic tract. When they arrive in the pretectal region, the axons destined for the dorsomedial part of the tectum may enter the medial brachium of the optic tract, while fibers destined for the ventrolateral part of the tectum may enter the lateral brachium (M. Jacobson, 1960*a,* 1961*a,b,* 1966; Arora and Sperry, 1962; Attardi and Sperry, 1963). The problem that is posed here is the general problem of how growing nerve fibers select the proper pathway, and especially how fibers that have grown along the same pathway are able to diverge into separate pathways at the proper branching points. Evidence of branching and of guidance is indirect and inadequate. Attempts to discover intermediate stages in the regeneration of the optic nerve in adult frogs showed that the earliest visuotectal projection map is random in both axes, that some cases also show a map that is organized in the nasotemporal axis but random in the dorsoventral axis, and that, finally, the order of the map is restored in both axes (M. Jacobson, 1960*a,* 1961*a,b;* Gaze and Jacobson, 1963*a*). This may indicate that the selection of a target is made independently in two axes, or that the interaction between optic axons is stronger in the nasotemporal axis than in the dorsoventral axis, or it may mean neither the former nor the latter, but may merely indicate that the resolution of the mapping method is better in one axis than another. In any event, the results of such experiments are difficult to understand.

Attardi and Sperry (1963) tried to determine the route taken by regenerating optic axons in the tectum of adult goldfish by examining serial sections of the tectum. They observed that optic axons grow through deafferented regions of the tectum to reach their correct destinations, and concluded that the optic axons "appear to be not only rather specifically destination bound, but also definitely inclined to follow particular routes to their respective destinations." Such observations might lead one to suspect that the nerve fibers are guided by preformed chemical markers along their routes or are attracted by specific chemicals emanating from their final destinations. The observations of DeLong and Coulombre

(1968) showing that optic axons appear to grow preferentially toward their correct destinations from retinal grafts placed on the surface of the tectum of the chick embryo have been shown by S. Goldberg (1974) to be the result of passive displacement of the grafts relative to the underlying tectum rather than of selective growth of optic axons toward their correct tectal targets, as was first supposed.

9.9.3. Assembly of the Retinotectal Map after Surgical Removal of Parts of the Retinotectal System

Interpretation of the retinotectal map after surgical removal of parts of both the retina and tectum is a matter so esoteric that I am glad that my present task does not involve an exhaustive analysis. I have been relieved of that obligation by reviews of the obstacles and pitfalls that impede the way to any understanding of the results of such experiments (M. Jacobson, 1974*a,b,* 1976*a;* R. K. Hunt and Jacobson, 1974*c*). I shall, therefore, confine my remarks to a few generalities.

The question posed by the finding that removal of brain tissue results in a reorganization of the residual structures is "What is changing or being reorganized?" Are the structures themselves replaced? If not, are the properties or specificities of the residual cells replaced or changed so that new cellular associations can form on the basis of the new specificities? Alternatively, do none of the above occur, but instead do the residual structures merely make different associations on the basis of their original properties and specificities? The reader will realize that these questions merely pose the problem, alluded to in Section 9.1, of what components of the system are sensitive to changes in their context: are cell deployment, cellular properties, or operations of cells sensitive to the change in context produced by such surgical operations? The question has not been possible to answer. To assert, as many authors have done, that one rather than another of the former alternatives actually occurs, is to claim to have proved what is at present unprovable.

When we consider the experimental strategies that have been used to study specificity and plasticity in the nervous system, we are struck by the lack of critical appreciation of the **limitations of the methodology.** For example, a classical strategy is to make size disparities between neuron set A and set B, by removing parts, for example, of retina or tectum during embryonic development and ultimately mapping the final configuration of connections or projections between the two sets. "Specificity" in the system is assayed by determining whether the final map is normal or compressed, expanded or distorted in any other way. Unfortunately, this strategy is intrinsically limited because the result can never be interpreted unambiguously. One cannot ever tell, without other controls, whether the set of elements present in the altered map is the same as the set that would have developed without surgical interference. Thus the cells in set A (retina) and/or set B (tectum) might have been replaced by new cells. Or the cells might have changed their properties; or, if their properties were retained, their expression might have been altered in the novel context produced by the experimental situation.

Attempts to force such maps to reveal the rules governing connectivity between two sets of nerve cells lead inevitably to circular arguments: the map is an operational indication of the relatively orderly expression of position-dependent properties in a set of elements, but after experimental surgery neither the identity of the set nor the expression of its properties can be determined from the map. It is not known whether the same elements are present or the same properties persist, nor whether the expression of the properties has been altered under the experimental conditions. Realization of these limitations of the experimental methods reduces confidence in many of the conclusions that have been reached about neuronal specificity and the mechanism of formation of synaptic connections in the retinotectal system or in other neural systems in which uncontrolled changes may result from ablation of part of the nervous system.

The main experimental results of producing size disparities in the retinotectal system can now be reviewed in the light of these considerations of the limitations of the methodology. In the initial study of the effects of making size disparities in the retinotectal system, Attardi and Sperry (1963) removed part of the retina and cut the optic nerve in the goldfish. They showed histologically that after 3–67 days the optic nerve fibers grow back only to the appropriate parts of the tectum. They concluded that the regenerating optic nerve fibers are "destination bound" and that the optic nerve fibers grow by the most direct pathway to their proper synaptic sites in the tectum, bypassing inappropriate sites on the way. In such studies, each animal is studied at only one postoperative stage, and whether the system has arrived at a steady state or is at an intermediate state cannot be known. A similar criticism can be leveled at the study of retinotectal size disparities in the goldfish by M. Jacobson and Gaze (1965). We did two kinds of experiments; in the first, the entire population of optic nerve fibers were allowed to regenerate into a residual lateral or medial part of the tectum; in the second, we studied the regeneration of about half the normal number of optic nerve fibers to the intact tectum. In both experiments, it seemed as if, by 139 days, the optic fibers had returned only to the appropriate positions in the tectum, and the assumption was made that the system had reached its final state.

The first strong suggestion of plasticity in the retinotectal system of the goldfish appeared after regeneration of the optic nerve into a residual rostral half-tectum (Gaze and Sharma, 1970). In such studies on goldfish, the entire retina is found to send its fibers into the residual part of the tectum: the optic fibers are deployed in the correct order, but are compressed by a factor of about 2 into the rostrocaudal axis of the tectum (Yoon, 1971; Sharma, 1972*a*). Yoon (1972*a,b*) showed that such compression of the optic nerve fibers into the residual part of the tectum can occur into either mediolateral or rostrocaudal axis of the tectum, and is reversible (Fig. 9.25).

There is some evidence that the result of removing a part of the tectum may depend on the time after the operation. Thus Sharma (1972*b*) found that a few weeks after removing the central part of the goldfish tectum and crushing the optic nerve, the regenerated optic nerve fibers return to their correct places in the tectum, leaving a large central scotoma in the visual field. In other fish, examined months after removal of the central part of the tectum, the scotoma is not present and the fibers from the entire retina seem to be compressed into the residual tectum. These results suggest that the optic nerve fibers initially return to their proper places in the tectum (as shown by Attardi and Sperry in 1963 and by M. Jacobson and Gaze in 1965), but later the optic nerve terminals are repositioned in order to accommodate all the regenerating optic fibers into the residual part of the tectum, as found by Yoon (1971, 1972*a,b*).

Two different mechanisms have been invoked to explain the phenomena of compression and expansion of the retinotectal map after removal of part of the tectum or part of the retina. The first type of mechanism invokes regulation of tectal or retinal position-dependent properties of the reduced set of retinal and tectal elements—after surgical reduction of the set, the residual elements assume the full range of properties of an entire set. The second type of hypothesis invokes interaction between the optic axons which results in their orderly deployment to form a map in the available tectal space. Neither mechanism alone can account for all the observations. Anybody who states that the evidence clearly favors either one

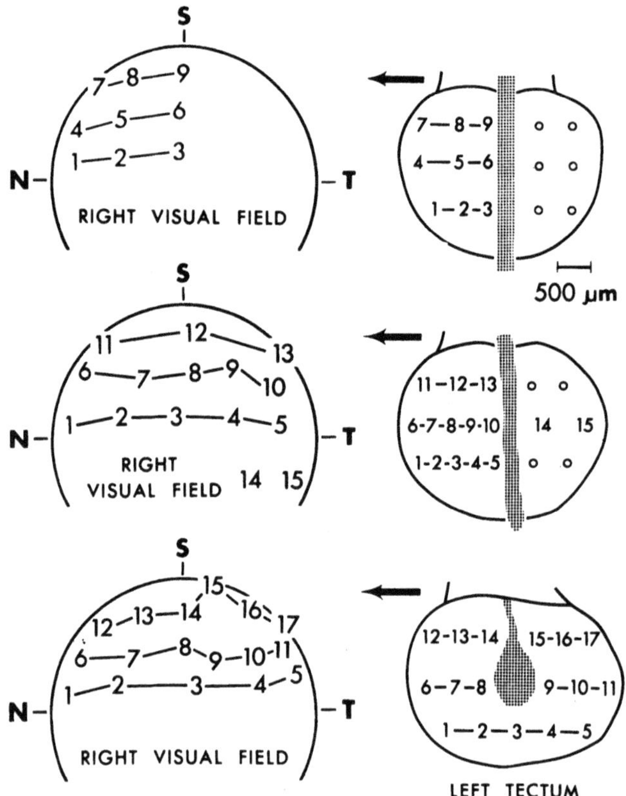

Figure 9.25. Reversible compression of the retinotectal map in goldfish. The top map was made immediately after insertion of a gelatin film in a mediolateral cut bisecting the tectum. The middle map, made 67 days later, shows the compression of the entire visual field into the rostral half-tectum. The bottom map, obtained 184 days postoperatively, after resorption of the gelatin film, shows expansion of the projection to the caudal half-tectum. The arrow points rostrally in the midsaggital plane of the tectum. N,S,T, Nasal, superior, and temporal visual fields. From M. G. Yoon, *Exp. Neurol. 35:*565–577 (1972).

or the other mechanism shows that by "clear" they mean anything that has the same degree of confusion as their own thoughts on the subject.

There is evidence for and against tectal regulation, and the conflict is unlikely to be resolved before the cellular mechanisms of regulation are better understood. Evidence for regulation is provided by Yoon (1976), who showed that when the map reforms rapidly, within a few weeks after removal of the caudal half-tectum plus section of the optic nerve, a partial map forms initially, appropriate to the residual part of the tectum, and compression of the entire map into the residual tectum occurs later, at 40–90 days postoperative. However, when optic nerve regeneration is delayed for more than 40 days after removal of the caudal half-tectum, an entire but compressed map forms from the start. Yoon concludes that tectal regulation is delayed for about 3–6 weeks after removal of part of the tectum.

In conflict with Yoon's conclusion is the evidence that when the optic nerve is cut after compression or expansion of the map has occurred, regeneration of the optic nerve results at first in assembly of a partial map appropriate to the residual part of the retinotectal system, and only later does the map compress or expand, as appropriate (J. E. Cook and Horder, 1974). It seems impossible to conceive of a single variable, namely regulation, that could be responsible for such widely divergent results. The conclusion seems inescapable that regulation (however broadly the term is defined) is not the *only* means of altering the spatial dimensions of the retinotectal map without altering its topological pattern. However, it also seems that axon–axon interactions cannot be the only mechanism of setting up the retinotectal map. This is not to imply that axonal interactions have no role to play, as they certainly do, but that they are insufficient to account for the evidence, for example, of mapping to grafted patches of tectum (see Section 9.8).

The notion that optic axons can assemble themselves in retinotopic order as a result of their affinities and disaffinities has been frequently proposed, largely as a theoretical possibility, for there is little direct evidence to support the notion. The possibility that axonal interactions play a role in assembly of the retinotectal map has been advanced in several forms, ranging from little more than a mere statement of the possibility (M. Jacobson, 1966, p. 371; Gaze and Keating, 1972; R. E. Cook and Horder, 1974; R. Levine and Jacobson, 1974, 1975) to more detailed models replete with computer simulations (Prestige and Willshaw, 1975; Willshaw and von der Malsberg, 1976; Hope *et al.*, 1976). These models are considerably weakened by the evidence that fragments of tectum rotated or transplanted to different positions in the tectum of frogs and fish serve as targets for optic axons independently of the surrounding tectum, and that compression of part of the map onto a rotated fragment of the tectum occurs independently of compression of the map to the surrounding part of the tectum of the goldfish (Yoon, 1977). Interactions between optic axons alone are insufficient to explain such results, and interactions between axons and tectal targets must also be invoked.

The phenomena of compression and expansion of the retinotectal map that occur easily and rapidly in adult goldfish occur very slowly if at all in amphibians and in the chick embryo. Removal of part of the tectum and section of the optic nerve in frogs are followed by regeneration of the optic nerve fibers only to the correct positions in the tectum (Straznicky, 1973; Meyer and Sperry, 1973). No compression occurs after removal of the caudal part of the tectum without section of the optic nerve in frogs, but if the optic nerve is cut, compression of the entire retinal projection to the residual half-tectum occurs in 260–414 days in frogs (Udin, 1975, 1976). Because of the long postoperative interval before any compression of the map is seen, it is unlikely that the compression results from tectal regulation or from interactions between the fibers themselves. Rather, slow reorganization of the retinotectal map in the frog probably involves death of the disconnected retinal ganglion cells whose tectal targets have been removed and their replacement by new retinal and tectal cells. No expansion of the retinotectal projection occurs in the chick embryo after the third day of incubation. Removal of a retinal quadrant after the third day of incubation results in permanent deafferentation of the corresponding area of the tectum (DeLong and Coulombre, 1965; Crossland *et al.,* 1974*a*).

Another serious limitation of all the experiments in which the retinal projection is mapped electrophysiologically by recording from presynaptic terminals of optic axons is that they do not show whether the regenerated optic nerve fibers form functional synaptic connections in the tectum either at the correct positions or at anomalous positions. Doubts about the formation of functional synaptic connections by optic fibers at anomalous positions in the tectum are increased by a report that, in the rabbit, optic nerve fibers which can be seen sprouting into tectal locations that they do not normally occupy do not activate tectal cells at anomalous positions but drive tectal neurons only at the normal positions (Chow *et al.,* 1973). In the retinal mapping assay (as used in the goldfish, e.g., by M. Jacobson and Gaze, 1965; Yoon, 1971, 1972*a,b;* Sharma, 1972*a,b*), the presynaptic potentials, indicating the positions of optic fibers in the tectum, may originate from a sessile nerve terminal that has arrived at its final position or from one that is moving about; or the presynaptic potentials may come from a fiber that ends in a nonfunctional synapse, or as we usually assume, from a fiber that terminates in a functional synapse at the position at which we record the potentials.

Whatever the final configuration of connections, we want to know whether it was produced *ab initio* or only after a period of trial and error—and, if so, whether malconnections were eliminated by error elimination, error correction, or error neutralization. To study the kinetics of regrowth of the optic nerve fibers in the tectum will require repeated mapping of the retinotectal projection in the same animal at close intervals during the process of regeneration of the optic nerve. To determine whether the regenerated optic nerve fibers have formed functional connections in the tectum will require postsynaptic recording (Skarf and Jacobson, 1974). Tests of visual behavior are of limited value in this regard for a number of reasons: First, there are other visual centers besides the tectum that might mediate the behavior in the absence of functional retinotectal connections. Second, abnormal behavior might occur even if the optic axons form functional synaptic connections in the tectum, either because the sensory map has expanded or contracted and is not congruent with the motor map or because malconnections have been made in other visual centers. Finally, although tests of visual function in fish and amphibians are relatively crude, the presence of visually guided behavior shows that at least some reflex circuits function normally, and a loss of visual function after a tectal lesion, followed by recovery of vision, shows that either the reflex circuits through the tectum have been restored or an alternative reflex pathway has developed. For example, M. Y. Scott (1977) has shown that the blind region produced in the goldfish immediately after removal of the caudal half of the tectum is gradually filled in as the entire retinal projection compresses onto the residual rostral half of the tectum.

Removal of part of a neuronal population during the time of histogenesis of that population may produce results that are difficult to interpret. The difficulty arises because "regulation" of the residual part may involved changes in nerve cell production and cell migration as well as changes in the genesis and expression of neuronal specificity. Therefore, whenever an experiment requires removal of part of a proliferating nerve cell population, adequate control experiments are required to determine the changes that occur in cell production. These controls have often been omitted or have been inadequate in experiments in which retinotectal size disparities have been produced by removing part of the retina and/or tectum in fish and amphibians at stages of development before cell proliferation has ceased. Surgical operations on such cell populations may result in changes in the rate of cell production, in the spatial pattern of cell proliferation, and in the rate and spatial pattern of cell death. Thus, after removal of the nasal or the temporal half of an eye rudiment in the tailbud frog embryo, and replacement with a temporal or nasal half-eye, respectively, double-nasal (NN) or double-temporal (TT) eyes could be constructed—so-called compound eyes (Gaze *et al.*, 1963, 1965). Similarly, double-ventral (VV) and double-dorsal (DD) compound eyes can be made, but only the former project to the tectum (Straznicky *et al.*, 1974), the DD eyes failing to form an optic nerve. When the projection of the compound eye to the tectum is mapped in the adult frog, each half-eye projects to the entire tectum (Fig 9.26). In the initial interpretation of this result, we made the assumption that each half-eye had expressed the properties of half the set of elements normally present in an entire eye, but no control experiments were done to justify such an assumption. One cannot know from those experiments whether the elements in each half-eye might have been replaced by a full set of elements, whether the properties of the elements might have altered to those of a full set of properties, or whether the properties of the half-set of elements in the retina might have been expressed as a full set of elements in the development of the retinotectal map. J. D. Feldman and Gaze (1972) reported that the pattern of

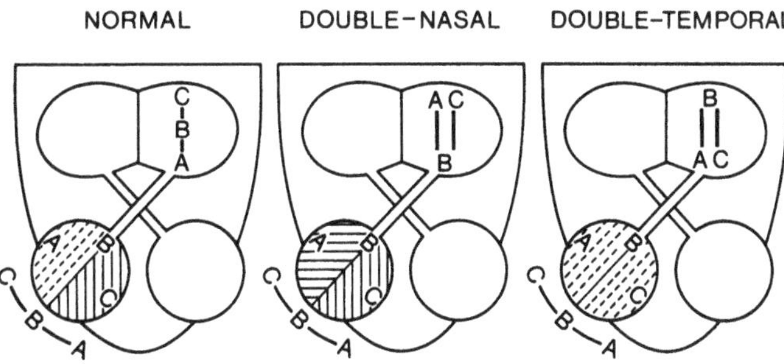

Figure 9.26. Relationship among visual field, retina, and tectum in *Xenopus* with normal retina, double-nasal compound retina, and double-temporal compound retina. Normally points A,B, and C in the visual field project in the same order rostrocaudally on the tectum. In the compound retina, the projection from each half-retina has spread over the whole contralateral tectum. The order of tectal projection from the compound retina is correct for the original half of the retina, but is reversed for the grafted half-retina. From R. M. Gaze, M. Jacobson, and G. Székely, *J. Physiol. (London) 165:*484–499 (1963).

histogenesis is not altered in compound eyes, but their observations were limited to embryonic and early larval stages. Studies of histogenesis of the retina from the embryo to the adult show that the pattern of retinal histogenesis of normal and compound eyes is markedly asymmetrical (M. Jacobson, 1976*a;* D. H. Beach and Jacobson, 1978; Straznicky and Tay, 1978). In the compound eye, the pattern of histogenesis in each half-retina conforms to the pattern of that half in the intact eye (D. H. Beach and Jacobson, 1978; Straznicky and Tay, 1977). Although the rate of retinal cell production and the final total number of ganglion cells in the compound eye have not been measured, rough estimates suggest that they are within the normal limits.

More recently, we made other kinds of compound eyes (M. Jacobson and Hunt, 1973; R. K. Hunt and Jacobson, 1973*b*, 1974*a*) which were constructed from different retinal halves: a nasal half-retina and a ventral half-retina were fused together, or a right nasal half-retina was combined with an inverted left temporal half-retina, for example. In all cases, the half-eye, regardless of its site of origin in the retina, projects to the entire tectum. The most likely explanation of these results is that embryonic regulation has occurred, which could mean that either the half-eye acquires a full set of properties or that the half-set of properties is expressed as a full set in the formation of a retinotectal map. Without knowing the mechanisms of expression of the ganglion cell locus specificities during formation of the retinotectal map, we cannot deduce from the map which specificities are present in the retina as a whole or at any particular retinal position. The elementary strategy, then, of partially excising or reconstituting the retina or tectum, making retinotectal size disparities, which on the face of it appears to be quite simple to interpret, is in reality highly ambiguous. Methods which may resolve some of the ambiguities inherent in the retinotectal mapping assay of neuronal specificity are outlined below.

Postsynaptic recording from tectal cells that are visually driven from both eyes assays the specificity of functional retinotectal synaptic connections. If two neurons with different locations of their cell bodies and different presynaptic trajectories converge to form synaptic connections on the same postsynaptic element, the presynaptic neurons must share the same specificity as regards the selection of a specific synaptic locus. The normal development of such converging inputs is in itself evidence of a shared specificity, but the evidence of a common specificity is much more compelling if the convergence onto a specific target occurs experimentally, for example, after eye rotation and optic nerve regeneration (Skarf and Jacobson, 1974) or after growth of both optic nerves into the same tectum.

Because there is no absolute measure of the specific properties of the elements that compose a neuronal set—the set of ganglion cells in the retina, for example—we are compelled to use some form of comparative or relative measure. The retinotectal map, for example, gives only a relative measure of some parameters within a set, and permits us to map the relative order of elements within the set, but provides no information about the identity of individual elements. Inversions or translocations may be detected directly, but deletions or additions that do not alter the relative order of the elements in the map can be detected only by comparing the unknown set directly with a neuron set of known composition. Thus we lose information about the completeness of the set of nerve fibers projecting from the retina to the tectum because there is nothing in the tectum to compare with an unknown set of optic nerve fibers. One method of avoiding this theoretical impasse is to project two sets of optic nerve fibers into the same tectum, one from a test eye and another from a normal or reference eye grafted into the same socket. The way in which the two sets of optic nerve fibers mingle in the tectum may provide a measure of their shared locus specificities, while the regions of tectum in which the two sets of optic fibers do not mingle may show which specificities are not common to both sets (M. Jacobson, 1973; M. Jacobson and Hunt, 1973; R. K. Hunt and Jacobson, 1974*c*). This can be done either by grafting an additional eye into the same socket as a normal eye in the frog embryo so that both sets of optic nerve fibers grow into the tectum at the same time or, alternatively, by deflecting one optic nerve at the chiasm so that both eyes innervate the tectum on the same side. The latter can be done in adult frogs and goldfish, and can be combined with surgical operations to one or both eyes or to the tectum. This comparative or competitive retinotectal mapping assay must be used with adequate controls to deal with the effects of experimental surgery on cell proliferation, cell migration, and cell death in the retina and tectum, and is potentially able to give information about the completeness and range of the set of locus specificities in a retina that has been surgically reduced or deranged in any other way. By using this strategy with presynaptic retinotectal mapping, we assay the set of retinal locus specificities in the operated eye and compare it directly with the normal set. An experimental result of this kind in a frog is shown in Fig. 9.27.

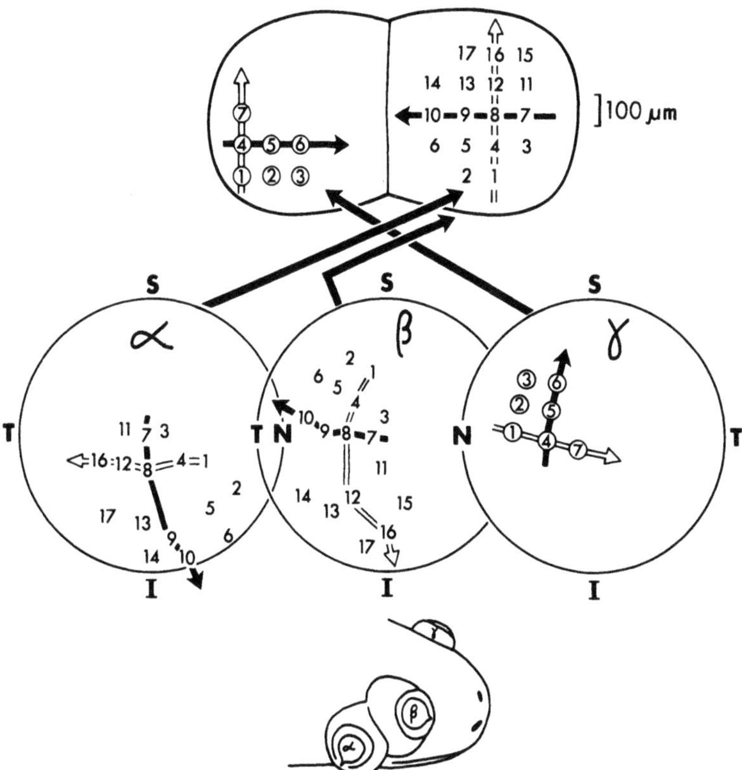

Figure 9.27. Competitive retinotectal innervation assay in a three-eyed frog which compares the set of locus specificities in an experimental retina (α) with that in a normal retina (β) when both sets compete for the same set of tectal targets. That both eyes project in register to the entire tectum shows that the experimental retina, in spite of axial inversion and transplantation from left to right eye socket, has a normal set of locus specificities.

Sperry (1945*b*) showed that vision recovered in frogs after he uncrossed the optic nerves, thus demonstrating that the set of tectal locus specificities on left and right sides are equivalent but mirror-imaged across the midline. More recently, M. Jacobson and Hirsch (1973) found that removal of one eye in frog tadpoles frequently results in formation of complete visuotectal maps to both sides of the midbrain, apparently as a result of branching of the optic axons at the chiasm. Sharma (1972*a,d*) has found that after removal of the tectum on one side in the adult goldfish, the optic axons that normally project to it grow to the tectum on the other side and form a complete projection in register with the projection from the normal eye. However, optic axons from both eyes do not always share the same tectal space. We have found, by microelectrode recording as well as by autoradiographic tracing of the pathways from retina to tectum, that after removal of the tectum on one side the two eyes may project to mutually exclusive zones of the retinotectal map, or both eyes may project, in register, to the same tectal zone (R. Levine and Jacobson, 1975). The map is complete and orderly, although it is composed of irregular patches projecting from one or both eyes, and no part of the map is duplicated. This shows that the orderly deployment of optic axons must be under tectal control, for if it was not there would be cases of duplication of parts of the map. Absence of some regenerating optic axons would result in a discontinuity in the map from the regenerating set of axons, but absence of parts of the map from the normal eye indicates that interaction between the two sets of optic axons may result in functional suppression and even in elimination of some axons from the normal set.

The observations of growth of optic nerve fibers, destined for one tectum, to the other tectum, if the latter is deafferented, or of growth of optic axons to the residual tectum after removal of the tectum to which they are normally destined, seem to imply an action of the tectum on the optic axons at a distance. However, there are alternatives that do not invoke action at a distance. For example, after removal of their tectal targets, optic axons may simply sprout collaterals into all available pathways, including the ipsilateral optic tract, at the chiasm, and the posterior and intertectal commissures, and so reach targets in the residual tectum. Removal of one eye at developmental stages before all the optic axons have arrived at the chiasm may leave the way open to both sides at the chiasm, and axons from the residual eye that were destined for the contralateral side may enter the ipsilateral or both sides. This appears to occur after removal of one eye in frog tadpoles (M. Jacobson and Hirsch, 1973) and in young rats (R. D. Lund *et al.*, 1973). How axons grow selectively to the correct side at the chiasm is not known.

9.10. Expression of Neuronal Specificity of Retinal Ganglion Cells in Albino Mammals

Some of the temporal retinal ganglion cells in albino mammals project their axons across the optic chiasm to the opposite side of the brain, whereas in normal animals those axons do not cross at the chiasm but grow into the same side of the brain, as shown in Fig. 9.28 (Guillery, 1969, 1974). The congenital defect in the routing of optic nerve fibers has been found in all albino animals that have been examined but is most marked in animals that have an extensive binocular visual field and thus a large percentage of optic axons that do not cross at the chiasm.

The relation of the albino gene to the defect found in the visual pathways is not known. Defects have not been found in other parts of the central nervous system of albinos: the commissures and nerve fiber pathways appear to be normal. The albino gene is not the only gene that produces the misrouting of the optic nerve fibers. In the mink, a number of different mutants that result in deficient retinal pigmentation are also associated with misrouting of optic axons. The more severe the retinal pigment defect, the greater the anomalous visual projection (Sanderson *et al.,* 1974). This shows that the retinal pigment deficiency is in some way related to the misrouting of optic axons. It is tempting to suggest that the pigment epithelium of the retina is the source of the positional information obtained by retinal ganglion cells, a suggestion that appears to be reasonable because the entire neural retina can regenerate from the pigment epithelium in amphibians (R. Levine, 1975) and in the chick embryo (Coulombre and Coulombre, 1965). However, in flecked mice, in which the pigment epithelium consists of patches without pigment and normally pigmented patches, the spatial pattern of deficient retinal pigment does not coincide with the abnormal visual projection (Guillery *et al.,* 1973). Therefore, it is most likely that the deficient pigmentation and the abnormal visual pathways result from the same defect rather than that the pathway abnormality is the direct result of the lack of pigment.

In normal mammals the input from the two eyes is first brought into alignment in the laminae of the lateral geniculate nucleus (LGN). The laminae (there may be from two to six in different mammalian species) form two sets, each set receiving input from one eye. The visual field projection maps to each lamina are in register with the maps in the other laminae so that "lines of projection" that represent single points in the visual field can be drawn through the LGN, roughly perpendicular to the laminae. Although the misrouted optic nerve fibers end in

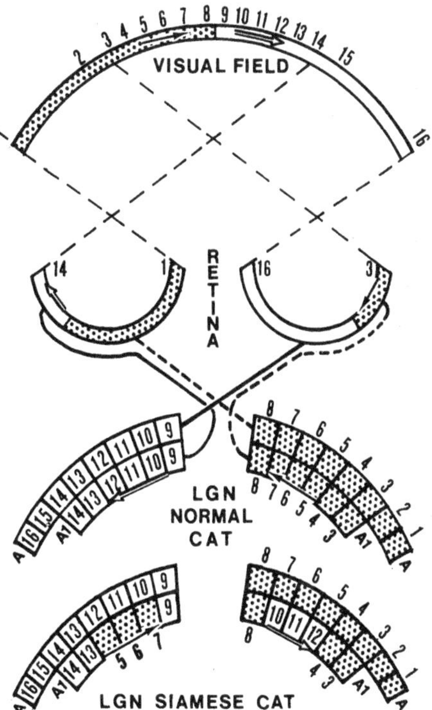

Figure 9.28. Visual projection from the retina to the lateral geniculate nucleus in the normal cat and in the Siamese cat. Modified from R. W. Guillery and J. H. Kaas, *J. Comp. Neurol. 143:*73–100 (1971), and R. W. Guillery and V. A. Casagrande, *Cold Spring Harbor Symp. Quant. Biol. 15:*611–617 (1975).

the wrong side of the brain, they terminate in the proper part of the LGN. As this occurs bilaterally, the result is a left-to-right exchange of some optic news fibers, and a left-to-right reversal of the order of their projection to the LGN (Guillery and Kaas, 1971). This shows that there is no error made by the retinal fiber in selection of a terminal locus, and that the locus specificity of the retinal ganglion cells is normal in albinos. The initial abnormality of development is in the selection of the side of the brain into which optic nerve fibers are routed at the optic chiasm, and the anomalous projections to the visual centers probably arise secondarily during development.

In normal cats, the nasal part of the retina sends its axons across the chiasm to end in laminae A, C_1, and C_2 of the LGN on the opposite side of the brain. The temporal part of the retina sends its axons into laminae A_1 and C_1 of the LGN on the same side. In the Siamese cat, the nasal retinal fibers cross normally to end in lamina A and apparently also in C_1 and C_2 (Hickey and Guillery, 1974). However, a segment of temporal retina, representing some part of the first 20° of the ipsilateral projection, projects its axons aberrantly across the chiasm to end in lamina A_1, in reversed retinotopic order. Thus the retinal axons projecting anomalously to the wrong side of the brain of the Siamese cat simply insert themselves into the positions that are left vacant by the nerve fibers that would normally have come from the ipsilateral retina. The resulting projection is as one would expect on the basis of a strict specificity relationship between retinal ganglion cells and LGN cells (Guillery and Kaas, 1971).

The projection from the lateral geniculate nucleus to the striate cortex also forms a continuous and orderly map in which the projection from the anomalous geniculate laminae can be dealt with in two different ways. In "midwestern" Siamese cats Kaas and Guillery (1973) found that the anomalous inputs from lamina A_1 tend to be suppressed, while in "Boston" Siamese cats Hubel and Wiesel (1971) showed that the input from lamina A_1 is reversed and inserted as a separate projection at the border between areas 17 and 18 of the cortex (Fig. 9.29). These patterns of geniculostriate projections are relatively unaffected by postnatal binocular visual deprivation (Hubel and Wiesel, 1971). However, the fact that monocular visual deprivation can unmask the anomalous projection to the cortex from the experienced eye in midwestern Siamese cats shows that the suppression of this projection to the cortex is due to competition between eyes (Guillery and Casagrande, 1975*a*,*b*).

The anomalous retinal projection to the lateral geniculate nucleus shows that misrouted optic axons express their locus specificities in selecting targets in lamina A_1 independently of the neighboring normal axons. By contrast, the projection to the cerebral cortex in Boston Siamese cats may reflect a contextual form of mapping, in which interactions between geniculostriate axons themselves as well as between the axons and their postsynaptic targets determine that the order and continuity of the map is reestablished at the visual cortex. These anomalous projections illustrate the principle that even a detailed knowledge of the final product gives little insight into the processes of its development. To obtain that insight requires much more information about the intermediate stages of development of the anomalous visual projections as well as information about the corresponding stages of development of the visual system in normal mammals.

Any discussion of the development of the mammalian visual system has to take into account the fact that there are three different types of retinal ganglion cells, named W, X, and Y, which have different functional properties, different sizes, and different distributions in the retina, and behave differently in decussating at the chiasm and also in selecting targets in the visual centers. These three types of ganglion cells have been most thoroughly studied in the cat, but similar classes of cells have been found in the monkey and rabbit, and they probably occur in most, if not all, mammals. However, the following description of these ganglion cells applies to the cat. They are not evenly distributed in the retina, and they differ in morphology and functions. The W cells are small ganglion cells found mainly in the central retina (Rowe and Stone, 1976). The X cells are larger than W cells, and they are also found in the area centralis. The Y cells have the largest cell bodies, are sparse in the central retina, and are concentrated in the retinal periphery (Enroth-Cugell and Robson, 1966; Fukuda and Stone, 1974).

The functional properties of the three types of ganglion cells can be summarized briefly as follows (Hirsch and Leventhal, 1978): X cells have axons with moderately fast conduction (20–25 m/sec); they have a high rate of maintained discharge, have small receptive fields, sum the excitation of different parts of their receptive fields linearly, have a sustained response to a stationary stimulus situated in the receptive field, and respond best to slowly moving stimuli. Y cells have the most rapidly conducting (35–45 m/sec) axons; they have a low rate of maintained discharge, have large receptive fields, have a transient response to stimulation, sum excitation in different regions of the receptive field nonlinearly, and respond to a wider range of stimulus velocities. W cells have axons with the slowest conduction velocity (3–15 m/sec); they lack the antagonistic center-surround organization found in other ganglion cells and have large receptive fields. W cells are heterogeneous: tonic W cells have sustained discharges, while phasic W cells have transient discharges in response to appropriate stimulation; some are selectively sensitive to stimuli moving in a particular direction; many W cells respond best to rapidly moving stimuli.

The central projections of these three classes of ganglion cells are different (Hoffmann, 1973; Fukuda and Stone, 1974; Hoffmann and Sherman, 1975). The Y cells project mainly to the lateral geniculate nucleus (LGN), but some project to the superior colliculus. The Y cells in the LGN connect mainly with complex cells

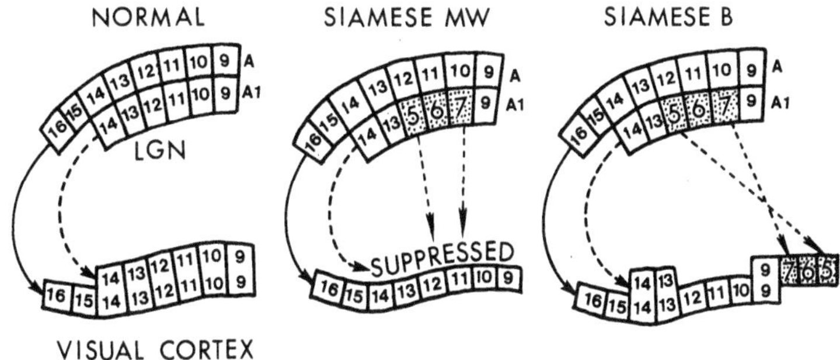

Figure 9.29. Projection from the left lateral geniculate nucleus (LGN) to the left visual cortex of the midwestern Siamese cat and the Boston Siamese cat. In the midwestern cat the anomalous projection to the cortex from lamina A_1 is largely suppressed. In the Boston cat the projection of the anomalous segment of the LGN to the cortex restores the order of the projection, but the anomalous projection to the incorrect side of the brain persists. Modified from J. H. Kaas and R. W. Guillery, *Brain Res.* *59:*61–95 (1973).

in the visual cortex, and those cortical cells project to the superior colliculus. X cells project mainly to the LGN and virtually none project to the superior colliculus. W cells project mainly to the superior colliculus and midbrain.

The neurons in the LGN that receive direct inputs from X, Y, and W ganglion cells have response characteristics similar to those of the homonymous retinal ganglion cells. The response properties of the cells in the visual cortex also, to a large extent, reflect the characteristics of their afferents from the LGN (Hoffmann and Stone, 1971; J. Stone and Dreher, 1973; W. Singer *et al.,* 1975; J. R. Wilson and Sherman, 1976). Cortical cells with X-type afferents (Sa cells) have small receptive fields, respond to slowly moving stimuli, respond to specific stimulus orientation, have receptive fields with parallel excitatory and inhibitory zones, and generally resemble the simple cortical cells described initially by Hubel and Wiesel (1962). Cortical cells that appear to receive input from Y cells (Ifa and Fa cells) have large receptive fields with "on–off" types of responses, respond to fast-moving stimuli, and have less orientation selectivity than simple cells. These cortical cells resemble the complex cells described by Hubel and Wiesel (1962).

It has been shown that the W, X, and Y retinal ganglion cells behave differently in their tendency to cross at the optic chiasm (Fukuda and Stone, 1974; J. Stone and Fukuda, 1974*a,b*). X cells project to both sides of the brain; those on the nasal side of the vertical median project contralaterally, while those on the temporal side of the retinal vertical meridian project ipsilaterally. Y cells also project into both sides, but the line of decussation is 1–2° temporal to that of the X cells, and about 5 percent of Y cells in the temporal retina project contralaterally. In addition, the phasic W cells from the entire retina project contralaterally, although the tonic W cells, which are confined to the temporal retina, project ipsilaterally. Thus, in normal cats, the X cells and the tonic W cells respect the vertical meridian of the retina as the line of decussation, but the Y cells and the phasic W cells do not. It is conceivable that the defect of decussation of optic axons that occurs in albino mammals is due to a change in the retinal distribution of W, X, and Y cells, and especially of the last (R. K. Lund, 1975).

Analysis of this anomaly, whether by anatomical tracing of fibers or by electrical recording, is severely limited by inadequate knowledge of the normal mechanisms that control the routes taken by growing axons and by ignorance of the factors that determine whether optic axons cross or do not cross over at the optic chiasm. In mammals in which some optic axons do not cross at the chiasm, there is a boundary (line of decussation) between the temporal region of the retina which projects its optic fibers ipsilaterally and the more nasal retinal region that projects contralaterally. This line would be at the boundary of a developmental element of the retina according to the hypothesis discussed in Section 9.6. One can conceive of the anomaly resulting from a temporal shift in the position of the boundary between ganglion cells that project to the same side and those that project to the opposite side of the brain, and in terms of the hypothesis of developmental elements the minimal shift would occur over a single retinal element and larger shifts would occur over distances equivalent to multiples of a retinal element. The problem is complicated by the fact that the line of decussation for each type of retinal ganglion cell (W, X, Y) is different. At present, it is not possible to say whether the misrouting of optic nerve fibers in albino mammals is a primary defect of the optic axon growth mechanism or whether the primary defect is in the specification of the retinal ganglion cells.

9.11. Role of Visual Experience in the Development of the Frog's Visual System

Observations of the visuomotor behavior of amphibians in which one eye has been surgically inverted during larval development have established that these animals consistently misdirect their responses to visual stimuli, and that this maladaptive behavior is never corrected by visual experience (Sperry, 1943, 1944; L. S. Stone, 1953). There is no behavioral evidence that neuronal reorganization has occurred anywhere in the visual system to compensate for inversion of the eye.

That the projection from the retina to the contralateral tectum undergoes no compensatory reorganization after eye inversion has also been shown by electrophysiological mapping of the retinotectal projection (M. Jacobson, 1968*a;* M. Jacobson and Hirsch, 1973; Skarf, 1973; Skarf and Jacobson, 1974). The retinotectal map also develops normally in frogs (*Rana pipiens* and *Xenopus*) raised in the dark (M. Jacobson, 1971*b;* Keating and Feldman, 1975) and in frogs raised with skin grafts over one or both eyes that prevent pattern vision but not light stimulation (M. Jacobson and Hirsch, 1973; Skarf and Jacobson, 1974). Moreover, the retinotectal projection in *Rana pipiens* develops normally from the remaining eye after one eye has been removed in the embryo, although in some animals the retinal axons are misrouted at the chiasm to the ipsilateral tectum, where they form a map with its axes properly aligned with that tectum. These aberrant fibers blindly obey the rules of retinotectal mapping and pay no heed to the fact that abnormal visual functions result from their connections to the wrong side of the brain (Hirsch and Jacobson, 1973).

The intertectal projection also does not require visual experience for its development. The intertectal visual projection subserves the binocular region of the visual field. The image of any point in the binocular visual field falls on corresponding positions in the two retinae; these each project to the corresponding positions in the contralateral tectum. These corresponding tectal positions are linked reciprocally across the midline by the intertectal projection, as shown in Figs. 9.9 and 9.30 (Gaze and Jacobson, 1962, 1963*a;* Keating and Gaze, 1970*b*). Thus, when a frog looks at an object in the binocular visual field, nerve impulses originating in both eyes traverse separate pathways which converge onto binocularly driven tectal neurons (Fite, 1969; Skarf, 1973; Skarf and Jacobson, 1974).

The suggestion has been made that simultaneous stimulation of both eyes by objects in the binocular part of the visual field, giving rise to corresponding patterns of impulse traffic from both eyes, might be the factor controlling the convergence of inputs from both eyes to a common terminus in the tectum (Keating, 1968; Keating and Gaze, 1970*a*). However, the supposition that binocular visual stimulation is responsible for the development of intertectal linkages cannot stand against the observation that intertectal connections develop normally in frogs (*Rana* and *Xenopus*) raised through metamorphosis in darkness (M. Jacobson, 1971*b;* Keating and Feldman, 1975) and in *Rana pipiens* raised through metamorphosis with a skin graft over one or both eyes or with one inverted eye (M. Jacobson and Hirsch, 1973; Hirsch and Jacobson, 1973). These various forms of visual deprivation do not prevent the intertectal projection from developing on time, starting at Stage 61 in *Xenopus* (Beazley *et al.,* 1972) and at Stage XIX in *Rana pipiens* (M. Jacobson, 1971*b*).

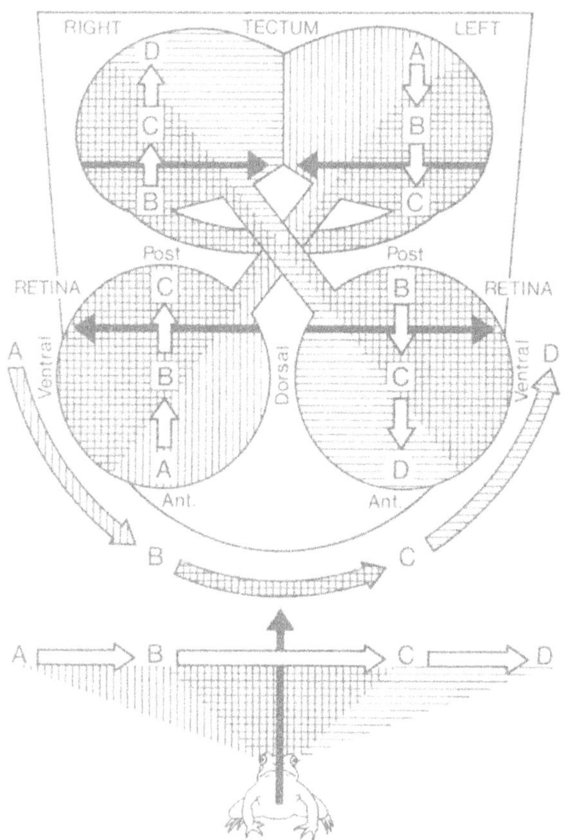

Figure 9.30. The retinotectal projection of the frog consists of a monocular projection (A-B from the right eye, and C-D from the left eye), which crosses at the optic chiasm to the tectum on the opposite side, and a binocular projection (B–C) from each eye to the tectum on the same side. Corresponding points in the binocular projection are connected by intertectal pathways (B to B and C to C).

In support of the hypothesis that visual experience can reorganize the intertectal projection is the observation that 90° or 180° rotation of one eye of the *Xenopus* tadpole results in rearrangement of the intertectal projection so as to bring it back into register with the contralateral retinotectal projection (Keating and Gaze, 1970*a*). This compensatory rearrangement occurs in 8–12 days after 90° rotation of one eye of *Xenopus* at Stage 63 as shown in Fig. 9.31 (Keating, 1975*b*). The rearrangement, known as "functional adaptation," is prevented by keeping the animal in the dark, thus showing that it requires visual experience (Keating and Feldman, 1975). The functional significance of this rearrangement of intertectal linkages is obscure for several reasons, notably because it does not result in amelioration of the animal's maladaptive visual behavior. The phenomenon is not seen in *Rana pipiens:* rotation of one eye by any angle between 15° and 180° produces a permanent disparity between the retinotectal projection and intertectal projection, and no evidence of compensation of the intertectal projection is seen. Binocularly driven tectal neurons develop in such frogs with visual disparities, but, after eye rotation, these neurons are activated by a stimulus at one position viewed by the normal eye and at a different position viewed by the rotated eye (Skarf, 1973; Skarf and Jacobson, 1974). If the eye of *Rana pipiens* is inverted before larval Stage XIV, the intertectal projection develops normally, starting at Stage XIX, but after several months the intertectal receptive fields gradually enlarge and the intertectal electrical responses to visual stimulation become weaker and may disappear (M. Jacobson and Hirsch, 1973). Intertectal responses also become markedly abnormal in *Rana pipiens* after monocular eye occlusion (M. Jacobson and Hirsch, 1973). The effect may be due to a functional competition between the eyes, perhaps analogous to the effect in mammals after monocular visual deprivation.

The lack of functional adaptation of the intertectal projection after misalignment of the eyes in *Rana* and its presence in *Xenopus* may be correlated with the movement of the eyes during metamorphosis—the change in position of the eyes is large in *Xenopus* but small in *Rana* (P. Grobstein and Comer, 1976). Therefore, functional adaptation would be necessary in *Xenopus* in order to maintain the intertectal connections between tectal neurons that receive inputs from corresponding points in the two retinae, as the relative position of the eyes change during metamorphosis.

The extent of reorganization of the intertectal projection that has been reported to occur after inversion of one eye of *Xenopus,* or even the extent of the change that would be required to compensate for the movements of the eyes relative to one another during development, is far greater than most cases of sprouting of axons to form anomalous connections (see Section 5.8). Those sprouts rarely extend more than 250 μm from their normal positions, whereas in *Xenopus* the intertectal axons have been reported to have moved almost a millimeter in order to adapt to inversion of one eye.

The mechanism of such a radical change in the pattern of connections is unknown. Keating (1968, 1974) and Gaze *et al.* (1970*b*) have suggested that "those positions on the two tecta that are simultaneously receiving a similar spatiotem-

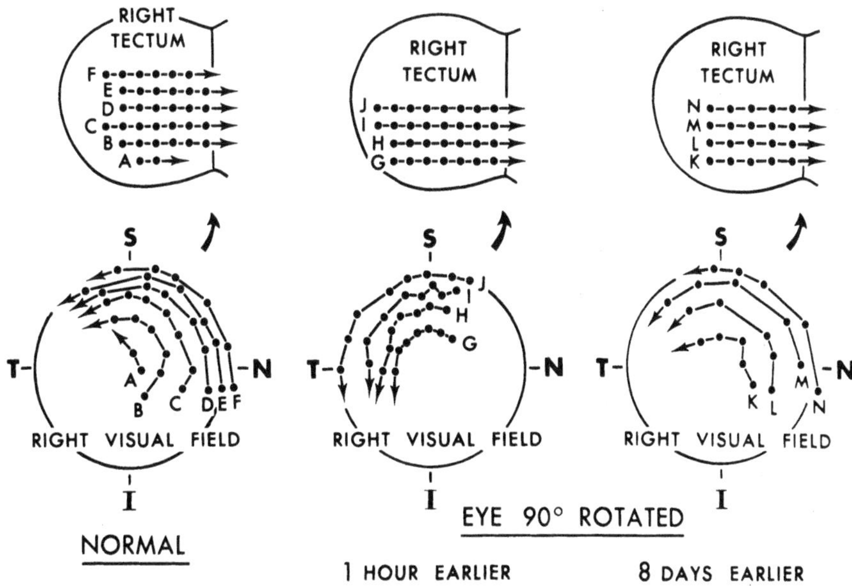

Figure 9.31. Functional adaptation of the ipsilateral visuotectal projection in *Xenopus,* which is mediated through intertectal connections. Shown are the normal ipsilateral visuotectal map in a young frog (left diagram), the map made immediately after 90° anticlockwise rotation of the right eye at Stage 63 (middle diagram), and the map 8 days postoperative (right diagram). From M. J. Keating, *Proc. Roy. Soc. (London) B Ser. 189:*603–610 (1975).

poral pattern of impulses through the two eyes from a stimulus at one position in the binocular field, become neuronally linked together" (Gaze *et al.*, 1970*b*). This would, if proven, be the first evidence of the formation of new neuronal connections as the result of sensory experience. The hypothesis of association of neurons that have correlated activities is an extension of the psychological theory of association of ideas. That theory, deriving from the epistemology of John Locke and David Hume, was first given a neurological explanation by David Hartley. In his *Observations on Man* (first published in 1749), he proposed that mental associations form as a result of corresponding vibrations in nerves (an idea that Newton had thrown out in the last paragraph of his *Principia*). The step from a psychological to a neurophysiological theory of association appears to have been made before the mid-nineteenth century, as evidenced by Herbert Spencer's statement: "As every student of the nervous system knows, the combination of any set of impressions, or motions, or both, implies a ganglion in which the various nerve-fibres concerned are put into connection" (*Principles of Psychology,* 1855). The hypothesis that synapses form or become altered between neurons whose electrical activities coincide has become widely accepted in approximately the way in which it is formulated by Ariëns Kappers (1907) and is stated by Ariëns Kappers *et al.* (1936) that "the relationships which determine connections are synchronic or immediately successive functional activities." The general idea that learning is predicated by synaptic changes (Ramón y Cajal, 1895) has become accepted in various forms (Hebb, 1949, 1966; J. Z. Young, 1951; Eccles, 1964; Konorski, 1967; Beritoff, 1969; Anokhin, 1968).

All these neurophysiological theories of strengthening of synapses between neurons that have corresponding functional activities imply that linkages are extensive initially and become more restricted, functionally and anatomically, as a result of functional activity. In this view, the final arrangement is the result of cooperative interactions between neurons. This view has been extended to include competitive functional interactions between neurons—neurons with equal activities being able to maintain connections with a shared postsynaptic target, while functional imbalance results in the more active neuron excluding the less active neuron from a share of the postsynaptic space (Guillery, 1972*a;* Sherman *et al.,* 1974; Sherman and Wilson, 1975; C. Blakemore *et al.,* 1975). This concept is expanded in the following section.

9.12. Role of Visual Experience in Development of the Visual System in Mammals

Recent evidence has indicated that the mammalian visual system contains three functional projections to the visual centers originating from three classes of retinal ganglion cells, named X, Y, and W (see Section 9.10). These projections are affected differently by visual stimulation during development. Development of Y cells and their central projections is sensitive to visual stimulation during a critical period shortly after birth, while the development of X and W cells and their projections may not require visual stimulation. Several reviews of the role of visual stimulation on development of the visual system have appeared recently (C. Blakemore, 1974; Barlow, 1975; Hirsch and Jacobson, 1975; P. Grobstein and Chow, 1975, 1976; Daniels and Pettigrew, 1976; Hirsch and Leventhal, 1978).

Before considering how visual stimulation or deprivation may affect the developing mammalian visual system, it is necessary to review the relevant aspects of functional organization of the mammalian visual system.

These findings, which will be described in greater detail below, support the concept that "neurons develop in two complementary modes which together permit all possible functions to be represented: functions that are innately predetermined as well as those that develop as a result of individual experience. In the first mode of development, neurons can express their functions only in a predetermined way as highly predictable patterns of behavior which are characteristic of each species. In the second mode of development, neurons form populations with such diverse functional potentials that all possible contingencies of functions can be realized. . . . From this *plenum formarum* some neuronal functions and not others will be actualized" (M. Jacobson, 1974*b*, p. 152). The invariant component of the system provides the intrinsically determinate, innate framework within which the variable component can achieve the flexibility to enable the organism to adapt to its individual visual input. To some extent the conflicting reports on the effect of visual deprivation or of restricted visual experience on development of the visual system come from failure to recognize that there is an invariant as well as a variable component, and that the relative effects of experimental conditions on those two components of the visual system are different in different species (Hirsch and Leventhal, 1978).

The effects of visual deprivation on the *lateral geniculate* nucleus depend on whether the deprivation is monocular or binocular. Binocular deprivation appears to affect the Y cells selectively in all parts of the LGN (Sherman *et al.*, 1972). The effect is clearly less severe than the effects of monocular deprivation, and there have been several reports of failure to find any effects of binocular deprivation (Chow and Stewart, 1972; Guillery, 1973*a,b;* Hendrickson and Boothe, 1976). By contrast, monocular deprivation results in severe shrinking of the affected segments of the LGN. Because these effects of monocular deprivation are confined to the binocular segments of the LGN while the monocular segment to which the deprived eye projects is virtually unaffected (except after prolonged deprivation, lasting more than 6 months), the effects must be due to interaction between the two eyes (Wiesel and Hubel, 1963*a,* 1965; Guillery, 1972*a,* 1973*a,b,* 1974). Guillery (1972*a*) demonstrated this very elegantly by showing that no apparent effects of visual deprivation occur in an artificial monocular segment of the LGN made by destroying a small area of temporal retina in one eye shortly after birth and then occluding the intact eye (Fig. 9.32). Because interactions between laminae of the LGN are very weak, the interactions between LGN cells must occur at their endings in the visual cortex. The shrinkage of LGN cell bodies is a retrograde effect, originating in the striate cortex.

Earlier reports that visual deprivation has no effect on the functions of LGN neurons (Wiesel and Hubel, 1963*a,* 1965; Chow and Stewart, 1972) have been contradicted by the reports that considerable reduction in the number of Y cells but not X cells in the cat LGN results from binocular as well as monocular deprivation and that Y cell reponses can be recorded from an artificial monocular segment but not from the binocular segment of the LGN of the cat after monocular deprivation (Sherman *et al.,* 1972, 1975; Hoffmann and Cynader, 1975).

The effect of visual deprivation on the superior colliculus in newborn cats, first shown by Wickelgren and Sterling (1969), has recently been shown to be mediated by the indirect Y cell projection from the complex cells of the visual cortex to the superior colliculus. These cells respond to fast-moving stimuli, and are directionally selective and binocular. Reduction of their activity after visual deprivation is due to absence of Y cells in the LGN (Hoffmann and Sherman, 1974, 1975). The binocularly driven cells in the superior colliculus require visual stimulation for their normal development: they cannot be recorded in newborn kittens. Their activity normally increases during the first few weeks after birth, but this is prevented by visual deprivation (Hoffmann and Sherman, 1974, 1975).

The role of visual stimulation in the development of the visual cortex varies according to species and according to the type of neuron in question. Some types of neurons develop largely or entirely under intrinsic control, while others require sensory stimulation. These may be termed "invariant" and "variable" components, and their proportions vary in different species so that results cannot be freely generalized from one species to others. Thus, in the mouse, rat, and rabbit, development of the visual cortex is completed in the absence of visual stimulation, although the rate of development is slowed by visual deprivation. In these species, after a short period of visual deprivation the striate cortex is found to be less mature structurally and functionally than in normal controls, but after about 6–8 months in the dark the structure and function of the visual cortex are virtually indistinguishable from normal (Boas *et al.,* 1969; Vrensen and de Groot, 1974; P. Grobstein and Chow, 1975; P. Grobstein *et al.,* 1975).

In principle, it may seem relatively easy to record all the functional types of neurons that are present in the visual cortex of visually naive animals and to

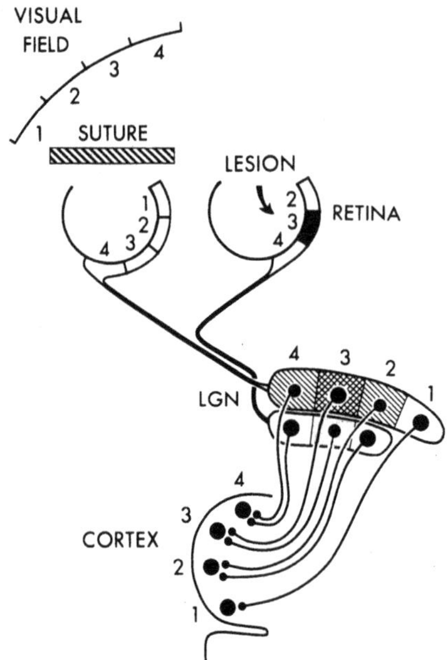

Figure 9.32. Binocular competition between neurons of the lateral geniculate nucleus (LGN) for cortical synaptic space is shown in this experiment. Left eyelid closure (shown by oblique shading) produces cell shrinkage in segments 2, 3, and 4 of lamina A of the right LGN. When an additional lesion is made in the right temporal retina, resulting in atrophy of cells in segment 3 of lamina A_1, the cells in the corresponding segment (segment 3) of lamina A grow more than the cells in segments 2 and 4. From R. W. Guillery, *J. Comp. Neurol. 144:*117–130 (1972).

determine whether new functions develop as a result of visual experience. In practice, the experiments are restricted by the sampling problem, by possible differential effects of anesthetics on different functional types of neurons, by optical aberrations and cloudiness of the ocular media, and by the fact that any assay of functional maturation of cortical neurons is limited by the stage of maturation of neurons in the retina and lateral geniculate nucleus. In addition, the functional maturation of the neurons under investigation may occur during the several hours that the animal is exposed to visual stimulation while its visual cortex is being explored by the microelectrode. These are some of the variables that may be responsible for the different results that have been reported.

There are conflicting reports of the proportion of visual cortical cells in the cat and monkey that have normal functional properties at birth or develop normally in the absence of visual stimulation. In the original report on the types of cells in the visually naive kitten striate cortex, Hubel and Wiesel (1963*a*) found examples of all types of cells found in adult cats. They therefore concluded that striate cortical cells can develop normal functional capacities in the absence of normal stimulation. The presence of cells with adult types of functions has also been found in the visually deprived kitten by Sherk and Stryker (1976) and in the monkey by Wiesel and Hubel (1974). In those studies, some cortical cells in visually naive kittens and young monkeys were shown to be driven binocularly, to respond to lines at a specific orientation, and to be arranged in columns according to their ocular dominance and preferred orientation. In conflict with the last results are reports that there are few orientation-selective cells in the cortex of visually naive kittens (Barlow and Pettigrew, 1971; Pettigrew, 1974*a,b*). The differences between investigations may reflect real differences in the functions of the cells, or they may merely reflect sampling differences or differences in the criteria of normal functions of cortical neurons that are adopted by different workers—Barlow and Pettigrew apparently adopting stricter criteria than Wiesel and Hubel.

To some extent, these conflicting results may be resolved by the findings that some cortical cells retain their orientation preferences while other cells appear to lose them in cats that have been raised in the dark for up to a year after birth (Hirsch and Leventhal, 1976). In such visually naive cats, some of the so-called simple type of cell, which receives X cell inputs, retain orientation selectivity, while the so-called complex type of cell, which receives Y cell inputs, has no orientation preference. These results should also be considered in relation to the anatomical changes in the visual cortex of cats reared in the dark (see Fig. 5.10). The fact that dendritic spines of pyramidal cells in the striate cortex are particularly vulnerable to visual deprivation while stellate cells appear less affected is significant in the light of the evidence that pyramidal cells have been identified as the "complex" cells while stellate cells have been identified as "simple" cells (Van Essen and Kelly, 1973; Kelly and Van Essen, 1974), and that complex cortical cells receive input from retinal Y cells while simple cells receive input from X cells.

The majority of cells in the striate cortex of the normal monkey and about 80 percent of striate cortical cells in the cat are binocularly driven, although most binocular cells are dominated by one eye (Fig. 9.33). Segregation of the geniculostriate fibers into columns can be demonstrated by autoradiography after injection of [^{3}H]proline into one eye in a series of newborn kittens at different ages (Fig. 9.34). Cells with the same ocular dominance are arranged in walls or columns about 500 μm wide and several millimeters long, alternating with the columns of cortical cells dominated by the other eye. If the pattern of ocular dominance columns could be seen at the surface of the cortex it would resemble a zebra's stripes. Ocular dominance columns in the striate cortex of the cat develop gradually from 2 to 16 weeks after birth, but appear to be fully formed at the time of birth in the superior colliculus. In the rhesus monkey, ocular dominance columns start appearing more than 3 weeks before birth in the superior colliculus and striate cortex (Rakic, 1977). Those in the superior colliculus of the rhesus monkey appear to be fully developed at birth (Rakic, 1977), but those in the striate cortex continue developing postnatally, and are then vulnerable to monocular visual deprivation (Fig. 9.36).

The effects of monocular deprivation are known to be different from those of binocular deprivation. The type of deprivation may also affect the result; the conditions are obviously different when animals are reared in complete darkness than when they are deprived of pattern vision by closing the eyelids with sutures. After binocular suture of the eyelids of the kitten for the first 3 months after birth, most neurons in the visual cortex respond to visual stimuli, and more than half are quite normal (Wiesel and Hubel, 1965). By contrast, monocular lid suture for 2–3 months after birth results in a significant reduction, although not complete absence, of cells in the striate cortex that can be driven by the deprived eye (Fig. 9.35). Those that can be driven by the deprived eye have very abnormal receptive fields. The reduction of binocularly driven cortical neurons that occurs after monocular visual deprivation during the neonatal period has been found in the

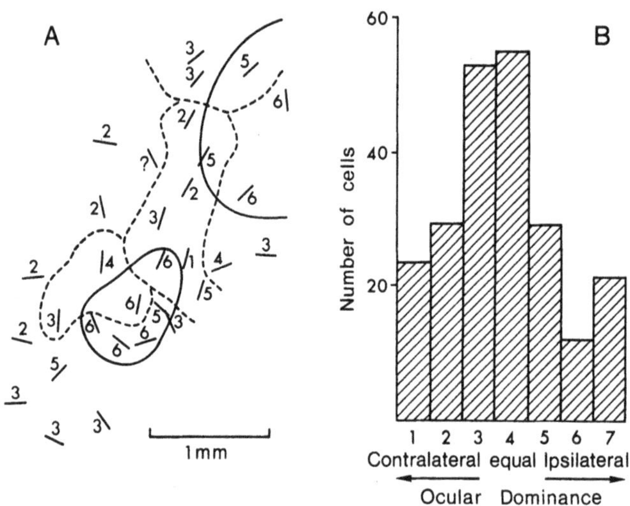

Figure 9.33. A: Surface view of a region of the right striate cortex in normal adult cat, showing receptive field orientations and ocular dominance of the first cells, encountered near the surface, in 31 microelectrode penetrations. Dashed lines separate regions of relatively constant receptive field orientation. The numbers refer to ocular dominance groups. Continuous lines separate areas of strong ipsilateral dominance from areas of mixed or contralateral dominance. From D. H. Hubel and T. N. Wiesel, *J. Neurophysiol. 28:*1041–1059 (1965). B: Ocular dominance distribution of 223 cells recorded from striate cortex of normal adult cats in a series of 45 penetrations. Cells in group 1 receive input only from the contralateral eye; cells in group 7 receive input only from the ipsilateral eye; and cells in groups 2–6 receive input in different proportions from both eyes. From D. H. Hubel and T. N. Wiesel, *J. Physiol. (London) 160:*106–154 (1962).

cat, monkey, rabbit, rat, mouse, and owl (Wiesel and Hubel, 1963*b*, 1965; Hubel and Wiesel, 1970; Shaw *et al.*, 1974; Van Sluyters and Stewart, 1974; Dräger, 1976; Pettigrew and Konishi, 1976). Monocular visual deprivation of monkeys from birth results in an increase in width of the cortical ocular dominance columns of the normal eye and a commensurate decrease in width of the ocular dominance

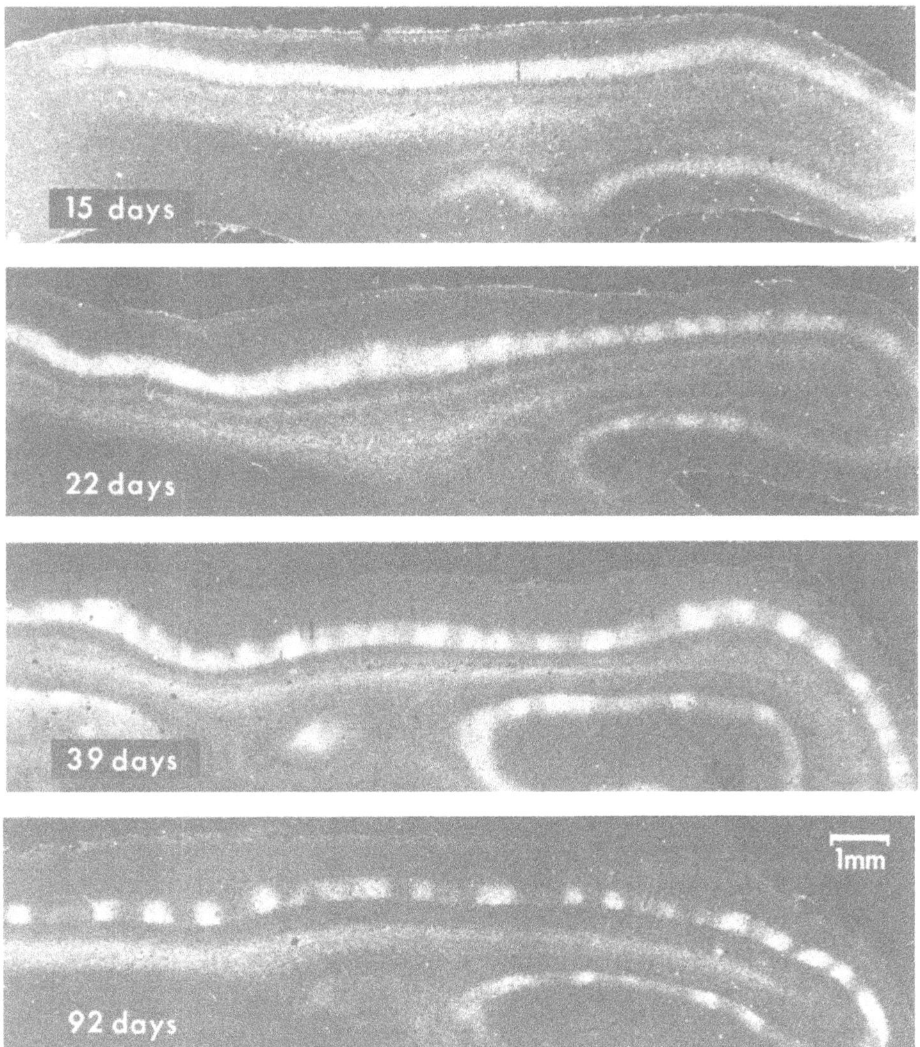

Figure 9.34. Postnatal development of ocular dominance columns in the cat. Darkfield autoradiographs of the visual cortex at four different ages, ipsilateral to an eye which was injected with [^{3}H]proline. Horizontal sections, midline at the top in each figure, anterior to the left. The geniculocortical afferents serving the ipsilateral eye are labeled by transneuronal transport. At 15 days of age the afferents are spread uniformly along layer IV, completely intermingled with the (unlabeled) afferents serving the contralateral eye. At later ages the afferents progressively aggregate into clumps—the anatomical basis for the physiologically described ocular dominance columns. The gaps are occupied by unlabeled afferents serving the other eye. Physiological recordings show that in young kittens neurons in layer IV may be influenced readily by stimulation of either eye, but at later ages they come to be strongly dominated by one eye or the other. Courtesy of S. LeVay, M. P. Stryker, and C. J. Shatz.

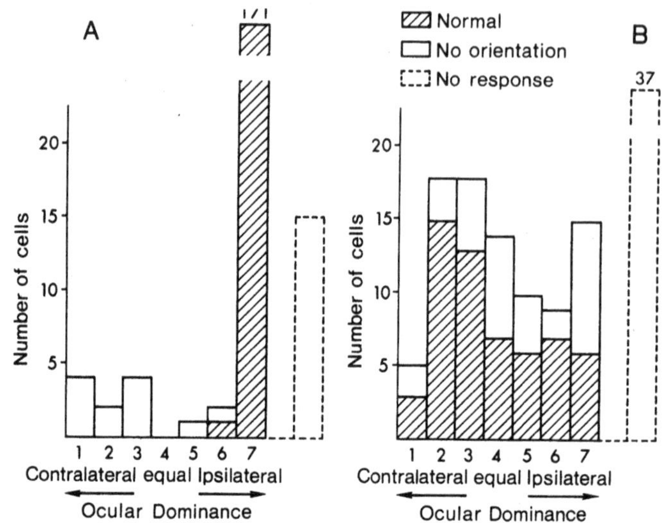

Figure 9.35. Ocular dominance distribution of cells in the striate cortex of kittens deprived of pattern vision in one eye (A) compared with kittens deprived of pattern vision in both eyes (B) by suturing the eyelids of one or both eyes from about 4 weeks to 8–14 weeks of age. A shows the ocular dominance distribution of 199 cells recorded in the striate cortex of five monocularly deprived kittens, and B shows the ocular dominance distribution of 126 striate cortical cells recorded in four binocularly deprived kittens. Shading indicates that cells had normal specific responses to visual stimulation; absence of shading indicates that cells lacked orientation specificity; dashed lines indicate that cells did not respond to visual stimulation of either eye. From T. N. Wiesel and D. H. Hubel, *J. Neurophysiol. 28:*1029–1040 (1965).

columns of the deprived eye (Hubel *et al.,* 1975), as shown in Fig. 9.36. Development of ocular dominance columns and orientation columns occurs in animals deprived of visual experience in both eyes (Hubel and Wiesel, 1974*c*), and it is only when visual deprivation is monocular that the columns develop abnormally.

Considerable reduction in the number of binocularly driven cortical neurons without any reduction in orientation selectivity is found in kittens 3 months after strabismus is produced by cutting the medial rectus muscle shortly after birth (Hubel and Wiesel, 1965*b*). It seems that, for each neuron, the dominant eye has taken over. The effect is not due to visual deprivation but to lack of correspondence or cooperation between the two eyes. A similar effect can be produced by placing an opaque shield over the left or right eye on alternate days (Hubel and

Figure 9.36. Ocular dominance columns in a normal rhesus monkey (a) and in monkeys deprived of vision in one eye from shortly after birth (b,c). These are montages made from serial tangential sections through layer IV of primary visual cortex (area 17), processed for autoradiography and photographed with darkfield illumination. Each monkey had one eye injected with tritiated proline 10 days prior to death: the bright bands correspond to the terminal fields of transneuronally labeled geniculocortical afferents serving the injected eye. In (b) the injection was made into the eye which was left open, in (c) it was made into the closed eye. The autoradiographs show that in monkeys raised with one eye closed the ocular dominance columns for the open eye are wider than normal, while those for the closed eye are narrowed. The combined width of a left- and right-eye pair is the same as normal. From D. H. Hubel, T. N. Wiesel, and S. LeVay, Plasticity of ocular dominance columns in monkey striate cortex, *Phil. Trans. Roy. Soc. London Ser. B* (1977), in press.

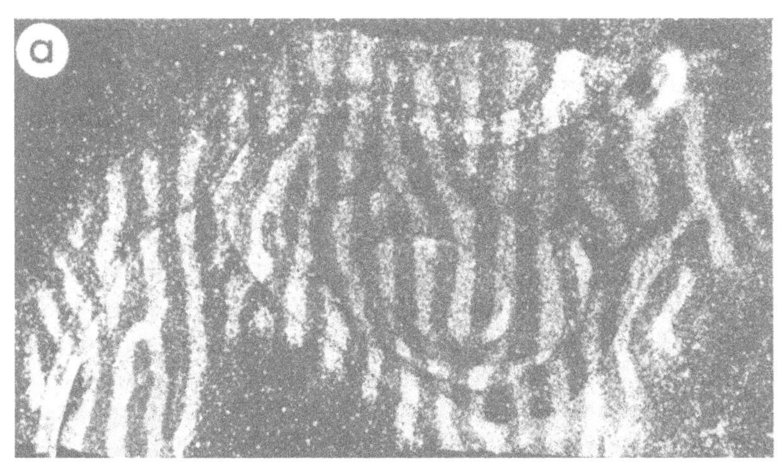
a

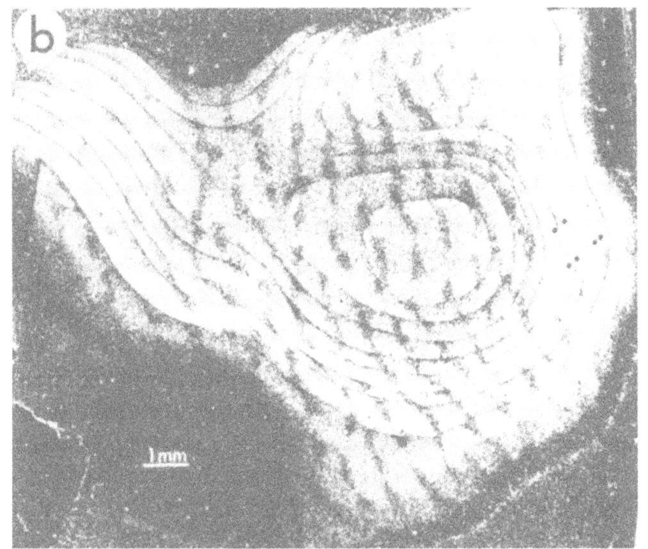
b
1mm

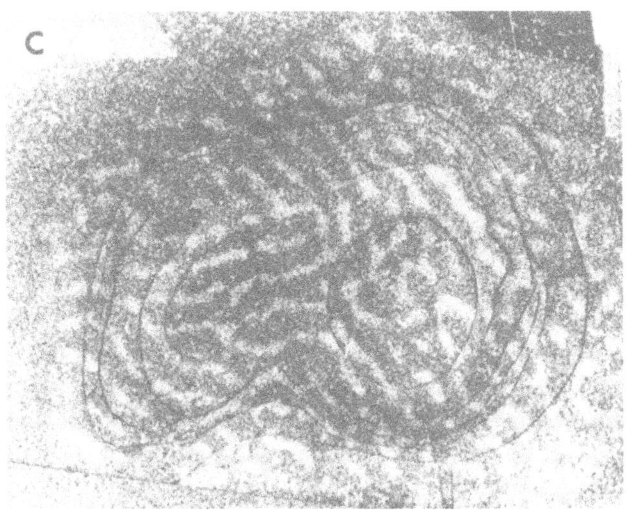
c

Wiesel, 1965*b;* Blake and Hirsch, 1975). Neurons in the visual cortex appear to require congruent inputs from corresponding points on the two retinae: if the inputs are incongruent, the neurons that were binocularly connected at birth lose the ability to respond to stimulation of one eye but retain the input from the other eye. The physiological basis of this change from binocularity to monocularity appears to be an inhibition of the input from one eye. This can be inferred from the evidence that the binocularity can be partially restored in monocularly deprived cats immediately after intravenously injected bicuculine, a drug which blocks the action of the inhibitory synaptic transmitter γ-aminobutyric acid (GABA) (Sillito, 1975*a,b;* Duffy *et al.,* 1976). A similar rapid restoration of function of the deprived eye occurs after removal of the experienced eye (Kratz and Spear, 1976).

The loss of binocularity can occur after a few days of monocular deprivation during the critical period, which extends into the third postnatal month (Hubel and Wiesel, 1970). A brief exposure of the binocularly deprived cat to a short period (6–20 hours) of monocular stimulation is sufficient to reduce the number of binocularly driven cortical neurons (Peck and Blakemore, 1975; C. R. Olson and Freeman, 1975).

The effects of selective visual stimulation on orientation selective neurons can be studied by fitting kittens with goggles which allow one eye to view vertical lines and the other to view horizontal lines (Hirsch, 1970; Hirsch and Spinelli, 1970, 1971; Leventhal and Hirsch, 1975; Stryker *et al.,* 1976). Kittens that have worn these goggles for the first 12 weeks of life have a majority of cortical neurons whose orientation selectivity matches the orientation of the stimulus to which the eye was exposed. However, some neurons respond best to orientations at right angles to the lines to which the eye was exposed (Leventhal and Hirsch, 1975). After selective exposure of kittens to diagonal lines, cortical cells are found that respond selectively to horizontal or vertical as well as other cells that respond best to the diagonal orientation to which the eye was exposed (Leventhal and Hirsch, 1975). These observations suggest that some neurons are inherently predisposed to develop vertical or horizontal orientation selectivity, while others require appropriate visual stimulation. Another method of selective visual exposure, by raising kittens in cylinders decorated inside with either vertical or horizontal stripes, results in development of visual cortical cells whose orientation selectivity matches the orientation of the stripes which the animal was allowed to see (C. Blakemore and Cooper, 1970; C. Blakemore, 1974). Failure to confirm these results shows that the striped cylinder is a less reliable method of restricting visual experience than goggles attached to the head (Stryker and Sherk, 1975; Daw and Wyatt, 1976).

The embryo and fetus are buffered against the effects of the external environment. Although susceptibility of the fetus to normal environmental conditions starts, to a limited extent, shortly before birth, it reaches a peak only after birth. The period during which development of the nervous system is sensitive to external conditions is termed the *sensitive period,* or the *vulnerable period,* if the effect of external conditions or agents is harmful. If a specific condition or stimulus is required for the normal development of the system, the condition or stimulus is termed *critical,* and the period during which its action is required is termed the *critical period.* The times when various critical conditions or stimuli are effective are concentrated in the same relatively short period, shortly after birth in birds and mammals, the animals in which critical periods have been studied extensively (reviews by Thorpe, 1961, 1964; G. Gottlieb, 1973, 1976; J. P. Scott *et al.,* 1974).

Although the critical periods for various systems and conditions overlap in time, it is unlikely that they all share the same underlying mechanisms. For example, the vulnerability of the nervous system to nutritional deficiency affects cellular differentiation and growth, synaptogenesis, and myelination, depending on the time and duration of the deprivation. Quite different effects are produced by sensory deprivation, depending on the quality and quantity, time and duration of the deprivation. In general, however, the critical period is fairly specific for each form of deprivation in a particular species. Thus, in the cat, the critical period for development of binocular vision, for which the use of both eyes is required, extends from 3 to 16 weeks of age, after which the vulnerability to monocular visual deprivation is greatly diminished. The comparable critical period in the human infant, during which both eyes must work together to ensure development of binocularity, can be determined from studies of the effect of strabismus originating in children at different ages. The maximal deleterious effect is produced if the strabismus starts before the age of 2½ years (Hohmann and Creutzfeldt, 1975), and the effect is greatly diminished thereafter, although some deleterious effects may be produced by strabismus starting at up to 6 years of age (Banks *et al.,* 1975). The ability of the system to recover from deprivation diminishes with age: the capacity for recovery falls off sharply after the critical period. This may be a reflection of the progressive loss with age of the capacity for growth and differentiation of nerve cells. An apparently similar loss of functional recovery occurs after brain injury sustained at later ages. For example, the cerebral lateralization of functions such as language is already present at birth in man (see Section 7.11), but recovery of function occurs after removal of or damage to the dominant cerebral hemisphere provided that the damage occurs before the age of 3 or 4 years. The importance of age on the capacity to recover, whether from sensory deprivation, undernutrition, or loss of brain tissue, is well known, but the reasons for this age dependence are still open to conjecture. The resemblances between recovery from brain damage and recovery from sensory deprivation may be only formal, and there is no reason, *a priori,* for the same mechanisms to operate in both types of recovery. There is also so little evidence regarding the neuronal and developmental mechanisms underlying critical periods that it is impossible to determine whether different critical periods have the same or different underlying mechanisms.

At present, virtually nothing is known about the mechanisms by which the critical conditions produce changes in the development of nerve cells that result in permanent changes in neuronal function and behavior. The mechanisms are also unknown by means of which neuronal modifiability increases during the critical period and later diminishes or disappears. In those neurons in which the final stage of development is contingent on adequate sensory stimulation, there must be a mechanism by which the activity evoked in the neuron by sensory stimulation may control the synthesis or assembly of materials required for neuronal differentiation and growth. Either the effect may be simply proportional to the total quantity of nervous activity, or qualitative differences in the effect on the neuron may be produced by different spatiotemporal patterns of neuronal activity. The latter is implied in all theories of the formation or stabilization of neuronal connections as a result of "association," "concomitance," or "functional interaction" of nerve impulses (see Section 9.11). Whatever the mechanism of stimulation of the final differentiation of the neuron by functional activity, the last is not regarded as the primary formative agent in the development of nerve connections and circuits, but the stimulation is believed to constitute a **functional validation or modification of preexisting neuronal structures.** Development of those structures is determined by genetic and developmental mechanisms that are relatively unaffected by the normal range of environmental conditions. To understand how an appropriate combination of genetic determination and sensory stimulation interacts to control the final stages of development of some types of neurons is one of the most important tasks for the future.

The importance of early experience for the development of normal behavior has been repeatedly confirmed in many species from birds to man, but the underlying mechanisms are unknown. The effects of early experience are greatest in those species in which large-scale development of the brain continues after birth. While imprinting occurs even in precocial animals, the altricial animals are far more susceptible to a larger range of environmental conditions. This reaction range is greatest in man, less in other mammals, and least in submammals (Fig. 9.37). The increased reaction range is gained at the risk of increased vulnerability of the brain to unfavorable conditions during the neonatal period.

This book is only a preliminary reconnaissance along the trail leading to an understanding of the development of the human brain and mind. Although all the problems that have been considered here have relevance for human development, we are far from understanding why the rate of development of the human brain, particularly in the postnatal period, so greatly exceeds that of the other mammals. Why do no residues remain in later life of the experiences of infancy? Psychoanalysis notwithstanding, this period of life seems to be totally beyond recall. As Tolstoy described in his *Recollections,* jotted down between the ages of 74 and 80, "from the day I was born until I was three years old, all the time I was nursing and being weaned, beginning to crawl and walk and talk, however I rack my brains, I can remember nothing. . . . From the child of five to me is only a step. From the newborn babe to the child of five is a great leap. From the embryo to the newborn child is an abyss." Why are the memories of infancy beyond recall? Are

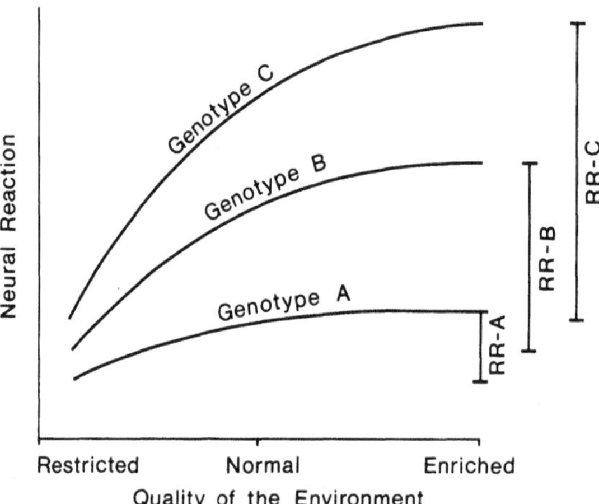

Figure 9.37. Scheme of reaction range concept for three hypothetical genotypes, either of the same or of different species. RR denotes the range of neural reaction to the quality of the environment. Neural reaction may be measured in such terms as biochemical changes in the brain, alterations in brain weight or size of individual neurons, changes in connectivity, or variations in behavior.

they obliterated by the growth of dendrites and development of synapses that occur in the cerebral cortex during the first years after birth? What part do those early experiences play in the postnatal development of the human brain? I believe that research on the development of the nervous system will eventually provide answers to such questions and that these answers will be the means of arriving at a deeper understanding of the nature of man.

References

This bibliography includes all references cited in the text but it is not exhaustive. To have included all known references, like a pack of little dogs yapping at the heels of each statement in the text, would have proved more annoying than useful to the reader.

Abbott, J., and H. Holtzer. (1968) *Proc. Natl. Acad. Sci. U.S.A.* **59:**1144–1151. The loss of phenotypic traits by differentiated cells. V. The effect of 5-bromodeoxyuridine on cloned chondrocytes.

Abeles, M., and M. H. Goldstein, Jr. (1970) *J. Neurophysiol.* **33:**172–187. Functional architecture in cat primary auditory cortex. Columnar organization and organization according to depth.

Abercrombie, M. (1946) *Anat. Rec.* **94:**239–247. Estimation of nuclear population from microtome sections.

Abercrombie, M. (1950) *Phil. Trans. Roy. Soc. (London) Ser. B* **234:**317–338. The effects of antero-posterior reversal of lengths of the primitive streak in the chick.

Abercrombie, M. (1970) *In Vitro* **6:**128–142. Contact inhibition in tissue culture.

Abercrombie, M., and R. Bellairs. (1954) *J. Embryol. Exp. Morphol.* **2:**55–72. The effects in chick blastoderms of replacing the primitive node by a graft of the posterior primitive streak.

Abercrombie, M., and J. Heaysman. (1954) *Exp. Cell Res.* **6:**293–306. Observations on the social behavior of cells in tissue culture. II. "Monolayering" of fibroblasts.

Abercrombie, M., and M. L. Johnson. (1942) *J. Exp. Biol.* **19:**266–278. The outwandering of cells in tissue cultures of nerves undergoing Wallerian degeneration.

Abercrombie, M., and M. L. Johnson. (1946) *J. Anat. (London)* **80:**37–47. Quantitative histology of Wallerian degeneration. I. Nuclear population in rabbit sciatic nerve.

Abercrombie, M., and J. E. Santler. (1957) *J. Cell. Comp. Physiol.* **50:**429–450. An analysis of growth in nuclear population during Wallerian degeneration.

Abercrombie, M., M. L. Johnson, and G. A. Thomas. (1949) *Proc. Roy. Soc. (London) Ser. B* **136:**448–460. The influence of nerve fibres on Schwann cell migration investigated in tissue culture.

Acheson, G., and J. Remolina. (1955) *J. Physiol. (London)* **127:**602–616. The temporal course of the effects of postganglionic axotomy on the inferior mesenteric ganglion of the cat.

Achúcarro, N. (1915) *Trab. Lab. Invest. Biol. (Madrid).* 169–212. De l'evolution de la névroglie et spécialment de ses relation avec l'appareil vasculaire.

Adams, R. D., and J. M. Foley. (1953) *Res. Pub. Assoc. Res. Nerv. Ment. Dis.* **32:**198–237. The neurological disorder associated with liver disease.

Adams Smith, W. N. (1967) *J. Embryol. Exp. Morphol.* **17:**1–10. The ovary and sexual maturation of the brain.

Addison, W. H. F. (1911) *J. Comp. Neurol.* **21:**459–485. The development of the Purkinje cells and of the cortical layers in the cerebellum of the albino rat.

Adinolfi, A. M. (1972*a*) *Exp. Neurol.* **34:**372–382. Morphogenesis of synaptic junctions in layers I and II of the somatic sensory cortex.

Adinolfi, A. M. (1972*b*) *Exp. Neurol.* **34:**383–393. The organization of paramembranous densities during postnatal maturation of synaptic junctions in the cerebral cortex.

Adler, J. (1966) *Science* **153:**708–716. Chemotaxis in bacteria.

Adler, J., and W.-W. Tso. (1974) *Science* **184:**1292–1294. "Decision"-making in bacteria: Chemotactic response of *Escherichia coli* to conflicting stimuli.

Adolph, E. F. (1949) *Science* **109:**579–585. Quantitative relations in the physiological constitution of mammals.

Adrian, E. K., and R. D. Smothermon (1970) *Anat. Rec.* **166:**99–116. Leukocytic infiltration into the hypoglossal nucleus following injury to the hypoglossal nerve.

Adrian, E. K., and B. E. Walker. (1962) *J. Neuropathol. Exp. Neurol.* **21:**597–609. Incorporation of thymidine-H^3 by cells in normal and injured mouse spinal cord.

Adrian, E. K., and M. G. Williams. (1973*a*) *Anat. Rec.* **175:**261–262. An electron microscopic study of reactive cells in the spinal cord labeled with ^{3}H-thymidine before spinal cord injury.

Adrian, E. K. and M. G. Williams. (1973*b*). *J. Comp. Neurol.* **151:**1–24. Cell proliferation in injured spinal cord. An electron microscopic study.

Aghajanian, G. K., and F. E. Bloom. (1967) *Brain Res.* **6:**716–727. The formation of synaptic junctions in developing rat brain: A quantitative electron microscopic study.

Aguayo, A. J., J. Epps, J. Charron, and G. M. Bray. (1976*a*) *Brain Res.* **104:**1–20. Multipotentiality of Schwann cells in cross-anastomosed and grafted unmyelinated nerves—Quantitative microscopy and radioautography.

Aguayo, A. J., L. Charron, and G. M. Bray. (1976*b*) *J. Neurocytol.* **5:**565–573. Potential of Schwann cells from unmyelinated nerves to produce myelin: A quantitative ultrastructural and radiographic study.

Aguayo, A. J., M. Attiwell, J. Trecarten, C. S. Perkins, and C. M. Bray. (1976*c*) *Clin. Res.* **24:**688A. Schwann cell transplantation: Evidence for a primary disorder of myelination in Trembler mouse nerves.

Aguayo, A. J., M. Attiwell, J. Trecarten, S. Perkins, and G. M. Bray. (1977) *Nature* **265:**73–75. Abnormal myelination in transplanted Trembler mouse Schwann cells.

Aguilar, C. E., M. A. Bisby, E. Cooper, and J. Diamond. (1973) *J. Physiol. (London)* **234:**449–464. Evidence that axoplasmic transport of trophic factors is involved in the regulation of peripheral nerve fields in salamanders.

Aitken, J. T. (1950) *J. Anat. (London)* **84:**38–49. Growth of nerve implants in voluntary muscle.

Aitken, J. T., M. Sharman, and J. Z. Young. (1947) *J. Anat. (London)* **81:**1–22. Maturation of regenerating nerve fibers with various peripheral connexions.

Akert, K., K. Pfenninger, C. Sandri, and H. Moor. (1972) Freeze-etching and cytochemistry of vesicles and membrane complexes in synapses of the CNS. In *Structure and Function of Synapse* (G. D. Pappas and D. P. Purpura, eds.), Raven Press, New York.

Albuquerque, E. X., and S. Thesleff. (1968) *Acta Physiol. Scand.* **73:**471–480. A comparative study of membrane properties of innervated and chronically denervated fast and slow skeletal muscles of the rat.

Albuquerque, E. X., J. E. Warnick, J. R. Tasse, and F. M. Sansone. (1972) *Exp. Neurol.* **37:**607–634. Effects of vinblastine and colchicine on neural regulation of the fast and slow skeletal muscles of the rat.

Alderman, A. L. (1935) *J. Exp. Zool.* **70:**205–232. The determination of the eye in the anuran *Hyla regilla.*

Alfert, M. (1950) *J. Cell. Comp. Physiol.* **36:**381–409. A cytochemical study of oogenesis and cleavage in the mouse.

Allara, E. (1952) *Riv. Biol.* **44:**209–229. Sull' influenza esercitata dagli ormoni sulla stattura dell formazioni gustative di mus rattus albinus.

Allbrook, D. B., and J. T. Aitken. (1951) *J. Anat.* **85:**376–390. Reinnervation of striated muscle after acute ischaemia.

Allen, B. M. (1924) *Endocrinology* **8:**639–651. Brain development in anuran larvae after thyroid or pituitary gland removal.

Allen, F. (1912) *J. Comp. Neurol.* **22:**547–568. The cessation of mitosis in the central nervous system of the rat.

Alley, K. E. (1973) *Anat. Rec.* **177:**49–60. Quantitative analysis of the synaptogenic period in the trigeminal mesencephalic nucleus.

Alley, K. E. (1974) *J. Embryol. Exp. Morphol.* **31:**99–121. Morphogenesis of the trigeminal mesencephalic nucleus in the hamster: Cytogenesis and neurone death.

Alouf, J. (1929) *J. Psychol. Neurol.* **38:**5–41. Die vergleichende Cytoarchitektonik der Area striata.

Alpers, B. J., and W. Haymaker. (1934) *Brain* **57:**195–205. The participation of the neuroglia in the formation of myelin in prenatal infantile brain.

Altman, J. (1962*a*) *Exp. Neurol.* **5:**302–318. Autoradiographic study of degenerative and regenerative proliferation of neuroglia cells with tritiated thymidine.

Altman, J. (1962*b*) *J. Comp. Neurol.* **119:**77–96. Some fiber projections to the superior colliculus in the cat.

Altman, J. (1963) *Anat. Rec.* **145:**573–591. Autoradiographic investigation of cell proliferation in the brains of rats and cats.

Altman, J. (1966*a*) *Exp. Neurol.* **16:**263–278. Proliferation and migration of undifferentiated precursor cells in the rat during postnatal gliogenesis.

Altman, J. (1966*b*) *J. Comp. Neurol.* **128:**431–474. Autoradiographic and histological studies of postnatal neurogenesis. II. A longitudinal investigation of the kinetics, migration and transformation of cells incorporating tritiated thymidine in infant rats, with special reference to postnatal neurogenesis in some brain regions.

Altman, J. (1967) Postnatal growth and differentiation of the mammalian brain, with implications for a morphological theory of memory. In *The Neurosciences: A Study Program* (G. Quarton, T. Melnechuk, and F. O. Schmitt, eds.), Rockefeller University Press, New York.

Altman, J. (1969) *J. Comp. Neurol.* **136:**269–294. Autoradiographic and histological studies of postnatal neurogenesis. III. Dating the time of production and onset of differentiation of cerebellar microneurons in rats.

Altman, J. (1972*a*) *J. Comp. Neurol.* **145:**353–398. Postnatal development of the cerebellar cortex in the rat. I. The external germinal layer and the transitional molecular layer.

Altman, J. (1972*b*) *J. Comp. Neurol.* **145:**399–464. Postnatal development of the cerebellar cortex in the rat. II. Phases in the maturation of Purkinje cells and of the molecular layer.

Altman, J. (1972*c*) *J. Comp. Neurol.* **145:**465–514. Postnatal development of the cerebellar cortex in the rat. III. Maturation of the components of the granular layer.

Altman, J., and W. J. Anderson. (1972) *J. Comp. Neurol.* **146:**355–406. Experimental reorganization of the cerebellar cortex. I. Morphological effects of elimination of all microneurons with prolonged x-irradiation started at birth.

Altman, J., and S. L. Chorover. (1963) *J. Physiol. (London)* **169:**770–779. Autoradiographic investigation of the distribution and utilization in intraventricularly injected adenine-^{3}H, uracil-^{3}H and thymidine-^{3}H in the brains of cats.

Altman, J., and G. D. Das. (1964) *Nature* **204:**1161–1165. Autoradiographic examination of the effects of enriched environment on the rate of glial multiplication in the adult rat brain.

Altman, J., and G. D. Das. (1965*a*) *Nature* **207:**953–956. Post-natal origin of microneurones in the rat brain.

Altman, J., and G. D. Das. (1965*b*) *J. Comp. Neurol.* **124:**319–336. Autoradiographic and histological evidence of postnatal hippocampal neurogenesis in rats.

Altman, J., and G. D. Das. (1966) *J. Comp. Neurol.* **126:**337–390. Autoradiographic and histological studies of postnatal neurogenesis. I.

Altman, J., and G. D. Das. (1967) *Nature* **214:**1098–1101. Postnatal neurogenesis in the guinea-pig.

Altman, J., and A. T. Winfree. (1977) *J. Comp. Neurol.* **171:**1–16. Postnatal development of the cerebellar cortex in the rat. V. Spatial organization of Purkinje cell perikarya.

Altman, J., W. J. Anderson, and K. A. Wright. (1968) *Exp. Neurol.* **22:**52–74. Differential radiosensitivity of stationary and migratory primitive cells in the brains of infant rats.

Altman, J., W. J. Anderson, and K. A. Wright. (1969) *Exp. Neurol.* **24:**196–216. Early effects of X-irradiation of the cerebellum in infant rats: Decimation and reconstitution of the external granular layer.

Alvarez, J., and M. Püschel. (1972) *Brain Res.* **37:**265–278. Transfer of material from efferent axons to sensory epithelium in goldfish vestibular system.

Ancel, P., and P. Vintemberger. (1948) *Bull. Biol. Fr. Belg. Suppl.* **31**:1–182. Recherches sur le déterminisme de la symétrie bilatérale dans l'oeuf des amphibiens.

Anders, H. E. (1921) *Arch. Entw.-Mech. Organ.* **114**:272–363. Die entwicklungsmechanische Bedeutung der Doppelbildungen nebst Untersuchungen über den Einfluss des Zentralnervensystems auf die quergestreifte Muskulatur des Embryo.

Andersen, P., J. C. Eccles, and Y. Loyning. (1963) *Nature* **198**:541–542. Recurrent inhibition in the hippocampus with identification of the inhibitory cell and its synapses.

Andersen, P., T. W. Blackstad, and T. Lomo. (1966) *Exp. Brain Res.* **1**:236–248. Location and identification of excitatory synapses on hippocampal pyramidal cells.

Anderson, K.-E., A. Edström, and M. Hanson. (1972) *Brain Res.* **43**:299–302. Heavy water reversibly inhibits fast axonal transport of proteins in frog sciatic nerves.

Andres, G. (1953) *J. Exp. Zool.* **122**:507–540. Experiments on the fate of dissociated embryonic cells (chick) disseminated by the vascular route. Part II. Teratomas.

Andres, K. H. (1964) *Z. Zellforsch.* **64**:63–73. Mikropinozytose in Zentralnervensystem.

Andres, K. H., and M. Von Düring. (1966) *Naturwissenschaften* **23**:615–616. Mikropinozytose in motorische Endplatten.

Andrews, A. (1970) *J. Anat. (London)* **108**:169–184. The origin of intramural ganglia. IV. The origin of enteric ganglia: A critical review.

Andy, O. J., and H. Stephan. (1966) *J. Comp. Neurol.* **126**:157–171. Septal nuclei in primate phylogeny; A quantitative investigation.

Angeletti, R. H., and R. A. Bradshaw (1971) *Proc. Natl. Acad. Sci. U.S.A.* **68**:2417–2420. Nerve growth factor from mouse submaxillary gland: Amino acid sequence.

Angeletti, P. U., and R. Levi-Montalcini. (1970) *Proc. Natl. Acad. Sci. U.S.A.* **65**:114–121. Sympathetic nerve cell destruction in newborn mammals by 6-hydroxydopamine.

Angeletti, P. U., A. Liuzzi, and R. Levi-Montalcini. (1964*a*) *Biochim. Biophys. Acta* **84**:778–781. Stimulation of lipid biosynthesis in sympathetic and sensory ganglia by a specific nerve growth factor.

Angeletti, P. U., A. Liuzzi, R. Levi-Montalcini, and D. G. Gandini-Attardi. (1964*b*) *Biochim. Biophys. Acta* **90**:445–450. Effect of a nerve growth factor on glucose metabolism by sympathetic and sensory nerve cells.

Angeletti, P. U., D. Gandini-Attardi, G. Toschi, M. L. Salvi, and R. Levi-Montalcini. (1965) *Biochim. Biophys. Acta* **95**:111–120. Metabolic aspects of the effect of nerve growth factor on sympathetic and sensory ganglia: Protein and ribonucleic acid synthesis.

Angeletti, P. U., R. Levi-Montalcini, and P. Calissano. (1968) *Adv. Enzymol.* **31**:51–75. The nerve growth factor: Chemical properties and metabolic effects.

Angeletti, P. U., L. Levi-Montalcini, and F. Caramia. (1971*a*) *Brain Res.* **27**:343–355. Analysis of the effects of the antiserum to the nerve growth factor in adult mice.

Angeletti, P. U., R. Levi-Montalcini, and F. Caramia. (1971*b*) *J. Ultrastruct. Res.* **36**:24–36. Ultrastructural changes in sympathetic neurons of newborn and adult mice treated with nerve growth factor.

Angeletti, P. U., R. Levi-Montalcini, R. Kettler, and H. Thoenen. (1972) *Brain Res.* **44**:197–206. Comparative studies on the effect of the nerve growth factor on sympathetic ganglia and adrenal medulla in newborn rats.

Angevine, J. B. (1965) *Exp. Neurol. Suppl.* **2**:1–70. Time of neuron origin in the hippocampal region: An autoradiographic study in the mouse.

Angevine, J. B., Jr. (1968) *Anat. Rec.* **160**:308. Autoradiographic study of neuronal proliferation gradients in the diencephalon of the mouse.

Angevine, J. B., Jr. (1970*a*) *J. Comp. Neurol.* **139**:129–187. Time of neuron origin in the diencephalon of the mouse.

Angevine, J. B., Jr. (1970*b*) Critical cellular events in the shaping of the neural centers. In *The Neurosciences*, Vol. II (F. O. Schmitt and T. Melnechuck, eds.), Rockefeller University Press, New York.

Angevine, J. B., Jr., and R. L. Sidman. (1961) *Nature* **192**:766–768. Autoradiographic study of cell migration during histogenesis of cerebral cortex in the mouse.

Angevine, J. B., Jr., and R. L. Sidman. (1962) *Anat. Rec.* **142**:210. Autoradiographic study of histogenesis in the cerebral cortex of the mouse.

Angulo y Gonzalez, A. W. (1929) *J. Comp. Neurol.* **48**:459–464. Is myelogeny an absolute index of behavioral capacity?

Angulo y Gonzalez, A. W. (1932) *J. Comp. Neurol.* **55**:395–442. The prenatal development of behavior in the albino rat.

Anokhin, P. K. (1968) *The Biology and Neurophysiology of the Conditioned Reflex* (in Russian), Meditsina, Moscow.

Appeltauer, G. S. L., C. Benech, A. Levitas, and C. M. Franchi. (1965) *Exp. Neurol.* **12**:215–229. Uptake of C^{14}-L-Lysine into segments of normal rat sciatic nerve.

Arey, L. B., M. J. Tremaine, and F. L. Monzingo. (1935) *Anat. Rec.* **64**:9–25. The numerical and topographical relations of taste buds to human circumvallate papillae throughout the life span.

Ariëns Kappers, C. U. (1907) *Folia Neurobiol.* **1**:507–534. Weitere Mitteilungen über Neurobiotaxis. Die Selektivität der Zellwanderung: Die Bedeutung synchronischer Reizwandschaft.

Ariëns Kappers, C. U. (1917) *J. Comp. Neurol.* **27**:261–298. Further contributions on neurobiotaxis. IX. An attempt to compare the phenomenon of neurobiotaxis with other phenomena of taxis and tropism. The dynamic polarization of the neuron.

Ariëns Kappers, C. U. (1921) *Brain* **44**:125–149. On the structural laws in the nervous system: The principles of neurobiotaxis.

Ariëns Kappers, C. U. (1932) Principles of development of the nervous system (neurobiotaxis), pp. 43–89. In *Cytology and Cellular Pathology of the Nervous System* Vol. I (W. Penfield, ed.), Hoeber, New York.

Ariëns Kappers, C. U., G. C. Huber, and E. C. Crosby. (1936) *The Comparative Anatomy of the Nervous System of Vertebrates Including Man.* 2 vols., 1845 pp. Macmillan, New York.

Arora, H. L., and R. W. Sperry. (1957) *J. Embryol. Exp. Morphol.* **5**:256–263. Myotypic respecification of regenerated nerve fibres in cichlid fishes.

Arora, H. L., and R. W. Sperry. (1962) *Am. Zool.* **2**:61. Optic nerve regeneration after surgical cross-union of medial and lateral optic tracts.

Asbury, A. L. (1967) *J. Cell Biol.* **34**:735–743. Schwann cell proliferation in developing mouse sciatic nerve.

Athias, M. (1897*a*) *J. Anat. Physiol. (Paris)* **33**:372–404. L'histogénese de l'ecorce du cervelet.

Athias, M. (1897*b*) *Bibl. Anat.* **5**:58–89. Structure histologique de la moelle épinière du têtard de la grenouille.

Atlas, M., and V. P. Bond. (1965) *J. Cell Biol.* **26**:19–24. The cell generation cycle of the eleven-day mouse embryo.

Attardi, B., and E. Ruoslahti. (1976) *Nature* **263**:685–687. Foetoneonatal oestradiol-binding protein in mouse brain cytosol is α foetoprotein.

Attardi, D. G., and R. W. Sperry. (1963) *Exp. Neurol.* **7**:46–64. Preferential selection of central pathways by regenerating optic fibers.

Auerbach, R. (1960) *Dev. Bio.* **2**:271–284. Morphogenetic interactions in the development of the mouse thymus gland.

Aufsess, A. von. (1941) *Arch. Entw.-Mech. Organ.* **141**:248–339. Defeckt und Isolationsversuche an der Medullarplatte und ihrer Unterlagerung an Triton alpestris- und Amblystoma-Keimen, mit besonderer Berücksichtigung der Rumpf- und Schwantzregion.

Austin, L., and I. Morgan. (1967) *J. Neurochem.* **14**:377–387. Incorporation of radioactively labelled leucine into synaptosomes from rat cerebral cortex *in vitro.*

Autilio-Gambetti, L., P. Gambetti, and B. Shafer. (1973) *Brain Res.* **53**:387–398. RNA and axonal flow, biochemical and autoradiographic study in the rabbit optic system.

Axelsson, J., and S. Thesleff. (1959) *J. Physiol. (London)* **149**:178–193. A study of supersensitivity in denervated mammalian skeletal muscle.

Bacher, B. E. (1973) *J. Exp. Zool.* **185**:209–216. The peripheral dependency of Rohon-Beard cells.

Baden, V. (1936) *J. Morphol.* **60**:159–190. Embryology of the nervous system in the grasshopper, *Melanoplus differentialis.*

Baffoni, G. M. (1953) *Rend. Accad. Nazl. Lincei, Ser. 8,* **14**:138–144. Azione dell' attivitá mitotica e modificazioni cellulari nel prosencefalo e nel mesencefalo di Anfibi.

Baffoni, G. M. (1957*a*) *Rend. Accad. Nazl. Lincei, Ser. 8,* **23**:90–96. Tardiva determinazione numerica di cellule nervose nel rombencefalo di *Anfibi.*

Baffoni, G. M. (1957*b*) *Rend. Accad. Nazl. Linci, Ser. 8,* **23**:495–503. Influenza dell' ormone tiroideo sull' attivita mitotica del rombencephalo di un *Anfibio anuro.*

Baffoni, G. M. (1959) *Rend. Accad. Nazl. Lincei, Ser. 8* **27**:427–435. Effetti dell' ormone tiroidea sul midollo spinale di larve di *Anfibi anuri.*

Baffoni, G. M. (1960) *Rend. Accad. Nazl. Lincei, Ser. 8* **28**:102–108. Variazioni dell' attivitá mitotica e modificazioni cellulari nel presencefalo e nel mesencefalo di larve di *Anfibi anuri* trattate con ormone tiroideo.

Baffoni, G. M., and G. Catte. (1950) *Rend. Acad. Nazl. Lincei, Ser. 8,* **9:**282–287. Il comportamento della cellula di' Mauthner di raganella nella metamorfosi accelerata con somministrazione di tiroide.

Baffoni, G. M., and G. Catte. (1951) *Riv. Biol.* **43:**373–397. La citomorfosi della cellula di Mauthner in *Hyla arborea savignyi* (nello sviluppo normale e nella metamorfosi sperimentalmente anticipata).

Baffoni, G. M., and E. Elia. (1957) *Rend. Accad. Nazl. Lincei, Ser. 8* **22:**109–114. L'attivitata mitotica durante la morfogenesi cerebellare in un *Anfibio anuro.*

Bagust, J., D. M. Lewis, and R. A. Westerman. (1973) *J. Physiol. (London)* **229:**241–255. Polyneuronal innervation of kitten skeletal muscle.

Bailey, P., and G. von Bonin. (1951) *The Isocortex of Man,* University of Illinois Press, Urbana, Ill.

Baird, H. W., III, M. Chavez, J. Adams, H. T. Wycis, and E. A. Spiegel. (1957) *Confin. Neurol.* **17:**288–299. Studies in stereoencephalotomy. VII. Variations in the position of the globus pallidus.

Baker, F. H., P. Grigg, and G. K. von Noorden. (1974) *Brain Res.* **66:**185–208. Effects of visual deprivation and strabismus on the response of neurons in the visual cortex of the monkey, including studies on the striate and prestriate cortex in the normal animal.

Baker, P. C., and T. E. Schroeder. (1967) *Dev. Biol.* **15:**432–450. Cytoplasmic filaments and morphogenetic movement in the amphibian neural tube.

Baker, R. C., and G. O. Graves. (1939) *J. Comp. Neurol.* **71:**389–415. The behavior of the neural crest in the forebrain region of *Amblystoma.*

Baker, R. E. and M. Jacobson. (1970) *Dev. Biol.* **22:**476–494. Development of reflexes from skin grafts in *Rana pipiens:* Influence of size and position of grafts.

Baker, R. E., A. P. J. Richter, and N. Piller. (1976) *Neuroscience* **1:**367–370. A light and electron microscopic examination of dorsal root afferent development in three species of anurans.

Balázs, R. (1974) *Br. Med. Bull.* **30:**126–134. Influence of metabolic factors on brain development.

Balázs, R., and W. A. Cocks. (1967) *J. Neurochem.* **14:**1035–1055. RNA metabolism in subcellular fractions of brain tissue.

Balázs, R., S. Kovacs, P. Teichgraber, W. A. Cocks, and J. T. Eayrs. (1968) *J. Neurochem.* **15:**1335–1349. Biochemical effects of thyroid deficiency on the developing brain.

Balázs, R., B. W. L. Brooksbank, A. N. Davison, J. T. Eayrs, and D. A. Wilson. (1969) *Brain Res.* **15:**219–232. The effect of neonatal thyroidectomy on myelination in the rat brain.

Balázs, R., S. Kovács, W. A. Cocks, A. L. Johnson, and J. T. Eayrs. (1971) *Brain Res.* **25:**555–570. Effect of thyroid hormone on the biochemical maturation of rat brain: Postnatal cell formation.

Ballard, K. J., and S. J. Holt. (1968) *J. Cell Sci.* **3:**245–262. Cytological and cytochemical studies on cell death and digestion in foetal rat foot; the role of macrophages and hydrolytic enzymes.

Bamburg, J. R., E. M. Shooter, and L. Wilson. (1973) *Biochemistry* **12:**1476–1482. Developmental changes in microtubule protein of chick brain.

Banerjee, S. P., S. H. Snyder, P. Cuatrecasas, and L. A. Greene. (1973) *Proc. Natl. Acad. Sci. U.S.A.* **70:**2519–2523. Binding of nerve growth factor receptor in sympathetic ganglia.

Banks, M. S., R. N. Aslin, and R. D. Letson. (1975) *Science* **190:**675–677. Sensitive period for the development of human binocular vision.

Banks, P., D. Mangnall, and D. Mayor. (1969) *J. Physiol. (London)* **200:**745–762. The re-distribution of cytochrome oxidase, noradrenaline and adenosine triphosphate in adrenergic nerves constricted at two points.

Bär, T., and J.-R. Wolff. (1972) *Z. Zellforsch. Mikrosk. Anat.* **133:**231–248. The formation of capillary basement membranes during internal vascularization of the rat's cerebral cortex.

Bär, T., and J.-R. Wolff. (1973) *Z. Anat. Entwicklungsqesch.* **141:**207–221. Quantitative Beziehungen zwischen der Verzweigungsdichte und Länge von Capillaren im Neocortex der Ratte während der postnatalen Entwicklung.

Barber, R. P., J. E. Vaughn, R. E. Wimer, and C. C. Wimer. (1974) *J. Comp. Neurol.* **156:**417–434. Genetically associated variations in the distribution of dentate granule cell synapses upon the pyramidal cell dendrites in mouse hippocampus.

Barbera, A. J. (1975) *Dev. Biol.* **46:**167–191. Adhesive recognition between developing retinal cells and optic tecta of the chick embryo.

Barbera, A. J., R. B. Marchase, and S. Roth. (1973) *Proc. Natl. Acad. Sci. U.S.A.* **70:**2482–2486. Adhesive recognition and retinotectal specificity.

Bard, J., and I. Lauder. (1974) *J. Theor. Biol.* **45:**501–531. How well does Turing's theory of morphogenesis work?

Barker, D. (1974) The morphology of muscle receptors, pp. 1–190. In *Handbook of Sensory Physiology,* Vol. III/2 (C. C. Hunt, ed.), Springer-Verlag, New York.

Barker, D., and M. C. Ip. (1966) *Proc. R. Soc. (London) Ser. B* **163:**538–554. Sprouting and degeneration of mammalian motor axons in normal and deafferented skeletal muscle.

Barker, D., and A. Milburn. (1972) *J. Physiol. (London)* **222:**159–160. Increase in number of intrafusal muscle fibres during the development of muscle spindles in the rat.

Barlow, H. B. (1975) *Nature* **258:**199–204. Visual experience and cortical development.

Barlow, H. B., and J. D. Pettigrew. (1971) *J. Physiol. (London)* **218:**98–100P. Lack of specificity of neurones in the visual cortex of young kittens.

Barlow, R. M. (1969) *J. Comp. Neurol.* **135:**249–262. The foetal sheep: Morphogenesis of the nervous system and histochemical aspects of myelination.

Barnard, E. A., J. Wieckowski, and T. H. Chiu. (1974) *Nature* **234:**207. Cholinergic receptor molecules and cholinesterase molecules at mouse skeletal junctions.

Barnes, B. G. (1961) *J. Ultrastruct. Res.* **5:**453–467. Ciliated secretory cells in the pars distalis of the mouse hypophysis.

Barnes, R. H., S. R. Cunnold, R. R. Zimmerman, H. Simmons, R. B. MacCleod, and L. Krook. (1966) *J. Nutr.* **89:**399–410. Influence of nutritional deprivation in early life on learning behavior as measured by performance in a water maze.

Barnicot, N. A. (1964) Biological variation in modern populations. In *Human Biology* (G. A. Harrison, J. S. Weiner, J. M. Tanner, and N. A. Barnicot, eds.), Clarendon, Oxford.

Barondes, S. H. (1966) *J. Neurochem.* **13:**221–227. On the site of synthesis of the mitochondrial protein of nerve endings.

Barr, M. L., and E. G. Bertram. (1951) *J. Anat. (London)* **85:**171–181. The behaviour of nuclear structures during depletion and restoration of Nissl material in motor neurons.

Barron, D. H. (1943) *J. Comp. Neurol.* **78:**1–26. The early development of the motor cells and columns in the spinal cord of the sheep.

Barron, D. H. (1946) *J. Comp. Neurol.* **85:**149–169. Observations on the early differentiation of the motor neuroblasts in the spinal cord of the chick.

Barron, D. H. (1948) *J. Comp. Neurol.* **88:**93–127. Some effects of amputation of the chick wing bud on the early differentiation of the motor neuroblasts in the associated segments of the spinal cord.

Barron, D. H. (1950) *J. Exp. Zool.* **113:**553–573. An experimental analysis of some factors involved in the development of the fissure pattern of the cerebral cortex.

Barron, D. H., and J. Barcroft. (1938) *J. Physiol. (London)* **93:**29P. A case of amputation of leg, 90 days before birth.

Barron, K. D., and T. O. Tuncbay. (1962) *Am. J. Pathol.* **40:**637–652. Histochemistry of acid phosphatase and thiamine pyrophosphatase during axon reaction.

Barron, K. D., and T. O. Tuncbay, (1964) *J. Neuropathol. Exp. Neurol.* **23:**368–386. Phosphatase histochemistry of feline cervical spinal cord after brachial plexectomy.

Barth, L. G. (1965) *Biol. Bull.* **129:**471–481. The nature of the action of ions as inductors.

Barth, L. G., and L. J. Barth. (1969) *Dev. Biol.* **20:**236–262. The sodium dependence of embryonic induction.

Barth, L. G., and L. J. Barth. (1972) *Dev. Biol.* **28:**18–34. ^{22}Sodium and ^{45}calcium uptake during embryonic induction in *Rana pipiens.*

Bate, C. M. (1976) *J. Embryol Exp. Morphol.* **35:**107–123. Embryogenesis of an insect nervous system. I. A map of the thoracic and abdominal neuroblasts in *Locusta migratoria.*

Bate, C. M. (1978) The development of sensory systems in arthropods. In *Handbook of Sensory Physiology,* Vol. IX: *Development of Sensory Systems* (M. Jacobson, ed.), Springer-Verlag, New York.

Batten, E. H. (1958) *J. Embryol. Exp. Morphol.* **6:**597–615. The origin of the acoustic ganglion in the sheep.

Bauer, V. (1904) *Zool. Jahrb. Abt. Anat. Ontog. Tiere* **20:**123–150. Zur inneren Metamorphose des Zentralnervensystems der Insekten.

Baumann, L., and W. Landauer. (1943) *J. Comp. Neurol.* **79:**153–163. Polydactyly and anterior horn cells in fowl.

Bautzmann, H. (1933) *Arch. Entw.-Mech. Organ.* **128:**666–765. Über Determinationsgrad und Wirkungsbezeichungen der Randzonenteilanlagen (Chorda, Ursegmente, Seitenplatte und Kopfdarmanlage) bei Urodelen und Anuren.

Bautzmann, H. (1955) *Naturwissenschaften* **42:**286–294. Die Problemlage des Spemannschen Organisators.

Baylor, D. A., and J. G. Nicholls. (1971) *Nature* **237:**268–270. Patterns of regeneration between individual nerve cells in the central nervous system of the leech.

Beach, D. H., and M. Jacobson. (1978) *J. Comp. Neurol.* (in preparation). The pattern of cell proliferation in the developing neural retina of *Xenopus laevis.*

Beach, F. A. (1975) *Psychoneuroendocrinology* **1**:3–23. Hormonal modification of sexually dimorphic behavior.

Beaudoin, A. R. (1955) *Anat. Rec.* **121**:81–96. The development of lateral motor column cells in the lumbo-sacral cord in *Rana pipiens.* I. Normal development and development following unilateral limb ablation.

Beaudoin, A. R. (1956) *Anat. Rec.* **125**:247–259. The development of lateral motor column cells in the lumbo-sacral cord in *Rana pipiens.* II. Development under the influence of thyroxine.

Beazley, L., M. J. Keating, and R. M. Gaze. (1972) *Vision Res.* **12**:407–410. The appearance, during development, of responses in the optic tectum following stimulation of the ipsilateral eye in *Xenopus laevis.*

Begliomini, A., and A. Moriconi. (1960) *Riv. Biol.* **51**:517–530. Sull'epoca della comparsa e sulla localizzazione della colinesterasi nel muscolo striato dell'embrione di pollo.

Behnke, O. (1975) *Nature* **257**:709–710. An outer component of microtubules.

Beidler, L. M. (1963) Dynamics of taste cells, pp. 133–148. In *Olfaction and Taste* (Y. Zotterman, ed.), Pergamon, Oxford.

Beidler, L. M., and R. L. Smallman. (1965) *J. Cell Biol.* **27**:263–272. Renewal of cells within taste buds.

Bekoff, A. (1976) *Brain Res.* **106**:271–291. Ontogeny of leg motor output in the chick embryo: A neural analysis.

Bellairs, R. (1959) *J. Embryol. Exp. Morphol.* **7**:94–115. The development of the nervous system in chick embryos studied by electron microscopy.

Benes, F. M., T. N. Parks, and E. W. Rubel. (1975) *Neurosci. Abstr.* **1**:669. Dendritic atrophy following deafferentation in nucleus laminaris of the chicken: An E. M. morphometric analysis.

Benjamin, P. R. (1976) *Nature* **260**:338–340. Interganglionic variation in cell body location of snail neurones does not affect synaptic connections or central axonal projections.

Bennett, E. L., M. L. Diamond, D. Krech, and M. R. Rosenzweig. (1964) *Science* **146**:610–619. Chemical and anatomical plasticity of brain.

Bennett, G., L. DiGiamberardino, H. L. Koenig, and B. Droz. (1973) *Brain Res.* **60**:129–146. Axonal migration of protein and glycoprotein to nerve endings. II. Radioautographic analysis of the renewal of glycoproteins in nerve endings of chicken ciliary ganglion after intracerebral injection of [^{3}H] fucose and [^{3}H] glucosamine.

Bennett, M. R. (1972) *Autonomic Neuromuscular Transmission,* Cambridge University Press, London.

Bennett, M. R., and A. G. Pettigrew. (1974) *J. Physiol. (London)* **241**:547–573. The formation of synapses in reinnervated and cross-reinnervated striated muscle during development.

Bennett, M. R., and J. Raftos. (1977) *J. Physiol. (London)* **265**:261–295. The formation and regression of synapses during the re-innervation of axolotl striated muscles.

Bennett, M. R., E. M. McLachlan, and R. S. Taylor. (1973*a*) *J. Physiol. (London)* **233**:501–518. The formation of synapses in reinnervated mammalian striated muscle.

Bennett, M. R., E. M. McLachlan, and R. S. Taylor. (1973*b*) *J. Physiol. (London)* **241**:547–573. The formation of synapses in mammalian striated muscle reinnervated with autonomic preganglionic nerves.

Bennett, M. R., A. G. Pettigrew, and R. S. Taylor. (1973*c*) *J. Physiol. (London)* **230**:331–357. The formation of synapses in reinnervated and cross-reinnervated adult avian muscle.

Benoit, P., and J.-P. Changeux. (1975) *Brain Res.* **99**:354–358. Consequences of tenotomy on the evolution of multiinnervation in developing rat soleus muscle.

Bensted, J. P. M., J. Dobbing, R. S. Morgan, R. T. W. Reid, and G. P. Wright. (1957) *J. Embryol. Exp. Morphol.* **5**:428–437. Neuroglial development and myelination in the spinal cord of the chick embryo.

Bentley, D. R., and R. R. Hoy. (1970) *Science* **170**:1409–1411. Postembryonic development of adult motor patterns in crickets: A neural analysis.

Benton, J. W., H. W. Moser, P. R. Dodge, and S. Carr. (1966) *Pediatrics* **38**:801–807. Modification of the schedule of myelination in the rat by early nutritional deprivation.

Benzer, S. (1973) *Sci. Am.* **229**:24–37. Genetic dissection of behavior.

Berg, D. K., R. B. Kelly, P. B. Sargent, P. Williamson, and Z. Hall. (1972) *Proc. Natl. Acad. Sci. U.S.A.* **69**:147. Binding of α-bungarotoxin to acetylcholine receptor in mammalian muscle.

Berger, H. (1921) *Z. Ges. Neurol. Psychiat.* **69**:46–59. Untersuchungen uber den Zellgehalt der menschlichen Grosshirnrinde.

Bergey, G. K., R. K. Hunt, and H. Holtzer. (1973) *Anat. Rec.* **175:**271. Selective effects of bromodeoxyuridine on developing *Xenopus laevis* retina.

Bergquist, H. (1960) *J. Embryol. Exp. Morphol.* **8:**69–72. Volumetric investigation on overgrowth (hypermorphosis) in chick embryo brains.

Beritoff, J. S. (1969) *Structure and Functions of the Cerebral Cortex* (in Russian), Nauka, Moscow.

Berl, S., S. Puszkin, and W. K. Nicklas. (1973) *Science* **179:**441–446. Actomyosin-like protein in brain.

Berlinrood, M., S. M. McGee-Russell, and R. D. Allen. (1972) *J. Cell Sci.* **II:**875–886. Patterns of particle movement in nerve fibres *in vitro*—An analysis by photokymography and microscopy.

Bernfield, M. R., and N. K. Wessells. (1970) *Dev. Biol. Suppl.* **4:**195–249. Intra- and extracellular control of epithelial morphogenesis.

Bernstein, J. J., and L. Guth. (1961) *Exp. Neurol.* **4:**262–275. Nonselectivity in establishment of neuromuscular connections following nerve regeneration in the rat.

Berry, M., and J. T. Eayrs. (1963) *Nature* **197:**884–885. Histogenesis of the cerebral cortex.

Berry, M., and J. T. Eayrs. (1966) *J. Anat. (London)* **100:**707–722. The effects of X-irradiation on the development of the cerebral cortex.

Berry, M., and A. C. Riches. (1974) *Br. Med. Bull.* **30:**135–140. An immunological approach to regeneration in the central nervous system.

Berry, M., and A. W. Rogers. (1965) *J. Anat. (London)* **99:**691–709. The migration of neuroblasts in the developing cerebral cortex.

Berry, M., and A. W. Rogers. (1966) Histogenesis of mammalian neocortex, pp. 197–205. In *Evolution of the Forebrain* (R. Hassler and H. Stephan, eds.), Plenum, New York.

Berry, M., A. W. Rogers, and J. T. Eayrs. (1964*a*) *Nature* **203:**591–593. Pattern of cell migration during cortical histogenesis.

Berry, M., A. W. Rogers, and J. T. Eayrs. (1964*b*) *J. Anat. (London)* **98:**291–292. The pattern and mechanism of migration of the neuroblasts of the developing cerebral cortex.

Bielschowsky, M. (1923) *J. Psychol. Neurol.* **30:**29–76. Über die Oberflächengestaltung des Grosshirnmantels bei Mikrogyrie und bei normaler Entwicklung.

Bignami, A., and D. Dahl. (1973) *Brain Res.* **49:**393–402. Differentiation of astroycytes in the cerebellar cortex and the pyramidal tracts of the newborn rat: An immunofluorescence study with antibodies to a protein specific to astrocytes.

Bignami, A., and D. Dahl. (1974*a*) *Nature* **252:**55–56. Astrocyte-specific protein and radial glia in the cerebral cortex of newborn rat.

Bignami, A., and D. Dahl. (1974*b*) *J. Comp. Neurol.* **153:**27–38. Astrocyte-specific protein and neuroglial differentiation: An immunofluorescence study with antibodies to the glial fibrillary acidic protein.

Bignami, A., and D. Dahl. (1974*c*) *J. Comp. Neurol.* **155:**219–230. The development of Bergmann glia in mutant mice with cerebellar malformations: Reeler, staggerer and weaver. Immunofluorescence study with antibodies to the glial fibrillary acidic protein.

Bignami, A., and D. Dahl. (1975) *Dev. Biol.* **44:**204–209. Astroglial protein in the developing spinal cord of the chick embryo.

Billings, S. M., and F. J. Swartz. (1969) *Z. Anat. Entwicklungsgeschichte* **129:**14–23. DNA content of Mauthner cell nuclei in *Xenopus laevis:* A spectrophotometric study.

Billings-Gagliardi, S., H. deF. Webster, and M. F. O'Connell. (1974) *Am. J. Anat.* **141:**375–392. *In vivo* and electron microscopic observations on Schwann cells in developing tadpole nerve fibers.

Binder, L. I., W. L. Dentler, and J. L. Rosenbaum. (1975) *Proc. Natl. Acad. Sci. U.S.A.* **72:**1122–1126. Assembly of chick brain tubulin onto flagellar microtubules from *Chlamydomonas* and sea urchin sperm.

Biondi, R. J., M. J. Levy, and P. A. Weiss. (1972) *Proc. Natl. Acad. Sci. U.S.A.* **69:**1732–1736. An engineering study of the peristaltic drive of axonal flow.

Birks, R. I. (1966) *Ann. N.Y. Acad. Sci.* **135:**8–19. The fine structure of motor nerve endings at frog myoneural junctions.

Birks, R. I., M. C. Mackey, and P. R. Weldon. (1972) *J. Neurocytol.* **I:**311–340. Organelle formation from pinocytotic elements in neurites of cultured sympathetic ganglia.

Birnstiel, M. L., M. I. H. Chipchase, and B. B. Hyde. (1963) *Biochim. Biophys. Acta* **76:**454–462. The nucleolus, a source of ribosomes.

Birren, J. E., and P. D. Wall. (1956) *J. Comp. Neurol.* **104:**1–16. Age changes in conduction velocity, refractory period, number of fibers, connective tissue space and blood vessels in sciatic nerve of rats.

Birse, S. C., and G. D. Bittner. (1976) *Brain Res.* **113**:575–581. Regeneration of giant axons in earthworms.

Bisby, M. A. (1975) *Exp. Neurol.* **47**:481–489. Inhibition of axonal transport in nerves chronically treated with local anesthetics.

Bisconte, J. C., and R. Marty. (1975) *Exp. Brain Res.* **22**:37–56. Etude quantitative du marquage radioautographique dans le système nerveux du Rat. II. Caractéristiques finales dans le cerveau de l'animal adulte: Lois d'interprétation et concept de chronoarchitectonic corticale.

Bishop, G. H. (1959) *J. Nerv. Ment. Dis.* **128**:89–114. The relation between nerve fiber size and sensory modality: Phylogenetic implications of the afferent innervation of cortex.

Bittner, G. D. (1973) *Am. Zool.* **13**:379–408. Degeneration and regeneration in crustacean neuromuscular systems.

Bjerre, B., A. Björklund, and U. Stenevi. (1973) *Brain Res.* **60**:161–176. Stimulation of growth of new axonal sprouts from lesioned monoamine neurones in adult rat brain by nerve growth factor.

Bjerre, B., A. Björklund, and D. C. Edwards. (1974) *Cell Tissue Res.* **148**:441–476. Axonal regeneration of peripheral adrenergic neurons: Effects of antiserum to nerve growth factor in mouse.

Bjerre, B., L. Wiklund, and D. C. Edwards. (1975*a*) *Brain Res.* **92**:257–278. A study of the de- and regenerative changes in the sympathetic nervous system of the adult mouse after treatment with the antiserum to nerve growth factor.

Bjerre, B., A. Björklund, W. Mobley, and E. Rosengren. (1975*b*) *Brain Res.* **94**:263–277. Short- and long-term effects of nerve growth factor on the sympathetic nervous system in the adult mouse.

Björklund, A., and U. Stenevi. (1972) *Science* **175**:1251–1253. Nerve growth factor: Stimulation of regenerative growth of central noradrenergic neurons.

Black, I. B., and S. C. Green. (1973) *Brain Res.* **63**:291–302 Trans-synaptic regulation of adrenergic neuron development: Inhibition of ganglionic blockade.

Black, I. B., and C. Mytilineou. (1976*a*) *Brain Res.* **101**:503–521 Trans-synaptic regulation of the development of end organ innervation by sympathetic neurons.

Black, I. B., and C. Mytilineou. (1976*b*) *Brain Res.* **108**:199–204. The interaction of nerve growth factor and trans-synaptic regulation in the development of target organ innervation by sympathetic neurons.

Black, I. B., E. M. Bloom, and R. W. Hamill. (1976) *Proc. Natl. Acad. Sci. U.S.A.* **73**:3575–3578. Central regulation of sympathetic neuron development.

Blackshaw, S. E., and A. E. Warner. (1976*a*) *J. Physiol. (London)* **255**:231–247. Alterations in resting membrane properties during neural plate stages of development of the nervous system.

Blackshaw, S., and A. Warner. (1976*b*) *Nature* **262**:217–218. Onset of acetylcholine sensitivity and endplate activity in developing myotome muscles of *Xenopus.*

Blackstad, T. W. (1956) *J. Comp. Neurol.* **105**:417–538. Commissural connections of the hippocampal region in the rat, with special reference to their mode of termination.

Blackstad, T. W., and P. R. Flood. (1963) *Nature* **198**:542–543. Ultrastructure of hippocampal axosomatic synapses.

Blake, R., and H. V. B. Hirsch. (1975) *Science* **190**:1114–1116. Deficits in binocular depth perception in cats after alternating monocular deprivation.

Blakemore, C. (1974) *Br. Med. Bull.* **30**:152–157. Development of functional connexions in the mammalian visual system.

Blakemore, C., and G. F. Cooper. (1970) *Nature* **228**:477–478. Development of the brain depends on visual experience.

Blakemore, C., and R. C. Van Sluyters. (1974) *J. Physiol. (London)* **237**:195–216. Reversal of the physiological effects of monocular deprivation in kittens: Further evidence for a sensitive period.

Blakemore, C., and R. C. Van Sluyters. (1975) *J. Physiol. (London)* **248**:663–716. Innate and environmental factors in the development of the kitten's visual cortex.

Blakemore, C., R. C. Van Sluyters, and J. A. Movshon. (1975) *Cold Spring Harbor Symp. Quant. Biol.* **40**:601–609. Synaptic competition in the kitten's visual cortex.

Blakemore, W. F. (1969) *J. Anat.* **104**:423–433. The ultrastructure of the subependymal plate in the rat.

Blakemore, W. F., and R. D. Jolly. (1972) *J. Neurocytol.* **I**:69–84. The subependymal plate and associated ependyma in the dog: An ultrastructural study.

Blaurock, A. E. (1976) *Biophys. J.* **16**:491–501. Myelin x-ray patterns reconciled.

Blenkinsopp, W. K. (1967) *J. Cell Sci.* **2**:305–308. Effect of tritiated thymidine on cell proliferation.

Blinkov, S. M., and I. Glezer. (1968) *The Human Brain in Figures and Tables,* Plenum, New York.

Blinzinger, K. H., and G. W. Kreutzberg. (1968) *Z. Zellforsch. Mikrosk. Anat.* **85:**145–157. Displacement of synaptic terminals from regenerating motoneurons by microglial cells.

Bliss, T. V. P., and S. H. Chung. (1974) *Nature* **252:**153–155. An electrophysiological study of the hippocampus of the "reeler" mutant mouse.

Block, J. B., and W. B. Essman. (1965) *Nature* **205:**1136–1137. Growth hormone administration during pregnancy: A behavioral difference in offspring rats.

Bloom, B. S. (1964) *Stability and Change in Human Characteristics,* Wiley, New York.

Bloom, E. M., and R. Tompkins. (1976) *J. Exp. Zool.* **195:**237–246. Selective reinnervation in skin rotation grafts in *Rana pipiens.*

Bloom, F. E. (1972) The formation of synaptic junctions in developing rat brain, pp. 101–120. In *Structure and Function of Synapses* (G. D. Pappas and D. P. Purpura, eds.), Raven Press, New York.

Bloom, F. E., and G. K. Aghajanian. (1968) *J. Ultrastruct. Res.* **22:**361–375. Fine structural and cytochemical analysis of the staining of synaptic junctions with phosphotungstic acid.

Blunt, M. J., C. P. Wendell-Smith, P. B. Paisley, and F. Baldwin. (1967) *J. Anat. (London)* **101:**13–26. Oxidative enzyme activity in macroglia and axons of cat optic nerve.

Blunt, M. J., F. Baldwin, and C. P. Wendell-Smith. (1972) *Z. Zellforsch. Mikrosk. Anat.* **124:**293–310. Gliogenesis and myelination in kitten optic nerve.

Boas, J. A. R., R. L. Ramsey, A. J. Riesen, and J. P. Walker. (1969) *Psychon. Sci.* **15:**251–252. Absence of change in some measures of cortical morphology in dark-reared adult rats.

Bodenstein, D. (1957) *J. Exp. Zool.* **136:**89–115. Studies on nerve regeneration in *Periplaneta americana.*

Bodian, D. (1947) *Symp. Soc. Exp. Biol.* **1:**163–178. Nucleic acid in nerve-cell regeneration.

Bodian, D. (1952) *Cold Spring Harbor Symp. Quant. Biol.* **17:**1–13. Introductory survey of neurons.

Bodian, D. (1964) *Bull. Johns Hopkins Hosp.* **114:**13–40. An electron-microscopic study of the monkey spinal cord. I. Fine structure of normal motor column. II. Effects of retrograde chromatolysis. III. Cytologic effects of mild and virulent poliovirus infection.

Bodian, D. (1966*a*) *Bull. Johns Hopkins Hosp.* **119:**129–149. Development of fine structure of spinal cord in monkey foetuses. I. Motoneuron neuropil at time of onset of reflex activity.

Bodian, D. (1966*b*) *Bull. Johns Hopkins Hosp.* **119:**217–234. Spontaneous degeneration in the spinal cord of monkey foetuses.

Bodian, D., and H. A. Howe. (1941*a*) *Bull. Johns Hopkins Hosp.* **68:**248–267. Experimental studies on intraneural spread of poliomyelitis virus.

Bodian, D., and H. A. Howe. (1941*b*) *Bull. Johns Hopkins Hosp.* **69:**79–85. The rate of progression of poliomyelitis virus in nerves.

Bodian, D., and R. C. Mellors. (1945) *J. Exp. Med.* **81:**469–488. The regeneration cycle of motoneurons, with special reference to phosphatase activity.

Boerema, I. (1929) *Arch. Entw.-Mech. Organ.* **115:**601–615. Die Dynamik des Medullarrohrschlusses.

Bok, S. T. (1915) *Folia Neurobiol.* **9:**475–565. Die Entwicklung der Hirnnerven und ihrer zentralen Bahnen. Die stimulogene Fibrillation.

Bok, S. T. (1959) *Histonomy of the Cerebral Cortex,* Elsevier, Amsterdam.

Bondareff. W. (1965) *Anat. Rec.* **152:**119–128. The extracellular compartment of the cerebral cortex.

Bondareff, W. (1966) *Z. Zellforsch. Mikrosk. Anat.* **72:**487–495. Electron microscopic evidence for the existence of an intercellular substance in rat cerebral cortex.

Bondareff, W. (1967*a*) *Anat. Rec.* **157:**527–536. An intercellular substance in rat cerebral cortex: Submicroscopic distribution of ruthenium red.

Bondareff, W. (1967*b*) *Z. Zellforsch. Mikrosk. Anat.* **81:**366–373. Demonstration of an intercellular substance in mouse cerebral cortex.

Bondareff, W., and J. J. Pysh. (1968) *Anat. Rec.* **160:**773–780. Distribution of the extracellular space during postnatal maturation of rat cerebral cortex.

Bondy, S. C. (1972) *J. Neurochem.* **19:**1769–1776. Axonal migration of various ribonucleic acid species along the optic tract of the chick.

Bondy, S. C., and C. J. Madsen. (1971) *J. Neurobiol.* **2:**279–286. Development of rapid axonal flow in the chick embryo.

Bondy, S. C., and C. J. Madsen. (1973) *J. Neurobiol.* **4:**535–542. Axoplasmic transport of RNA.

Bondy, S. C., and C. J. Madsen. (1974) *J. Neurochem.* **23:**905–910. The extent of axoplasmic transport during development, determined by migration of various radioactively-labelled materials.

Bondy, S. C., and P. C. Marchisio. (1973) *Exp. Neurol.* **41:**29–37. Development of axonal transport of RNA and its precursors in the optic pathway of the chick embryo.

Bone, Q. (1964) *Int. Rev. Neurobiol.* **6:**99–147. Patterns of muscular innervation in the lower chordates.

Bonner, J. T. (1947) *J. Exp. Zool.* **106:**1–26. Evidence for the formation of cell aggregates by chemotaxis in the development of slime mould *Dictyostelium discoideum.*

Bonner, J. T. (1959) *The Cellular Slime Molds,* Princeton University Press, Princeton, N.J.

Borisy, G. G., and E. W. Taylor. (1967*a*) *J. Cell Biol.* **34:**525–533. The mechanism of action of colchicine: Binding of colchicine-^{3}H to cellular protein.

Borisy, G. G., and E. W. Taylor. (1967*b*) *J. Cell Biol.* **34:**535–548. The mechanism of action of colchicine: Colchicine binding to sea urchin eggs and the mitotic apparatus.

Borisy, G. G., J. B. Olmsted, J. M. Marcum, and C. Allen. (1974) *Fed. Proc.* **33:**167–174. Microtubule assembly *in vitro.*

Bornstein, M. B., and M. R. Murray. (1958) *J. Biophys. Biochem. Cytol.* **4:**499–504. Serial observations on patterns of growth, myelin formation, maintenance and degeneration in cultures of newborn rat and kitten cerebellum.

Bornstein, M. B., H. Iwanami, G. M. Lehrer, and L. Breitbart. (1968) *Z. Zellforsch. Mikrosk. Anat. Abt. Histochem.* **92:**197–206. Observations on the appearance of neuromuscular relationships in cultured mouse tissues.

Boulder Committee: Angevine, J. B., Jr., D. Bodian, A. J. Coulombre, M. V. Edds, Jr., V. Hamburger, M. Jacobson, K. M. Lyser, M. C. Prestige, R. L. Sidman, S. Varon, and P. Weiss. (1970) *Anat. Rec.* **166:**257–262. Embryonic vertebrate central nervous system: Revised terminology.

Bowman, W. C., and M. W. Nott. (1969) *Pharmacol. Rev.* **21:**27–72. Actions of sympathomimetic amines and their antagonists on skeletal muscle.

Boyd, J. D. (1960) Development of striated muscle, pp. 63–85. In *Structure and Functions of Muscle,* Vol. 1 (G. H. Bourne, ed.), Academic Press, New York.

Boyd, W. C. (1974) *Science* **186:**846. How specific is specific?

Bradley, P. B., J. T. Eayrs, and K. Schmalbach. (1960*a*) *Electroencephalog. Clin. Neurophysiol.* **12:**467–477. The electroencephalogram of normal and hypothyroid rats.

Bradley, P. B., J. T. Eayrs, A. Glass, and R. W. Heath. (1960*b*) *Electroencephalog. Clin. Neurophysiol.* **12:**759–760. The recruiting response in neonatal hypothyroidism.

Bradley, R. M. (1972) Development of the taste bud and gustatory papillae in human fetuses, pp. 137–162. In *Third Symposium on Oral Sensation and Perception: The Mouth of the Infant* (J. F. Bosma ed.), Thomas, Springfield, Ill.

Bradley, R. M. (1975) *Physiol. Rev.* **55:**352–382. Fetal sensory receptors.

Bradley, R. M., and C. M. Mistretta. (1973) *J. Physiol. (London)* **231:**271–282. The gustatory sense in foetal sheep during the last third of gestation.

Bradley, R. M., and C. M. Mistretta. (1975) *Physiol. Rev.* **55:**352–382. Fetal sensory receptors.

Bradley, R. M., and I. B. Stern. (1967) *J. Anat.* **101:**743–752. The development of the human taste bud during the foetal period.

Bradom, W. F. (1960) *J. Exp. Zool.* **143:**323–345. Gene-dosage studies in polyploid hybrids of California newts.

Bradom, W. F. (1962) *Biol. Bull.* **123:**253–263. Karyoplasmic studies in haploid, androgenetic hybrids of California newts.

Braekevelt, C. R., and M. J. Hollenberg. (1970) *Am. J. Anat.* **102:**281–302. The development of the retina of the albino rat.

Braitenberg, V., and M. Kemali. (1970) *J. Comp. Neurol.* **138:**137–146. Exceptions to bilateral symmetry in the epithalamus of lower vertebrates.

Brattgard, S.-O., J. E. Edström, and H. Hydén. (1957) *J. Neurochem.* **I:**316–325. The chemical changes in regenerating neurons.

Braus, H. (1905) *Anat. Anz.* **26:**433–479. Experimentelle Beiträge zur Frage nach der Entwicklung peripherer Nerven.

Bray, D. (1970) *Proc. Natl. Acad. Sci. U.S.A.* **65:**905–910. Surface movements during the growth of single explanted neurons.

Bray, D. (1973*a*) *Nature* **244:**93–96. Model for membrane movements in the neural growth cone.

Bray, D. (1973*b*) *J. Cell. Biol.* **56:**702–712. Branching patterns of individual sympathetic neurons in culture.

Bray, D. (1974) *Endeavour* **33:**131–136. The fibrillar proteins of nerve cells.

Bray, D., and M. B. Bunge. (1973) The growth cone in neurite extension, pp. 195–209. In *Locomotion of Tissue Cells,* Ciba Foundation Symposium 14 (new series), Elsevier, Amsterdam.

Bray, J. J., and L. Austin. (1968) *J. Neurochem.* **15:**731–740. Flow of protein and ribonucleic acid in peripheral nerve.

Bray, J. J., and L. Austin. (1969) *Brain Res.* **12:**230–233. Axoplasmic flow of ^{14}C proteins at two rates in chicken sciatic nerve.

Bremermann, H. J. (1963) *IEEE Trans.* **MIL7:**200–205. Limits of genetic control.

Brenner, S. (1974) *Genetics* **77:**71–94. The genetics of *Caenorhabditis elegans.*

Brightman, M. W. (1965) *J. Cell Biol.* **26:**99–123. The distribution within the brain of ferritin injected into cerebrospinal fluid compartments. I. Ependymal distribution.

Brightman, M. W., and S. L. Palay. (1963) *J. Cell Biol.* **19:**415–439. The fine structure of ependyma in the brain of the rat.

Britten, R. J., and E. H. Davidson. (1969) *Science* **165:**349–357. Gene regulation for higher cells: A theory.

Britten, R. J., and E. H. Davidson. (1971) *Quart. Rev. Biol.* **46:**111–138. Repetitive and non-repetitive DNA sequences and a speculation on the origins of evolutionary novelty.

Brizzee, K. R. (1949) *J. Comp. Neurol.* **91:**129–146. Histogenesis of the supporting tissue in the spinal and sympathetic trunk ganglia in the chick.

Brizzee, K. R., and L. A. Jacobs. (1959) *Growth* **23:**337–347. Early postnatal changes in neuron packing density and volumetric relationships in the cerebral cortex of the white rat.

Brizzee, K. R., J. Vogt, and X. Kharetchko. (1964) *Progr. Brain. Res.* **4:**136–149. Postnatal changes in glia-neuron index with a comparison of methods of cell enumeration in the white rat.

Brizzee, K. R., N. Sherwood, and P. S. Timiras. (1968) *J. Gerontol.* **23:**289–291. A comparison of cell populations at various depth levels in cerebral cortex of young adult and aged Long-Evans rats.

Brockes, J. P. and Z. W. Hall. (1975) *Proc. Natl. Acad. Sci. U.S.A.* **72:**1368–1372. Synthesis of acetylcholine receptor by denervated rat diaphragm muscle.

Brodal, A. (1940*a*) *Arch. eurol. Psychiat. (Chicago)* **43:**46–58. Modification of Gudden method for study of cerebral localization.

Brodal, A. (1940*b*) *Z. Ges. Neurol. Psychiat.* **169:**1–153. Experimenteller Untersuchungen über die olivo-cerebellare Lokalisation.

Brody, H. (1955) *J. Comp. Neurol.* **102:**511–556. Organization of the cerebral cortex. III. A study of aging in the human cerebral cortex.

Brown, A. G., and A. Iggo. (1962) *J. Physiol. (London)* **165:**28–29P. The structure and function of cutaneous "touch corpuscles" after nerve crush.

Brown, D. L., and W. L. Salinger. (1975) *Science* **189:**1011–1012. Loss of X-cells in lateral geniculate nucleus with monocular paralysis: Neural plasticity in the adult cat.

Brown, G. L., ad J. E. Pascoe. (1954) *J. Physiol. (London)* **123:**565–573. The effect of degenerative section of ganglionic axons on transmission through the ganglion.

Brown, I. R., and R. B. Church. (1972) *Dev. Biol.* **29:**73–84. Transcription of nonrepeated DNA during mouse and rabbit development.

Brown, M. C., J. K. Jansen, and D. Van Essen. (1976) *J. Physiol. (London)* **261:**387–422. Polyneuronal innervation of skeletal muscle in new-born rats and its elimination during maturation.

Brown, M. E. (1946) *Am. J. Anat.* **78:**79–113. The histology of the tadpole tail during metamorphosis, with special reference to the nervous system.

Brown-Séquard, E. (1853) *Experimental Researches Applied to Physiology and Pathology,* H. Ballière, New York.

Brugal, G. (1971) *Arch. Entw.-Mech. Organ.* **168:**205–225. Etude autoradiographique de l'influence de la température sur la prolifération cellulaire ches les embryones âgés de *Pleurodeles waltlii* Michah.

Brummelkamp. R. (1939) *Acta Morphol. Neerl. Scand.* **2:**268–271. Das Wachstum der Gehirnmasse mit kleinen Cephalisierungssprungen (sog. $\sqrt{2}$-Sprungen) bei Amphibien und Fischen.

Brustowicz, R. J., and J. W. Kernohan. (1952) *Arch Neurol. Psychiat.* **67:**592. Cell rests in the region of the 4th ventricle.

Bryan, J. (1974) *Fed. Proc.* **33:**152–157. Biochemical properties of microtubules.

Bryans, W. A. (1959) *Anat. Rec.* **133:**65–71. Mitotic activity in the brain of the adult rat.

Bryant, P. J., and H. A. Schneiderman. (1969) *Dev. Biol.* **20:**263–290. Cell lineage, growth, and determination in the imaginal leg discs of *Drosophila melanogaster.*

Bücher, V. M., and S. M. Bürgi. (1950) *J. Comp. Neurol.* **93:**139–172. Some observations on the fiber connections of the di- and mesencephalon in the cat.

Bueker, E. D. (1943) *J. Exp. Zool.* **93:**99–129. Intracentral and peripheral factors in the differentiation of motor neurons in transplanted lumbo-sacral cords of chick embryos.

Bueker, E. D. (1944) *Science* **100:**169. Differentiation of the lateral motor column in the avian spinal cord.

Bueker, E. D. (1945*a*) *J. Comp. Neurol.* **82:**335–361. The influence of a growing limb on the differentiation of somatic motor neurons in transplanted avian spinal cord segments.

Bueker, E. D. (1945*b*) *Anat. Rec.* **93:**323–331. Hyperplastic changes in the nervous system of a frog *(Rana)* as associated with multiple functional limbs.

Bueker, E. D. (1948) *Anat. Rec.* **102:**369–390. Implantation of tumors in the hindlimb field of the embryonic chick and developmental response of the lumbosacral nervous system.

Bueker, E. D., I. Schenkein, and J. L. Bane. (1960) *Cancer Res.* **20:**1220–1228. The problem of distribution of a nerve growth factor specific for spinal and sympathetic ganglia.

Buller, A. J. (1966) *Br. Med. Bull.* **22:**45–48. Developmental physiology of the neuromuscular system.

Buller, A. J., and D. M. Lewis. (1946) *J. Physiol. (London)* **176:**355–370. Further observations on the differentiation of skeletal muscles in the kitten hindlimb.

Buller, A. J., and D. M. Lewis (1965) *J. Physiol. (London)* **178:**343–358. Further observations on mammalian cross-innervated skeletal muscle.

Buller, A. J., J. C. Eccles, and R. M. Eccles. (1960*a*) *J. Physiol. (London)* **150:**399–416. Differentiation of fast and slow muscles in the cat hindlimb.

Buller, A. J., J. C. Eccles, and R. M. Eccles. (1960*b*) *J. Physiol. (London)* **150:**417–439. Interactions between motoneurons and muscles in respect of the characteristic speeds of their responses.

Bullock, T. H., and G. A. Horridge. (1965) *Structure and Function in the Nervous Systems of Invertebrates,* 2 vols., Freeman, San Francisco.

Bunge, M. B. (1973*a*) *Anat. Rec.* **175:**280. Uptake of peroxidase by growth cones of cultured neurons.

Bunge, M. B. (1973*b*) *J. Cell Biol.* **56:**713–735. Fine structure of nerve fibers and growth cones of isolated sympathetic neurons in culture.

Bunge, M. B., R. P. Bunge, and G. D. Pappas. (1962) *J. Cell Biol.* **12:**448–453. Electron microscopic demonstration of connections between glia and myelin sheaths in the developing mammalian nervous system.

Bunge, M. B., R. P. Bunge, and E. R. Peterson. (1967) *Brain Res.* **6:**728–749. The onset of synapse formation in spinal cord cultures as studied by electron microscopy.

Bunge, R. P. (1968) *Physiol. Rev.* **48:**197–251. Glial cells and the central myelin sheath.

Bunt, A. H., R. D. Lund, and J. S. Lund. (1974) *Brain Res.* **73:**215–228. Retrograde axonal transport of horseradish peroxidase by ganglion cells of the albino rat retina.

Burdick, M. L. (1968) *J. Exp. Zool.* **167:**1–20. A test of the capacity of chick embryo cells to home after vascular dissemination.

Burdman, J. A. (1967) *J. Neurochem.* **14:**367–371. Early effects of a nerve growth factor on the RNA content and base ratios of isolated chick embryo sensory ganglia neuroblasts in tissue culture.

Burdwood, W. O. (1965) *J. Cell Biol.* **27:**115A. Rapid bidirectional particle movement in neurons.

Burger, M. M. (1974) Role of the cell surface in growth and transformation, pp. 3–24. In *Macromolecules Regulating Growth and Development* (E. D. Hay, T. J. King, and J. Papaconstantinou, eds.), Academic Press, New York.

Burger, M. M., R. S. Turner, W. J. Kuhns, and G. Weinbaum. (1975) *Phil. Trans. Roy. Soc. London Ser. B.* **271:**379–393. A possible model for cell–cell recognition via surface macromolecules.

Burgess, P. R., and K. W. Horch. (1973) *J. Neurophysiol.* **36:**101–114. Specific regeneration of cutaneous fibers in the cat.

Burgess, P. R., K. B. English, K. W. Horch, and L. J. Stensaas. (1974) *J. Physiol. (London)* **236:**57–82. Patterning in the regeneration of Type I cutaneous receptors.

Bürgi, S. (1957) *Deutsch. Z. Nervenheilk.* **176:**701–729. Das Tectum opticum. Seine Verbindungen bei der Katze und seine Bedeutung beim Menschen.

Burke, W., and W. R. Hayhow. (1968) *J. Physiol. (London)* **194:**495–519. Disuse in the lateral geniculate nucleus of the cat.

Burleigh, I. G. (1974) *Biol. Rev.* **49:**267–320. On the cellular regulation of growth and development in skeletal muscle.

Burnham, P., and S. Varon. (1973) *Neurobiology.* **3:**232–245. *In vitro* uptake of active nerve growth factor by dorsal root ganglia of embryonic chick.

Burnham, P., and S. Varon. (1974) *Neurobiology.* **4:**57–70. Biosynthetic activities of dorsal root ganglia *in vitro* and the influence of nerve growth factor.

Burnham, P., C. Raiborn, and S. Varon. (1972) *Proc. Natl. Acad. Sci. U.S.A.* **69:**3556–3560. Replacement of nerve growth factor by ganglionic non-neuronal cells for the survival *in vitro* of dissociated ganglionic neurons.

Burnside, B. (1971) *Dev. Biol.* **26:**416–441. Microtubules and microfilaments in newt neurulation.

Burnside, B. (1973) *Am. Zool.* **13:**989–1006. Microtubules and microfilaments in amphibian neurulation.

Burnside, B. (1975) *Ann. N.Y. Acad. Sci.* **253:**14–26. The form and arrangement of microtubules: An historical, primarily morphological, review.

Burnside, B., and A. G. Jacobson. (1968) *Dev. Biol.* **18:**537–552. Analysis of morphogenetic movements in the neural plate of the newt *Taricha torosa.*

Burr, H. S. (1916) *J. Exp. Zool.* **20:**27–57. The effects of the removal of the nasal pits in *Amblystoma* embryos.

Burr, H. S. (1920) *J. Exp. Zool.* **30:**159–169. The transplantation of the cerebral hemispheres of *Amblystoma.*

Burr, H. S. (1924) *J. Comp. Neurol.* **37:**455–479. Some experiments on the transplantation of the olfactory placode in *Amblystoma.* I. An experimentally produced aberrant cranial nerve.

Burr, H. S. (1930) *J. Exp. Zool.* **55:**171–191. Hyperplasia in the brain of *Amblystoma.*

Burr, H. S. (1932) *J. Comp. Neurol.* **56:**347–371. An electro-dynamic theory of development suggested by studies of proliferation rates in the brain of *Amblystoma.*

Burr, H. S. (1947) *Sci. Month.* **64:**217–225. Field theory in biology.

Burt, A. M., and C. H. Narayanan. (1970) *Exp. Neurol.* **29:**201–210. Effect of extrinsic neuronal connections on development of acetylcholinesterase and choline acetyltransferase activity in the ventral half of the chick spinal cord.

Burton, H., and R. M. Benjamin. (1971) Central projections of the gustatory system, pp. 148–164. In *Handbook of Sensory Physiology,* Vol. IV, Part 2: *Chemical Senses,* 2: *Taste* (L. M. Beidler, ed.), Springer-Verlag, New York.

Burton, P. R., and H. L. Fernandez. (1973) *J. Cell Sci.* **12:**567–583. Delineation by lanthanum staining of filamentous elements associated with the surfaces of axonal microtubules.

Byers, M. R. (1974) *Brain Res.* **75:**97–113. Structural correlates of rapid axonal transport: Evidence that microtubules may not be directly involved.

Cabak, V., and R. Najdanvic. (1965) *Arch. Dis. Child.* **40:**532–534. Effect of undernutrition in early life on physical and mental development.

Cabak, V., R. Najdanvic, B. Curcic, E. Serstnev, and L. Skoric. (1967) The long-term prognosis of infantile malnutrition, pp. 521–532. In *Proceedings of the First Congress of the International Association for Scientific Study of Mental Deficiency* (B. W. Richards, ed.), Michael Jackson, Montpellier, France.

Calaresu, F. R., and J. L. Henry. (1971) *Science* **173:**343–344. Sex difference in the number of sympathetic neurons in the spinal cord of the cat.

Caley, D. W., and D. S. Maxwell. (1968*a*) *J. Comp. Neurol.* **133:**17–44. An electron microscopic study of neurons during postnatal development of the rat cerebral cortex.

Caley, D. S., and D. S. Maxwell. (1968*b*) *J. Comp. Neurol.* **133:**45–70. An electron microscopic study of the neuroglia during postnatal development of the rat cerebrum.

Caley, D. W., and D. S. Maxwell. (1970) *J. Comp. Neurol.* **138:**31–48. Development of the blood vessels and extracellular spaces during postnatal maturation of rat cerebral cortex.

Cameron, I. L. (1964) *J. Cell Biol.* **20:**185–188. Is the duration of DNA synthesis in somatic cells of mammals and birds a constant?

Cammermeyer, J. (1963) *J. Neuropathol. Exp. Neurol.* **12:**594–616. Differential response of two neuron types to facial nerve transection in young and old rabbits.

Cammermeyer, J. (1965*a*) *Ergeb. Anat. Entwicklungsgesch.* **38:**1–22. Juxtavascular karyokinesis and microglia cell proliferation during retrograde reaction in the mouse facial nucleus.

Cammermeyer, J. (1965*b*) *Ergeb. Anat. Entwicklungsgesch.* **38:**195–229. Histiocytes, juxtavascular mitotic cells and microglia cells during retrograde changes in the facial nucleus of rabbits of varying age.

Cammermeyer, J. (1965*c*) *A. Anat. Entwicklungsgesch.* **124:**543–561. The hypo-ependymal microglial cell.

Cammermeyer, J. (1970) The life history of the microglial cell: A light microscopic study, pp. 43–129. In *Neurosciences Research,* Vol. 3 (S. Ehrenpreis and O. Z. Solnitzky, eds.), Academic Press, New York.

Campbell, A. C. P. (1939) *Arch Neurol. Psychiat. (Chicago)* **41:**223–242. Variation in vascularity and oxidase content in different regions of the brain of the cat.

Capps-Covey, P., and D. L. McIlwain. (1975) *J. Neurochem.* Bulk isolation of large ventral spinal neurons.

Carlson, B. M. (1973) *Am. J. Anat.* **137:**119–150. The regeneration of skeletal muscle—a review.

Carmel, P. W., and B. M. Stein. (1969) *J. Comp. Neurol.* **135:**145–166. Cell changes in sensory ganglia following proximal and disal nerve section in the monkey.

Carmichael, L. (1926) *Psychol. Rev.* **33:**51–58. The development of behavior in vertebrates experimentally removed from the influence of external stimulation.

Carmichael, L. (1927) *Psychol. Rev.* **34:**34–47. A further study of the development of behavior in vertebrates experimentally removed from the influence of external stimuli.

Carpenter, F. G., and R. M. Bergland. (1957) *Am. J. Physiol.* **190:**371–376. Excitation and conduction in immature nerve fibers of the developing chick.

Carr, V. McM. (1975) *Neurosci. Abstr.* **1:**749. Peripheral effects on early development of chick spinal ganglia.

Carr, V. McM. (1976) Ph.D. thesis, Northwestern University, Evanston, Ill.

Carr, V. McM., and S. Simpson. (1975) *Neurosci. Abstr.* **1:**749. Peripheral effects on early development of chick spinal ganglia

Carter, S. B. (1972) *Endeavour* **3:**77–82. The cytochalasins as research tools in cytology.

Casola, L., G. A. Davis, and R. E. Davis. (1969) *J. Neurochem.* **16:**1037–1041. Evidence for RNA transport in rat optic nerve.

Caspar, D. L. D., and D. A. Kirschner. (1971) *Nature New Biol* **231:**46–52. Myelin membrane structure at 10 Å resolution.

Caspersson, T. (1940) *J. Roy. Microsc. Soc.* **60:**8–25. Methods for the determination of the absorption spectra of cell structures.

Caspersson, T. (1950) *Cell Growth and Cell Function,* Norton, New York, 185 pp.

Cass, D. T., T. J. Sutton, and R. F. Mark. (1973) *Nature* **243:**201–203. Competition between nerves for functional connexions with axolotl muscles.

Causey, G. (1960) *The Cell of Schwann,* Livingston, Edinburgh and London.

Cavanagh, J. B. (1974) *Res. Publ. Assoc. Nerv. Ment. Dis.* **53:**13–38. Liver bypass and the glia.

Cavanagh, J. B., and M. H. Kyu. (1971) *J. Neurol. Sci.* **12:**241–261. On the mechanism of type I Alzheimer abnormality in the nuclei of astrocytes.

Cavanaugh, J. B. (1970) *J. Anat.* **106:**471–487. The proliferation of astrocytes around a needle wound in the rat brain.

Cavanaugh, M. W. (1951) *J. Comp. Neurol.* **94:**181–219. Quantitative effects of the peripheral innervation area on nerves and spinal ganglion cells.

Caviness, V. S. Jr. (1976) *J. Comp Neurol.* **170:**435–448. Patterns of cell and fiber distribution in the neocortex of the reeler mutant mouse.

Caviness, V. S., Jr., and R. L. Sidman. (1972) *J. Comp. Neurol.* **145:**85–104. Olfactory structures of the forebrain in the reeler mutant mouse.

Caviness, V. S. Jr., and R. L. Sidman. (1973) *J. Comp. Neurol.* **148:**141–152. Time of origin of corresponding cell classes in the cerebral cortex of normal and reeler mutant mice: An autoradiographic analysis.

Caviness, V. S. Jr., and C. H. Yorke, Jr. *J. Comp. Neurol.* **170:**449–460. Interhemispheric neocortical connections of the corpus callosum in the reeler mutant mouse: A study based on anterograde and retrograde methods.

Ceccarelli, B., F. Clementi, and P. Mantegazza. (1971) *J. Physiol. (London)* **216:**87–98. Synaptic transmission in the superior cervical ganglion of the cat after reinnervation by vagus fibers.

Cerf, J. A., and L. W. Chacko. (1958) *J. Comp. Neurol.* **109:**205–216. Retrograde reaction in motoneuron dendrites following ventral root section in the frog.

Chambers, W. W., C. N. Liu, and G. P. McCouch. (1973) *Brain, Behav. Evol.* **8:**5–26. Anatomical and physiological correlates of plasticity in the central nervous system.

Chamley, J. H., I. Goller, and G. Burnstock. (1973) *Dev. Biol.* **31:**362–379. Selective growth of sympathetic nerve fibers to explants of normally densely innervated autonomic effector organs in tissue culture.

Chanda, R., D. J. Woodward, and S. Griffin. (1973) *J. Neurochem.* **21:**547–555. Cerebellar development in the rat after early postnatal damage by methylazoxymethanol: DNA, RNA and protein during recovery.

Chang, C. (1972) *J. Cell Biol.* **55:**37. Effect of colchicine and cytochalasin B on axonal particle movement and outgrowth *in vitro.*

Chang, C. C., and M. C. Huang. (1975) *Nature* **253:**643–644. Turnover of junctional and extrajunctional acetylcholine receptors of the rat diaphragm.

Changeux, J.-P., and A. Danchin. (1976) *Nature* **264:**705–711. Selective stabilization of developing synapses as a mechanism for the specification of neuronal networks.

Chan-Palay, V. (1972) *Z. Anat. Entwicklungsgesch.* **139:**11–20. Arrested granule cells and their synapses with mossy fibers in the molecular layer of the cerebellar cortex.

Chan-Palay, V. (1973) *Z. Anat. Entwicklungsgesch.* **142:**23–35. Neuronal plasticity in the cerebellar cortex and lateral nucleus.

Chase, H. B. (1945) *J. Comp. Neurol.* **83:**121–140. Studies on an anophthalmic strain of mice. V. Associated cranial nerve and brain centers.

Chase, H. P., J. Dorsey, and G. M. McKhann. (1967) *Pediatrics* **40:**551–559. The effect of malnutrition on the synthesis of a myelin lipid.

Chaube, S. (1959) *J. Exp. Zool.* **140:**29–78. On axiation and symmetry in transplated wing of the chick.

Chernenko, G. A. and R. W. West. (1976) *J. Comp. Neurol.* **167:**49–62. A re-examination of anatomical plasticity in the rat retina.

Chiakulas, J. J., and J. E. Pauly. (1965) *Anat. Rec.* **152:**55–61. A study of postnatal growth of skeletal muscle in the rat.

Chibon, P. (1967) *J. Embryol. Exp. Morphol.* **18:**343–358. Marquage nucléaire par la thymidine tritíee des dérivés de la crête neurale chez l'Amphibien urodèle *Pleurodeles waltlii* Michah.

Child, C. M. (1911) *Science* **39:**73–76. Susceptibility gradients in animals.

Child, C. M. (1928) *Protoplasma* **5:**447–476. The physiological gradients.

Child, C. M. (1936) *Arch. Entw.-Mech. Organ.* **135:**426–451. Differential reduction of vital dyes in the early development of echinoderms.

Child, C. M. (1941) *Patterns and Problems of Development,* University of Chicago Press, Chicago, 811 pp.

Child, C. M. (1946) *Physiol. Zool.* **19:**89–148. Organizers in development and the organizer concept.

Child, C. M. (1947) *J. Exp. Zool.* **104:**153–193. Oxidation and reduction of indicators by *Hydra.*

Choinowski, H. (1958) *Zool. Anz.* **161:**259–279. Vergleichende Messungen an Gehirnen von Wild-und Hauskaninchen.

Chouchkov, H. N. (1971) *Z. Mikrosk. Anat. Forsch.* **86:**33–46. Ultrastructure of Pacinian corpuscle after the section of nerve fibers.

Chow, K. L., and J. H. Dewson, (1966) *J. Comp. Neurol.* **128:**63–74. Numerical estimates of neurons and glia in lateral geniculate body during retrograde degeneration.

Chow, K. L., and N. Randall. (1964) *Psychon. Sci.* **1:**259–260. Learning and retention in cats with lesions in reticular formation.

Chow, K. L., and P. D. Spear. (1974) *Exp. Neurol.* **42:**Morphological and functional effects of visual deprivation on the rabbit visual system.

Chow, K. L., and D. S. Stewart. (1972) *Exp. Neurol.* **43:**409–433. Reversal of structural and functional effects of long-term visual deprivation in cats.

Chow, K. L., L. H. Mathers, and P. D. Spear. (1973) *J. Comp. Neurol.* **151:**307–322. Spreading of uncrossed retinal projection in superior colliculus of neonatally enucleated rabbits.

Christensen, B. N. (1973) *Science* **182:**1255–1256. Procion brown: An intracellular dye for light and electron microscopy.

Chung, S. H., and J. Cooke. (1975) *Nature* **258:**126–132. Polarity of structure and of ordered nerve connections in the developing amphibian brain.

Chung, S. H., T. V. P. Bliss and M. J. Keating. (1974*a*) *Proc. Roy. Soc. London (Biol.)* **187:**421–447. The synaptic organization of optic afferents in the amphibian tectum.

Chung, S. H., M. J. Keating, and T. V. P. Bliss. (1974*b*) *Proc. Roy. Soc. London (Biol.)* **187:**449–459. Functional synaptic relations during the development of the retino-tectal projection in amphibians.

Church, J. C. T. (1969) *J. Anat.* **105:**419–438. Satellite cells and myogenesis: A study in the fruit bat web.

Church, J. C. T. (1970) *J. Embryol. Exp. Morphol.* **23:**531–537. Cell populations in skeletal muscle after regeneration.

Churchill, J. A., J. W. Neff, and D. F. Caldwell. (1966) *Obstet. Gynecol.* **28:**425–429. Birth weight and intelligence.

Cicero, T. J., and R. R. Provine. (1972) *Brain Res.* **44:**294–298. The levels of the brain-specific proteins, S-100 and 14-3-2, in the developing chick spinal cord.

Clark, W. G. (1973*a*) *Plant Physiol* **12:**409–440. Electrical polarity and auxin transport.

Clark, W. G. (1938) *Plant Physiol.* **13:**529–552. Polar transport of auxin and electrical polarity in the coleoptile of *Avena.*

Clarke, E. (1968) The doctrine of the hollow nerve in the seventeenth and eighteenth centuries, pp. 123–141. In *Medicine, Science and Culture* (L. G. Stevenson and R. P. Multhauf, eds.), Johns Hopkins Press, Baltimore.

Clarke, E., and C. D. O'Malley. (1968) *The Human Brain and Spinal Cord. A Historical Study Illustrated by*

Writings from Antiquity to the Twentieth Century, University of California Press, Berkeley and Los Angeles.

Clarke, P. G. H. (1975) *J. Physiol. (London)* **256:**44–45P. Neuronal death as an error-correcting mechanism in the development of the chick's isthmo-optic nucleus.

Clarke, P. G. H., and W. M. Cowan. (1975) *Proc. Natl. Acad. Sci. U.S.A.* **72:**4455–4458. Ectopic neurons and aberrant connections during neural development.

Clarke, P. G. H., and W. M. Cowan (1976) *J. Comp. Neurol.* **167:**143–164. The development of the isthmo-optic tract in the chick, with special reference to the occurrence and correction of developmental errors in the location and connections of isthmo-optic neurons.

Clarke, P. G. H., L. A. Rogers, and W. M. Cowan. (1976) *J. Comp Neurol.* **167:**125–142. The time of origin and the pattern of survival of neurons in the isthmo-optic nucleus of the chick.

Claxton, J. H. (1964) *J. Theoret. Biol.* **7:**302–317. The determination of patterns with special reference to that of the central primary skin follicles in sheep.

Cleaver, J. E. (1967) *The Frontiers of Biology,* Vol 6: *Thymidine Metabolism and Cell Kinetics,* p. 45, North-Holland, Amsterdam.

Cleaver, J. E., G. H. Thomas, and H. J. Burki. (1972) *Science* **177:**996–998. Biological damage from intranuclear tritium: DNA strand breaks and their repair.

Clementi, C. (1964) *Int. Rev. Neurobiol.* **6:**257–301. Regeneration in the vertebrate central nervous system.

Clendinnen, B. G., and J. T. Eayrs. (1961) *J. Endocrinol.* **22:**183–193. The anatomical and physiological effects of prenatally administered somatotrophin on cerebral development.

Clos, J., and J. Legrand. (1969) *Arch. Anat. Mikrosk. Morphol. Exp.* **58:**339–354. Influence de la déficience thyroidienne et de la sous-alimentation sur la croissance et la myélinisation des fibres nerveuses de la moelle cervicale et du nerf sciatique chez le jeune rat blanc.

Clos, J., and J. Legrand. (1970) *Brain Res.* **22:**285–297. Influence de la déficience thyroïdienne et de la sous-alimentation sur la croissance et la myélinisation des fibres nerveuses du nerf sciatique chez le jeune rat blanc: Étude au microscope électronique.

Clos, J., F. Crépel, C. Legrand, J. Legrand, J. Rabié, and E. Vigourouz. (1974) *Gen. Comp. Endocrinol.* **23:**178–192. Thyroid physiology during the postnatial period in the rat: A study of the development of thyroid function and of the morphogenetic effects of thyroxine with special references to cerebellar maturation.

Close, R. (1964) *J. Physiol. (London)* **173:**74–95. Dynamic properties of fast and slow skeletal muscles of the rat during development.

Close, R. (1965) *Nature* **206:**831–832. Effects of cross-union of motor nerves to fast and slow skeletal muscles.

Close, R. (1967) *J. Physiol. (London)* **193:**45–55. Properties of motor units in fast and slow skeletal muscles of the rat.

Coërs, C. (1967) *Int. Rev. Cytol.* **22:**239–267. Structure and organization of the myoneural junction.

Coërs, C., and A. L. Woolf. (1959) *The Innervation of Muscle,* Blackwell, Oxford.

Coggeshall, R. E. (1967) *J. Neurophysiol.* **30:**1263–1287. A light and electron microscopic study of the abdominal ganglion of *Aplysia californica.*

Coghill, G. E. (1924) *J. Comp. Neurol.* **37:**71–120. Correlated anatomical and physiological studies of the growth of the nervous system of *Amphibia.* IV. Rates of proliferation and differentiation in the central nervous system of *Amblystoma.*

Coghill, G. E. (1933) *J. Comp. Neurol.* **57:**327–358. Correlated anatomical and physiological studies of the growth of the nervous system of *Amphibia.* XI. The proliferation of cells in the spinal cord as a factor in the individuation of the hing leg of *Amblystoma punctatum.*

Cohen, A. M. (1972) *J. Exp. Zool.* **179:**167–182. Factors directing the expression of sympathetic nerve traits in cells of neural crest origin.

Cohen, A. M., and I. R. Konigsberg. (1975) *Dev. Biol.* **46:**262–280. A clonal approach to the problem of neural crest determination.

Cohen, J., Mareš, and Z. Lodin. (1973) *J. Neurochem.* **20:**651–657. DNA content of purified preparations of mouse Purkinje neurons isolated by a velocity sedimentation technique.

Cohen, M. H., and A. Robertson. (1971) *J. Theor. Biol.* **31:**119–130. Chemotaxis and the early stages of aggregation in cellular slime molds.

Cohen, M. J. (1967) Correlations between structure function and RNA metabolism in central neurons of insects, pp. 65–78. In *Invertebrate Nervous Systems* (C. A. G. Wiersma, ed.), University of Chicago Press, Chicago.

Cohen, M. J., and J. W. Jacklet. (1965) *Science* **148:**1237–1239. Neurons of insects: RNA changes during injury and regeneration.

Cohen, M. J., and J. W. Jacklet. (1967) *Philos. Trans. R. Soc. (London) Ser. B* **781:**561–572. The functional organization of motor neurons in an insect ganglion.

Cohen, M. W. (1972) *Brain Res.* **41:**457–463. The development of neuromuscular connexions in the presence of D-tubocurarine.

Cohen, S. (1958) A nerve growth-promoting protein, pp. 665–679. In *The Chemical Basis of Development* (W. D. McElroy and B. Glass, eds.), Johns Hopkins Press, Baltimore.

Cohen, S. (1959) *J. Biol. Chem.* **234:**1129–1137. Purification and metabolic effects of a nerve growth-promoting protein from snake venom.

Cohen, S. (1960) *Proc. Natl. Acad. U.S.* **46:**302–311. Purification of a nerve-growth promoting protein from the mouse salivary gland and its neurocytotoxic antiserum.

Cohen, S. (1964) *Natl. Cancer Inst. Monogr.* **13:**14–37. Isolation and biological effects of an epidermal growth-stimulating protein.

Cohen, S. (1965) *Dev. Biol.* **12:**394–407. The stimulation of epidermal proliferation by a specific protein (EGF).

Cohen, S., and R. Levi-Montalcini. (1956) *Proc. Natl. Acad. Sci. U.S.A.* **42:**571–574. A nerve growth stimulating factor isolated from snake venom.

Cohen, S., and M. Stastny. (1968) *Biochim. Biophys. Acta* **166:**427–437. Epidermal growth factor. 3. Stimulation of polysome formation in chick embryo epidermis.

Cohen, S., and J. M. Taylor. (1974) Epidermal growth factor: Chemical and biological characterisation, pp. 25–42. In *Macromolecules Regulating Growth and Development* (E. D. Hay, T. J. King, and J. Papaconstantinous, eds.), Academic Press, New York.

Cohen, S., R. Levi-Montalcini, and V. Hamburger, (1954) *Proc. Natl. Acad. Sci. U.S.A.* **40:**1014–1018. A nerve growth-stimulating factor isolated from sarcomas 37 and 180.

Cole, M. (1968) Retrograde degeneration of axon and soma in the central nervous system, pp. 269–300. In *The Structure and Function of Nervous Tissue* (G. H. Bourne, ed.), Academic Press, New York.

Coleman, P. D., and A. H. Riesen, (1968) *J. Anat. (London)* **102:**363–374. Environmental effects on cortical dendritic fields: I. Rearing in the dark.

Collin, R. (1906) *Névraxe* **8:**181–308. Recherches cytologiques sur le développement de la cellule nerveuse.

Colonnier, M. (1968) *Brain Res.* **9:**268–287. Synaptic patterns on different cell types in the different laminae of the cat visual cortex. An electron microscope study.

Colonnier, M. (1964) *J. Anat. (London)* **98:**327–344. The tangential organization of the visual cortex.

Colonnier, M. (1966) The structural design of the neocortex, pp. 1–23. In *Brain and Conscious Experience* (J. C. Eccles ed.), Springer-Verlag, Berlin.

Concalon, P., and L. M. Beidler. (1975) *Brain Res.* **89:**225–244. Distribution along the axon and into various subcellular fractions of molecules labeled with [^{3}H]leucine and rapidly transported in the garfish olfactory nerve.

Conel, J. L. (1939–1963) *The Postnatal Development of the Human Cerebral Cortex,* 6 vols., Harvard University Press, Cambridge, Mass.

Conger, A. D., and M. A. Wells. (1969) *Radiat. Res.* **37:**31–49. Radiation and aging effect on taste structure and function.

Connolly, C. J. (1950) *External Morphology of the Primate Brain,* 378 pp., Thomas, Springfield, Ill.

Conradi, S., and L.-O. Ronnevi. (1975) *Brain Res.* **92:**505–510. Spontaneous elimination of synapses on cat spinal motoneurons after birth: Do half of the synapses on the cell bodies disappear?

Constantine-Paton, M., and R. R. Capranica, (1975) *Science* **189:**480–482. Central projection of optic tract from translocated eyes in the leopard frog (*Rana pipiens*).

Constantine-Paton, M., and R. R. Capranica, (1976*a*) *J. Comp. Neurol.* **170:**17–31. Axonal guidance of developing optic nerves in the frog. I. Anatomy of the projection from transplanted eye primordia.

Constantine-Paton, M., and R. R. Capranica. (1976*b*) *J. Comp. Neurol.* **170:**33–51. Axonal guidance of developing optic nerves in the frog. II. Electrophysiological studies of the projection from transplanted eye primordia.

Cook, J. E., and T. J. Horder. (1974) *J. Physiol. (London)* **241:**89–90P. Interactions between optic fibres in their regeneration to specific sites in the goldfish tectum.

Cook, L. M. (1971) *Coefficients of Natural Selection,* Hutchinson, London.

Cook, W. H., J. H. Walker, and M. L. Barr. (1951) *J. Comp. Neurol.* **94:**267–292. A cytological study of transneuronal atrophy in the cat and the rabbit.

Cooke, J. (1973*a*) *J. Embryol. Exp. Morphol.* **30:**49–62. Properties of the primary organization field in the embryo of *Xenopus laevis.* IV. Pattern formation and regulation following early inhibition of mitosis.

Cooke, J. (1973*b*) *J. Embryol. Exp. Morphol.* **30:**283–300. Properties of the primary organization field in the embryo of *Xenopus laevis.* V. Regulation after removal of the head organizer, in normal early gastrulae and in those already possessing a second implanted organizer.

Cooke, J. (1973*c*) *Nature* **242:**55–57. Morphogenesis and regulation in spite of continued mitotic inhibition in *Xenopus* embryos.

Cooper, E., and J. Diamond. (1977) *J. Physiol. (London)* **264:**695–723. A quantitative study of the mechanosensory innervation of the salamander skin.

Cooper, E., J. Diamond, and C. Turner. (1977) *J. Physiol. (London)* **264:**725–749. The effects of nerve section and of colchicine treatment on the density of mechanosensory nerve endings in salamander skin.

Cooper, G. W. (1965) *Dev. Biol.* **12:**185–212. Induction of somite chondrogenesis by cartilage and notochord: A correlation between inductive activity and specific stages of cytodifferentiation.

Cooper, P. D., and R. S. Smith. (1974) *J. Physiol. (London)* **242:**77–97. The movement of optically detectable organelles in myelinated axons of *Xenopus laevis.*

Corliss, C. E., and G. C. Robertson. (1963) *J. Exp. Zool.* **153:**125–140. The pattern of mitotic density in the early chick neural epithelium.

Corner, M. A. (1963) *J. Exp. Zool.* **153:**301–311. Development of the brain of *Xenopus laevis* after removal of parts of the neural plate.

Corner, M. A. (1964) *J. Comp. Neurol.* **123:**243–256. Localization of capacities for functional development in the neural plate of *Xenopus laevis.*

Corner, M. A., and S. M. Crain. (1964) *Experientia* **21:**1–7. Spontaneous contractions and bioelectric activity after differentiation in culture of presumptive neuromuscular tissues in the early frog embryo.

Corner, M. A., J. P. Achadé, J. Sedlaček, and A. P. C. Bot. (1967) *Progr. Brain Res.* **26:**145–192. Developmental patterns in the central nervous system of birds. I. Electrical activity in the cerebral hemisphere, optic lobe and cerebellum.

Cotman, C. W., D. Taylor, and G. Lynch. (1973) *Brain Res.* **63:**205–213. Ultrastructural changes in synapses in the dentate gyrus of the rat during development.

Cotterrell, M., R. Balázs, and A. L. Johnson. (1972) *J. Neurochem.* **19:**2151–2167. Effects of corticosteroids on the biochemical maturation of rat brain: Postnatal cell formation.

Coughlin, M. D. (1975) *Dev. Biol.* **43:**140–158. Target organ stimulation of parasympathetic nerve growth in the developing mouse submandibular gland.

Coulombre, J. L., and A. J. Coulombre. (1965) *Dev. Biol.* **12:**79–92. Regeneration of neural retina from the pigmented epithelium in the chick embryo.

Count, E. W. (1947) *Ann. N.Y. Acad. Sci.* **46:**993–1122. Brain and body weight in man: their antecedents in growth and evolution.

Coursin, D. B. (1967) *Fed. Proc.* **26:**134–138. Relationship of nutrition to central nervous system development and function.

Couteaux, R. (1963) *Proc. Roy Soc. (London) Ser. B* **158:**457–480. The differentiation of synaptic areas.

Cowan, W. M. (1970) Anterograde and retrograde transneuronal degeneration in the central and peripheral nervous system, pp. 217–251. In *Contemporary Research Methods in Neuroanatomy* (W. J. H. Nauta and S. O. E. Ebbesson, eds.), Springer-Verlag, New York.

Cowan, W. M. (1973) Neuronal death as a regulative mechanism in the control of cell number in the nervous system, pp. 19–41. In *Development and Aging in the Nervous* System (M. Rockstein, ed.), Academic Press, New York.

Cowan, W. M., and P. G. H. Clarke. (1976) *Brain Behav. Evol.* **13:**345–375. The development of the isthmo-optic nucleus.

Cowan, W. M., and E. Wenger. (1967) *J. Exp. Zool.* **164:**265–280. Cell loss in the trochlear nucleus of the chick during normal development and after radical extirpation of the optic vesicle.

Cowan, W. M., and E. Wenger. (1968*a*) *J. Comp. Neurol.* **133:**207–239. The development of the nucleus of origin of centrifugal fibers to the retina in the chick.

Cowan, W. M., and E. Wenger. (1968*b*) *J. Exp. Zool.* **168:**105–124. Degeneration in the nucleus of origin of the preganglionic fibers to the chick ciliary ganglion following early removal of the optic vesicle.

Cowan, W. M., A. H. Martin, and E. Wenger. (1968) *J. Exp. Zool.* **169:**71–92. Mitotic patterns in the optic tectum of the chick during normal development and after early removal of the optic vesicle.

Cowan, W. M., D. I. Gottlieb, A. E. Hendrickson, J. L. Price, and T. A. Woolsey. (1972) *Brain Res.* **37:**21–51. The autoradiographic demonstration of axonal connections in the central nervous system.

Cowdry, E. V. (1914) *Am. J. Anat.* **15:**389–429. The development of the cytoplasmic constituents of the nerve cells of the chick. I. Mitochondria and neurofibrils.

Cowdry, E. V. (1932) *Special Cytology,* 2nd ed., 3 vols., Hoeber, New York.

Cowley, J. J., and R. D. Griesel. (1963) *J. Genet. Psychol.* **103:**233–242. Development of second generation low protein rats.

Cragg, B. G. (1967) *J. Anat.* **101:**639–654. The density of synapses and neurons in the motor and visual areas of the cerebral cortex.

Cragg, B. R. (1969) *Brain Res.* **13:**53–67. The effects of vision and dark-rearing on the size and density of synapses in the lateral geniculate nucleus measured by electron microscopy.

Cragg, B. G. (1970) *Brain Res.* **23:**1–21. What is the signal for chromatolysis?

Cragg, B. G. (1972*a*) *Brain* **95 (1):**143–150. The development of cortical synapses during starvation in the rat.

Cragg, B. G. (1972*b*) *Invest. Ophthalmol.* **11:**377–385. The development of synapses in cat visual cortex.

Cragg, B. G. (1972*c*) Plasticity of synapses, pp. 1–66. In *Structure and Function of Nervous Tissue,* Vol. IV (G. H. Bourne, ed.), Academic Press, New York.

Cragg, B. G. (1975*a*) *Exp. Neurol.* **46:**445–451. The development of synapses in kitten visual cortex during visual deprivation.

Cragg, B. G. (1975*b*) *Exp. Neurol.* **49:**858–862. Absence of barrels and disorganization of thalamic afferent distribution in the sensory cortex of reeler mice.

Cragg, B. G. (1975*c*) *J. Comp. Neurol.* **160:**147–166. The development of synapses in the visual system of the cat.

Craigie, E. H. (1925) *J. Comp. Neurol.* **39:**301–324. Postnatal changes in vascularity in the cerebral cortex of the male albino rat.

Craigie, E. H. (1938) *Res. Publ. Assoc. Res. Nerv. Men. Dis.* **18:**3–28. The comparative anatomy and embryology of the capillary bed of the central nervous system.

Crain, B., C. Cotman, D. Taylor, and G. Lynch. (1973) *Brain Res.* **63:**195–204. A quantitiative electron microscopic study of synaptogenesis in the dentate gyrus of the rat.

Crain, S. M. (1964) *Anat. Rec.* **148:**273–274. Electrophysiological studies of cord-innervated skeletal muscle in long-term tissue cultures of mouse embryo myotomes.

Crain, S. M. (1966) *Int. Rev. Neurobiol.* **9:**1–43. Development of "organotypic" bioelectric activities in central nervous tissues during maturation in culture.

Crain, S. M. (1968) *Anat. Rec.* **160:**466. Development of functional neuromuscular connections between separate explants of fetal mammalian tissues after maturation in culture.

Crain, S. M. (1974) Tissue culture models of developing brain functions, pp. 69–114. In *Studies on the Development of Behavior and the Nervous System,* Vol. 2: *Aspects of Neurogenesis* (G. Gottlieb, ed.), Academic Press, New York.

Crain, S. M. (1976) *Neurophysiologic Studies in Tissue Culture,* Raven Press, New York.

Crain, S. M., and E. R. Peterson, (1967) *Brain Res.* **6:**750–762. Onset and development of functional interneuronal connections in explants of rat spinal cord ganglia during maturation in culture.

Crain, S. M., and E. R. Peterson. (1974) *Ann. N.Y. Acad. Sci.* **228:**6–34. Development of neural connections in culture.

Crain, S. M., H. Benitez, and A. E. Vatter. (1964*a*) *Ann. N.Y. Acad. Sci.* **118:**206–231. Some cytologic effects of salivary nerve-growth factor on tissue cultures of peripheral ganglia.

Crain, S. M. B. P. Bunge, and E. R. Peterson. (1964*b*) *J. Cell Biol.* **23:**114A–115A. Bioelectric and electron microscope evidence for development of synapses in spinal cord cultures.

Crain, S. M., M. B. Bornstein, and E. R. Peterson. (1968) *Brain Res.* **8:**363–372. Maturation of cultured embryonic CNS tissues during chronic exposure to agents which prevent bioelectrical activity.

Crain, S. M., L. Alfei, and E. Peterson. (1970) *J. Neurobiol.* **1:**471–489. Neuromuscular transmission in cultures of adult human and rodent skeletal muscle after innervation *in vitro* by fetal rodent spinal cord.

Cravioto, J. (1966) Malnutrition and behavioral development in the preschool child. In *Preschool Child Malnutrition,* National Health Science Publ. No. 1282.

Cravioto, J., and E. R. DeLicardi. (1972) *Environmental Correlates of Severe Clinical Malnutrition, and Language Development in Survivors from Kwashiorkor and Marasmus,* Pan American Health Organization, Scientific Publ. No. 251, Washington, D.C.

Cravioto, J., E. R. DeLicardi and H. G. Birch. (1966) *Pediatrics* **38:**319–372. Nutrition, growth and neurointegrative development: An experimental and ecologic study.

Creasey, W. A. (1968) *Cancer Chemother. Rep.* **52:**501–507. Modifications in biochemical pathways produced by the vinca alkaloids.

Crelin, E. S. (1952) *J. Exp. Zool.* **120:**547–578. Excision and rotation of the developing *Amblystoma* optic tectum and subsequent visual recovery.

Creps, E. S. (1974*a*) *J. Comp. Neurol.* **157:**139–160. Time of neuron origin in the anterior olfactory nucleus and nucleus of the lateral olfactory tract of the mouse: An autoradiographic study.

Creps, E. S. (1974*b*) *J. Comp. Neurol.* **157:**161–244. Time of neuron origin in preoptic and septal areas of the mouse: An autoradiographic study.

Crick, F. (1970) *Nature* **225:**420–422. Diffusion in embryogenesis.

Crick, F. H. C. (1971) *Symp. Soc. Exp. Biol.* **25:**429–438. The scale of pattern formation.

Crile, G. W., and D. P. Quiring. (1940) *Ohio J. Sci.* **40:**219–259. A record of body weight and certain organ and gland weights of 3,690 animals.

Crome, L., and J. Stern. (1972) *Pathology of Mental Retardation,* 2nd ed., Churchill, Livingstone, Edinburgh.

Crome, L., V. Tymms, and L. I. Woolf. (1962) *J. Neurol. Neurosurg. Psychiat.* **25:**143–153. A chemical investigation of the defects of myelination in phenylketonuria.

Cronkite, E. P., T. M. Fliedner, S. A. Killmann, and J. R. Rubini. (1962) Tritium-labelled thymidine (H^3-TdR): Its somatic toxicity and use in the study of growth rates and potentials in normal and malignant tissue of man and animals, pp. 198–206. In *Tritium in the Physical and Biological Sciences,* Vol. 2, International Atomic Energy Agency, Vienna.

Croskerry, P. G., and G. K. Smith. (1975) *Science* **189:**648–650. Prolongation of gestation by growth hormone: A confounding factor in the assessment of its prenatal action.

Croskerry, P. G., G. K. Smith, B. J. Shepard, and K. B. Freeman. (1973) *Brain Res.* **52:**413–418. Perinatal brain DNA in the normal and growth hormone-treated rat.

Crossland, W. J., W. M. Cowan, and J. P. Kelly. (1973) *Brain Res.* **56:**77–105. Observations on the transport of radioactively labeled proteins in the visual system of the chick.

Crossland, W. J., W. M. Cowan, L. A. Rogers, and J. P. Kelly. (1974*a*) *J. Comp. Neurol.* **155:**127–164. The specification of the retino-tectal projection in the chick.

Crossland, W. J., J. R. Currie, L. A. Rogers, and W. M. Cowan. (1974*b*) *Brain Res.* **78:**483–489. Evidence for a rapid phase of axoplasmic transport at early stages in the development of the visual system of the chick and frog.

Crowther, J. G. (1940) *British Scientists of the Nineteenth Century,* 2 vols., Penguin Books, London.

Cruce, W. L. R. (1974) *J. Comp. Neurol.* **153:**59–76. The anatomical organization of hindlimb motoneurons in the lumbar spinal cord of the frog, *Rana catesbiana.*

Cuajunco, F. (1927*a*) *Anat. Rec.* **35:**8–9. The embryology of the neuromuscular spindles.

Cuajunco, F. (1927*b*) *Contrib. Embryol. Carnegie Inst.* **19:**45–72. Embryology of the neuromuscular spindle.

Cuatrecasas, P. (1969) *Proc. Natl. Acad. Sci. U.S.A.* **63:** 450–457. Interaction of insulin with the cell membrane: The primary action of insulin.

Cuénod, M., and J. Schönbach. (1971) *J. Neurochem.* **18:**809–816. Synaptic proteins and axonal flow in the pigeon visual pathway.

Cull, R. E. (1974) *Exp. Brain Res.* **20:**307–310. Rôle of nerve–muscle contact in maintaining synaptic connections.

Culley, W. J., and E. T. Mertz. (1965) *Proc. Soc. Exp. Biol. N.Y.* **118:**233–235. Effect of restricted food intake on growth and composition of preweaning rat brain.

Currie, J., and W. M. Cowan (1974*a*) *Brain Res.* **71:**133–139. Evidence for the late development of the uncrossed retinothalamic projections in the frog. *Rana pipiens.*

Currie, J., and W. M. Cowan. (1974*b*) *J. Comp. Neurol.* **156:**123–142. Some observations on the early development of the optic tectum in the frog (*Rana pipiens*), with special reference to the effects of early eye removal on mitotic activity in the larval tectum.

Currie, J., and W. M. Cowan. (1975) *Dev. Biol.* **46:**103–119. The development of the retinotectal projection in *Rana pipiens.*

Curtis, A. S. G. (1960) *J. Embryol. Exp. Morphol.* **8:**163–173. Cortical grafting in *Xenopus laevis.*

Curtis, A. S. G. (1962) *Biol. Rev.* **37:**82–129. Cell contact and adhesion.
Curtis, A. S. G. (1967) *The Cell Surface: Its Molecular Role in Morphogenesis,* Logos, London.
Curtis, A. S. G. (1973) Cell adhesion, pp. 315–383. In *Progress in Biophysics and Molecular Biology,* Vol. 27 (J. A. V. Butler and D. Noble, eds.), Pergamon, Oxford.
Cuzner, M. L., and A. N. Davison, (1968) *Biochem. J.* **106:**29–34. The lipid composition of rat brain myelin and subcellular fractions during development.
Czéh, G., and G. Székely. (1971) *Acta Physiol. Acad. Sci. Hung.* **40:**287–302. Muscle activities recorded simultaneously from normal and supernumerary forelimbs in *Ambystoma.*
Dahl, D., and A. Bignami. (1973) *Brain Res.* **61:**279–293. Immunochemical and immunofluorescence studies of the glial fibrillary acidic protein in vertebrates.
Dahl, D. R., and F. E. Samson, Jr. (1959) *Am. J. Physiol.* **196:**470–472. Metabolism of rat brain mitochondria during postnatal development.
Dahl, H. A. (1963) *Z. Zellforsch. Mikrosk. Anat. Abt. Histochem.* **60:**369–386. Fine structure of cilia in rat cerebral cortex.
Dahlström, A. (1967*a*) *Acta Physiol. Scand.* **69:**158–166. The transport or noradrenaline between two simultaneously performed ligations of the sciatic nerves of rat and cat.
Dahlström, A. (1967*b*) *Acta Physiol. Scand.* **69:**167–179. The effect of reserpine and tetrabenazine on the accumulation of noradrenaline in the rat sciatic nerve after ligation.
Dahlström, A. (1968) *Eur. J. Pharmacol.* **5:**111–113. Effect of colchicine on transport of amine storage granules in sympathetic nerves of rat.
Dahlström, A., and J. Häggendal. (1966) *Acta Physiol. Scand.* **67:**278–288. Transport and life-span of amine storage granules in peripheral adrenergic neuron system.
Dahlström, A., and J. Häggendal. (1967) *Acta Physiol. Scand.* **69:**153–157. Studies on the transport and life-span of amine storage granules in the adrenergic neuron system of the rabbit sciatic nerve.
Dale, H. (1935) *Proc. Roy. Soc. Med.* **28:**319–332. Pharmacology and nerve-endings.
Dalton, M. M., O. R. Hommes, and C. P. Leblond. (1968) *J. Comp. Neurol.* **134:**397–400. Correlation of glial proliferation with age in the mouse brain.
Daneo, L. S., and G. Filogamo. (1974) *J. Submicrosc. Cytol.* **6:**219–228. Ultrastructure of developing myo-neural junctions: Evidence for two patterns of synaptic area differentiation.
Daniel, P. M., and D. Whitteridge. (1961) *J. Physiol. (London)* **159:**203–221. The representation of the visual field on the cerebral cortex in monkeys.
Daniels, J. D., and J. D. Pettigrew. (1976) Development of neuronal responses in the visual system of cats, pp. 195–232. In *Studies on the Development of Behavior and the Nervous System,* Vol. 3: *Neuronal and Behavioral Specificity* (G. Gottlieb, ed.), Academic Press, New York.
Daniels, M. P. (1972) *J. Cell Biol.* **53:**164–176. Colchicine inhibition of nerve fiber formation *in vitro.*
Daniels, M. P. (1973) *J. Cell Biol.* **58:**463–470. Ultrastructural changes in neurons and nerve fibers associated with colchicine inhibition of nerve fiber formation *in vitro.*
Daniels M. P. (1975) *Ann. N.Y. Acad. Sci.* **253:**535–544. The role of microtubules in the growth and stabilization of nerve fibers.
D'Arcy Thompson, W. (1942) *On Growth and Form,* 2d ed., 1116 pp., Cambridge University Press, London.
Darwin, C. (1868) *The Variation of Animals and Plants under Domestication,* 2 vols., John Murray, London.
Darwin, F. (1888) *The Life and Letters of Charles Darwin,* 3 vols., John Murray, London.
Davidoff, M. (1973) *Z. Zellforsch.* **141:**427–442. Über die Glia in Hypoglossuskern der Ratte nach Axotomie.
Davidson, E. H., and R. H. Britten. (1973) *Quart. Rev. Biol.* **48:**565–613. Organization, transcription, and regulation in the animal genome.
Davidson, J. M., and S. Levine. (1972) Annu. Rev. Physiol. **34:**375–408. Endocrine regulation of behavior.
Davidson, R. L. (1973) Control of the differentiated state in somatic cell hybrids, pp. 295–328. In *Genetic Mechanisms of Development* (F. H. Ruddle, ed.), Academic Press, New York.
Davies, P. A., and A. L. Stewart. (1975) *Br. Med. Bull.* **31:**85–91. Low-birth-weight infants: Neurological sequelae and later intelligence.
Davis, C. J. F. (1970) Prolonged nembutal narcosis of the cat and its effects upon the isometric contraction characteristics of fast twitch and slow twitch skeletal muscle. Ph.D. thesis, University of Bristol.
Davison, A. N., and J. Dobbing. (1960*a*) *Biochem. J.* **75:**565–570. Phospholipid metabolism in nervous tissue. 2. Metabolic stability.

Davison, A. N., and J. Dobbing. (1960*b*) *Biochem. J.* **75:**571–574. Phospholipid metabolism in nervous tissue, 3. The anatomical distribution of metabolically inert phospholipid in the central nervous system.

Davison, A. N., and M. B. Dobbing, (1966) *Br. Med. Bull.* **22:**40–44. Myelination as a vulnerable period in brain development.

Davison, A. N., M. L. Cuzner, N. L. Banik, and J. Oxberry. (1966) *Nature* **212:**1373–1374. Myelinogenesis in the rat brain.

Davison, P. F., and B. Winslow. (1974) *J. Neurobiol.* **5:**119–133. The protein subunit of calf brain neurofilament.

Daw, N. W., and H. J. Wyatt. (1976) *J. Physiol. (London)* **257:**155–170. Kittens reared in a unidirectional environment: Evidence for a critical period.

Dawson, D. M., and F. C. A. Romanul. (1964) *Arch. Neurol.* **11:**369–378. Enzymes in muscle. II. Histochemical and quantitative studies.

Dawydoff, C. (1928) *Traité d'Embryologie Comparée des Invertébrés,* Masson, Paris, 930 pp.

Dayton, D. H., L. J. Filer, and C. Canosa. (1969) *Fed. Proc.* **28:**488. Cellular changes in placentas of undernourished mothers in Guatamala.

De Anda, G., M. A. Rebollo, and M. Achaval. (1963) *Acta Neurol. Latinoam.* **9:**93–101. Differentiation of the skeletal muscle in the chicken. II. Development of the myoneural synapse.

De Brabander, M., F. Aerts, R. Van de Veire, and M. Borgers. (1975) *Nature* **253:**119–120. Evidence against interconversion of microtubules and filaments.

Decker, R. S. (1976) *Dev. Biol.* **49:**101–118. Influence of thyroid hormones on neuronal death and differentiation in larval *Rana pipiens.*

Defendi, Va., and L. A. Manson. (1963) *Nature* **198:**359–361. Analysis of the life cycle in mammalian cells.

DeHan, R. S., and P. Graziadei. (1973) *Life Sci.* **13:**1435–1449. The innervation of frog's taste organ: "A histochemical study."

Deitch, A. D., and M. R. Murray. (1956) *J. Biophys. Biochem. Cytol.* **2:**433–444. The Nissl substance of living and fixed spinal ganglion cells.

Dekaban, A. (1956) *Anat. Rec.* **126:**111–122. Oligodendroglia and axis cylinders in rabbits before, during, and after myelination.

Del Castillo, J., and A. D. Vizoso. (1953) *J. Physiol. (London)* **122:**33–34P. The electrical activity of embryonic nerves.

Del Cerro, M. (1974) *J. Comp. Neurol.* **157:**245–280. Uptake of tracer proteins in the developing cerebellum, particularly by the growth cones and blood vessels.

Del Cerro, M. P., and R. S. Snider. (1967) *J. Microsc.* **133:**515–518. Cilia in the cerebellum of immature and adult rats.

Del Cerro, M. P., and R. S. Snider. (1968) *J. Comp. Neurol.* **133:**341–362. Studies on the developing cerebellum. Ultrastructure of the growth cones.

Del Cerro, M. P., and R. S. Snider, (1969) *Anat. Rec.* **165:**127–140. The Purkinje cell cilium.

Del Cerro, M. P., R. S. Snider, and M. L. Oster. (1968) *Experientia* **24:**929–930. Evolution of the extracellular space in immature neurons.

DeLong, G. R., and A. J. Coulombre. (1965) *Exp. Neurol.* **13:**351–363. Development of the retinotectal topographic projection in the chick embryo.

DeLong, G. R., and A. J. Coulombre. (1968) *Dev. Biol.* **16:**513–531. The specificity of retino-tectal connections studied by retinal grafts onto the optic tectum in chick embryos.

DeLong, G. R., and R. L. Sidman. (1962) *J. Comp. Neurol.* **118:**205–224. Effects of eye removal at birth on histogenesis of the mouse superior colliculus: An autoradiographic analysis with tritiated thymidine.

Del Rio-Hortega, P. (1916) *Trabajos Lab. Invest. Biol. Univ. Madrid* **14:**117–153. Estudios sobre el centrosoma de las células nerviosas y neuróglias de los vertebrados, en sus formas normal y anormales.

Del Rio-Hortega, P. (1919) *Bol. Soc. Espan. Biol.* **9:**68–83. El tercer elemento de los centros nerviosos.

Del Rio-Hortega, P. (1921) *Mem. Soc. Espan. Hist. Nat.* **11:**213–268. Histogénesis y evolución normal exodo y distribución regional de la microglia.

Del Rio-Hortega, P. (1924) *Compt. Rend. Soc. Biol.* **9:**818–820. La glie à radiations peu nombreuses et la cellule de Schwann sont elles homologables?

Del Rio-Hortega, P. (1928) *Mem. Real. Soc. Espan. Hist. Nat.* **14:**5–122. Tercera aportación conocimiento morfologico e interpretación funcional de la oligodendroglia.

Del Rio-Hortega, P. (1932) Microglia, pp. 483–534. In *Cytology and Cellular Pathology of the Nervous System,* Vol. II (W. Penfield, ed.), Hoeber, New York.

Denny-Brown, D. (1929) *Proc. Roy. Soc. London Ser. B.* **104:**371–411. The histological features of striped muscle in relation to its functional activity.

Denham, S. (1967) *J. Embryol. Exp. Morphol.* **18:**53–66. A cell proliferation study of the neural retina in the two-day rat.

Dentler, W. L., S. Granett, G. B. Witman, and J. L. Rosenbaum. (1974) *Proc. Natl. Acad. Sci. U.S.A.* **71:**1710–1714. Directionality of brain microtubule assembly *in vitro.*

Deol, M. S. (1967) *J. Embryol. Exp. Morphol.* **17:**533–541. The neural crest and the acoustic ganglion.

Deol, M. S. (1970) *J. Embryol. Exp. Morphol.* **23:**773–784. The origin of the acoustic ganglion and effects of the gene dominant spotting (W^v) in the mouse.

De Robertis, E. D. P., and H. M. Gershenfeld. (1961) *Int. Rev. Neurobiol.* **3:**1–65. Submicroscopic morphology and function of glial cells.

Derrick, G. E. (1937) *J. Morphol.* **61:**257–284. An analysis of the early development of the chick by means of the mitotic index.

de Solla Price, D. J. (1964) *Technol. Culture* **5:**9–23. Automata and the origins of mechanism and mechanistic philosophy.

Detwiler, S. R. (1920*a*) *J. Exp. Zool.* **31:**117–169. Experiments on the transplantation of limbs in *Amblystoma:* The formation of nerve plexuses and the function of the limbs.

Detwiler, S. R. (1920*b*) *Proc. Natl. Acad. Sci. U.S.A.* **6:**96–101. On the hyperplasia of nerve centers resulting from excessive peripheral loading.

Detwiler, S. R. (1923) *J. Exp. Zool.* **37:**339–393. Experiments on the transplantation of the spinal cord in *Amblystoma* and their bearing upon the stimuli involved in differentiation of nerve cells.

Detwiler, S. R. (1924) *J. Comp. Neurol.* **37:**1–14. The effects of bilateral extirpation of the anterior limb rudiments in *Amblystoma* embryos.

Detwiler, S. R. (1925) *J. Comp. Neurol.* **38:**461–490. Coordinated movements in supernumerary transplanted limbs.

Detwiler, S. R. (1930*a*) *J. Exp. Zool.* **55:**319–379. Observations upon the growth, function and nerve supply of limbs when grafted to the head of salamander embryos.

Detwiler, S. R. (1930*b*) *J. Exp. Zool.* **57:**183–203. Some observations upon the growth, innervation, and funciton of heteroplastic limbs.

Detwiler, S. R. (1933*a*) *Biol. Rev.* **8:**269–310. Experimental studies upon the development of the amphibian nervous system.

Detwiler, S. R. (1933*b*) *J. Exp. Zool.* **64:**405–414. On the time of determination of the antero-posterior axis of the forelimb on *Amblystoma.*

Detwiler, S. R. (1933*c*) *Anat. Rec.* **57:**81–98. Growth and cell proliferation in heterotopic spinal cord grafts.

Detwiler, S. R. (1934) *J. Exp. Zool.* **67:**395–441. An experimental study of spinal nerve segmentation in *Amblystoma* with reference to the plurisegmental contribution to the brachial plexus.

Detwiler, S. R. (1936) *Neuroembryology: An Experimental Study,* Macmillian, New York.

Detwiler, S. R. (1937*a*) *Am. J. Anat.* **61:**63–94. Observations upon the migration of neural crest cells, and upon the development of the spinal ganglia and vertebral arches in *Amblystoma.*

Detwiler, S. R. (1937*b*) *J. Exp. Zool.* **77:**109–122. Does the developing medulla influence cellular proliferation within the spinal cord?

Detwiler, S. R. (1940) *J. Exp. Zool.* **84:**13–22. Unilateral reversal of the anteroposterior axis of the medulla in *Amblystoma.*

Detwiler, S. R. (1943) *J. Exp. Zool.* **94:**169–179. Reversal of the medulla in *Amblystoma* embryos.

Detwiler, S. R. (1944) *J. Exp. Zool.* **96:**129–142. Restitution of the medulla following unilateral excision in the embryo.

Detwiler, S. R. (1947) *J. Exp. Zool.* **104:**53–68. Resitution of the brachial region of the cord following unilateral excision in the embryo.

Detwiler, S. R. (1949) *J. Exp. Zool.* **111:**79–93. The swimming capacity of *Amblystoma* larvae following reversal of the embryonic hind brain.

Detwiler, S. R. (1951) *J. Exp. Zool.* **116:**431–446. Structural and functional adjustments following reversal of the embryonic medulla in *Amblystoma.*

Detwiler, S. R., and R. L. Carpenter. (1929) *J. Comp. Neurol.* **47:**427–447. An experimental study of the mechanism of coordinated movements in heterotopic limbs.

Detwiler, S. R., and K. Kehoe. (1939) *J. Exp. Zool.* **81**:415–435. Further observations on the origin of the sheath cells of Schwann.

de Vellis, J. (1973) Mechanisms of enzymatic differentiation in the brain and in cultured cells, pp. 171–198. In *Development and Aging in the Nervous System* (M. Rockstein, ed.), Academic Press, New York.

de Vellis, J., and G. Kukes. (1973) *Tex. Rep. Biol. Med.* **31**:271–293. Regulation of glial cell functions by hormones and ions: A review.

Devine, C. E., and F. O. Simpson. (1968) *J. Cell Biol.* **38**:184–192. Localization of tritiated norepinephrine in vascular sympathetic axons of the rat intestine and mesentery by electron microscope radioautography.

De Vito, J. L., K. W. Clausing, and O. A. Smith. (1974) *Brain Res.* **82**:269–271. Uptake and transport of horseradish peroxidase by cut end of the vagus nerve.

Devor, M. (1975) *Science* **190**:998–1000. Neuroplasticity in the sparing or deterioration of function after early olfactory tract lesions.

Devor, M., V. S. Caviness, Jr., and P. Derer. (1975) *J. Comp. Neurol.* **164**:471–482. A normally laminated afferent projection to an abnormally laminated cortex: Some olfactory connections in the reeler mouse.

Devreotes, P. N., and D. M. Fambrough. (1976*a*) *Proc. Natl. Acad. Sci. U.S.A.* **73**:161–164. Synthesis of acetylcholine receptors by cultured chick myotubes and denervated mouse extensor digitorum longus muscles.

Devreotes, P. N., and D. M. Fambrough. (1976*b*) *Cold Spring Harbor Symp. Quant. Biol.* **40**:237–251. Turnover of acetylcholine receptors in skeletal muscle.

Deysson, G. (1968) *Int. Rev. Cytol.* **24**:99–148. Antimitotic substances.

Diamond, J., and R. Miledi. (1962) *J. Physiol. (London)* **162**:393–408. A study of foetal and new-born rat muscle fibers.

Diamond, J., E. Cooper, C. Turner, and L. Macintyre. (1976) *Science* **193**:371–377. Trophic regulation of nerve sprouting.

Diamond, M. C., D. Krech, and M. R. Rosenzweig. (1964) *J. Comp. Neurol.* **123**:111–119. The effects of an enriched environment on the histology of the rat cerebral cortex.

Diamond, M. C., F. Law, H. Rhodes, B. Lindner, M. R. Rosenzweig, D. Krech, and E. L. Bennett. (1966) *J. Comp. Neurol.* **128**:117–126. Increases in cortical depth and glia numbers in rats subjected to enriched environment.

Diamond, M. C., R. E. Johnson, C. Ingham, and B. Stone. (1969) *Exp. Neurol.* **23**:51–57. Lack of direct effect of hypophysectomy and growth hormone on postnatal rat brain morphology.

Dickie, M. M., J. Schneider, and P. J. Harman. (1952) *J. Hered.* **43**:283–286. A juvenile wabbler-lethal in the house mouse.

DiGiamberardino, L., G. Bennett, H. L. Koenig, and B. Droz. (1973) *Brain Res.* **60**:147–159. Axonal migration of protein and glycoprotein to nerve endings. III. Cell fraction analysis of chicken ciliary ganglion after intracerebral injection of labelled precursors of proteins and glycoproteins.

Dijkstra, C. (1933) *Z. Mikrosk. Anat. Forsch.* **34**:75–158. Die De- und Regeneration der sensiblen Endkörperchen des Entenschnabels (Grandry- und Herbst-Körperchen) nach Durchschneidung des Nerven, nach Fortnahme der ganzen Haut und nach Transplantation des Hautstückchens.

Diller, D. A., R. H. Brownson, and D. B. Suter. (1964) *J. Neuropathol. Exp. Neurol.* **23**:446–456. X-irradiation induced acute brain damage as a function of age.

Dixon, J. S., and J. R. Cronly-Dillon. (1972) *J. Embryol. Exp. Morphol.* **28**:659–666. The fine structure of the developing retina in *Xenopus laevis*.

Dobbing, J. (1963) *Proc. R. Soc. (London) Ser. B.*, **159**:503–509. The influence of early nutrition on the development and myelination of the brain.

Dobbing, J. (1971) *Psychiat. Neurol. Neurochir.* **74**:433–442. Undernutrition and the developing brain: The use of animal models to elucidate the human problem.

Dobbing, J. (1976) Vulnerable periods in brain growth and somatic growth, pp. 137–147. In *The Biology of Human Fetal Growth* (D. F. Roberts and A. M. Thomson, eds.), Taylor and Francis, London.

Dobbing, J., and J. Sands. (1970) *Nature* **226**:639–640. Timing of neuroblast multiplication in developing human brain.

Dobbing, J., and J. L. Smart. (1974) *Br. Med. Bull.* **30**:164–168. Vulnerability of developing brain and behaviour.

Dobbing, J., J. W. Hopewell, and A. Lynch. (1971) *Exp. Neurol.* **32**:439–447. Vulnerability of developing brain. VII. Permanent deficit of neurons in cerebral and cerebellar cortex following early mild undernutrition.

Dobzhansky, T. (1951) *Genetics and the Origin of Species,* 3rd ed., Columbia University Press, New York.

Donahue, S., and C. D. Pappas. (1961) *Am. J. Anat.* **115:**17–26. The fine structure of capillaries in the cerebral cortex of the rat at various stages of development.

Donaldson, H. H. (1925) *Arch. Neurol. Psychiat. (Chicago)* **13:**385–386. The significance of brain weight.

Donaldson, H. H., and G. Nagasaka. (1918) *J. Comp. Neurol.* **29:**529–552. On the increase in the diameter of nerve cell bodies and of the fibers arising from them during the later phases of growth (albino rat).

Donegani, G., and G. Gabella. (1967) *Boll. Soc. Ital. Biol. Sper.* **43:**1165–1167. Effetto della sezione intracranica del nervo glosso-faringeo sui corpuscoli gustativi nel coniglio.

Dorgan, W. J., and R. L. Schultz. (1971) *J. Exp. Zool.* **178:**497–512. An *in vitro* study of programmed death in rat placental giant cells.

Dörner, G., and J. Staudt. (1969) *Neuroendocrinology* **5:**103–106. Perinatal structural sex differentiation of the hypothalamus in rats.

Dorris, F. (1939) *J. Exp. Zool.* **86:**315–345. The production of pigment by chick neural crest in grafts to the 3-day limb bud.

Dougherty, T. F. (1944) *Am. J. Anat.* **74:**61–95. Studies on the cytogenesis of microglia and their relation to cells of the reticulo-endothelial system.

Drachman, D. B. (1965) *J. Physiol. (London)* **180:**735–740. The developing motor end-plate: curare tolerance in the chick embryo.

Drachman, D. B. (1967) *Arch. Neurol.* **17:**206–218. Is acetylcholine the trophic neuromuscular transmitter?

Drachman, D. B. (1972) *J. Physiol. (London)* **226:**619–627. Neurotrophic regulation of muscle cholinesterase: Effects of botulinum toxin and denervation.

Drachman, D. B. (1976) Trophic interactions between nerves and muscles: The role of cholinergic transmission (including usage) and other factors, pp. 161–186. In *Biology of Cholinergic Function* (A. M. Goldberg and I. Hanin eds.), Raven Press, New York.

Drachman, D. B. and F. C. A. Romanul. (1970) *Arch. Neurol.* **23:**85–89. Effect of neuromuscular blockade on enzymatic activities of muscles.

Drachman, D. B., and F. Witzke. (1972) *Science* **176:**514–516. Trophic regulation of acetylcholine sensitivity of muscle: Effect of electrical stimulation.

Dräger, U. C. (1976) The effects of monocular deprivation on mouse striate cortex. Paper presented at the Society for Neuroscience, Toronto.

Dribin, L., and M. Jacobson. (1978) *Brain Res.* (in press). Effects of 5-bromodeoxyuridine on development of Mauthner's neuron and neural retina of *Xenopus laevis* embryos.

Droz, B. (1973) *Brain Res.* **62:**383–394. Renewal of synaptic proteins.

Droz, B., H. L. Koenig, and L. DiGiamberardino. (1973) *Brain Res.* **60:**93–127. Axonal migration of protein and glycoprotein to nerve endings. I. Radioautographic analysis of the renewal of protein in nerve endings of chicken ciliary ganglion after intracerebral injection of [^{3}H]lysine.

Droz, B., A. Rambourg, and H. L. Koenig. (1975) *Brain Res.* **93:**1–13. The smooth endoplasmic reticulum: Structure and role in the renewal of axonal membrane and synaptic vesicles by fast axonal transport.

Dubey, P. N., D. K. Kadasne, and V. S. Gosavi. (1968) *J. Anat. (London)* **102:**407–414. The influence of the peripheral field on the morphogenesis of Hofmann's nucleus major of chick spinal cord.

Dubois, E. (1923) *Proc. Koninkl. Med. Akad. Wetenschap* (Amsterdam) **25:**230–255. Phylogenetic and ontogenetic increase of the volume of the brain in vertebrata.

Dubowitz, V. and A. G. E. Pearse. (1960) *Histochimie* **2:**105–117. A comparative histochemical study of oxidative enzyme and phosphorylase activity in skeletal muscle.

Duchen, L. W. (1971) *J. Neurol. Sci.* **14:**47–60. An electron microscopic study of the changes induced by botulinum toxin in the motor end-plate of slow and fast skeletal muscle fibres of the mouse.

Duchen, L. W. (1972) *Proc. Roy. Soc. Med.* **65:**10–11. Motor nerve growth induced by botulinum toxin as regenerative phenomenon.

Duchen, L. W., and S. J. Strich, (1968) *Quart. J. Exp. Physiol.* **53:**84–89. The effects of botulinum toxin on the pattern of innervation of skeletal muscle in the mouse.

Duckett, S., and A. G. E. Pearse. (1968) *J. Anat. (London)* **102:**183–187. The cells of Cajal-Retzius in the developing human brain.

Duffy, F. H., and S. R. Snodgrass, J. L. Burchfiel, and J. L. Conway. (1976) *Nature* **260:**256–257. Bicuculline reversal of deprivation amblyopia in the cat.

Duncan, D. (1934*a*) *J. Comp. Neurol.* **60:**437–472. A relation between axon diameter and myelination determined by measurement of myelinated spinal root fibers.

Duncan, D. (1934*b*) *Science* **79:**363. The importance of axon diameter as a factor in myelination.

Duncan, D. (1957) *Texas Rep. Biol. Med.* **15:**367–377. Electron microscope study of the embryonic neural tube and notochord.

Dunn, G. A. (1971) *J. Comp. Neurol.* **143:**491–508. Mutual contact inhibition of extension of chick sensory nerve fibres *in vitro.*

Dunnebacke, T. H. (1953) *J. Comp. Neurol.* **98:**155–177. The effects of the extirpation of the superior oblique muscle on the trochlear nucleus in the chick embryo.

Dunning, H. S., and H. G. Wolff. (1937) *J. Comp. Neurol.* **67:**433–450. The relative vascularity of various parts of the central and peripheral nervous system of the cat and its relation to function.

Dürken, B. (1911) *Z. Wiss. Zool.* **99:**189–355. Über frühzeitige Extirpation von Extremitätenanlagen beim Frosch.

Dürken, B. (1913) *Z. Wiss. Zool. Abt. A* **105:**192–242. Über einseitige Augenextirpation bei jungen Froschlarven.

Dürken, B. (1930) *Biol Generalis* **6:**511–552. Zur Frage nach der Wirkung einseitiger Augenextirpation bei Froschlarven.

Du Shane, G. P. (1935) *J. Exp. Zool.* **72:**1–31. An experimental study of the origin of pigment cells in Amphibia.

Du Shane, G. (1938) *J. Exp. Zool.* **78:**485–503. Neural fold derivatives in the amphibia: Pigment cells, spinal ganglia and Rohon-Beard cells.

Dustin, A. P. (1910) *Arch. Biol. Liège* **25:**269–388. Le rôle des tropismes et de l'odogenés dans la régéneration du système nerveux.

Eastlick, H. L. (1943) *J. Exp. Zool.* **93:**27–49. Studies on transplanted embryonic limbs of the chick. I. The development of muscle in nerveless and in innervated grafts.

Eastlick, H. L. and R. A. Wortham, (1947) *J. Morphol.* **80:**369–389. Studies on transplanted embryonic limbs of the chick. III. The replacement of muscle by adipose tissue.

Eayrs, J. T. (1955) *Acta Anat.* **25:**160–183. The cerebral cortex of normal and hypothyroid rats.

Eayrs, J. T. (1960) *Br. Med. Bull.* **16:**122–126. Influence of the thyroid on the central nervous system.

Eayrs, J. T., and B. Goodhead. (1959) *J. Anat. (London)* **93:**385–402. Postnatal development of the cerebral cortex in the rat.

Eayrs, J. T., and W. A. Lishman. (1953) Br. J. Animal Behav. **3:**17–24. The maturation of behaviour in hypothyroidism and starvation.

Ebendal, T., (1976*a*) *Exp. Cell Res.* **98:**159–169. The relative roles of contact inhibition and contact guidance in orientation of axons extending on aligned collagen fibrils *in vitro.*

Ebendal, T. (1976*b*) Experiments *in vitro* on neuron development and axon orientation in the chick embryo. Doctoral thesis, Uppsala University, Sweden.

Ebendal, T. (1977) *Cell Tiss. Res.* **175:**439–458. Extracellular matrix fibrils and cell contacts in the chick embryo.

Ebendal, T., and K.-O. Hedlund. (1975) *Zoon* **3:**33–47. Effects of nerve growth factor on the chick embryo trigeminal ganglion in culture.

Ebendal, T., and C.-O. Jacobson. (1975) *Zoon* **3:**169–172. Human glial cells stimulating outgrowth of axons in cultured chick embryo ganglia.

Ebendal, T., and C.-O. Jacobson. (1977) *Exp. Cell Res.* **105:**379–387. Tissue explants affecting extension and orientation of axons in cultured chick embryo ganglia.

Ebinger, P. (1974) *Z. Anat. Entwicklungsgesch.* **144:**267–302. A cytoarchitectonic volumetric comparison of brains in wild and domestic sheep.

Eccles, J. C. (1964) *The Physiology of Synapses,* Springer-Verlag, Berlin.

Eccles, J. C., R. M. Eccles, and A. Lundberg. (1958*a*) *J. Physiol (London)* **142:**275–291. The action potentials of the alpha motoneurones supplying fast and slow muscles.

Eccles, J. C., B. Libet, and R. R. Young. (1958*b*) *J. Physiol. (London)* **143:**11–40. The behavior of chromatolyzed motoneurones studied by intracellular recording.

Eccles, J. C., R. M. Eccles, and F. Magni. (1960) *J. Physiol. (London)* **154:**68–88. Monosynaptic excitatory action on motoneurones regenerated to antagonistic muscles.

Eccles, J. C., R. M. Eccles, and C. N. Shealy. (1962*a*) *J. Neurophysiol.* **25:**544–558. An investigation into the effect of degenerating primary afferent fibers on the monosynaptic innervation of motoneurons.

Eccles, J. C., R. M. Eccles, C. N. Shealy, and W. D. Willis. (1962*b*) *J. Neurophysiol.* **25:**559–580. Experiments utilizing monosynaptic excitatory action on motoneurons for testing hypotheses relating to specificity of neuronal connections.

Eccles, J. C., M. Ito, and J. Szentágothai. (1967) *The Cerebellum as a Neuronal Machine,* Springer, New York.

Ecker, A. (1869) *Die Hirnwindung des Menschen nach eigenen Untersuchungen insbesondere über die Entwicklung derselben beim Fötus,* Vieweg, Braunschweig. (English transl. 1873, by J. C. Galton, *On the Convolutions of the Human Brain,* Smith and Elder, London.)

Eckholm, R., and H. Hydén. (1965) *J. Ultrastruct. Res.* **13:**269–280. Polysomes from microdissected fresh neurons.

Edds, M. V., Jr. (1950*a*) *J. Exp. Zool.* **113:**517–552. Collateral regeneration of residual motor axons in partially denervated muscles.

Edds, M. V., Jr. (1950*b*) *J. Comp. Neurol.* **93:**258–276. Hypertrophy of nerve fibers to functionally overloaded muscles.

Edds, M. V., Jr. (1953) *Quart. Rev. Biol.* **28:**260–276. Collateral nerve regeneration.

Edström, A. (1964*a*) *J. Neurochem.* **11:**309–314. The ribonucleic acid in the Mauthner neuron of the goldfish.

Edström, A. (1964*b*) *J. Neurochem.* **11:**557–559. The effect of spinal cord transection on the base composition and content of RNA in the Mauthner nerve fibre of the goldfish.

Edström, A. (1966) *J. Neurochem.* **13:**315–321. Amino acid incorporation in isolated Mauthner nerve fibre components.

Edström, A. (1967) *J. Neurochem.* **14:**239–243. Inhibition of protein synthesis in Mauthner nerve fibre components by Actinomycin-D.

Edström, A., and J. Sjöstrand. (1969) *J. Neurochem.* **16:**67–82. Protein synthesis in the isolated Mauthner nerve fiber of the goldfish.

Edström, A., J.-E. Edström, and T. Hökfelt, (1969) *J. Neurochem.* **16:**53–66. Sedimentation analysis of ribonucleic acid extracted from isolated Mauthner nerve fiber components.

Edström, J.-E., D. Eichner, and A. Edström. (1962) *Biochim. Biophys. Acta* **61:**178–184. The ribonucleic acid of axons and myelin sheaths from Mauthner neurons.

Edwards, J. S., and J. Palka. (1973) Neural specificity as a game of cricket: Some rules of sensory regeneration in *Acheta domesticus,* pp. 131–146. In *Developmental Neurobiology of Arthropods* (D. Young, ed.), Cambridge University Press, London.

Edwards, J. S., and J. Palka. (1974) *Proc. Roy. Soc. London (Biol.)* **185:**83–103. The cerci and abdominal giant fibres of the house cricket, *Acheta domesticus.* 1. Anatomy and physiology of normal adults.

Edwards, J. S., and T. S. Sahota. (1967) *J. Exp. Zool.* **166:**387–396. Regeneration of a sensory system: The formation of central connections by normal and transplanted cerci of the house cricket *Acheta domesticus.*

Edwards, M. J. (1969) *Teratology* **2:**329–336. Congenital defects in guinea-pigs: Prenatal retardation of brain growth of guinea-pigs following hyperthermia during gestation.

Edwards, M. J., R. H. C. Penny, and I. Zevnik. (1971) *Brain Res.* **28:**341–345. A brain cell deficit in newborn guinea-pigs following prenatal hyperthermia.

Edwards, M. J., R. Mulley, S. Ring, and R. A. Wanner. (1974) *J. Embryol. Exp. Morphol.* **32:**593–602. Mitotic cell death and delay of mitotic activity in guinea-pig embryos following brief maternal hyperthermia.

Ehrhardt, A. A., and J. Money. (1967) *J. Sex Res.* **3:**83–100. Progestin-induced hermaphroditism: IQ and psychosexual identity in a study of ten girls.

Eichenwald, H. F., and P. C. Fry. (1969) *Science* **163:**644–648. Nutrition and learning.

Eichler, V. (1971) *J. Comp. Neurol.* **141:**375–396. Neurogenesis in the optic tectum of larval *Rana pipiens* following unilateral enucleation.

Eichhorn, D. H., and N. Bayley. (1962) *Child Dev.* **33:**257. Growth in head circumference from birth through young adulthood.

Eisenfeld, A. J., and J. Axelrod, (1965) *J. Pharmacol. Exp. Ther.* **150:**469–475. Selectivity of estrogen distribution in tissues.

Elam, J. S., and B. W. Agranoff. (1971) *J. Neurobiol.* **2:**379–390. Transport of proteins and sulfated mucopolysaccharides in the goldfish visual system.

Ellenberger, C., Jr., J. Hanaway, and M. G. Netsky. (1969) *J. Comp. Neurol.* **137:**71–88. Embryogenesis of the inferior olivary nucleus in the rat: A radioautographic study and re-evaluation of the rhombic lip.

Ellingson, R. J., and R. C. Wilcott. (1960) *J. Neurophysiol.* **23:**363–375. Development of evoked responses in visual and auditory cortices of kittens.

Elliott, B. J., and D. G. F. Harriman. (1974) *Nature* **251:**622–624. Growth of human muscle spindles *in vitro.*

Ellis, R. S., (1919) *J. Comp. Neurol.* **30:**229–252. A preliminary quantitiative study of the Purkinje cells in normal, subnormal and senescent human cerebella.

Ellia, R. S. (1920) *J. Comp. Neurol.* **32:**1–33. Norms for some structural changes in the human cerebellum from birth to old age.

Elsberg, C. A. (1917) *Science* **45:**318–320. Experiments on motor nerve regeneration and the direct neurotization of paralyzed muscles by their own and by foreign nerves.

Emmelin, N., and L. Malmfors. (1965) *Quart. J. Exp. Physiol.* **50:**142–145. Development of supersensitivity as dependent on the length of degenerating nerve fibers.

Engberg, I., and A. Lundberg. (1962) *Experientia* **18:**174–177. An electromyographic analysis of stepping in the cat.

Engel, W. K. (1961) *J. Histochem. Cytochem.* **9:**66–72. Cytological localization of cholinesterase in cultured skeletal muscle cells.

Enroth-Cugell, C., and J. G. Robson. (1966) *J. Physiol. London* **187:**517–552. The contrast sensitivity of retinal ganglion cells in the cat.

Epstein, H. T. (1973) *Am J. Phys. Anthropol.* **39:**135–136. Possible metabolic constraints on human brain weight at birth.

Erlanger, J., and G. M. Schoepfle. (1946) *Am. J. Physiol.* **147:**550–581. A study of nerve degeneration and regeneration.

Ernst, M. (1926). *Z. Anat. Entwicklungsgesch.* **79:**228–262. Über Untergang von Zellen während der normalen Entwicklung bei Wirbeltieren.

Ernyei, S., and M. R. Young. (1966) *J. Physiol. (London)* **183:**469–480. Pulsatile and myelin-forming activities of Schwann cells *in vitro.*

Eschner, J., and P. Glees. (1963) *Experientia* **19:**301–303. Free and membrane-bound ribosomes in maturing neurons of the chick and their possible functional significance.

Essick, C. R. (1907) *Am. J. Anat.* **7:**119–135. The corpus ponto-bulbare—a hitherto undescribed nuclear mass in the human hind brain.

Essick, C. R. (1909) *Anat. Rec.* **3:**254–257. On the embryology of the corpus ponto-bulbare and its relation to the development of the pons.

Essick, C. R. (1912) *Am. J. Anat.* **13:**25–34. The development of the nuclei pontis and the nucleus arcuatus in man.

Etkin. W. (1964) Metamorphosis, pp. 427–468. In *Physiology of the Amphibia* (J. A. Morre, ed.), Academic Press, New York.

Evans, D. H. L., and A. D. Vizoso. (1951). *J. Comp. Neurol.* **95:**429–461. Observations on the mode of growth of motor nerve fibers in rabbits during postnatal development.

Evans, H. E., and W. O. Sack. (1973) *Anat. Histol. Embryol.* **2:**11–45. Prenatal development of domestic and laboratory animals: Growth curves, external features and selected references.

Ewert, J.-P. (1974) *Sci. Am.* **230:**34–42. The neural basis of visually guided behavior.

Ewert, J.-P., and A. von Wietersheim. (1974) *Acta Anat.* **88:**56–66. Ganglienzellklassen in der retinotectalen Projection der Kröte *Bufo bufo* (L.).

Falconer, D. S. (1951) *J. Genet.* **50:**192–201. Two new mutations, trembler and reeler, with neurological action in the house mouse.

Fallon, J. F., and J. W. Saunders, Jr. (1968) *Dev. Biol.* **18:**553–570. *In vitro* analysis of the control of cell death in a zone of prospective necrosis from the chick wing bud.

Fambrough, D. M. (1970) *Science* **168:**372. Acetylcholine sensitivity of muscle fiber membranes: Mechanism of regulation by motoneurons.

Fambrough, D. M. (1974*a*) *J. Gen. Physiol.* **64:**468–472. Revised estimates of extrajunctional receptor density in denervated rat diaphragm.

Fambrough, D. M. (1974*b*) Cullular and developmental biology of acetylcholine receptors in skeletal muscle, pp. 85–113. In *Neurochemistry of Cholinergic Receptors* (E. de Robertis and J. Schact, eds.), Raven Press, New York.

Fambrough, D. M., and J. E. Rash, (1971) *Dev. Biol.* **26:**55–68. Development of acetylcholine sensitivity during myogenesis.

Fambrough, D. M., D. B. Drachman, and S. Satyamurti. (1973) *Science* **182:**293–295. Neuromuscular junction in myasthenia gravis: Decreased acetylcholine receptors.

Fankhauser, G. (1941) *J. Morphol.* **68:**161–177. Cell size, organ and body size in triploid newts (*Triturus viridescens*).

Fankhauser, G. (1945*a*) *J. Exp. Zool.* **100:**445–455. Maintenance of normal structure in heteroploid salamander larvae, through compensation of changes in cell size by adjustment of cell number and cell shape.

Fankhauser, G. (1945*b*) *Quart. Rev. Biol.* **20:**20–78. The effects of changes in chromosome number on amphibian development.

Fankhauser, G., J. A. Vernon, W. H. Frank, and W. V. Slack. (1955) *Science* **122:**692–693. Effect of size and number of brain cells on learning in larvae of the salamander, *Triturus viridescens.*

Farbman, A. I. (1965) *Dev. Biol.* **11:**110–135. Electron microscope study of the developing taste bud in rat fungiform papilla.

Farbman, A. I. (1971) Development of the taste bud, pp. 50–62 In *Handbook of Sensory Physiology,* Vol. IV/2: *Chemical Senses: Taste* (L. M. Beidler, ed.), Springer-Verlag, Heidelberg.

Farbman, A. I. (1972) *J. Cell Biol.* **52:**489–493. Differentiation of taste buds in organ culture.

Farbman, A. I., and M. Ziegner. (1968) *Anat. Rec.* **160:**347. Differentiation of fetal rat tongue grafts in the anterior chamber of the eye.

Farkas-Bargeton, E., O. Robain, and P. Mandel. (1972) *Acta Neuropathol.* **21:**272–281. Abnormal glial maturation in the white matter of Jimpy mice: An optical study.

Farquhar, M. G., and J. F. Hartmann. (1957) *J. Neuropathol. Exp. Neurol.* **16:**18–39. Neuroglial structure and relationships as revealed by electron microscopy.

Fautrez, J. (1942) *Acad. Roy. Belg. Bull. Classe Sci.* **28:**391–403. La Signification de la partie céphalique du bourrelet de la plaque médullaire chez les Urodèles. Localisation des ébauches présomptives des microplacodes des nerfs crâniens it de la crête ganglionnaire de la tête au stade neurula.

Feeney, J. F., and R. L. Watterson. (1946) *J. Morphol.* **78:**231–303. The development of the vascular pattern within the walls of the central nervous system of the chick embryo.

Feit, H., G. R. Dutton, S. H. Barondes, and M. L. Shelanski. (1971) *J. Cell Biol.* **51:**138–147. Microtubule protein. Identification in and transport to nerve endings.

Feldman, J. D., and R. M. Gaze. (1972) *J. Embroyol. Exp. Morphol.* **27:**381–387. The growth of the retina in *Xenopus laevis.* II. an autoradiographic study.

Feldman, M. L., and J. M. Harrison. (1969) *J. Comp. Neurol.* **137:**267–294. The projection of the acoustic nerve to the ventral cochlear nucleus of the rat: A Golgi study.

Feldman, M. L., and A. Peters. (1973) *Anat. Rec.* **175:**318–319. The significance of barrels in the cerebral cortex.

Feremutsch, K. (1952) *Bibliotheca Psychiat. Neurol. Suppl.* **91:**33–73. Die Morphogenese des Paleocortex und des Archicortex.

Feremutsch, K. (1960) *Z. Anat. Entwicklungsgesch.* **122:**155–172. Die cytoarchitektonische Hetermorphie.

Ferguson, T. (1966) *Gen. Comp. Endocrinol.* **7:**74–79. Thyroxine effects upon the mitotic activity of the medulla oblongata after unilateral excision in embryos of the frog.

Fernandez, H. L., F. C. Huneeus, and P. F. Davison. (1970) *J. Neurobiol.* **1:**395–409. Studies on the mechanism of axoplasmic transport in the crayfish cord.

Fernandez, H. L., P. R. Burton, and F. E. Samson. (1971) *J. Cell Biol.* **53:**258–263. Axoplasmic transport in the crayfish nerve cord.

Fernandez, V. (1969) *J. Comp. Neurol.* **136:**423–452. An autoradiographic study of the development of the anterior thalamic group and limbic cortex in the rabbit.

Fernando, D. A. (1971) *Brain Res.* **27:**365–368. A third glial cell seen in retrograde degeneration of the hypoglossal nerve.

Feulgen, R., and H. Rossenbeck. (1924) *Hoppe-Seylers Z. Physiol. Chem.* **135:**203–248. Mikroskopisch-chemischer Nachweis einer Nucleinsäure vom Typus der Thymonucleinsäure und die darauf beruhrende elektive Färbung von Zellkernen in mikroskopischen Präperaten.

Fex, S., and S. Thesleff. (1967) *Life Sci.* **6:**635–639. The time required for innervation of denervated muscles by nerve implants.

Fex, S., B. Sonesson, S. Thesleff, and J. Zelená. (1966) *J. Physiol. (London)* **184:**872–882. Nerve implants in botulinum poisoned mammalian muscle.

Feynman, R. P., Leighton, R. B., and Sands, M. (1964) *The Feynman Lectures in Physics,* Vol. 2, p. 12, Addison-Wesley, Reading, Mass.

Field, E. J., D. Hughes, and C. S. Raine. (1968*a*) *J. Neurol. Sci.* **8:**49–60. Electron microscopic observations on the development of myelin in cultures of neonatal rat cerebellum.

Field, E. J., C. S. Raine, and D. Hughes. (1968*b*) *J. Neurol. Sci.* **8:**129–141. Failure to induce myelin sheath formation around artificial fibers with a note on the toxicity of polyester fibers for nervous tissue *in vitro.*

Fifková, E. (1972) *Exp. Nuerol.* **35:**458–469. Effect of visual deprivation on the retina.

Fifková, E. (1973) *Experientia* **29:**851–854. Effect of light on the synaptic organization of the inner plexiform layer of the retina in albino rats.

Filogamo, G. (1950) *Riv. Biol. Coloniale (Rome)* **42:**73–79. Conseguenze della demolizione dell-abbozzo dell' occhio sullo sviluppo del lobo ottico nell' embrione di pollo.

Filogamo, G. (1960) *Arch. Biol. (Liège),* **71:**159–198. Recherches expérimentales sur l'activité des cholinestérases spécifique et non spécifique dans le développment du lobe optique du poulet.

Filogamo, G., and G. Gabella, (1967) *Arch. Biol. (Liège)* **78:**9–60. The development of neuro-muscular correlations in vertebrates.

Fine, R. E., and D. Bray. (1971) *Nature New Biol.* **234:**115–118. Actin in growing nerve cells.

Finger, S., B. Walbran, and D. G. Stein. (1973) *Brain Res.* **63:**1–18. Brain damage and behavioral recovery: Serial lesion phenomena.

Fischbach, G. D. (1972) *Dev. Biol.* **28:**407–429. Synapse formation between dissociated nerve and muscle cells in low density cell cultures.

Fischbach, G. D., and N. Robbins. (1969) *J. Physiol. (London)* **201:**305–320. Changes in contractile properties of disused soleus muscles.

Fischer, C. A., and P. Morell. (1974) *Brain Res.* **74:**51–65. Turnover of proteins in myelin and myelin-like material of mouse brain.

Fischer, K. (1967) *Acta Neuropathol.* **8:**242–252. Subependymale Zellproliferation und Tumordisposition brachycephaler Hunderassen.

Fish, H. S., D. D. Malone, and C. P. Richter. (1944) *Anat. Rec.* **89:**429–440. The anatomy of the tongue of the domestic Norway rat. I. The skin of the tongue, the various papillae, their number and distribution.

Fish, I., and M. Winick. (1969) *Exp. Neurol.* **25:**534–540. Effect of malnutrition on regional growth of the developing rat brain.

Fisher, S., and M. Jacobson. (1970) *Z. Zellforsch. Mikrosk. Anat.* **104:**165–177. Ultrasturctural changes during early development of retinal ganglion cells in *Xenopus.*

Fite, K. V. (1969) *Exp. Neurol.* **24:**475–486. Single-unit analysis of binocular neurons in the frog optic tectum.

Fitzgerald, M. J. T. (1961) *J. Anat. (London)* **95:**495–514. Developmental changes in epidermal innervation.

Fitzgerald, M. J. T. (1962) *J. Anat. (London)* **96:**189–208. On the structure and life history of bulbous corpuscles (corpuscula nervorum terminalia bulboidea).

Flamm, J. (1968) *Z. Anat. Entwicklungsgeschichte* **127:**359–366. Über die Beziehung zwischen der Dicke motorischer Nervenfasern und der Grösse der Endplatter.

Flechsig, P. (1876) *Die Leitungsbahnen im Gehirn und Rückenmark des Menschen auf Grund entwicklungsgeschichtlicher Untersuchungen,* Engelmann, Leipzig.

Flechsig, P. (1920) *Anatomie des menschlichen Gehirns und Rückenmarks,* Georg Thieme, Leipzig.

Flechsig, P. (1927) *Meine myelogenetische Hirnlehre mit biographischer Einleitung,* Springer, Berlin.

Fleischauer, K. (1966) *Z. Zellforsch. Mikrosk. Anat.* **75:**96–108. Über die postnatale Entwicklung der subependymalen und marginalen Gliafaserschichten im Gehirn der Katze.

Fleischauer, K. (1968) *Acta Neuropathol. Suppl.* **4:**20–32. Postnatale Entwicklung der Neuroglia.

Fleming, W. W. (1974) *Fed. Proc.* **34:**1969–1970. Supersensitivity in smooth muscle.

Flickinger, R. A., M. L. Freedman, and P. J. Stambrook. (1967) *Dev. Biol.* **16:**457–473. Generation times and DNA replication patterns of cells of developing frog embryos.

Flores, F., F. Naftolin, K. J. Ryan, and R. J. White. (1973) *Science* **180:**1074–1075. Estrogen formation by the isolated perfused rhesus monkey brain.

Flower, M., and C. Grobstein. (1967) *Dev. Biol.* **15:**193–205. Interconvertibility of induced morphogenetic responses of mouse embryonic somites to notochord and ventral spinal cord.

Foelix, R. F., and R. Oppenheim. (1974) *J. Neurocytol.* **3:**277–294. The development of synapses in the cerebellar cortex of the chick embryo.

Foerster, O. (1930) *Deutsch. Z. Nervenheilk.* **115:**248–314. Klinisches: Restitution der Motilität: Restitution der Sensibilität.

Ford, D. H., and G. Cohan, (1968) *Acta Anat.* **71:**311–319. Changes in weight and volume of rat spinal cord motor neurons with increasing age.

Forel, A. (1887) *Arch. Psychiat. Nerv. Krankh.* **18**:162–198. Einige hirnanatomische Betrachtungen und Ergebnisse.

Forman, D. S., B. S. McEwen, and B. Grafstein. (1971) *Brain Res.* **28**:119–130. Rapid transport of radioactivity in goldfish optic nerve following injections of labeled glucosamine.

Forssman, J. (1898) *(Ziegler's) Beitr. Pathol. Anat. Allgem. Pathol.* **24**:56–100. Ueber die Ursachen, welche die Wachstumsrichtung der peripheren Nervenfasern bei der Regeneration bestimmen.

Forssman, J., (1900) *(Ziegler's) Beitr. Pathol. Anat. Allgem. Pathol.* **27**:407–430. Zur Kenntnis des Neurotropismus.

Forströnen, P. F. (1963) *Acta Neurol. Scand.* **39**:314–316. The origin and the morphogenetic significance of the external granular layer of the cerebellum as determined experimentally in chick embryos.

Fouvet, P. B. (1973) *Arch. Anat. Microsc. Morphol. Exp.* **62**:269–280. Innervation et morphogenèse de la patte chez l'embryon de poulet. I. Mise en place de l'innervation normale.

Fox, C. A., D. E. Hillman, K. A. Siegesmund, and C. R. Dutta. (1967) *Progr. Brain Res.* **25**:174–225. The primate cerebellar cortex: A Golgi and electron microscopy study.

Fox, G. Q., G. D. Pappas, and D. P. Purpura. (1976) *Brain Res.* **101**:411–425. Fine structure of growth cones in medullary raphe nuclei in the postnatal cat.

Fox, H. (1973) *J. Embryol. Exp. Morphol.* **30**:377–396. Degeneration of the nerve cord in the tail of *Rana temporaria* during metamorphic climax: Study by electron microscopy.

Fox, H., and J. M. Moulton. (1968) *Arch. Anat. Microsc. Morphol. Exp.* **57**:107–120. Mauthner cells and the thyroid hormonal level in larvae of *Rana temporaria.*

Fox, J. H., M. A. Fishman, P. R. Dodge, and A. L. Prensky. (1972) *Neurology* **22**:1213–1216. The effect of malnutrition on human central nervous system myelin.

Fox, M. W., O. R. Inman, and W. A. Himwich. (1966) *J. Comp. Neurol.* **127**:199–206. The postnatal development of neocortical neurons in the dog.

Fox, M. W., O. Inman, and S. Glisson. (1968) *Dev. Psychobiol.* **1**:48–54. Age differences in central nervous effects of visual deprivation in the dog.

Francis-Williams, J., and P. A. Davies. (1974) *Dev. Med. Child Neurol.* **16**:709–728. Very low birthweight and later intelligence.

Frank, E., and J. K. S. Jansen. (1976) *J. Neurophysiol.* **39**:84–90. Interaction between foreign and original nerves innervating gill muscles in fish.

Frank, E., J. K. S. Jansen, T. Lömo, and R. Westgaard. (1974) *Nature* **247**:375–376. Maintained function of foreign synapses on hyperinnervated skeletal muscle fibres of the rat.

Frank, E., J. K. S. Jansen, T. Lömo, and R. H. Westgaard. (1975) *J. Physiol. (London)* **247**:725–743. The interaction between foreign and original motor nerves innervating the soleus muscle of rats.

Franson, P., and C. Hildebrand. (1975) *Neurobiology* **5**:8–22. Postnatal growth of nerve fibres in the pyramidal tract of the rabbit.

Frazier, W. A., R. A. Angeletti, and R. A. Bradshaw. (1972) *Science* **176**:482–488. Nerve growth factor and insulin.

Frazier, W. A., L. F. Boyd, and R. A. Bradshaw. (1973*a*) *Proc. Natl. Acad. Sci. U.S.A.* **70**:2931–2935. Interaction of nerve growth factor with surface membranes: Biological competence of insolubilized nerve growth factor.

Frazier, W. A., C. E. Ohlendorf, L. F. Boyd, L. Aloe, E. M. Johnson, J. A. Ferrendelli, and R. A. Bradshaw. (1973*b*) *Proc. Natl. Acad. Sci. U.S.A.* **70**:2448–2452. Mechanism of action of nerve growth factor and cyclic AMP on neurite outgrowth in embryonic chick sensory ganglia: Demonstration of independent pathways of stimulation.

Freeman, J. A., and J. Stone, (1969) A technique for current density analysis of field potentials and its application to the frog cerebellum, pp. 421–430. In *Neurobiology of Cerebellar Evolution and Development* (R. R. Llinás, ed.), American Medical Association, Chicago.

Freeman, R. D., and L. N. Thibos. (1973) *Science* **180**:876–878. Electrophysiological evidence that abnormal early visual experience can modify the human brain.

Freeman, R. D., D. E. Mitchell, and M. Millodot. (1972) *Science* **175**:1384–1386. A neural effect of partial visual deprivation in humans.

Freeman, S. S., A. G. Engel, and D. B. Drachman. (1976) *Ann. N.Y. Acad. Sci.* **274**:46–59. Experimental acetylcholine blockade of the neuromuscular junction: Effects on end-plate and muscle fiber ultrastructure.

Frick, H., and H.-J. Nord. (1963) *Anat. Anz.* **113**:307–316. Domestikation und Hirngewicht.

Friede, R. L. (1954) *Acta Anat.* **20**:290–296. Der quantitative Anteil der Glia an der Cortexentwicklung.

Friede, R. L. (1961) *J. Neurochem.* **8:**17–30. A histochemical study of DPN-diaphorase in human white matter, with some notes on myelination.

Friede, R. L. (1963) *Proc. Natl. Acad. Sci. U.S.A.* **49:**187–193. The relationship of body size, nerve cell size, axon length and glial density in the cerebellum.

Friede, R. L. (1966) *Topographic Brain Chemistry,* Academic Press, New York.

Friede, R. L. (1972) *J. Comp. Neurol.* **144:**233–252. Control of myelin formation by axon caliber (with a model of the control mechanism).

Friede, R. L. (1973*a*) *Z. Neurol.* **204:**243–254. Principles of quantitative organization of peripheral nerve fibers and their relation to growth and pathologic changes.

Friede, R. L. (1973) *Prog. Brain Res.* **40:**425–436. Mechanics of myelin sheath expansion.

Friede, R. L., and K.-C. Ho. (1977) *J. Physiol. (London)* **265:**507–519. The relation of axonal transport of mitochondria with microtubules and other axoplasmic organelles.

Friede, R. L., and T. Samorajski. (1968) *J. Neuropath. Exp. Neurol.* **27:**546–570. Myelin formation in the sciatic nerve of the rat: A quantitative electron microscopic, histochemical and radioautographic study.

Friede, R. L., and T. Samorajski. (1970) *Anat. Rec.* **167:**379–388. Axon caliber related to neurofilaments and microtubules in sciatic nerve fibers of rats and mice.

Friede, R. L., and W. H. van Houten. (1962) *Proc. Natl. Acad. Sci. U.S.A.* **48:**817–821. Neuron extension and glial supply: functional significance of glia.

Friedrich, V. L. Jr. (1975) *Anat. Embryol.* **147:**259–271. Hyperplasia of oligodendrocytes in quaking mice.

Frisch, R. E. (1971) *Psychiat. Neurol. Neurochir.* **74:**463–479. Does malnutrition cause permanent mental retardation in human beings?

Fry, F. J., and W. M. Cowan. (1972) *J. Comp. Neurol.* **144:**1–24. A study of retrograde cell degeneration in the lateral mammillary nucleus of the cat, with special reference to the role of axonal branching in the preservation of the cell.

Fujisawa, H. (1971) *Dev. Growth Differ.* **13:**25–36. A complete reconstruction of the neural retina of chick embryo grafted onto the chorio-allantoic membrane.

Fujisawa, H., H. Nakamura, and M. Chin. (1974) *J. Embryol. Exp. Morphol.* **31:**139–149. The fine structure of the reconstructed neural retina of chick embryos.

Fujita, H., and S. Fujita. (1963) *Z. Zellforsch. Mikrosk. Anat.* **60:**463–478. Electron microscopic studies on neuroblast differentiation in the central nervous system of domestic fowl.

Fujita, H., and S. Fujita. (1964) *Z. Zellforsch. Mikrosk. Anat.* **64:**262–272. Electron microscopic studies on the differentiation of the ependymal cells and the glioblast in the spinal cord of domestic fowl.

Fujita, S. (1962) *Exp. Cell Res.* **28:**52–60. Kinetics of cell proliferation.

Fujita, S. (1963) *J. Comp. Neurol.* **120:**37–42. The matrix cell and cytogenesis in the developing central nervous system.

Fujita, S. (1964) *J. Comp. Neurol.* **122:**311–328. Analysis of neuron differentiation in the central nervous system by tritiated thymidine autoradiography.

Fujita, S. (1965*a*) *Laval Med.* **36:**125–130. The matrix cell and histogenesis of the nervous system.

Fujita, S. (1965*b*) *J. Comp. Neurol.* **124:**51–60. An autoradiographic study on the origin and fate of the subpial glioblasts in the embryonic chick spinal cord.

Fujita, S. (1966) Application of light and electron microscopic autoradiography to the study of cytogenesis of the forebrain, pp. 180–196. In *Evolution of the Forebrain* (R. Hassler and H. Stephan, eds.), Plenum, New York.

Fujita, S. (1967) *J. Cell Biol.* **32:**277–287. Quantitative analysis of cell proliferation and differentiation in the cortex of the postnatal mouse cerebellum.

Fujita, S. (1974) *J. Comp. Neurol.* **155:**195–202. DNA constancy in neurons of the human cerebellum and spinal cord as revealed by Feulgen cytophotometry.

Fujita, S., and M. Horii. (1963) *Arch Histol. (Japan)* **23:**359–366. Analysis of cytogenesis in chick retina by tritiated thymidine autoradiography.

Fujita, S., and T. Kitamura. (1975) *Acta Neuropathol. (Suppl.) (Berl.)* **6:**291–296. Origin of brain macrophages and the nature of the so-called microglia.

Fujita, S., M. Shimada, and T. Nakamura. (1966) *J. Comp. Neurol.* **128:**191–208. ^{3}H-Thymidine autoradiographic studies on the cell proliferation and differentiation in the external and internal granular layers of the mouse cerebellum.

Fujita, S., S. Yoshida, and M. Fukuda. (1971) *Acta Histochem. Cytochem.* **4:**126–136. Improvement of technique to minimize non-specific absorption in microspectrophotometric measurement of nuclear DNA.

Fujita, S., M. Fukuda, T. Kitamura, and S. Yoshida. (1972) *Acta Histochem. Cytochem.* **5**:146–152. Two-wavelength-scanning method in Feulgen cytophotometry.

Fujita, S., T. Hattori, M. Fukuda, and T. Kitamura. (1974) *Dev. Growth Differ.* **16**:205–211. DNA contents in Purkinje cells and inner granule neurons in the developing rat cerebellum.

Fukuda, Y., and J. Stone. (1974) *J. Neurophysiol.* **37**:749–772. Retinal distribution and central projections of Y-, X-, and W-cells of the cat's retina.

Furmanski, P., D. L. Silverman, and M. Lubin. (1971) *Nature New Biol.* **233**:413–415. Expression of differentiated functions in mouse neuroblastoma mediated by dibutyryl cyclic monophosphate.

Gabella, G. (1969) *J. Neurol. Sci.* **9**:237–242. Taste buds and adrenergic fibres.

Gallera, J. (1967) *Experientia* **23**:461. L'induction neurogene chez les oiseaux passage du flux inducteur par le filtre millipore.

Gallera, J., G. Nicolet, and M. Baumann. (1968) *J. Embryol. Exp. Morph.* **19**:439–450. Induction neurale chez les oiseaux à travers un filtre millipore: Étude au microscope optique et électronique.

Garber, B. B., and A. A. Moscona. (1972*a*) *Dev. Biol.* **27**:217–234. Reconstruction of brain tissue from cell suspensions. I. Aggregation patterns of cells dissociated from different regions of the developing brain.

Garber, B. B., and A. A. Moscona. (1972*b*) *Dev. Biol.* **27**:235–243. Reconstruction of brain tissue from cell suspensions. II. Specific enhancement of aggregation of embryonic cerebral cells by supernatant from homologous cell cultures.

García-Bellído, A. (1975) Genetic control of wing disc development in *Drosophila,* pp. 161–178. In *Cell Patterning,* Ciba Foundation Symposium 29, Elsevier, New York.

García-Bellído, A., P. Ripoll, and G. Morata. (1973) *Nature New Biol.* **245**:251–253. Developmental compartmentalisation of the wing disk of *Drosophila.*

Garland, D., and D. Teller. (1973) *J. Cell Biol.* **59**:107a. Mechanism of colchicine binding.

Gaskell, G. H. (1889) *J. Physiol. (London)* **10**:153–211. On the relation between the structure, function, distribution and origin of the cranial nerves; together with a theory of the origin of the nervous system.

Gasser, H. S. (1958) Comparison of the structure, as revealed with the electron microscope, and the physiology of the unmedullated fibers in the skin nerves and in the olfactory nerves, pp. 3–17. In *The Submicroscopic Organization and Function of Nerve Cells* (H. Fernandez-Moran, ed.), Academic Press, New York.

Gause, G. (1932) *Quart. Rev. Biol.* **7**:27–46. Ecology of populations.

Gause, G. (1934) *The Struggle for Existence,* Williams and Wilkins, Baltimore (Reprinted, 1971, Dover, New York.)

Gaze, R. M. (1959) *Quart. J. Exp. Physiol.* **44**:209–308. Regeneration of the optic nerve in *Xenopus laevis.*

Gaze, R. M. (1960) *Int. Rev. Neurobiol.* **2**:1–40. Regeneration of the optic nerve in Amphibia.

Gaze, R. M. (1970) *Formation of Nerve Connections,* Academic Press, New York.

Gaze, R. M., and M. Jacobson. (1962) *Quart. J. Exp. Physiol.* **47**:273–280. The projection of the binocular visual field on the optic tecta of the frog.

Gaze, R. M., and M. Jacobson. (1963*a*) *Proc. Roy. Soc. (London) Ser. B* **157**:420–448. A study of the retino-tectal projection during regeneration of the optic nerve in the frog.

Gaze, R. M., and M. Jacobson. (1963*b*) *J. Physiol. (London)* **165**:73–74P. The path from the retina to the ipsilateral optic tectum of the frog.

Gaze, R. M., and M. J. Keating. (1969) *J. Physiol. (London)* **200**:128–129P. The depth distribution of visual units in the tectum of the frog following regeneration of the optic nerve.

Gaze, R. M., and M. J. Keating. (1972) *Nature* **237**:375–378. The visual system and "neuronal specificity."

Gaze, R. M., and A. Peters. (1961) *Quart. J. Exp. Physiol.* **46**:299–309. The development, structure and composition of the optic nerve of *Xenopus laevis* (Daudin).

Gaze, R. M., and S. C. Sharma. (1970) *Exp. Brain Res.* **10**:171–181. Axial differences in the reinnervation of the goldfish optic tectum by regenerating optic nerve fibres.

Gaze, R. M., M. Jacobson, and G. Székely. (1963) *J. Physiol. (London)* **165**:484–499. The retinotectal projection in *Xenopus* with compound eyes.

Gaze, R. M., M. Jacobson, and G. Székely. (1965) *J. Physiol. (London)* **176**:409–417. On the formation of connections by compound eyes in *Xenopus.*

Gaze, R. M., M. J. Keating, and K. Straznicky. (1970*a*) *J. Physiol. (London)* **207**:51P. The re-establishment of retinotectal projections after uncrossing the optic chiasma in *Xenopus laevis* with one compound eye.

Gaze, R. M., M. J. Keating, G. Székely, and L. Beazley. (1970*b*) *Proc. Roy. Soc. (London) Ser. B* **175:**107–147. Binocular interaction in the formation of specific intertectal neuronal connexions.

Gaze, R. M., S. H. Chung, and M. J. Keating. (1972) *Nature New Biol.* **236:**133–135. Development of the retinotectal projection in *Xenopus.*

Gaze, R. M., M. J. Keating, and S. H. Chung. (1974) *Proc. Roy. Soc. London (Biol.)* **185:**301–330. The evolution of the retinotectal map during development in *Xenopus.*

Gebhardt, D. O. E., and P. D. Nieuwkoop. (1963) *J. Embryol. Exp. Morphol.* **12:**317–331. The influence of lithium on the competence of the ectoderm in *Ambystoma mexicanum.*

Geel, S., and P. S. Timiras. (1967) *Brain Res.* **4:**135–142. The influence of neonatal hypothyroidism and of thyroxine on the ribonucleic acid and deoxyribonucleic acid concentrations of rat cerebral cortex.

Geel, S. E., and P. S. Timiras. (1970) *Brain Res.* **22:**63–72. Influence of growth hormone on cerebral cortical RNA metabolism in immature hypothyroid rats.

Geffen, L. B. (1969) *J. Neurochem.* **16:**469–474. Is there bidirectional transport of noradrenaline in sympathetic nerves?

Geist, F. D. (1933) *Arch. Neurol. Psychiat. (Chicago)* **29:**88–103. Chromatolysis of efferent neurons.

Gentschev, T., and C. Sotelo. (1973) *Brain Res.* **62:**37–60. Degenerative patterns in the ventral cochlear nucleus of the rat after primary deafferentation: An ultrastructural study.

George, S. A., and W. B. Marks. (1974) *Exp. Neurol.* **42:**467–482. Optic nerve terminal arborizations in the frog: Shape and orientation inferred from electrophysiological measurements.

Geren, B. B. (1954) *Exp. Cell Res.* **7:**558–562. The formation from the Schwann cell surface of myelin in the peripheral nerves of chick embryos.

Geren, B. B., and J. Raskind. (1953) *Proc. Natl. Acad. Sci. U.S.A.* **39:**880–884. Development of the fine structure of the myelin sheath in sciatic nerves of chick embryos.

Gerisch, G., D. Hülser, D. Malchow, and U. Wick. (1975) *Phil. Trans. Roy. Soc. London Ser. B* **272:**181–192. Cell communication by periodic cyclic-AMP pulses.

Geschwind, N. (1970) *Science* **170:**940–944. The organization of language and the brain.

Geschwind, N. (1972) *Sci. Am.* **226:**76–83. Language and the brain.

Geschwind, N., and W. Levitsky. (1968) *Science* **161:**186–187. Human brain: Left–right asymmetries in temporal speach region.

Giacobini, G., G. Filogamo, M. Weber, P. Bouquet, and J. P. Changeux. (1973) *Proc. Natl. Acad. Sci. U.S.A.* **70:**1708–1712. Effects of a snake α-neurotoxin on the development of innervated skeletal muscles in chick embryo.

Gierer, A., and H. Meinhardt. (1972) *Kybernetik* **12:**30–39. A theory of biological pattern formation.

Gillette, R. (1944) *J. Exp. Zool.* **96:**201–222. Cell number and cell size in the ectoderm during neurulation.

Gilliatt, R. W. (1961) *Proc. Soc. Med.* **54:**324–326. Sensory nerve conduction in man.

Gilmore, S. A. (1971) *Anat. Rec.* **171:**283–292. Neuroglial population in the spinal white matter of neonatal and early postnatal rats: An autoradiographic study on numbers of neuroglia and changes in their proliferative activity.

Gitlin, D., J. Kumate, and C. Morales. (1965) *J. Clin. Endocrinol.* **25:**1599–1608. Metabolism and maternofetal transfer of human growth hormone in the pregnant woman at term.

Giuditta, A., M. Libonati, A. Packard, and N. Prozzo. (1971) *Brain. Res.* **25:**55–62. Nuclear counts in the brain lobes of *Octopus vulgaris* as a function of body size.

Globus, A., and A. B. Scheibel. (1966) *Nature* **212:**463–465. Loss of dendrite spines as an index of presynaptic terminal patterns.

Globus, A., and A. B. Scheibel. (1967*a*) *Exp. Neurol.* **18:**116–131. Synaptic loci on visual cortical neurons of rabbit: Specific afferent radiation.

Globus, A., and A. B. Scheibel. (1967*b*) *Exp. Neurol.* **19:**331–345. The effect of visual deprivation on cortical neurons: A Golgi study.

Globus, A., and A. B. Scheibel. (1967*c*) *J. Comp. Neurol.* **131:**155–172. Pattern and field in cortical structure: The rabbit.

Globus, A., and A. B. Scheibel. (1967*d*) *Science* **156:**1127–1129. Synaptic loci on parietal cortical neurons: Terminations of corpus callosum fibers.

Globus, J. H., and H. Kuhlenbeck. (1944) *J. Neuropathol. Exp. Neurol.* **3:**1–35. The subependymal cell plate (matrix) and its relationship to brain tumors of the ependymal type.

Glücksmann, A. (1940) *Br. J. Ophthalmol.* **24:**153–178. Development and differentiation of the tadpole eye.

Glücksmann, A. (1951) *Biol. Rev.* **26:**59–86. Cell deaths in normal vertebrate ontogeny.

Glücksmann, A. (1965) *Arch. Biol. (Liège)* **76:**419–437. Cell death in normal development.

Gmitro, J. I., and L. E. Scriven. (1966) A physicochemical basis for pattern and rhythm, pp. 221. In *Intracellular Transport,* Academic Press, New York.

Goerke, H. (1973) *Linnaeus,* Scribners, New York.

Goerttler, K. (1925) *Arch. Entw.-Mech. Organ.* **106:**503–541. Die Formbildung der Medullaranlage bei Urodelen.

Goetsch, W. (1957) *The Ants,* University of Michigan Press, Ann Arbor, Mich.

Goldberg, S. (1974) *Dev. Biol.* **36:**24–43. Studies on the mechanics of development of the visual pathways in the chick embryo.

Goldberg, S. (1976*a*) *Dev. Biol.* **53:**126–127. Progressive fixation of morphological polarity in the developing retina.

Goldberg, S. (1976*b*) *J. Comp. Neurol.* **168:**379–392. Polarization of the avian retina: Ocular transplantation studies.

Goldberg, S., and A. J. Coulombre. (1972) *J. Comp. Neurol.* **146:**507–518. Topographical development of the ganglion cell fiber layer in the chick retina: A whole mount study.

Goldberg, S., and M. Kotani. (1967) *Anat. Rec.* **158:**325–331. The projection of optic nerve fibers in the frog *Rana catesbiana* as studied by radioautography.

Goldman, P. S. (1974) An alternative to developmental plasticity: Heterology of CNS structures in infants and adults, pp. 149–174. In *Plasticity and Recovery of Function in the Central Nervous System* (D. G. Stein, J. J. Rosen, and N. Butters, eds.), Academic Press, New York.

Goldstein, J. L., and J. D. Wilson. (1975) *J. Cell. Physiol.* **85:**365–378. Genetic and hormonal control of male sexual differentiation.

Goldstein, M. N., and J. A. Burdman. (1965) *Anat. Rec.* **151:**199–208. Studies of the nerve growth factor in submandibular glands of female mice treated with testosterone.

Golgi, C. (1886) Sulla fina anatomia degli organi centrali del sistema nervosa, Pavia.

Goll, W. (1967) *Z. Morphol. Oekol Tiere* **59:**143–210. Strukturuntersuchungen am Gehirn von *Formica.*

Golosow, N., and C. Grobstein. (1962) *Dev. Biol.* **4:**242–255. Epitheliomesenchymal interaction between embryonic mouse tissues separated by a transmembrane filter.

Gombos, G., W. Filipowicz, and G. Vincendon. (1971) *Brain Res.* **26:**475–479. Fast and slow components of S-100 protein fraction: Regional distribution in bovine central nervous system.

Gomez, C. J., N. E. Ghittoni, and J. M. Dellacha. (1966) *Life Sci.* **5:**243–246. Effects of L-thyroxine or somatotrophin on body growth and cerebral development in neonatally thyroidectomized rats.

Gona, A. G. (1972) *J. Comp. Neurol.* **146:**133–142. Morphogenesis of the cerebellum of the frog tadpole during spontaneous metamorphosis.

Gona, A. G. (1973) *Exp. Neurol.* **38:**494–501. Effects of thyroxine, thyrotropin, prolactin, and growth hormone on the maturation of the frog cerebellum.

Gona, A. G. (1975) *Brain Res.* **95:**132–136. Golgi studies of cerebellar maturation in frog tadpoles.

Gona, A. G. (1976) *J. Comp. Neurol.* **165:**77–88. Autoradiographic studies of cerebellar histogenesis in the bullfrog tadpole during metamorphosis: The external granular layer.

Gonatas, N. K., and E. Robbins. (1965) *Protoplasma* **59:**377–391. The homology of spindle tubules and neuro-tubules in the chick embryo retina.

Goodman, C. (1974) *J. Comp. Physiol.* **95:**185–201. Anatomy of locust ocellar interneurons: Constancy and variability.

Goodman, D. C., and J. A. Horel. (1966) *J. Comp. Neurol.* **127:**71–88. Sprouting of optic tract projections in the brain stem of the rat.

Goodman, D. C., R. S. Bogdasarian, and J. A. Horel. (1973) *Brain Behav. Evol.* **8:**27–50. Axonal sprouting of ipsilateral optic tract following opposite eye removal.

Goodwin, B. C., and M. H. Cohen. (1969) *J. Theor. Biol.* **25:**49–107. A phase-shift model for the spatial and temporal organization of developing systems.

Goosen, H. (1949) *Zool. Jahrb. Abt. Allgem. Zool. Physiol. Tiere* **62:**1–64. Untersuchungen an Gehirnen verschieden grosser, jeweils verwandter Coleopteren-und Hymenopterenarten.

Gorski, R. A. (1966) *J. Reprod. Fertil. Suppl.* **1:**67–88. Localization and sexual differentiation of the nervous structures which regulate ovulation.

Gottlieb, D. I., and W. M. Cowan. (1972) *Brain Res.* **41:**452–456. Evidence for a temporal factor in the occupation of available synaptic sites during development of the dentate gyrus.

Gottlieb, D. I., and W. M. Cowan. (1973) *J. Comp. Neurol.* **149:**393–422. Autoradiographic studies of the commissural and ipsilateral associational connections of the hippocampus and dentate gyrus of the rat. I. The commissural connections.

Gottlieb, D. I., K. Rock, and L. Glaser. (1976) *Proc. Natl. Acad. Sci. U.S.A.* **73:**410–414. A gradient of adhesive specificity in developing avian retina.

Gottlieb, G. (1973) Introduction to behavioral embryology, pp. 3–45. In *Studies on the Development of Behavior and the Nervous System: Behavioral Embryology,* Vol. 1 (G. Gottlieb, ed.), Academic Press, New York.

Gottlieb, G. (1976) The roles of experience in the development of behavior and the nervous system, pp. 25–54. In *Neural and Behavioral Specificity* (G. Gottlieb, ed.), Academic Press, New York.

Gouin, F. J. (1965) *Fortschr. Zool.* **17:**189–237. Morphologie, Histologie und Entwicklungsgeschichte der Myriapoden und Insekten. III. Das Nervensystem und die neurocrinen Systeme.

Gould, S. J. (1966) *Biol. Rev.* **41:**587–640. Allometry and size in ontogeny and phylogeny.

Gourden, J., J. Clos, C. Coste, J. Dainat, and J. Legrand. (1973) *J. Neurochem.* **21:**861–871. Comparative effects of hypothyroidism, hyperthyroidism and undernutrition on the protein and nucleic acid contents of the cerebellum in the young rat.

Grady, K. L., C. H. Phoenix, and W. C. Young. (1965) *J. Comp. Physiol. Psychol.* **59:**176–182. Role of the developing rat testes in differentiation of the neural tissues mediating mating behavior.

Grafstein, B. (1975) Axonal transport: The intracellular traffic of the neuron. In *Handbook of the Nervous System,* Vol. 1: *Cellular Biology of Neurones* (E. R. Kandel, ed.), American Physiological Society, Washington, D.C.

Grafstein, B., and R. Laureno. (1973) *Exp. Neurol.* **39:**44–57. Transport of radioactivity from eye to visual cortex in the mouse.

Graham, C. F., and R. W. Morgan. (1966) *Dev. Biol.* **14:**439–460. Changes in the cell cycle during early amphibian development.

Graham, G. (1964) Diet and bodily constitution, p. 11. In *Ciba Foundation Study Group No. 17,* Churchill, London.

Graham, R. C., and M. J. Karnovsky. (1966) *J. Histochem. Cytochem.* **14:**271–302. The early stages of absorption of injected horseradish peroxidase in the proximal tubules of mouse kidney: Ultrastructural cytochemistry by a new technique.

Grampp, W., and J.-E. Edström. (1963) *J. Neurochem.* **10:**725–732. The effect of nervous activity on ribonucleic acid of the crustacean stretch receptor neuron.

Grampp, W. J., J. B. Harris and S. Thesleff. (1972) *J. Physiol. London* **221:**743–748. Inhibition of denervation changes in skeletal muscle by blockers of protein synthesis.

Granick, S., and A. Gibor. (1967) *Prog. Nucl. Acid. Res. Mol. Biol.* **6:**143–168. The DNA of chloroplasts, mitochondria, and centrioles.

Granit, R., H. D. Henatsch, and G. Steg. (1956) *Acta Physiol. Scand.* **37:**114–126. Tonic and phasic ventral horn cells differentiated by post-tetanic potentiation in cat extensors.

Grant, G. (1965) *Experientia* **21:**1–4. Degenerative changes in dendrites following axonal transection.

Grant, G. (1970) Neuronal changes central to the site of axon transection: A method for the identification of regrograde changes in perikarya, dendrites and axons by silver impregnation, pp. 173–185. In *Contemporary Research Methods in Neuroanatomy* (W. J. H. Nauta and S. O. E. Ebbesson, eds.), Springer-Verlag, Berlin.

Grant, G., and J. Westman. (1968) *Experientia* **24:**169–170. Degenerative changes in dendrites central to axonal transection: Electron microscopical observations.

Grasso, A., and R. Pirazzi. (1975) *Brain Res.* **90:**324–328. Changes in the concentration of the brain specific protein 14-3-2, during the development of the superior cervical ganglion of the rat and effects of surgical decentralization.

Gray, E. G., and R. W. Guillery. (1961) *J. Physiol. (London)* **157:**581–588. The basis for silver staining of synapses of the mammalian spinal cord: A light and electron microscope study.

Gray, E. G., and R. W. Guillery. (1966) *Int. Rev. Cytol.* **19:**111–182. Synaptic morphology in the normal and degenerating nervous system.

Gray, J. (1950) The role of peripheral sense organs during locomotion in the vertebrates, pp. 112–126. In *Physiological Mechanisms in Animal Behaviour* (J. F. Danielli and J. Brown, eds.), Cambridge University Press, Cambridge.

Graybiel, A. M. (1976) *Brain Res.* **114:**318–327. Evidence for banding of the cat's ipsilateral retinotectal connection.

Graziadei, P. P. C. (1973) *Tissue Cell* **5:**113–131. Cell dynamics in the olfactory mucosa.

Graziadei, P. P. C. (1974) The olfactory organ of vertebrates: A survey, pp. 191–222. In *Essays on the Nervous System* (R. Bellairs and E. G. Gray, eds.), Clarendon, Oxford.

Graziadei, P. P. C., and R. S. DeHan. (1973) *J. Cell Biol.* **59:**525–530. Neuronal regeneration in frog olfactory system.

Graziadei, P. P. C., and G. A. Monti Graziadei. (1978) Continuous nerve cell renewal in the olfactory system. In *Handbook of Sensory Physiology*, Vol. IX: *Development of Sensory Systems* (M. Jacobson, ed.), Springer-Verlag, New York.

Greene, L. A., S. Varon, A. Piltch, and E. M. Shooter. (1971) *Neurobiology* **1**:37–48. Substructure of the β subunit of mouse 7S nerve growth factor.

Greene, W. F. (1947) *Anat. Rec.* **97**:389. Histogenesis of Mauthner's neurone in *Amblystoma.*

Greenough, W. T., and F. R. Volkmar. (1973) *Exp. Neurol.* **40**:491–504. Pattern of dendritic branching in occipital cortex of rats reared in complex environments.

Greenough, W. T., F. R. Volkmar, and J. M. Juraska. (1973) *Exp. Neurol.* **41**:371–378. Effects of rearing complexity on dendritic branching in frontolateral and temporal cortex of the rat.

Gregory, K. M., and M. C. Diamond. (1968*a*) *Exp. Neurol.* **20**:394–414. The effects of early hypophysectomy on brain morphogenesis in the rat.

Gregory, K. M., and M. C. Diamond. (1968*b*) *Exp. Neurol.* **21**:502–511. Acetylcholinesterase and cholinesterase activities, protein content and wet weight measures in the rat brain after early hypophysectomy.

Gregson, N. A., and J. M. Oxberry. (1972) *J. Neurochem.* **19**:1065–1071. The composition of myelin from the mutant mouse "Quaking."

Grenell, R., and R. Scammon. (1943) *J. Comp. Neurol.* **79**:329–354. An iconometrographic representation of the growth of the central nervous system in man.

Griglatti, T., D. T. Suzuki, and R. Williamson. (1972) *Dev. Biol.* **28**:352–371. Temperature-sensitive mutations in Drosophila. X. Developmental analysis of the paralytic mutation $para^{ts}$.

Grillner, S., and P. Zangger. (1974) *Acta Physiol. Scand.* **91**:38A. Locomotor movements generated by the deafferented spinal cord.

Grillo, M. A., and S. L. Palay. (1963) *J. Cell Biol.* **16**:430–436. Ciliated Schwann cells in the autonomic nervous system of the adult rat.

Grimes, G. J., and F. S. Barnes. (1973) *Exp. Cell Res.* **79**:375–385. A technique for studying chemotaxis of leucocytes in well-defined chemotactic fields.

Grimm, L. M. (1971) *J. Exp. Zool.* **178**:479–496. An evaluation of myotypic respecification in axolotls.

Grobstein, C. (1953) *Nature* **172**:869–871. Morphogenetic interaction between embryonic mouse tissues separated by a transmembrane filter.

Grobstein, C. (1957) *Exp. Cell Res.* **13**:575–587. Some transmission characteristics of the tubule inducing influence on mouse metanephrogenic mesenchyme.

Grobstein, C. (1959) *J. Exp. Zool.* **142**:203–213. Autoradiography of the interzone between tissues in inductive interaction.

Grobstein, C. (1967) *Natl. Cancer Inst. Monogr.* **26**:279–299. Mechanisms of organogenetic tissue interaction.

Grobstein, P., and K. L. Chow. (1975) *Science* **190**:352–358. Receptive field development and individual experience.

Grobstein, P., and K. L. Chow. (1976) Receptive field organization in the mammalian visual cortex: The role of individual experience in development, pp. 155–193. In *Studies on the Development of Behavior and the Nervous System.* Vol. 3 (G. Gottlieb, ed.), Academic Press, New York.

Grobstein, P., and C. Comer. (1976) *Neurosci. Abstr.* **2**:278. Differences in development of adult relative eye position in *Xenopus* and *Rana.*

Grobstein, P., K. L. Chow, P. D. Spear, and L. H. Mathers. (1973) *Science* **180**:1185–1187. Development of rabbit visual cortex: Late appearance of a class of receptive fields.

Grobstein, P., K. L. Chow, and P. C. Fox. (1975) *Proc. Natl. Acad. Sci. U.S.A.* **72**:1543–1545. Development of receptive fields in rabbit visual cortex: Changes in the course due to delayed eye-opening.

Grouse, L., M. D. Chilton, and B. J. McCarthy. (1972) *Biochemistry* **11**:798–805. Hybridization of ribonucleic acid with unique sequences of mouse deoxyribonucleic acid.

Gruner, J. E., and J. P. Zahnd. (1967) Sur la maturation synaptique dans le cortex visuel du lapin, pp. 125–133. In *Regional Development of the Brain in Early Life* (A. Minkowski, ed.), Blackwell, Oxford.

Grüsser, O. J., and U. Grüsser-Cornehls. (1968) *Z. Vergl. Physiol.* **59**:1–24. Neurophysiologische Grundlagen visueller angeborener Auslosemechanismen beim Frosch.

Grüsser, O.-J., and U. Grüsser-Cornehls. (1973) Neuronal mechanisms of visual movement preception and some psychophysical and behavioral correlations, pp. 333–429. In *Handbook of Sensory Physiology*, Vol. VII (H. Autrum, R. Jung, W. R. Loewenstein, D. M. MacKay, and H. L. Teuber, eds.), Springer-Verlag, Berlin.

Gudden, B. A. von (1869) *Arch. Psychiat.* **2**:693–723. Experimentaluntersuchungen über das periphere und centrale Nervensystem.

Guillery, R. W. (1965) *Prog. Brain Res.* **14:**57–76. Some electron microscopical observations of degenerative changes in central nervous synapses.

Guillery, R. W. (1969) *Brain Res.* **14:**739–741. An abnormal retinogeniculate projection in Siamese cats.

Guillery, R. W. (1970) Light- and electron-microscopical studies of normal and degenerating axons, pp. 77–105. In *Contemporary Research Methods in Neuroanatomy* (W. J. H. Nauta and S. O. E. Ebbesson, eds.), Springer-Verlag, New York.

Guillery, R. W. (1972*a*) *J. Comp. Neurol.* **144:**117–130. Binocular competition in the control of geniculate cell growth.

Guillery, R. W. (1972*b*) *J. Comp. Neurol.* **146:**407–420. Experiments to determine whether retinogeniculate axons can form translaminar collateral sprouts in the dorsal lateral geniculate nucleus of the cat.

Guillery, R. W. (1973*a*) *J. Comp. Neurol.* **148:**417–422. The effect of lid suture upon the growth of cells in the dorsal lateral geniculate nucleus of kittens.

Guillery, R. W. (1973*b*) *J. Comp. Neurol.* **149:**423–438. Quantitative studies of transneuronal atrophy in the dorsal lateral geniculate nucleus of cats and kittens.

Guillery, R. W. (1974) *Sci. Am.* **230(5):**44–54. Visual pathways in albinos.

Guillery, R. W., and V. A. Casagrande. (1975*a*) *Cold Spring Harbor Symp. Quant. Biol.* **15:**611–617. Adaptive synaptic connections formed in the visual pathways in response to congenitally aberrant inputs.

Guillery, R. W., and V. A. Casagrande. (1975*b*) *Anat. Rec.* **181:**366. On restoring visual functions to the temporal retina of Siamese cats.

Guillery, R. W., and J. H. Kaas. (1971) *J. Comp. Neurol.* **143:**73–100. A study of normal and congenitally abnormal retinogeniculate projections in cats.

Guillery, R. W. and D. J. Stelzner. (1970) *J. Comp. Neurol.* **139:**413–422. The differential effects of unilateral lid closure upon the monocular and binocular segments of the dorsal lateral geniculate nucleus in the cat.

Guillery, R. W., and G. L. Scott, B. M. Cattanach, and M. S. Deol. (1973) *Science* **179:**1014–1016. Genetic mechanisms determining the central visual pathways of mice.

Gurdon, J. B. (1959) *J. Exp. Zool.* **141:**519–543. Tetraploid frogs.

Gurdon, J. B. (1970) *Proc. Roy. Soc. London (Biol.)* **176:**303–314. Nuclear transplantation and the control of gene activity in animal development.

Gurdon, J. B. (1974) *The Control of Gene Expression in Animal Development,* Harvard University Press, Cambridge, Mass.

Gurdon, J. B., and H. R. Woodland. (1968) *Biol. Rev.* **43:**233–267. The cytoplasmic control of nuclear activity in animal development.

Gurtrecht, J. A. and P. J. Dyck. (1970) *J. Comp. Neurol.* **138:**117–129. Quantitative teased-fiber and histologic studies of human sural nerve during post natal development.

Guth, L. (1956*a*) *Am. J. Physiol.* **185:**205–208. Functional recovery following vagosympathetic anastomosis in the cat.

Guth, L. (1956*b*) *Physiol. Rev.* **36:**441–478. Regeneration in the mammalian peripheral nervous system.

Guth, L. (1958) *Anat. Rec.* **130:**25–38. Taste buds on the cat's circumvallate papilla after reinnervation by glossopharyngeal, vagus, and hypoglossal nerves.

Guth, L. (1962) *Exp. Neurol.* **6:**129–141. Neuromuscular function after regeneration of interrupted nerve fibers into partially denervated muscles.

Guth, L. (1963) *Exp. Neurol.* **8:**336–349. Histological changes following partial denervation of circumvallate papilla of the rat.

Guth, L. (1968) *Physiol. Rev.* **48:**645–687. "Trophic" influences of nerve on muscle.

Guth, L. (1971) Degeneration and regeneration of taste buds, pp. 63–74. In *Handbook of Sensory Physiology,* Vol, IV: *Chemical Senses,* Part 2, (L. M. Beidler, ed.) Springer-Verlag, New York.

Guth, L., and J. J. Bernstein. (1961) *Exp. Neurol.* **4:**59–69. Selectivity in the reestablishment of synapses in the superior cervical sympathetic ganglion of the cat.

Guth, L., and P. K. Watson. (1967) *Exp. Neurol.* **17:**107–117. The influence of innervation on the soluble proteins of slow and fast muscles of the rat.

Guth, L., and H. Yellin. (1971) *Exp. Neurol.* **31:**277–300. The dynamic nature of the so-called "fiber types" of mammalian skeletal muscle.

Guth, L., F. J. Samaha, and R. W. Albers. (1970) *Exp. Neurol.* **26:**126–135. The neural regulation of some phenotypic differences between the fiber types of mammalian skeletal muscle.

Guthrie, D. (1962) *J. Insect Physiol.* **8:**79–92. Regenerative growth in insect nerve axons.

Guthrie, D. (1967) *J. Insect Physiol.* **13:**1593–1611. The regeneration of motor axons in an insect.

Gutmann, E. (1945) *J. Anat. (London)* **79:**1–7. Reinnervation of muscles by sensory nerve fibers.

Gutmann, E., and L. Gutmann. (1942) *Lancet* **242:**169–170. Effect of electrotherapy on denervated muscles in rabbits.

Gutmann, E., Z. Vodička, and J. Zelená. (1955) *Physiol. Bohemoslav.* **4:**200–204. Changes in striated muscle after section of nerve, as a function of the length of the peripheral segment.

Gutmann, E., I. Hajek, and P. Horsky. (1969) *J. Physiol. (London)* **203:**47P. Effect of excessive use on contraction and metabolic properties of cross-striated muscle.

Gwyn, D. G., and J. T. Aitken. (1964) *J. Anat. (London)* **100:**111–126. The formation of new motor endplates in mammalian skeletal muscles.

Gyllensten, L. (1959) *Acta Morphol. Neerl.-Scand.* **2:**331–345. Postnatal development of the visual cortex in darkness (mice).

Gyllensten, L., T. Malmfors, and M.-L. Norrlin. (1965) *J. Comp. Neurol.* **124:**149–160. Effect of visual deprivation on the optic centers of growing and adult mice.

Gymer, A., and J. S. Edwards. (1967) *J. Morphol.* **123:**191–198. The development of the insect nervous system. I. An analysis of postembryonic growth in the terminal ganglion of *Acheta domesticus.*

Haddara, M. (1956) *J. Anat. (London)* **90:**494–501. A quantitative study of the postnatal changes in the packing density of the neurons in visual cortex of the mouse.

Haddara, M. A., and M. A. Nooreddin. (1966) *J. Comp. Neurol.* **128:**245–254. A quantitative study on the postnatal development of the cerebellar vermis of mouse.

Hagan, H. R. (1951) *Embryology of the Viviparous Insects*, Ronald Press, New York, 472 pp.

Haggar, R. A. (1957) *J. Comp. Neurol.* **108:**269–283. Behavior of the accessory body of Cajal during axon reaction.

Hahn, W. E., and C. D. Laird. (1971) *Science* **173:**158–161. Transcription of nonrepeated DNA in mouse brain.

Hale, A. J. (1966) Feulgen microspectrophotometry and its correlation with other cytochemical methods, pp. 183–199. In *Introduction to Quantitative Cytochemistry* (G. L. Wied, ed.), Academic Press, New York.

Hall, E. K. (1939) *J. Exp. Zool.* **82:**173–192. On the duration of the polarization process in the ear primordium of embryos of *Amblystoma punctatum (Linn.).*

Hall, E. K., and M. A. Schneiderhan. (1945) *J. Comp. Neurol.* **82:**19–34. Spinal ganglion hypoplasia after limb amputation in the fetal rat.

Halley, G. (1955) *J. Anat. (London)* **89:**133–152. The placodal relations of the neural crest in the domestic cat.

Halstead, D. C., and M. G. Larrabee. (1972) Early effects of antiserum to the nerve growth factor on metabolism and transmission in superior cervical ganglia of mice, pp. 221–236. In *Immunosympathectomy* (G. Steiner and E. Schönbaum, eds.), Elsevier, Amsterdam.

Hamberger, A., C. Bloomstrand, and A. L. Lehninger. (1970*a*) *J. Cell Biol.* **45:**221–234. Comparative studies on mitochondria isolated from neurone-enriched and glia-enriched fractions of beef brain.

Hamberger, A., H. A. Hansson, and J. Sjöstrand. (1970*b*) *J. Cell Biol.* **47:**319–331. Surface structure of isolated neurons: Detachment of nerve terminals during axon regeneration.

Hamburger, V. (1928) *Arch. Entw.-Mech. Organ.* **114:**272–363. Die Entwicklung experimentell erzeugter nervloser und schwach innervierter Extremitäten von Anuren.

Hamburger, V. (1934) *J. Exp. Zool.* **68:**449–494. The effects of wing bud extirpation on the development of the central nervous system in chick embryos.

Hamburger, V. (1939) *Physiol. Zool.* **12:**268–284. Motor and sensory hyperplasia following limb-bud transplantations in chick embryos.

Hamburger, V. (1946) *J. Exp. Zool.* **103:**113–142. Isolation of the brachial segments of the spinal cord of the chick embryo by means of tantalum foil blocks.

Hamburger, V. (1948) *J. Comp. Neurol.* **88:**221–283. The mitotic patterns in the spinal cord of the chick embryo and their relation to histogenetic processes.

Hamburger, V. (1958) *Am. J. Anat.* **102:**365–410. Regression versus peripheral control of differentiation in motor hypoplasia.

Hamburger, V. (1973) Anatomical and physiological basis of embryonic motility in birds and mammals, pp. 51–76. In *Studies on the Development of Behavior and the Nervous System,* Vol. 1 (G. Gottlieb, ed.), Academic Press, New York.

Hamburger, V. (1975) *J. Comp. Neurol.* **160:**535–546. Cell death in the development of the lateral motor column of the chick embryo.

Hamburger, V., and H. Hamilton. (1951) *J. Morphol.* **88:**49–92. A series of normal stages in the development of the chick embryo.

Hamburger, V., and E. L. Keefe. (1944) *J. Exp. Zool.* **96:**223–242. The effects of peripheral factors on the proliferation and differentiation in the spinal cord of the chick embryo.

Hamburger, V., and R. Levi-Montalcini, (1949) *J. Exp. Zool.* **111:**457–501. Proliferation, differentiation and degeneration in the spinal ganglia of the chick embryo under normal and experimental conditions.

Hamburger, V., and M. Waugh. (1940) *Physiol. Zool.* **13:**367–380. The primary development of the skeleton in nerveless and poorly innervated limb transplants in chick embryos.

Hamburger, V., E. Wenger, and R. Oppenheim. (1966) *J. Exp. Zool.* **162:**133–160. Motility in the chick embryo in the absence of sensory input.

Hamburgh, M. (1960) *Experientia* **16:**460. Observations on the neuropathology of "Reeler," a neurological mutation in the mouse.

Hamburgh, M. (1963) *Dev. Biol.* **8:**165–185. Analysis of the postnatal development of "reeler" a neurological mutation in mice. A study in developmental genetics.

Hamburgh, M. (1968) *Gen. Comp. Endocrinol.* **10:**198–213. An analysis of the action of thyroid hormone on development based on *in vivo* and *in vitro* studies.

Hamburgh, M. (1969) *Curr. Top. Dev. Biol.* **4:**109–148. The role of thyroid and growth hormones in neurogenesis.

Hamburgh, M., and R. P. Bunge. (1964) *Life Sci.* **3:**1423–1430. Evidence for a direct effect of thyroid hormone on maturation of nervous tissue grown *in vitro.*

Hamdi, F. A., and D. Whitteridge. (1954) *Quart. J. Exp. Physiol.* **39:**111–119. The representation of the retina on the optic lobe of the pigeon.

Hammond, W. S. (1949) *J. Comp. Neurol.* **91:**67–86. Formation of the sympathetic nervous system in the trunk of the chick embryo following removal of the thoracic neural tube.

Hammond, W. S., and C. L. Yntema. (1947) *J. Comp. Neurol.* **86:**237–265. Depletions in the thoracolumbar sympathetic system following removal of the neural crest in the chick.

Hanaway, J. (1967) *J. Comp. Neurol.* **131:**1–14. Formation and differentiation of the external granular layer of the chick cerebellum.

Hanaway, J., S. I. Lee, and M. G. Netsky. (1968) *Neurology* **18:**791–799. Pachygyria: Relation of findings to modern embryologic concepts.

Hanaway, J., J. McConnell, and M. G. Netsky. (1971) *J. Comp. Neurol.* **142:**59–74. Histogenesis of the substantia nigra, ventral tegmental area of Tsai and interpeduncular nucleus: An autoradiographic study of the mesencephalon in the rat.

Hannah, R. S., and E. J. H. Nathaniel. (1974) *Anat. Rec.* **178:**691–710. The post-natal development of blood vessels in the substantia gelatinosa of rat cervical cord: An ultrastructural study.

Hansson, H. A., and J. Sjöstrand. (1971) *Brain Res.* **35:**379–396. Ultrastructural effects of colchicine on the hypoglossal and dorsal vagal neurons of the rabbit.

Hanström, B. (1926) *Z. Mikrosk.-Anat. Forsch.* **7:**135–190. Untersuchungen über die relative Grösse der Gehirnzentren verschiedener Arthropoden unter Berücksichtigung der Lebensweise.

Harcombe Smith, E., and R. J. Wyman. (1970) *J. Exp. Biol.* **53:**255–263. Diagonal locomotion in deafferented toads.

Hardesty, I. (1904) *Am. J. Anat.* **3:**229–268. On the development and nature of the neuroglia.

Hare, W. K., and J. C. Hinsey. (1940) *J. Comp. Neurol.* **73:**489–502. Reaction of dorsal root ganglion cells to section of peripheral and central processes.

Harkmark, W. (1954) *J. Comp. Neurol.* **100:**115–209. Cell migrations from the rhombic lip to the inferior olive, the nucleus raphe and the pons: A morphological and experimental investigation on chick embryos.

Harkmark, W. (1956) *J. Exp. Zool.* **131:**333–371. The influence of the cerebellum on development and maintenance of the inferior olive and the pons: An experimental investigation on chick embryos.

Harms, J. W. (1927) *Zool. Anz.* **74:**249–256. Alterscheinungen im Hirn von Affen und Menschen.

Harris, A. (1972) *Acta Protozool.* **11:**145–151. Surface movement in fibroblast locomotion.

Harris, A., and G. Dunn. (1972) *Exp. Cell Res.* **73:**519–522. Centripetal transport of attached particles on both surfaces of moving fibroblasts.

Harris, A. J. (1974) *Annu. Rev. Physiol.* **36:**251–305. Inductive functions of the nervous system.

Harris, G. W. (1964) *Endocrinology* **75:**627–648. Sex hormones, brain development and brain function.

Harris, G. W., and S. Levine. (1962) *J. Physiol. (London)* **163:**42–43P. Sexual differentiation of the brain and its experimental control.

Harris, G. W., and S. Levine. (1965) *J. Physiol. (London)* **181**:379–400. Sexual differentiation of the brain and its experimental control.

Harris, H. (1954) *Physiol. Rev.* **34**:529–562. Role of chemotaxis in inflammation.

Harris, H., J. J. Watkins, C. E. Ford, and G. I. Schoefl. (1966) *J. Cell Sci.* **1**:1–30. Artificial heterokaryons of animal cells from different species.

Harris, J. B., and S. Thesleff. (1972) *Nature New Biol.* **236**:60–61. Nerve stump length and membrane changes in denervated skeletal muscle.

Harrison, R. G. (1901) *Arch. Mikrosk.-Anat.* **57**:354–444. Ueber die Histogenese des peripheren Nervensystems bei *Salmo salar.*

Harrison, R. G. (1903) *Arch. Mikrosk.-Anat.* **63**:35–149. Experimentelle Untersuchungen über die Entwicklung der Sinnesorgane der Seitenlinie bei den Amphibien.

Harrison, R. G. (1904) *Am. J. Anat.* **3**:197–220. An experimental study of the relation of the nervous system to the developing musculature in the embryo of the frog.

Harrison, R. G. (1906) *Am. J. Anat.* **5**:121–131. Further experiments on the development of peripheral nerves.

Harrison, R. G. (1907*a*) *J. Exp. Zool.* **4**:239–281. Experiments in transplanting limbs and their bearing upon the problem of the development of nerves.

Harrison, R. G. (1907*b*) *Anat. Rec.* **1**:116–118. Observations on the living developing nerve fiber.

Harrison, R. G. (1910) *J. Exp. Zool.* **9**:787–846. The outgrowth of the nerve fiber as a mode of protoplasmic movement.

Harrison, R. G. (1911) *Science* **34**:279. On the stereotropism of embryonic cells.

Harrison R. G. (1912) *Anat. Rec.* **6**:181–193. The cultivation of tissues in extraneous media as a method of morphogenetic study.

Harrison, R. G. (1914) *J. Exp. Zool.* **17**:521–544. The reaction of embryonic cells to solid structures.

Harrison, R. G. (1918) *J. Exp. Zool.* **25**:413–461. Experiments on the development of the fore limb of *Amblystoma,* a self-differentiating equipotential system.

Harrison, R. G. (1921) *J. Exp. Zool.* **32**:1–136. On relations of symmetry in transplanted limbs.

Harrison, R. G. (1924*a*) *J. Comp. Neurol.* **37**:123–205. Neuroblast versus sheath cell in the development of peripheral nerves.

Harrison, R. G. (1924*b*) *Proc. Natl. Acad. Sci. U.S.A.* **10**:69–74. Some unexpected results of the heteroplastic transplantation of limbs.

Harrison, R. G. (1925) *Arch. Entw.-Mech. Organ.* **106**:469–502. The effect of reversing the medio-lateral or transverse axis of the forelimb bud in the salamander embryo (*Amblystoma punctatum* Linn).

Harrison, R. G. (1929) *Arch. Entw.-Mech. Organ.* **120**:1–55. Correlation in the development and growth of the eye studied by means of heteroplastic transplantation.

Harrison, R. G. (1935) *Proc. Roy. Soc. (London) Ser. B* **118**:155–196. On the origin and development of the nervous system studied by the methods of experimental embryology.

Harrison, R. G. (1936) *Proc. Natl. Acad. Sci. U.S.A.* **22**:238–247. Relations of symmetry in the developing ear of *Amblystoma punctatum.*

Harrison, R. G. (1945) *Trans. Conn. Acad. Arts Sci.* **36**:277–330. Relations of symmetry in the developing embryo.

Harrison, R. G. (1947) *J. Exp. Zool.* **106**:27–83. Wound healing and reconstitution of the central nervous system of the amphibian embryo after removal of parts of the neural plate.

Hartzell, H. C., and D. M. Fambrough. (1972) *J. Gen. Physiol.* **60**:248–262. Acetylcholine receptors: Distribution and extrajunctional density in rat diaphragm after denervation correlated with acetylcholine sensitivity.

Harvey, S. C., and H. S. Burr. (1926) *Arch. Neurol. Psychiat.* **15**:545. The development of the meninges.

Harvey, S. C., H. S. Burr, and E. VanCampenhout. (1933) *Arch. Neurol. Psychiat.* **29**:683–690. Development of the meninges: Further experiments.

Hatai, S. (1901) *J. Comp. Neurol.* **11**:25–39. On the presence of the centrosome in certain nerve cells of the white rat.

Hatai, S. (1902) *J. Comp. Neurol.* **12**:291–296. On the origin of neuroglia tissue from the mesoblast.

Hatai, S. (1910) *J. Comp. Neurol.* **20**:19–47. On the length of the internodes in the sciatic nerve of *Rana temporaria* (fusca) and *Rana pipiens:* being a reexamination by biometric methods of the data studied by Boycott (1904) and Takahashi (1908).

Haug, H. (1956) *J. Comp. Neurol.* **104**:473–492. Remarks on the determination and significance of the grey-cell coefficient.

Haug, H. (1960) Die quantitative Zellvolumenverhaltnisse der Hirnrinde. In *Structure and Function of the Cerebral Cortex* (D. B. Tower and J. P. Schadé eds.), Elsevier, Amsterdam.

Haug, H. (1967*a*) *Z. Zellforsch. Mikrosk. Anat. Abt. Histochem.* **83:**265–278. Die Länge der Internodien der Markfasern im Bereich der Sehrinde der erwachsenen Katze.

Haug, H. (1967*b*) *Acta Anat.* **67:**53–73. Über die exakte Feststellung der Anzahl Nervenzellen pro Volumeneinheit des Cortex cerebri, zugleich ein Beispiel für die Durchführung genauer Zählungen.

Haug, H. (1972) *Z. Zellforsch. Mikrosk. Anat.* **123:**544–565. Die postnatale Entwicklung der Gliadeckschicht der Sehrinde der Katze: Eine electronenmikroskopische Studie über die Ausbildung von Lamellenstapeln.

Hausman, R. E., and A. A. Moscona. (1975) *Proc. Natl. Acad. Sci. U.S.A.* **72:**916–920. Purification and characterization of the retina-specific cell-aggregating factor.

Hausman, R. E., and A. A. Moscona. (1976) *Proc. Natl. Acad. Sci. U.S.A.* **73:**3594–3598. Isolation of the retina-specific cell-aggregating factor from membrane of embryonic neural retina tissue.

Hawkins, A., and J. Olszewski. (1957) *Science* **126:**76–77. Glia/nerve cell index for cortex of the whale.

Hayashi, M. (1924) *Deutsch. Z. Nervenheilk.* **81:**74–82. Einige wichtige Tatsachen aus der ontogenetischen Entwicklung des menschlichen Kleinhirns.

Hayes, B. P. (1976) *Anat. Embryol.* **150:**99–111. The distribution of intercellular gap junctions in the developing retina and pigment epithelium of *Xenopus laevis.*

Hayes, B. P., and A. Roberts. (1973) *Z. Zellforsch Mikrosk. Anat.* **137:**251–269. Synaptic junction development in the spinal cord of an amphibian embryo: An electron microscope study.

Hayes, B. P., and A. Roberts. (1974) *Cell Tiss. Res.* **153:**227–244. The distribution of synapses along the spinal cord of an amphibian embryo: An electron microscope study of junction development.

Hebb, D. H. (1949) *Organization of Behavior,* Wiley, New York.

Hebb, D. H. (1966) *A Textbook of Psychology,* 2nd ed., Saunders, Philadelphia.

Heller, I. H., and K. A. C. Elliott. (1954) *Can. J. Biochem. Physiol.* **32:**584–592. Desoxyribonucleic acid content and cell density in brain and human brain tumors.

Hendrickson, A., and R. Boothe. (1976) *Vision Res.* **16:**517–521. Morphology of the retina and dorsal lateral geniculate nucleus in dark-reared monkeys (*Macaca nemestrina*).

Hendrickson, A. E., and W. M. Cowan. (1971) *Exp. Neurol.* **30:**403–422. Changes in the rate of axoplasmic transport during postnatal development of the rabbit's optic nerve and tract.

Hendry, I. A. (1976) *J. Neurocytol.* **5:**337–349. A method to correct adequately for the change in neuronal size when estimating neuronal numbers after nerve growth factor treatment.

Hendry, I. A., and J. Campbell. (1976) *J. Neurocytol.* **5:**351–360. Morphometric analysis of rat superior cervical ganglion after axotomy and nerve growth factor treatment.

Hendry, I. A., and L. L. Iversen. (1971) *Brain Res.* **29:**159–162. Effect of nerve growth factor and its antiserum on tyrosine hydroxylase activity in mouse superior cervical sympathetic ganglion.

Hendry, I. A., and L. L. Iversen. (1973) *Nature* **243:**500–504. Reduction in the concentration of nerve growth factor in mice after sialectomy and castration.

Hendry, I. A., K. Stöckel, H. Thoenen, and L. L. Iversen. (1974*a*) *Brain Res.* **68:**103–121. The retrograde axonal transport of nerve growth factor.

Hendry, I. A., R. Stach, and K. Herrup. (1974*b*) *Brain Res.* **82:**117–128. Characteristics of the retrograde axonal transport system for nerve growth factor in the sympathetic nervous system.

Henkin, R. I., and L. J. Kopin. (1964) *Life Sci.* **3:**1319–1325. Abnormalities of taste and smell thresholds in familial dysautonomia: Improvement with methacholine.

Henneman, E., and C. B. Olson. (1965) *J. Neurophysiol.* **28:**581–598. Relations between structure and function in the design of skeletal muscles.

Henneman, E., G. Somjen, and D. O. Carpenter. (1965) *J. Neurophysiol.* **28:**560–580. Functional significance of cell size in spinal motoneurons.

Heringa, G. C. (1918) *Arch. Néerl. Sci. Ex. Nat.* **3:**235–315. Le développement des corpuscles de Grandry et de Herbst.

Herman, C. J., and L. W. Lapham. (1968) *Science* **160:**537. DNA content of neurons in the cat hippocampus.

Herman, C. J., and L. W. Lapham. (1969) *Brain Res.* **15:**35–48. Neuronal polyploidy and nuclear volumes in the cat central nervous system.

Herman, L., and S. L. Kauffman. (1966) *Dev. Biol.* **13:**145–162. The fine structure of the embryonic mouse neural tube with special reference to cytoplasmic microtubules.

Herndon, R. M. (1963) *J. Cell Biol.* **18:**167–180. The fine structure of the Purkinje cell.

Herndon, R. M. (1968) *Exp. Brain Res.* **6**:49–68. Thiophen induced granule cell necrosis in the rat cerebellum.

Herndon, R. M., G. Margolis, and L. Kilham. (1971*a*) *J. Neuropathol. Exp. Neurol.* **30**:196–205. The synaptic organization of the malformed cerebellum induced by perinatal infection with the feline panleukopenia virus (PLV). I. Elements forming the cerebellar glomeruli.

Herndon, R. M., G. Margolis, and L. Kilham. (1971*b*) *J. Neuropathol. Exp. Neurol.* **30**:557–570. The synaptic organization of the malformed cerebellum induced by perinatal infection with the feline panelukopenia virus (PLV). II. The Purkinje cell and its afferents.

Herre, W. (1936) *Verhandl. Deutsch. Zool. Ges. Freiburg,* 200–211. Untersuchungen an Hirnen von Wild- und Hausschweinen.

Herre, W. (1958) *Deutsch. Med. Wochenschr.* **83**:1568–1574. Einflüsse der Umwelt auf das Säugetiergehirn.

Herre, W. (1966) Einige Bemerkungen zur Modifikabilität, Vererbung und Evolution von Merkmalen des Vorderhirns bei Säugetieren, pp. 162–174. In *Evolution of the Forebrain* (R. Hassler and H. Stephan, eds.), Plenum, New York.

Herre, W., and U. Thiede. (1965) *Zool. Jahrb. Abt. Anat. Ontog. Tiere* **82**:155–176. Studien an Gehirnen südamerikanischer Tylopoden.

Herrick, C. J. (1925) *J. Comp. Neurol.* **39**:433–489. The amphibian forebrain. III. The optic tracts and centers of *Amblystoma* and the frog.

Herrick, C. J. (1948) *The Brain of the Tiger Salamander,* University of Chicago Press, Chicago.

Herrup, K., and E. M. Shooter. (1973) *Proc. Natl. Acad. Sci. U.S.A.* **70**:3884–3888. Properties of the β nerve growth factor receptor of avian dorsal root ganglia.

Herrup, K., R. Stickgold, and E. M. Shooter. (1974) *Ann. N.Y. Acad. Sci.* **228**:381–392. The role of the nerve growth factor in the development of sensory and sympathetic ganglia.

Hersh, A. H. (1941) *Growth Suppl.* **5**:113–145. Allometric growth: The ontogenic and phylogenetic significance of differential rates of growth.

Herzig, M. E., H. G. Birch, S. A. Richardson, and J. Tizard. (1972) *Pediatrics* **49**:814–824. Intellectual levels of school children severely malnourished during the first two years of life.

Heslop, J. P. (1975) *Adv. Comp. Physiol. Biochem.* **6**:75–161. Axonal flow and fast transport in nerves.

Hess, A., and J. Z. Young. (1949) *Nature* **164**:490. Correlation of internodal length and fibre diameter in the central nervous system.

Heuser, J. E., and T. S. Reese. (1973) *J. Cell Biol.* **57**:315–344. Evidence for recycling of synaptic vesicle membrane during transmitter release at the frog neuromuscular junction.

Heuser, J. E., T. S. Reese, and D. M. D. Landis, (1974) *J. Neurocytol.* **3**:109–131. Functional changes in frog neuromuscular junctions studied with freeze-fracture.

Hibbard, E. (1959) *J. Exp. Zool.* **141**:323–351. Central integration of developing nerve tracts from supernumerary grafted eyes and brain in the frog.

Hibbard, E. (1964) *Exp. Neurol.* **10**:271–283. Selective innervation and reciprocal functional suppression from grafted extra labyrinths in amphibians.

Hibbard, E (1965*a*) *Exp. Neurol.* **13**:289–301. Orientation and directed growth of Mauthner's cell axons from duplicated vestibular nerve roots.

Hibbard, E. (1965*b*) *Anat. Rec.* **151**:360–361. Innervation of intrinsic limb musculature by cranial nerves in *Pleurodeles waltlii.*

Hibbard, E. (1967) *Exp. Neurol.* **19**:350–356. Visual recovery following regeneration of the optic nerve through oculomotor nerve root in *Xenopus.*

Hickey, T. L. (1975) *J. Comp. Neurol.* **161**:359–382. Translaminar growth of axons in the kitten dorsal lateral geniculate nucleus following removal of one eye.

Hickey, T. L., and R. W. Guillery. (1974) *J. Comp. Neurol.* **156**:239–253. An autoradiographic study of retinogeniculate pathways in the cat and the fox.

Hicks, S. P. (1954) *J. Cell. Comp. Physiol.* **43**: *Suppl.* **1**:151–178. The effects of ionizing radiation, certain hormones, and radiomimetic drugs on the developing nervous system.

Hicks, S. P. (1958) *Physiol. Rev.* **38**:337–356. Radiation as an experimental tool in mammalian developmental neurology.

Hicks, S. P., and C. J. D'Amato. (1963) Malformation and regeneration of the mammalian retina following experimental radiation, pp. 45–51. In *Les Phakomatoses Cérébrales, Deuxième Colloque International Malformations Congénitales de l'Encéphale* (L. Michaux and M. Field, eds.), SPEI, Paris.

Hicks, S. P., and C. J. D'Amato. (1966) Effects of ionizing radiations on mammalian development, pp. 196–250. In *Advances in Teratology* (D. H. M. Woollam, ed.), Logos, London.

Hicks, S. P., and C. J. D'Amato. (1968) *Anat. Rec.* **160:**619–634. Cell migrations to the isocortex in the rat.

Hicks, S. P., C. J. D'Amato, and M. J. Lowe. (1959) *J. Comp. Neurol.* **113:**435–469. The development of the mammalian nervous system. I. Malformations of the brain, especially the cerebral cortex, induced in rats by radiation.

Hicks, S. P., C. J. D'Amato, M. C. Coy, E. D. O'Brien, J. M. Thurston, and D. L. Joftes. (1961) Migrating cells in the developing central nervous system studied by their radiosensitivity and tritiated thymidine uptake, pp. 246–261. In *Fundamental Aspects of Radiosensitivity,* Brookhaven Symposium in Biology, No. 14, Upton, N.Y.

Hier, D. B., B. G. W. Arnason, and M. Young. (1972) *Proc. Natl. Acad. Sci. U.S.A.* **69:**2268–2272. Studies on the mechanism of action of nerve growth factor.

Hilber, H. (1943) *Arch. Entw.-Mech. Organ.* **142:**100–120. Experimentelle Studien zum Schicksal des Rumpfganglienleistenmaterials.

Hild, W. (1957) *Z. Zellforsch. Mikrosk. Anat.* **46:**71–95. Myelogenesis in cultures of mammalian central nervous system.

Hild, W. (1966) *Z. Zellforsch. Mikrosk. Anat.* **69:**155–188. Cell types and neuronal connections in cultures of mammalian central nervous tissue.

Hildebrand, C. (1971) *Acta Physiol. Scand. Suppl.* **364:**109–144. Ultrastructural and light-microscopic studies of the developing feline spinal cord white matter. II. Cell death and myelin sheath disintegration in the early postnatal period.

Hildebrand, C., and S. Skoglund. (1971) *Acta Physiol. Scand. Suppl.* **364:**5–41. Caliber spectra of some fiber tracts in the feline central nervous system during postnatal development.

Hillman, D. E. (1969) *J. Neurophysiol.* **32:**818–846. Morphological organization of frog cerebellar cortex: A light and electron microscopic study.

Hinds, J. W. (1966) *Anat. Rec.* **154:**358–359. Autoradiographic study of histogenesis in the olfactory bulb and accessory olfactory bulb in the mouse.

Hinds, J. W. (1968*a*) *J. Comp. Neurol.* **134:**287–304. Autoradiographic study of histogenesis in the mouse olfactory bulb. I. Time of origin of neurons and neuroglia.

Hinds, J. W. (1968*b*) *J. Comp. Neurol.* **134:**305–322. Autoradiographic study of histogenesis in the mouse olfactory bulb. II. Cell proliferation and migration.

Hinds, J. W., and J. B. Angevine, Jr. (1965) *Anat. Rec.* **151:**456–457. Autoradiographic study of histogenesis in the area pyriformis and claustrum in the mouse.

Hinds, J. W., and P. L. Hinds. (1972) *J. Neurocytol.* **1:**169–187. Reconstruction of dendritic growth cones in neonatal mouse olfactory bulb.

Hinds, J. W., and P. L. Hinds. (1974) *Dev. Biol.* **37:**381–416. Early ganglion cell differentiation in the mouse retina: An electron microscopic analysis utilizing serial sections.

Hinds, J. W., and P. L. Hinds. (1976*a*) *J. Comp. Neurol.* **169:**15–40. Synapse formation in the mouse olfactory bulb. I. Quantitative studies.

Hinds, J. W., and P. L. Hinds. (1976*b*) *J. Comp. Neurol.* **169:**41–62. Synapse formation in the mouse olfactory bulb. II. Morphogenesis.

Hinds, J. W. and T. L. Ruffett. (1971) *Z. Zellforsch. Mikrosk. Anat.* **115:**226–264. Cell proliferation in the neural tube: An electron microscopic and Golgi analysis in the mouse cerebral vesicle.

Hinsey, J. C. (1934) *Physiol. Rev.* **14:**514–585. Innervation of skeletal muscle.

Hinsey, J. C., M. A. Krupp, and W. T. Lhamon. (1937) *J. Comp. Neurol.* **67:**205–214. Reaction of spinal ganglion cells to section of dorsal roots.

Hirano, A. (1968) *J. Cell Biol.* **38:**637–640. A confirmation of oligodendroglial origin of myelin in the adult rat.

Hirano, A., and H. M. Dembitzer. (1967) *J. Cell Biol.* **35:**555–567. A structural analysis of the myelin sheath in the central nervous system.

Hirano, A., and H. M. Dembitzer. (1973) *J. Cell Biol.* **56:**478–486. Cerebellar alterations in the weaver mouse.

Hirano, A., and H. M. Dembitzer. (1975) *J. Neuropath. Exp. Neurol.* **34:**1–11. The fine structure of staggerer cerebellum.

Hirano, A., H. M. Dembitzer, and M. Jones. (1972) *J. Neuropathol. Exp. Neurol.* **31:**113–125. An electron microscope study of cycasin- induced cerebellar alterations.

Hirano, H. (1967*a*) *Z. Zellforsch. Mikrosk. Anat.* **79:**198–208. Ultrastructural study on the morphogenesis of the neuromuscular junction in the skeletal muscle of the chick.

Hirano, H. (1967*b*) *Arch. Histol. (Japan)* **28:**89–101. A histochemical study of the cholinesterase activity in the neuromuscular junction in developing chick skeletal muscles.

Hirsch, H. V. B. (1970) Controlled visual stimulation and deprivation. In *Genesis of Neuronal Patterns* (M. V. Edds, Jr., ed.), NRP Work Session, Brookline, Mass.

Hirsch, H. V. B., and M. Jacobson. (1973) *Brain Res.* **49:** 67–74. Development and maintenance of connectivity in the visual system of the frog. II. The effects of eye removal.

Hirsch, H. V. B., and M. Jacobson (1975) The perfectible brain: Principles of neuronal development, pp. 107–137. In *Foundations of Psychobiology* (M. Gazzaniga and C. Blakemore, eds.), Academic Press, New York.

Hirsch, H. V. B., and A. G. Leventhal. (1976) X-cell and Y-cell influenced neurons in the cat's visual cortex following long-term pattern deprivation. Paper presented at ARVO, Sarasota, Fla.

Hirsch, H. V. B., and A. G. Leventhal. (1978) Functional modification of the developing visual system. In *Handbook of Sensory Physiology,* Vol, IX. *Development of Sensory Systems* (M. Jacobson, ed.), Springer-Verlag, New York.

Hirsch, H. V. B., and D. N. Spinelli. (1970) *Science* **168:**869–871. Visual experience modifies distribution of horizontally and vertically oriented receptive fields in cats.

Hirsch, H. V. B., and D. N. Spinelli. (1971) *Exp. Brain Res.* **13:**509–527. Modification of the distribution of receptive field orientation in cats by selective visual exposure during development.

His, W. (1887) *Arch. Anat. Physiol. Leipzig Anat. Abt.* **92:**368–378. Die Entwicklung der ersten Nervenbahnen beim menschlichen Embryo: Uebersichtliche Darstellung.

His, W. (1888*a*) *Abhandl. Kgl. Sachs. Ges. Wiss. Math. Phys. Kl.* **24:**341–392. Zur Geschichte des Gehirns sowie der centralen und peripherischen Nervenbahnen.

His, W. (1888*b*) *Proc. Roy. Soc. Edinburgh* **15:**287–297. On the principles of animal morphology.

His, W. (1889) *Abhandl. Kgl. Sachs. Ges. Wiss. Math. Phys. Kl.* **15:**313–372. Die Neuroblasten und deren Entstehung im embryonalen Mark.

His, W. (1890*a*) *Abhandl. Klg. Sachs. Ges. Wiss. Math. Phys. Kl.* **29:**1–74. Die Entwicklung des menschlichen Rautenhirns vom Ende des ersten bis zum Beginn des dritten Monats. I. Verlängertes Mark.

His, W. (1890*b*) *Arch. Anat. Physiol. Leipzig Anat. Abt. Suppl.* **95:**95–119. Histogenese und Zusammenhang der Nervenelemente.

His, W. (1894) *Arch. Anat. Physiol. Leipzig Anat. Abt.* 1–80. Über mechanische Grundvorgänge thierische Formenbildung.

His, W. (1904) *Die Entwicklung des menschlichen Gehirns waehrend der ersten Monate,* S. Hirzel, Leipzig.

His, W., Jr. (1897) *Arch. Anat. Physiol. (Leipzig) Suppl.,* 137–170. Ueber die Entwicklung des Bauchsympathicus beim Hühnchen und Menschen.

Hiscoe, H. B. (1947) *Anat. Rec.* **99:**447–475. Distribution of nodes and incisures in normal and regenerated nerve fibers.

Hník, P., I. Jirmanová, L. Vyklický, and J. Zelená. (1967) *J. Physiol. (London)* **193:**309–325. Fast and slow muscles of the chick after nerve cross-union.

Hoffman, H. (1950) *Aust. J. Exp. Biol. Med. Sci.* **28:**383–397. Local re-innervation in partially denervated muscle: a histophysiological study.

Hoffman, H. (1951*a*) *Aust. J. Exp. Biol. Med. Sci.* **29:**211–219. Fate of interrupted nerve fibers regenerating into partially denervated muscles.

Hoffman, H. (1951*b*) *Aust. J. Exp. Biol. Med. Sci.* **29:**289–307. A study of the factors influencing innervation of muscles by implanted nerves.

Hoffman, H., and P. H., Springell. (1951) *Aust. J. Exp. Biol. Med. Sci.* **29:**417–424. An attempt at the chemical identification of "neurocletin." (The substance evoking axon-sprouting.)

Hoffman, P. N., and R. J. Lasek. (1975) *J. Cell Biol.* **66:**351–366. The slow component of axonal transport: Identification of major structural polypeptides of the axon and their generality among mammalian neurons.

Hoffman, W. W., and J. H. Peacock. (1973) *Exp. Neurol.* **41:**345–356. Postjunctional changes induced by partial interruption of axoplasmic flow in motor nerves.

Hoffmann, K.-P. (1973) *J. Neurophysiol.* **36:**409–424. Conduction velocity in pathways from retina to superior colliculus in the cat: A correlation with receptive-field properties.

Hoffmann, K.-P., and M. Cynader. (1975) *Brain Res.* **85:**179. Recovery in the LGN of the cat after early visual deprivation.

Hoffmann, K.-P., and S. M. Sherman. (1974) *J. Neurophysiol.* **37:**1276–1286. Effects of early monocular deprivation on visual input to cat superior colliculus.

Hoffmann, K.-P., and S. M. Sherman. (1975) *J. Neurophysiol.* **38:**1049–1059. Effects of early binocular deprivation on visual input to cat superior colliculus.

Hoffmann, K.-P., and J. Stone. (1971) *Brain Res.* **32:**460–466. Conduction velocity of afferents to cat visual cortex: A correlation with cortical receptive field properties.

Hogan, E. L., D. M. Dawson, and F. C. A. Romanul. (1965) *Arch. Neurol.* **13:**274–282. Enzymic changes in denervated muscle. II. Biochemical studies.

Hoh, J. F. Y. (1971) *Exp. Neurol.* **30:**263–276. Selective reinnervation of fast-twitch and slow-graded muscle fibers in the toad.

Hohmann, A., and O. D. Creutzfeldt. (1975) *Nature* **254:**613–614. Squint and the development of binocularity in humans.

Hollyday, M., and V. Hamburger. (1975) *Neurosci. Abstr.* **1:**779. Reduction of normally occurring motor neuron depletion following supernumerary limb transplantation in chick embryo.

Hollyday, M., and V. Hamburger. (1976) *J. Comp. Neurol.* **170:**311–320. Reduction of the naturally occurring motor neuron loss by enlargement of the periphery.

Hollyday, M., and L. Mendell. (1975) *J. Comp. Neurol.* **162:**205–220. Area specific reflexes from normal and supernumerary limbs of *Xenopus laevis.*

Hollyday, M., and L. Mendell. (1976) *Exp. Neurol.* **51:**316–329. Analysis of moving supernumerary limbs of *Xenopus laevis.*

Hollyfield, J. G. (1968) *Dev. Biol.* **18:**163–179. Differential addition of cells to the retina in *Rana pipiens* tadpoles.

Hollyfield, J. G. (1971) *Dev. Biol.* **24:**264–286. Differential growth of the neural retina in *Xenopus laevis* larvae.

Hollyfield, J. G. (1972) *J. Comp. Neurol.* **144:**373–380. Histogenesis of the retina in the killifish.

Hollyfield, J. G., and R. Adler. (1970) *Exp. Cell Res.* **59:**76–84. Localization of embryonic cells and polystyrene particles within chick embryos after vascular dissemination.

Holmdahl, D. E. (1928) *Z. Mikrosk. Anat. Forsch.* **14:**99–298. Die Entstehung und weitere Entwicklung der Neuralleiste (Ganglienleiste) bei Vögeln und Säugetieren.

Holt, E. B. (1931) *Animal Drive and the Learning Process,* Holt, New York.

Holtfreter, J. (1933) *Arch. Entw.-Mech. Organ.* **137:**619–775. Der Einfluss von Wirtsalter und Verschiedenen Organbezirken auf die Differenzierung von angelagertem Gastrulaektoderm.

Holtfreter, J. (1938*a*) *Arch. Entw.-Mech. Organ.* **138:**163–196. Veränderungen der Reaktionsweise im alternden isolierten Gastrulaektoderm.

Holtfreter, J. (1938*b*) *Arch. Entw.-Mech. Organ.* **138:**522–656. Differenzierungspotenzen isolierter Teile der Urodelen gastrula.

Holtfreter, J. (1939) *Arch. Exp. Zellforsch.* **23:**169–209. Gewebeaffinität, ein Mittel der embryonalen Formbildung.

Holtfreter, J. (1944) *J. Exp. Zool.* **95:**307–343. Neural differentiation of ectoderm through exposure to saline solution.

Holtfreter, J. (1945) *J. Exp. Zool.* **98:**161–209. Neurulization and epidermization of gastrula ectoderm.

Holtfreter, J., and V. Hamburger. (1955) Amphibians, pp. 230–296. In *Analysis of Development* (B. H. Willier, P. A. Weiss, and V. Hamburger, eds.), Saunders, Philadelphia.

Holtzer, H. (1951) *J. Exp. Zool.* **117:**523–558. Reconstitution of the urodele spinal cord following unilateral ablation. Part I. Chronology of neuron regulation.

Holtzer, H. (1952) *J. Exp. Zool.* **119:**263–302. Reconstitution of the urodele spinal cord following unilateral ablation. Part II. Regeneration of the longitudinal tracts and ectopic synaptic unions of the Mauthner's fibers.

Holtzer, H. (1968) Induction of chondrogenesis: A concept in quest of mechanisms, pp. 152–164. In *Epithelial-Mesenchymal Interactions* (R. Fleischmajer, ed.), Williams and Wilkins, Baltimore.

Holtzman, E. (1971) *Phil. Trans. Roy. Soc. London Ser. B* **261:**407–421. Cytochemical studies of protein transport in the nervous system.

Holtzman, E., and E. R. Peterson. (1969) *J. Cell Biol.* **40:**863–869. Uptake of protein by mammalian neurons.

Holtzman, E., A. B. Novikoff, and H. Villaverde. (1967) *J. Cell Biol.* **33:**419–435. Lysosomes and GERL in normal and chromatolytic neurons of the rat ganglion nodosum.

Holtzman, E., A. R. Freeman, and L. A. Kashner. (1971) *Science* **173:**733–736. Stimulation-dependent alterations in peroxidase uptake at lobster neuromuscular junctions.

Hommes, O. R., and C. P. Leblond. (1967) *J. Comp. Neurol.* **129:**269–278. Mitotic division of neuroglia in the normal adult rat.

Hoober, J. K., and S. Cohen. (1967) *Biochim. Biophys. Acta* **138:**347–356. Epidermal growth factor. I. The stimulation of protein and ribonucleic acid synthesis in chick embryo epidermis.

Hooker, D. (1911) *J. Exp. Zool.* **11:**159–186. The development and function of voluntary and cardiac muscle in embryos without nerves.

Hope, R. A., B. J. Hammond, and R. M. Gaze. (1976) *Proc. Roy. Soc. London (Biol.)* **194:**447–466. The arrow model: Retinotectal specificity and map formation in the goldfish visual system.

Höpker, W. (1951) *Z. Alternforsch.* **5:**256–279. Das Altern des Nucleus dentatus.

Horder, T. J. (1974*a*) *Brain Res.* **72:**41–52. Changes of fibre pathways in the goldfish optic tract following regeneration.

Horder, T. J. (1974*b*) *J. Physiol. (London)* **241:**84–85P. Electron microscopic evidence in goldfish that different optic nerve fibres regenerate selectively through specific routes into the tectum.

Hörstadius, S. (1950) *The Neural Crest,* Oxford University Press, London.

Horstmann, E., and H. Meves. (1959) *Z. Zellforsch. Mikrosk. Anat. Abt. Histochem.* **49:**569–589. Die Feinstruktur des molekularen Rindengraus und ihre physiologische Bedeutung.

Hoshino, K., T. Matsuzawa, and U. Murakami. (1973) *Exp. Cell Res.* **77:**89–94. Characteristics of the cell cycle of matrix cells in the mouse embryo during histogenesis of telencephalon.

Hotta, Y., and S. Benzer. (1970) *Proc. Natl. Acad. Sci. U.S.A.* **67:**1156–1163. Genetic dissection of the *Drosophila* nervous system by means of mosaics.

Hotta, Y., and S. Benzer. (1972) *Nature* **240:**527–535. Mapping of behavior in *Drosophila* mosaics.

Hotta, Y., and S. Benzer. (1973) Mapping of behavior of *Drosophila* mosaics, pp. 129–167. In *Genetic Mechanisms of Development* (F. H. Ruddle, ed.), Academic Press, New York.

Howard, A., and S. R. Pelc. (1953) *Heredity* **6:**261–273. Synthesis of deoxyribonucleic acid in normal and irradiated cells and its relation to chromosome breakage.

Howard, E. (1965) *J. Neurochem.* **12:**181–191. Effects of corticosterone and food restriction on growth and on DNA, RNA and cholesterol contents of the brain and liver in infant mice.

Howard, E. (1968) *Exp. Neurol.* **22:**191–208. Reductions in size and total DNA of cerebrum and cerebellum in adult mice after corticosterone treatment in infancy.

Howard, E. (1973) *Prog. Brain Res.* **40:**91–114. DNA content of rodent brains during maturation and aging, and autoradiography of postnatal DNA synthesis in monkey brain.

Howard, E., and D. M. Granoff. (1968) *J. Nutr.* **95:**111–121. Effect of neonatal food restriction in mice on brain growth, DNA and cholesterol, and on adult delayed response learning.

Howard, E., D. M. Granoff, and P. Bujnovszky. (1969) *Brain Res.* **14:**697–706. DNA, RNA, and cholesterol increases in cerebrum and cerebellum during development of human fetus.

Hoy, R. R. (1973) The curious nature of degeneration and regeneration in motor neurons and central connectives of the crayfish, pp. 203–232. In *Developmental Neurobiology of Arthropods* (D. Young, ed.), Cambridge University Press, London.

Hoy, R. R., G. D. Bittner, and D. Kennedy. (1967) *Science* **156:**251–252. Regeneration in crustacean motoneurons: evidence for axonal fusion.

Hsu, T. C., and C. E. Somer. (1961) *Proc. Natl. Acad. Sci. U.S.A.* **47:**396–403. Effect of 5-bromodeoxyuridine on mammalian chromosomes.

Hubel, D. H., and T. N. Wiesel. (1962) *J. Physiol. (London)* **160:**106–154. Receptive fields, binocular interaction and functional architecture in the cat's visual cortex.

Hubel, D. H., and T. N. Wiesel. (1963*a*) *J. Neurophysiol.* **26:**994–1002. Receptive fields of cells in striate cortex of very young, visually inexperienced kittens.

Hubel, D. H., and T. N. Wiesel. (1963*b*) *J. Physiol. (London)* **165:**559–568. Shape and arrangement of columns in the cat's striate cortex.

Hubel, D. H., and T. N. Wiesel. (1965*a*) *J. Neurophysiol.* **28:**229–289. Receptive fields and functional architecture in two nonstriate areas (18 and 19) of the cat.

Hubel, D. H., and T. N. Wiesel. (1965*b*) *J. Neurophysiol.* **28:**1041–1059. Binocular interaction in striate cortex of kittens reared with artificial squint.

Hubel, D. H., and T. N. Wiesel. (1968) *J. Physiol. (London)* **195:**215–243. Receptive fields and functional architecture of monkey striate cortex.

Hubel, D. H., and T. N. Wiesel. (1970) *J. Physiol. (London)* **206:** 419–436. The period of susceptibility to the physiological effects of unilateral eye closure in kittens.

Hubel, D. H., and T. N. Wiesel. (1971) *J. Physiol. (London)* **218:**33–62. Aberrant visual projections in the Siamese cat.

Hubel, D. H., and T. N. Wiesel. (1972) *J. Comp. Neurol.* **146:**421–450. Laminar and columnar distribution of geniculo-cortical fibers in the macaque monkey.

Hubel, D. H., and T. N. Wiesel. (1974*a*) *J. Comp. Neurol.* **158:**267–294. Sequence regularity and geometry of orientation columns in the monkey striate cortex.

Hubel, D. H., and T. N. Wiesel. (1974*b*) *J. Comp. Neurol.* **158:**295–306. Uniformity of monkey striate cortex: A parallel relationship between field size, scatter and magnification factor.

Hubel, D. H., and T. N. Wiesel. (1974*c*) *J. Comp. Neurol.* **158:**307–318. Ordered arrangement of orientation columns in monkeys lacking visual experience.

Hubel, D. H., T. N. Wiesel, and S. LeVay. (1975) *Cold Spring Harbor Symp. Quant. Biol.* **15:**581–590. Functional architecture of area 17 in normal and monocularly deprived macaque monkeys.

Huber, G. C., and E. C. Crosby. (1933) *Psychiat. Neurol. Bladen* **4:**459–474. The influences of afferent paths on the cytoarchitectonic structure of the submammalian optic tectum.

Hudson, R. C. L. (1969) *J. Exp. Biol.* **50:**47–67. Polyneuronal innervation of the fast muscles of the marine teleost *Cottus scorpius L.*

Hughes, A. F. (1934) *Phil. Trans. Roy. Soc. London B Ser.* **224:**75–129. On the development of the blood vessels in the head of the chick.

Hughes, A. F. (1952) *The Mitotic Cycle, the Cytoplasm and Nucleus during Interphase and Mitosis,* Academic Press, New York.

Hughes, A. F. (1953) *J. Anat. (London)* **87:**150–162. The growth of embryonic neurites. A study on cultures of chick neural tissue.

Hughes, A. F. (1955) *J. Embryol. Exp. Morphol.* **3:**305–325. The development of the neural tube of the chick embryo: A study with the ultraviolet microscope.

Hughes, A. F. (1957) *J. Anat. (London)* **91:**323–338. The development of the primary sensory system in *Xenopus laevis* (Daudin).

Hughes, A. F. (1961) *J. Embryol. Exp. Morphol.* **9:**269–284. Cell degeneration in the larval ventral horn of *Xenopus laevis* (Daudin).

Hughes, A. F. (1966) *J. Embryol. Exp. Morphol.* **16:**401–430. The thyroid and the development of the nervous system in *Eleutherodactylus martinicensis:* An experimental study.

Hughes, A. F. (1968*a*) *Aspects of Neural Ontogeny,* Logos, London.

Hughes, A. F. (1968*b*) Development of limb innervation, pp. 110–117. In *Ciba Foundation Symposium on Growth of the Nervous System* (G. E. W. Wolstenholme and M. O'Connor, eds), Churchill, London.

Hughes, A. F. (1968*c*) *Adv. Morphogenesis* **7:**79–113. The development of innervation in tetrapod limbs.

Hughes, A. F. (1973) *J. Embryol. Exp. Morphol.* **30:**359–376. The development of dorsal root ganglia and ventral horns in the opossum.

Hughes, A. F. (1974) Endocrines, neural development and behavior, pp. 223–243. In *Aspects of Neurogenesis,* Vol. 2: *Studies on the Development of Behavior and the Nervous System* (G. Gottlieb, ed,), Academic Press, New York.

Hughes, A. F., and V. McM. Carr. (1978) The interaction of periphery and center in the development of dorsal root ganglia, In *Handbook of Sensory Physiology,* Vol IX: *Development of Sensory Systems* (M. Jacobson, ed.), Springer-Verlag, New York.

Hughes, A. F., and M. Egar. (1972) *J. Embryol. Exp. Morphol.* **27:**389–412. The innervation of the hindlimb of *Eleutherodactylus martinicensis:* Further comparison of cell and fiber number during development.

Hughes, A. F., and M. C. Prestige. (1967) *J. Zool. (London)* **152:**347–359. Development of behaviour in the hindlimb of *Xenopus laevis.*

Hughes, A. F., and P.-A. Tschumi. (1958) *J. Anat. (London)* **92:**498–527. The factors controlling the development of the dorsal root ganglia and ventral horn in *Xenopus laevis.*

Hui, R. W., and A. A. Smith. (1972) *Exp. Neurol.* **34:**331–341. Degeneration of taste buds and lateral line organs in the salamander treated with cholinolytic drugs.

Huizinga, J. (1955) *Homo Ludens,* Beacon Press, Boston.

Humphreys, T. (1967) The cell surface and specific cell aggregation, pp. 195–210. In *The Specificity of Cell Surfaces* (B. D. Davis and L. Warren, eds.), Prentice-Hall, Englewood Cliffs, N.J.

Huneeus, F. C., and P. F. Davison, (1970) *J. Mol. Biol.* **52:**415–428. Fibrillar proteins of the squid axoplasm. I. Neurofilament protein.

Hunt, C. C. (1974) The physiology of muscle receptors, pp. 191–234. In *Handbook of Sensory Physiology,* Vol. III/2 (C. C. Hunt, ed.), Springer-Verlag, New York.

Hunt, C. C., and W. K. Riker. (1966) *J. Neurophysiol.* **29:**1096–1114. Properties of frog sympathetic neurones in normal ganglia and after axon section.

Hunt, E. A. (1932) *J. Exp. Zool.* **62:**57–91. The differentiation of the chick limb bud in chorio-allantoic grafts, with special reference to the muscle.

Hunt, R. K. (1975) Developmental programming for retinotectal patterns, pp. 131–150. In *Cell Patterning,* Ciba Foundation Symposium 29, Elsevier, New York.

Hunt, R. K., and E. Frank. (1975) *Science* **189:**563–565. Neuronal locus specificity: Trans-repolarization of *Xenopus* embryonic retina after the time of axial specification.

Hunt, R. K., and M. Jacobson. (1970) *Science* **170:**342–344. Brain enhancement in tadpoles: Increased DNA concentration after somatotrophin or prolactin.

Hunt, R. K., and M. Jacobson. (1971) *Dev. Biol.* **26:**100–124. Neurogenesis in frogs after early larval treatment with somatotropin or prolactin.

Hunt, R. K., and M. Jacobson. (1972*a*) *Proc. Natl. Acad. Sci. U.S.A.* **69:**780–783. Development and stability of positional information in *Xenopus* retinal ganglion cells.

Hunt, R. K., and M. Jacobson. (1972*b*) *Proc. Natl. Acad. Sci. U.S.A.* **69:**2860–2864. Specification of positional information in retinal ganglion cells of *Xenopus:* Stability of the unspecified state.

Hunt, R. K., and M. Jacobson. (1973*a*) *Proc. Natl. Acad. Sci. U.S.A.* **70:**507–511. Specification of positional information in retinal ganglion cells of *Xenopus:* Assay systems for analysis of the unspecified state.

Hunt, R. K., and M. Jacobson. (1973*b*) *Science* **180:**509–511. Neuronal locus specificity: Altered pattern of spatial deployment in fused fragments of embryonic *Xenopus* eyes.

Hunt, R. K. and M. Jacobson. (1974*a*) *Dev. Biol.* **40:**1–15. Development of neuronal locus specificity in *Xenopus* retinal ganglion cells after surgical eye transection or after fusion of whole eyes.

Hunt, R. K., and M. Jacobson. (1974*b*) *Proc. Natl. Acad. Sci. U.S.A.* **71:**3616–3620. Specification of positional information in retinal ganglion cells of *Xenopus laevis:* Intra-ocular control of the time of specification.

Hunt, R. K., and M. Jacobson. (1974*c*) Neuronal specificity revisited, pp. 203–258. In *Current Topics in Developmental Biology,* Vol. 8 (A. Moscona and A. Monroy, eds.), Academic Press, New York.

Hunt, R. K., and M. Jacobson. (1974*d*) *J. Physiol. (London)* **241:**90–91P. Rapid reversal of retinal axes in embryonic *Xenopus* eyes.

Hunt, S. P., and K. E. Webster. (1975) *J. Comp. Neurol.* **162:**433–446. The projection of the retina upon the optic tectum of the pigeon.

Hursh, J. B. (1939) *Am. J. Physiol.* **127:**131–139. Conduction velocity and diameter of nerve fibers.

Huttenlocher, P. R. (1966) *Nature* **211:**91–92. Development of neuronal activity in neocortex of the kitten.

Huttenlocher, P. R. (1967) *Exp. Neurol.* **17:**247–262. Development of cortical neuronal activity in the neonatal cat.

Huttenlocher, P. R. (1970) *Exp. Neurol.* **29:**405–415. Myelination and the development of function in immature pyramidal tract.

Huxley, A. F., and R. Stämpfli. (1949) *J. Physiol. (London)* **108:**315–339. Evidence for saltatory conduction in peripheral myelinated nerve fibres.

Huxley, J. S. (1932) *Problems of Relative Growth,* Methuen, London.

Huxley, J. S., and G. R. De Beer. (1934) *The Elements of Experimental Embryology,* Cambridge University Press, London, 514 pp.

Hydén, H. (1943) *Acta Physiol. Scand. Suppl.* **176:**1–136. Protein metabolism in the nerve cell during growth and function.

Hydén, H. (1960) The neuron, pp. 215–323. In *The Cell,* Vol. IV (J. Brachet and A. E. Mirsky, eds.), Academic Press, New York.

Hydén, H. (1962) *Endeavour* **21:**144–155. The neuron and its glia—A biochemical and functional unit.

Hyyppä, M. (1969) *Z. Anat. Entwicklungsgesch.* **129:**41–52. Differentiation of the hypothalamic nuclei during ontogenetic development in the rat.

Ifft, J. D. (1972) *J. Comp. Neurol.* **144:**139–204. An autoradiographic study of the time of final division of neurons in rat hypothalamic nuclei.

Ikeda, K., and W. D. Kaplan (1970*a*) *Proc. Natl. Acad. Sci. U.S.A.* **66:**765–772. Patterned activity of a mutant *Drosophila melanogaster.*

Ikeda, K., and W. D. Kaplan. (1970*b*) *Proc. Natl. Acad. Sci. U.S.A.* **67:**1480–1487. Unilaterally patterned neural activity of gynandromorphs, mosaic for a neurological mutant of *Drosophila melanogaster.*

Iles, J. F., and B. Mulloney. (1971) *Brain Res.* **30:**397–400. Procion yellow staining of cockroach motor neurons without the use of microelectrodes.

Ilyinsky, O. B., N. C. Chalisova, and V. F. Kuznetsov. (1973) *Experientia* **29:**1129–1131. Development of the new Pacinian corpuscles: Studies on the foreign innervation of mesentery.

Ingvar, D. (1947) *Acta Physiol. Scand.* **13:**150–154. Experiments on the influence of electric currents upon growing nerve cell processes *in vitro.*

Ingvar, S. (1920) *Proc. Soc. Exp. Biol. Med. N.Y.* **17:**198–199. Reaction of cells to galvanic current in tissue cultures.

Inouye, E. (1970) *Jpn. J. Hum. Genet.* **15:**1–25. Twin studies and human behavioral genetics.

Inukai, T. (1928) *J. Comp. Neurol.* **45:**1–31. On the loss of Purkinje cells, with advancing age, from the cerebellar cortex of the albino rat.

Jacklet, J. W., and M. J. Cohen. (1967*a*) *Science* **156:**1638–1640. Synaptic connections between a transplanted insect ganglion and muscles of the host.

Jacklet, J. W., and M. J. Cohen. (1967*b*) *Science* **156:**1640–1643. Nerve regeneration: correlation of electrical, histological, and behavioral events.

Jacobs, H. L., and K. N. Sharma. (1969) *Ann. N.Y. Acad. Sci.* **157:**1084–1125. Taste versus calories: Sensory and metabolic signals in the control of food intake.

Jacobson, C.-O. (1959) *J. Embryol. Exp. Morphol.* **7:**1–21. The localization of the presumptive cerebral regions in the neural plate of the axolotl larva.

Jacobson, C.-O. (1962) *Zool. Bidrag. Uppsala* **35:**433–449. Cell migration in the neural plate and the process of neurulation in the axototl larva.

Jacobson, C.-O. (1964) *Zool. Bidrag. Uppsala* **36:**73–160. Motor nuclei, cranial nerve roots, and fibre pattern in the medulla oblongata after reversal experiments on the neural plate of Axolotl. larvae. I. Bilateral operations.

Jacobson, C.-O. (1969) *Zool. Bidrag. Uppsala* **38:**241–247. Production of artificial heterokaryons from mammalian neurons and various undifferentiated cells.

Jacobson, M. (1960*a*) Studies in the organization of visual mechanisms in amphibians. Ph.D. thesis, Edinburgh University.

Jacobson, M. (1960*b*) *J. Physiol. (London)* **154:**31–32P. The representation of the visual field on the optic tectum of the frog: Evidence for the presence of an area centralis retinae.

Jacobson, M. (1961*a*) *J. Physiol. (London)* **157:**27–29P. The recovery of electrical activity in the optic tectum of the frog during early regeneration of the optic nerve.

Jacobson, M. (1961*b*) *Proc. Roy. Phys. Soc. Edinburgh* **28:**131–137. Recovery of electrical activity in the optic tectum of the frog during early regeneration of the optic nerve.

Jacobson, M. (1962) *Quart. J. Exp. Physiol.* **47:**170–178. The representation of the retina on the optic tectum of the frog: Correlation between retinotectal magnification factor and retinal ganglion cell count.

Jacobson, M. (1966) Starting points for research in the ontogeny of behavior, pp. 339–383. In *Major Problems in Developmental Biology* (M. Locke, ed.), Academic Press, New York.

Jacobson, M. (1967) *Science* **155:**1106–1108. Retinal ganglion cells: specification of central connections in larval *Xenopus laevis.*

Jacobson, M. (1968*a*) *Dev. Biol.* **17:**202–218. Development of neuronal specificity in retinal ganglion cells of *Xenopus.*

Jacobson, M. (1968*b*) *Dev. Biol.* **17:**219–232. Cessation of DNA synthesis in retinal ganglion cells correlated with the time of specification of their central connections.

Jacobson, M. (1969) *Science* **163:**543–547. Development of specific neuronal connections.

Jacobson, M. (1970*a*) Development, specification and diversification of neuronal connections. In *The Neurosciences: Second Study Program* (F. O. Schmitt, ed.-in-chief), Rockefeller University Press, New York.

Jacobson, M. (1970*b*) *Developmental Neurobiology,* Holt, Rinehart and Winston, New York.

Jacobson, M. (1971*a*) Formation of neuronal connections in sensory systems. In *Handbook of Sensory Physiology,* Vol. 1, Chap. 6 (W. Loewenstein, ed.), Springer-Verlag, New York.

Jacobson, M. (1971*b*) *Proc. Natl. Acad. Sci. U.S.A.* **68:**528–532. Absence of adaptive modification in developing retinotectal connections in frogs after visual deprivation or disparate stimulation of the eyes.

Jacobson, M. (1973) Genesis of neuronal specificity, pp. 105–119. In *Development and Ageing in the Nervous System* (M. Rockstein, ed.), Academic Press, New York.

Jacobson, M. (1974*a*) Neuronal plasticity: Concepts in pursuit of cellular mechanisms, pp. 31–43. In *Plasticity and Recovery of Function in the Central Nervous System* (D. G. Stein, J. J. Rosen, and N. Butler, eds.), Academic Press, New York.

Jacobson, M. (1974*b*) A plentitude of neurons, pp. 151–166. In *Studies on the Development of Behavior and the Nervous System,* Vol. 2 (G. Gottlieb, ed.), Academic Press, New York.

Jacobson, M. (1974*c*) *Ann. N.Y. Acad. Sci.* **228:**63–67. Through the jungle of the brain: Neuronal specificity and typology re-explored.

Jacobson, M. (1975*a*) Development and evolution of Type II neurons: Conjectures a century after Golgi. In *Golgi Centennial Symposium* (M. Santini, ed.), Raven Press, New York.

Jacobson, M. (1975*b*) Differentiation and growth of nerve cells. In *Differentiation and Growth of Cells in Vertebrate Tissues,* Chap. 2 (G. Golspink, ed.), Chapman and Hall, London.

Jacobson, M. (1975*c*) Brain development in relation to language, pp. 105–119. In *Foundations of Language Development,* Vol. 1 (E. H. Lenneberg and E. Lenneberg, eds.), UNESCO and Academic Press, Paris and New York.

Jacobson, M. (1976*a*) *Brain Res.* **103:**541–545. Histogenesis of retina in the clawed frog with implications for the pattern of development of retinotectal connections.

Jacobson, M. (1976*b*) *Science* **191:**288–290. Premature specification of the retina in embryonic *Xenopus* eyes treated with ionophore X537A.

Jacobson, M. (1976*c*) Neuronal recognition in the retinotectal system. In *Neuronal Recognition* (S. Barondes, ed.), Plenum, New York.

Jacobson, M. (1977) *Brain Res.* **127:**55–67. Mapping the developing retino-tectal projection in frog tadpoles by a double label autoradiographic technique.

Jacobson, M., and R. E. Baker. (1968) *Science* **160:**543–545. Neuronal specification of cutaneous nerves through connections with skin grafts in the frog.

Jacobson, M., and R. E. Baker. (1969) *J. Comp. Neurol.* **137:**121–142. Development of neuronal connections with skin grafts in frogs: Behavioral and electrophysiological studies.

Jacobson, M., and R. M. Gaze. (1964) *Quart. J. Exp. Physiol.* **49:**199–209. Types of visual response from single units in the optic tectum and optic nerve of the goldfish.

Jacobson, M., and R. M. Gaze. (1965) *Exp. Neurol.* **13:**418–430. Selection of appropriate tectal connections by regenerating optic nerve fibres in adult goldfish.

Jacobson, M., and H. V. B. Hirsch. (1973) *Brain Res.* **49:**47–65. Development and maintenance of connectivity in the visual system of the frog. I. The effects of eye rotation and visual deprivation.

Jacobson, M., and R. K. Hunt. (1973) *Sci. Am.* **228:**26–35. Origins of neuronal specificity.

Jacobson, M., and R. L. Levine. (1975*a*) *Brain Res.* **88:**339–345. Plasticity in the adult frog brain: Filling the visual scotoma after excision or translocation of parts of the optic tectum.

Jacobson, M., and R. Levine. (1975*b*) *Brain Res.* **92:**468–471. Stability of implanted duplicate tectal positional markers serving as targets for optic axons in adult frogs.

Jacobson, S. (1963) *J. Comp. Neurol.* **121:**5–29. Sequence of myelinization in the brain of the albino rat. A. Cerebral cortex, thalamus and related structures.

Jaffe, L. (1955) *Proc. Natl. Acad. Sci. U.S.A.* **41:**267–270. Do *Fucus* eggs interact through a CO_2-pH gradient?

Jaffe, L. (1968) *Adv. Morphogen.* **7:**295–328. Localization in the developing *Fucus* egg and the general role of localizing currents.

Jahn, T. L., and E. C. Bovee. (1969) *Physiol. Rev.* **49:**793–862. Protoplasmic movements within cells.

James, D. W., and R. L. Tresman. (1969) *Z. Zellforsch. Mikrosk. Anat. Abt. Histochem.* **100:**126–140. An electron microscopic study of the *de novo* formation of neuromuscular junctions in tissue culture.

Jansen, J. K. S., and J. G. Nicholls. (1972) *Proc. Natl. Acad. Sci. U.S.A.* **69:**636–639. Regeneration and changes in synaptic connections between individual nerve cells in the central nervous system of the leech.

Jansen, J. K. S., T. Lömo, K. Nicolaysen, and R. H. Westgaard. (1973) *Science* **181:**559–561. Hyperinnervation of skeletal muscle fibers: Dependence on muscle activity.

Jarlstedt, J., and J.-O. Karlsson. (1973) *Exp. Brain Res.* **16:**501–506. Evidence for axonal transport of RNA in mammalian neurons.

Jeffrey, P. L., and L. Austin. (1973) *Prog. Neurobiol.* **2:**207–255. Axoplasmic transport.

Jeffrey, P. L., K. A. C. James, A. D. Kidman, A. M. Richards, and L. Austin. (1972) *J. Neurobiol.* **3:**199–208. The flow of mitochondria in chicken sciatic nerve.

Jelínek, R. (1959) *Csk. Morfol.* **7:**163–173. Proliferace v centrálním nervovém kuřecich zárodku. I. Doba trvání mitosy v germinální zonĕ míchy od 2. do 6. dne zárodečného vývoje.

Jellinger, K. (1972) *Z. Anat. Entwicklungsgesch.* **138:**145–154. Embryonal cell nests in human cerebellar nuclei.

Jerison, H. J. (1963) *Hum. Biol.* **35:**263–291. Interpreting the evolution of the brain.

Jerison, H. J. (1969) *Am. Nat.* **103:**575–588. Brain evolution and dinosaur brains.

Jerison, H. J. (1970) *Science* **170:**1224–1225. Brain evolution: New light on old principles.

Jirminová, I., and S. Thesleff. (1972) *Z. Zellforsch.* **131:**77–97. Ultrastructural study of experimental muscle degeneration and regeneration in the adult rat.

Jirmanová, I., and J. Zelená. (1970) *Z. Zellforsch. Mikrosk. Anat.* **106:**333–347. Effect of denervation and tenotomy on slow and fast muscles of the chicken.

Jirmanová, I., and J. Zelená. (1973) *Z. Zellforsch. Mikrosk. Anat.* **146:**103–121. Ultrastructural transformation of fast chicken muscle fibres induced by nerve cross-union.

Jirmanová, I., and J. Zelená, (1974) *Folia Morphol. (Praha)* **22:**270–272. Ultrastructural transformation of fast chicken muscles reinnervated with slow-type nerves.

Johannsen, O. A., and F. H. Butt. (1941) *Embryology of Insects and Myriapods,* McGraw-Hill, New York.

Johnen, A. G. (1964) *Arch. Entwmech. Organ.* **155:**302–313. Experimentelle Untersuchungen über die Bedeutung des Zeitfaktors beim Vorgang der neuralen Induktion.

Johns, T. R., and S. Thesleff. (1961) *Acta Physiol. Scand.* **51:**136–141. Effects of motor inactivation on the chemical sensitivity of skeletal muscle.

Johnson, R., and M. Armstrong-James. (1970) *Z. Zellforsch Mikrosk. Anat.* **110:**540–558. Morphology of superficial postnatal cerebral cortex with special reference to synapses.

Johnston, M. C. (1966) *Anat. Rec.* **156:**143–156. A radioautographic study of the migration and fate of cranial neural crest cells in the chick embryo.

Jones, D. G. (1973) *Z. Zellforsch. Mikrosk. Anat.* **143:**301–312. Some factors affecting the PTA staining of synaptic junctions: A preliminary comparison of PTA stained junctions in various regions of the CNS.

Jones, D. G., M. M. Dittmer, and L. C. Reading. (1974) *Brain Res.* **70:**245–259. Synaptogenesis in guinea-pig cerebral cortex: A glutaraldehyde-PTA study.

Jones, E. G., H. Burton, and R. Porter. (1975) *Science* **190:**572–574. Commissural and cortico-cortical "columns" in the somatic sensory cortex of primates.

Joseph, B., and D. Whitlock. (1968) *Anat. Rec.* **160:**279–288. Central projections of selected spinal dorsal roots in anuran amphibians.

Joseph, J. (1948) *J. Anat. (London)* **82:**146–152. Changes in nuclear population following twenty-one days degeneration in a nerve consisting of small myelinated fibers.

Jouan, P., S. Samperez, M. L. Thieulant, and L. Mercier. (1971) *J. Steroid Biochem.* **2:**223–236. Etude du récepteur cytoplasmique de la [1,2-^{3}H]testostérone dan l'hypothalamus du rat.

Jouan, P., S. Samperez, and M. L. Thieulant. (1973) *J. Steroid Biochem.* **4:**65–74. Testosterone "receptors" in purified nuclei of rat anterior hypophysis.

Juntunen, J. (1973*a*) *Z. Anat. Entwicklungsgesch.* **143:**1–12. Morphogenesis of the myoneural junctions after immobilization of the muscle in the rat.

Juntunen, J. (1973*b*) *Z. Zellforsch. Mikrosk. Anat.* **142:**193–204. Effects of colchicine and vinblastine on neurotubules of the sciatic nerve and cholinesterases in the developing myoneural junction of the rat.

Kaas, J. H., and R. W. Guillery. (1973) *Brain Res.* **59:**61–95. The transfer of abnormal visual field representations from the dorsal lateral geniculate nucleus to the visual cortex in Siamese cats.

Kadanoff, D. (1925) *Arch. Entw.-Mech. Organ.* **106:**249–278. Untersuchungen über die Regeneration der sensiblen Nervenendigungen nach Vertauschung verschieden innervierten Hautstücke.

Kahn, A. J. (1973) *Brain Res.* **63:**285–290. Ganglion cell formation in the chick neural retina.

Kahn, A. J. (1974) *Dev. Biol.* **38:**30–40. An autoradiographic analysis of the time of appearance of neurons in the developing chick neural retina.

Kahn, M. A., and S. Ochs. (1975) *Brain Res.* **96:**267–277. Slow axoplasmic transport of mitochondria (MAO) and lactic dehydrogenase in mammalian nerve fibers.

Kalil, R. E., (1973) *Anat. Rec.* **175:**353. Formation of new retino-geniculate connections in kittens: Effects of age and visual experience.

Kalil, R. E., and G. E. Schneider. (1975) *Brain Res.* **100:**690–698. Abnormal synaptic connections of the optic tract in the thalamus after midbrain lesions in newborn hamster.

Källén, B. (1955) *J. Anat. (London)* **85:**153–161. Cell degeneration during normal ontogenesis of the rabbit brain.

Källén, B. (1958) *Z. Zellforsch, Mikrosk. Anat. Abt. Histochem.* **47:**469–480. Studies on the differentiation capacity of neural epithelium cells in chick embryos.

Källén, B. (1961) *Z. Anat. Entwicklungsgesch.* **122:**388–401. Studies on cell proliferation in the brain of chick embryos with special reference to the mesencephalon.

Källén, B. (1962) *Z. Anat. Entwicklungsgesch.* **123:**309–319. Mitotic patterning in the central nervous system of chick embryos studied by a colchicine method.

Källén, B. (1965) *Prog. Brain Res.* **14:**77–96. Degeneration and regeneration in the vertebrate central nervous system during embryogenesis.

Kalter, H. (1968) *Teratology of the Central Nervous System,* University of Chicago Press, Chicago, 483 pp.

Kalugina, M. A. (1956) *Ark. Anat. Gistol. Embriol.* **33**:59–63. On the question of the development of proprioceptors in the striated muscle of mammals. (In Russian.)

Kamrin, R. P., and M. Singer. (1953) *Am. J. Physiol.* **174**:146–148. Influence of sensory neurons isolated from central nervous system on maintenance of taste buds and regeneration of barbels in the catfish.

Kankel, D. R., and J. C. Hall. (1976) *Dev. Biol.* **48**:1–24. Fate mapping of nervous system and other internal tissues in genetic mosaics of *Drosophila melanogaster.*

Karfunkel, P. (1971) *Dev. Biol.* **25**:30–56. The role of microtubules and microfilaments in neurulation in *Xenopus.*

Karfunkel, P. (1972) *J. Exp. Zool.* **181**:289–302. The activity of microtubules and microfilaments in neurulation in the chick.

Karfunkel, P. (1974) *Int. Rev. Cytol.* **38**:245–271. The mechanisms of neural tube formation.

Karlin, A. (1974) *Life Sci.,* **14**:1385–1415. The acetylcholine receptor: Progress report.

Karlsson, J.-O., and J. Sjöstrand. (1968) *Brain Res.* **11**:431–439. Transport of labelled protein in the optic nerve and tract of the rabbit.

Karlsson, J.-O., and J. Sjöstrand. (1969) *Brain Res.* **13**:617–619. The effect of colchicine on the axonal transport of protein in the optic nerve and tract of the rabbit.

Karlsson, J.-O., and J. Sjöstrand (1971*a*) *J. Neurochem.* **18**:749–767. Synthesis, migration and turnover of protein in retinal ganglion cells.

Karlsson, J.-O., and J. Sjöstrand. (1971*b*) *J. Neurochem.* **18**:975–982. Transport of microtubular protein in axons of retinal ganglion cells.

Karlsson, J.-O., and J. Sjöstrand (1971*c*) *J. Neurochem.* **18**:2209–2216. Rapid intracellular transport of fucose-containing glycoproteins in retinal ganglion cells.

Karlsson, J.-O., H.-A. Hansson, and J. Sjöstrand. (1971) *Z. Zellforsch. Mikrosk. Anat.* **115**:265–283. Effect of colchicine on axonal transport and morphology of retinal ganglion cells.

Karlsson, U. (1966*a*) *J. Ultrastruct. Res.* **16**:429–481. Three-dimensional studies of neurons in the lateral geniculate nucleus of the rat. I. Organelle organization in the perikaryon and its proximal branches.

Karlsson, U. (1966*b*) *J. Ultrastruct. Res.* **16**:482–504. Three-dimensional studies of neurons in the lateral geniculate nucleus of the rat. II. Environment of perikarya and proximal parts of their branches.

Karlsson, U. (1967) *J. Ultrastruct. Res.* **17**:158–175. Observations on the postnatal development of neuronal structures in the lateral geniculate nucleus of the rat by electron microscopy.

Karpati, G., and W. K. Engel. (1967) *Nature* **215**:1509. Transformation of the histochemical profile of skeletal muscle by "foreign" innervation.

Karssen, A., and B. Sager. (1934) *Arch. Exp. Zellforsch.* **16**:255–259. Sur l'influence du courant électrique sur la croissance des neuroblastes *in vivo.*

Kater, S. B., C. Nicholson, and W. J. Davis. (1973) A guide to intracellular staining techniques, pp. 307–325. In *Intracellular Staining in Neurobiology* (S. B. Kater and C. Nicholson, eds.), Springer-Verlag, New York.

Kato, J., and T. Onouchi. (1973) *Endocrinol. Jpn.* **20**:429–432. 5d-Dihydrotestosterone "receptor" in the rat hypothalamus.

Kato, J., and C. A. Villee. (1967) *Endocrinology* **80**:567–575. Preferential uptake of estradiol by the anterior hypothalamus of the rat.

Katz, B., and R. Miledi. (1964) *J. Physiol. (London)* **170**:389–396. The development of acetylcholine sensitivity in nerve free segments of skeletal muscle.

Kauffman, R. C., J. E. Warnick, and E. X. Albuquerque. (1974) *Exp. Neurol.* **44**:404–416. Uptake of [^{3}H]colchicine from silastic implants by mammalian nerves and muscles.

Kauffman, S. L. (1968) *Exp. Cell Res.* **49**:420–424. Lengthening of the generation cycle during embryonic differentiation of the mouse neural tube.

Kawana, E., C. Sandri, and K. Akert. (1971) *Z. Zellforsch. Mikrosk. Anat.* **115**:284–298. Ultrastructure of growth cones in the cerebellar cortex of the neonatal rat and cat.

Keating, M. J. (1968) *J. Physiol. (London)* **198**:75P. Functional interaction in the development of specific nerve connexions.

Keating, M. J. (1974) *Br. Med. Bull.* **30**:145–151. The role of visual function in the patterning of binocular visual connexions.

Keating, M. J. (1975*a*) *J. Physiol. (London)* **248:**36–37P. Plasticity of intertectal connexions in adult *Xenopus.*

Keating, M. J. (1975*b*) *Proc. Roy. Soc. London (Biol.)* **189:**603–610. The time course of experience-dependent synaptic switching of visual connections in *Xenopus laevis.*

Keating, M. J., and J. D. Feldman. (1975) *Proc. Roy. Soc. London (Biol.)* **191:**467–474. Visual deprivation and intertectal neuronal connections in *Xenopus laevis.*

Keating, M. J., and R. M. Gaze. (1970*a*) *Brain Behav. Evol.* **3:**102–120. Rigidity and plasticity in the amphibian visual system.

Keating, M. J., and R. M. Gaze. (1970*b*) *Am. J. Exp. Physiol.* **55:**284–292. The ipsilateral retinotectal pathway in the frog.

Keene, M. F. L., and E. E. Hewer. (1931) *J. Anat. (London)* **66:**1–13. Some observations on myelination in the human central nervous system.

Keene, M. F. L., and E. E. Hewer. (1933) *J. Anat. (London)* **67:**522–536. The development and myelination of the posterior longitudinal bundle in the human.

Keller, H. U., and E. Sorkin. (1968) *Experientia* **24:**641–652. Chemotaxis of leucocytes.

Keller, R. E. (1975) *Dev. Biol.* **42:**222–241. Vital dye mapping of the gastrula and neurula of *Xenopus laevis.*

Kelly, A. M., and S. I. Zacks. (1969) *J. Cell Biol.* **42:**154–169. The fine structure of motor endplate morphogenesis.

Kelly, J. P., and W. M. Cowan. (1972) *Brain Res.* **42:**263–288. Studies on the development of the chick optic tectum. III. Effects of early eye removal.

Kelly, J. P., and D. C. Van Essen. (1974) *J. Physiol. (London)* **238:**515–547. Cell structure and function in the visual cortex of the cat.

Kelton, D. E. and H. Rauch (1962) *Exp. Neurol.* **6:**252–262. Myelination and myelin degeneration in the central nervous system of dilute–lethal mice.

Kemali, M. (1976) *Experientia* **32:**747–748. An "ultra" rapid Golgi method for vertebrate neuroanatomy.

Kemali, M., and V. Braitenberg. (1969) *Atlas of the Frog's Brain,* Springer-Verlag, Berlin, 74 pp.

Kennard, D. W. (1959) *J. Comp. Neurol.* **111:**447–467. The anatomical organization of neurons in the lumbar region of the spinal cord of the frog (*Rana temporaria*).

Kennard, M. A. (1940) *Arch. Neurol. Psychiat.* **44:**377–397. Relation of age to motor impairment in man and in subhuman primates.

Kennard, M. A. (1942) *Arch. Neurol. Psychiat.* **48:**227–240. Cortical reorganization of motor function: Studies on series of monkeys of various ages from infancy to maturity.

Kerkut, G. A., A. Shapira, and R. J. Walker. (1967) *Comp. Biochem Physiol.* **23:**729–748. The transport of ^{14}C-labelled material from CNS$\leftrightarrows$muscle along a nerve trunk.

Kerns, J. M., and E. J. Hinsman (1973*a*) *J. Comp. Neurol.* **151:**237–254. Neuroglial response to sciatic neurectomy. I. Light microscopy and autoradiography.

Kerns, J. M., and E. J. Hinsman. (1973*b*) *J. Comp. Neurol.* **151:**255–280. Neuroglial response to sciatic neurectomy. II. Electron microscopy.

Kerr, F. W. L. (1972) *Brain Res.* **43:**547–560. The potential of cervical primary afferents to sprout in the spinal nucleus of V following long term trigeminal denervation.

Kerr, F. W. L. (1975*a*) *Exp. Neurol.* **48:**16–31. Structural and functional evidence of plasticity in the central nervous system.

Kerr, F. W. L. (1975*b*) *J. Comp. Neurol.* **163:**305–328. Neuro plasticity of primary afferents in the neonatal cat and some results of early deafferentation of the trigeminal spinal nucleus.

Kershman, J. (1938) *Arch. Neurol. Psychiat. (Chicago)* **40:**937–967. The medulloblast and the medulloblastoma; a study of human embryos.

Kershman, J. (1939) *Arch. Neurol. Psychiat. (Chicago)* **41:**24–50. Genesis of microglia in the human brain.

Khan, M. A., and S. Ochs. (1974) *Brain Res.* **81:**413–426. Magnesium or calcium activated ATPase in mammalian nerve.

Kicliter, E., L. J. Misantone, and D. J. Stelzner. (1974) *Brain Res.* **82:**293–297. Neuronal specificity and plasticity in frog visual system: Anatomical correlates.

Kiehlman, B. A. (1966) *The Actions of Chemicals on Dividing Cells,* Prentice-Hall, Englewood Cliffs, N.J.

Kilham, L., and G. Margolis. (1964) *Science* **143:**1047–1048. Cerebellar ataxia in hamsters inoculated with rat virus.

Kilham, L., and G. Margolis. (1965) *Science* **148:**244–246. Cerebellar disease in cats induced by inoculation of rat virus.

Kilham, L., and G. Margolis. (1966*a*) *Am. J. Pathol.* **48:**991–1011. Viral etiology of spontaneous ataxia of cats.

Kilham, L., and G. Margolis. (1966*b*) *Am. J. Pathol.* **49:**457–485. Spontaneous hepatitis and cerebellar "hypoplasia" in suckling rats due to congenital infections with rat virus.

Killackey, H. P., G. Belford, R. Ryugo, and D. K. Ryugo. (1976) *Brain Res.* **104:**309–315. Anomalous organization of thalamomocortical projections consequent to vibrissae removal in the newborn rat and mouse.

Kim, S. U. (1975) *Brain Res.* **88:**52–58. Formation of unattached spines of Purkinje cell dendrite in organotypic cultures of mouse cerebellum.

Kimmel, C. B., and R. C. Eaton. (1976) Development of the Mauthner cell, pp. 186–302. In *Simpler Networks and Behavior* (J. C. Fentress, ed.), Sinauer, Sunderland, Mass.

Kimmel, C. B., and E. Schabtach. (1974) *J. Comp. Neurol.* **156:**49–80. Patterning in synaptic knobs which connect with Mauthner's cell (*Ambystoma mexicanum*).

King. T. J., and R. Briggs. (1956) *Cold Spring Harbor Symp. Quant. Biol.* **21:**271–290. Serial transplantation of embryonic nuclei.

Kirsche, W., and K. Kirsche. (1961) *Z. Mikrosk. Anat. Forsch.* **67:**140–182. Experimentelle Untersuchungen zur Frage der Regeneration und Funktion des Tectum opticum von Carassius carassius L.

Kitchin, I. C. (1949) *J. Exp. Zool.* **112:**393–415. The effects of notochordectomy in *Amblystoma mexicanum.*

Klatzko, I., and J. Miquel. (1960) *J. Neuropathol. Exp. Neurol.* **19:**475–487. Observations on pinocytosis in nervous tissue.

Kleihues, P., P. L. Lantos, and P. N. Magee. (1976) *Int. Rev. Exp. Pathol.* **15:**153–232. Chemical carcinogenesis in the nervous system.

Kleinfeld, R. G., and J. E. Sisken. (1966) *J. Cell Biol.* **31:**369. Morphological and kinetic aspects of mitotic arrest by and recovery from colcemid.

Klingman, G. I., and J. D. Klingman. (1967) *Int. J. Neuropharmacol.* **6:**501–508. Catecholamines in peripheral tissues of mice and cell counts of sympathetic ganglia after the prenatal and postnatal administration of the nerve growth factor antiserum.

Knobler, R. L., and J. G. Stempak. (1973) *Prog. Brain Res.* **40:**407–423. Serial section analysis of myelin development in the central nervous system of the albino rat: An electron microscopical study of early axonal ensheathment.

Kobayashi, T., O. R. Inman, W. Buno, and H. E. Himwich. (1964) *Prog. Brain Res.* **9:**87–88. Neurohistological studies of developing mouse brain.

Koch, W. E. (1967) *J. Exp. Zool.* **165:**155–170. *In vitro* differentiation of tooth rudiments of embryonic mice. I. Transfilter interaction of embryonic incisor tissues.

Koch, W. E., and C. Grobstein. (1963) *Dev. Biol.* **7:**303–323. Transmission of radioisotopically labeled materials during embryonic induction *in vitro.*

Koda, L. Y., and L. M. Partlow. (1976) *J. Neurobiol.* **7:**157–172. Membrane marker movement on sympathetic axons in tissue culture.

Koeke, H. U. (1960) *Arch. Entw.-Mech. Organ.* **151:**612–659. Untersuchungen über die regionalen Potenzen der Neuralleiste zur Bildung von Melanoblasten bei der Hausente (*Anas domestica*).

Koelliker, A. (1896) *Handbuch der Gewebelehre des Menschen,* Bd. 2: *Nervensystem des Menschen und der Thiere,* 6, Aufl., W. Engelmann, Leipzig.

Koenig, E. (1965) *J. Neurochem.* **12:**357–361. Synthetic mechanisms in the axon. II. RNA in myelin-free axons of the cat.

Koenig, E. (1967) *J. Neurochem.* **14:**437–446. Synthetic mechanisms in the axon. IV. *In vitro* incorporation of [^{3}H] precursors into axonal protein and RNA.

Koenig, H. L., L. DiGiamberardino, and G. Bennett. (1973) *Brain Res.* **62:**413–417. Renewal of proteins and glycoproteins of synaptic constituents by means of axonal transport.

Koenig, J. (1971) *Arch. Anat. Microsc. Morphol. Exp.* **60:**1–26. Contribution a l'étude de la réaformation expérimentale des plaques motrices de rat.

Koenig, J. (1973) *Brain Res.* **62:**361–365. Morphogenesis of motor end-plates "*in vivo*" and "*in vitro.*"

Kollros, J. J. (1942) *Proc. Soc. Exp. Biol. Med.* **49:**204–206. Localized maturation of lid-closure reflex mechanism by thyroid implants into tadpole hindbrain.

Kollros, J. J. (1943*a*) *Physiol. Zool.* **16:**269–279. Experimental studies on the development of the corneal reflex in Amphibia. II. Localized maturation of the reflex mechanism effected by thyroxin-agar implants into the hindbrain.

Kollros, J. J. (1943*b*) *J. Exp. Zool.* **92:**121–142. Experimental studies on the development of the corneal reflex in amphibia. III. The influence of the periphery upon the reflex center.

Kollros, J. J. (1953) *J. Exp. Zool.* **123:**153–187. The development of the optic lobes in the frog. I. The effects of unilateral enucleation in embryonic stages.

Kollros, J. J. (1958) *Science* **128:**1505. Hormonal control of onset of corneal reflex in the frog.

Kollros, J. J. (1968*a*) Endocrine influences in neural development, pp. 179–199. In *Growth of the Nervous System,* Ciba Found. Symp. (G. E. W. Wolstenholme and M. O'Connor, eds.), Little, Brown, Boston.

Kollros, J. J. (1968*b*) *Dev. Biol. Suppl.* **2:**274–305. Order and control of neurogenesis (as exemplified by the lateral motor column).

Kollros, J. J., and V. M. McMurray. (1956) *J. Exp. Zool.* **131:**1–26. The mesencephalic V nucleus in anurans. II. The influence of thyroid hormone on cell size and cell number.

Kollros, J. J., and V. Pepernik. (1952) *Anat. Rec.* **113:**527. Hormonal control of the size of mesencephalic V nucleus cells in *Rana pipiens.*

Kollros, J. J., and J. Race, Jr. (1960) *Anat. Rec.* **136:**224. Hormonal control of development of the lateral motor column cells in the lumbo-sacral cord in *Rana pipiens* tadpoles.

Konigsmark, B. W. (1970) Methods for the counting of neurons. In *Contemporary Research Methods in Neuroanatomy* (W. J. H. Nauta and S. O. E. Ebbeson, eds.). Springer-Verlag, New York.

Konigsmark, B. W., and E. A. Murphy. (1970) *Nature* **228:**1335–1336. Neuronal populations in the human brain.

Konigsmark, B. W., and E. A. Murphy. (1972) *J. Neuropathol. Exp. Neurol.* **31:**304–306. Volume of the ventral cochlear nucleus in man—Its relationship to neuronal population and age.

Konigsmark, B. W., and R. L. Sidman. (1963*a*) *J. Neuropathol Exp. Neurol.* **22:**327–328. Origin of gitter cells in the mouse brain.

Konigsmark, B. W., and Sidman, R. L. (1963*b*) *J. Neuropathol. Exp. Neurol.* **22:**643–676. Origin of brain macrophages in the mouse.

Konijn, T. M., D. S. Barkley, Y. Y. Chang, and J. T. Bonner. (1968) *Am. Nat.* **102:**225–233. Cyclic AMP: a naturally occurring acrasin in the cellular slime molds.

Konorski, J. (1967) *Integrative Activity of the Brain,* University of Chicago Press, Chicago.

Koppisch, E. (1935) *Z. Hyg. Infektionskrankh.* **117:**386–398. Zur Wanderungsgeschwindigkeit neurotroper Virusarten in peripheren Nerven.

Korneliussen, H. K. (1967) *J. Hirnforsch.* **9:**151–185. Cerebellar corticogenesis in Cetacea, with special reference to regional variations.

Korner, A. (1968) *Prog. Biophys. Mol. Biol.* **17:**63–98. Ribonucleic acid and hormonal control of protein synthesis.

Korner, A. (1970) *Proc. Roy. Soc. London Ser. B* **176:**287–290. Hormonal control of protein synthesis.

Kornguth, S. E., and G. Scott. (1972) *J. Comp. Neurol.* **146:**61–82. The role of climbing fibers in the formation of Purkinje cell dendrites.

Kornguth, S. E., J. W. Anderson, and G. Scott. (1967) *J. Comp. Neurol.* **130:**1–24. Observations on the ultrastructure of the developing cerebellum of the *Macaca mulatta.*

Kornguth, S. E., J. W. Anderson, and G. Scott. (1968) *J. Comp. Neurol.* **132:**531–546. The development of synaptic contacts in the cerebellum of *Macaca mulatta.*

Korr, H. (1968) *Z. Morphol. Oekol. Tiere* **62:**389–422. Das postembryonale Wachstum verschiedener Hirnbereiche by *Orchesella villosa* L. (Ins. Collembola).

Korr, H., B. Schultze, and W. Maurer. (1973) *J. Comp. Neurol.* **150:**169–176. Autoradiographic investigations of glial proliferation in the brain of adult mice. I. The DNA synthesis phase of neuroglia and endothelial cells.

Korr, I. M., and G. S. L. Appeltauer. (1974) *Exp. Neurol.* **43:**452–463. The time-course of axonal transport of neuronal proteins to muscle.

Korr, I. M., P. N. Wilkinson, and F. W. Chornock. (1967) *Science* **155:**342–346. Axonal delivery of neuroplasmic components to muscle cells.

Koshtoyantz, C., and A. Ryabinovskaya. (1935) *Pfluegers Arch. Ges. Physiol.* **235:**416–421. Beitrag zur Physiologie der Skelettmuskeln der Säugetiere in verschiedenen Stadien ihrer individuellen Entwicklung.

Kosunen, T. U., and B. H. Waksman. (1963) *J. Neuropath. Exp. Neurol.* **22:**324–326. Radioautographic studies of experimental allergic encephalomyelitis (EAE) in rats.

Kosunen, T. U., B. H. Waksman, and I. K. Samuelson. (1963) *J. Neuropath. Exp. Neurol.* **22:**367–380. Radio-autographic study of cellular mechanisms in delayed hypersensitivity. II. Experimental allergic encephalomyelitis in the rat.

Koyré, A. (1956) *Bull. Soc. Fr. Phil.* **50:**59–97. L'hypothèse et l'expérience chez Newton.

Kratz, K. E., and P. D. Spear. (1976) *J. Comp. Neurol.* **170:**141–151. Effects of visual deprivation and alterations in binocular competition on responses of striate cortex neurons in the cat.

Kreutzberg, G. W. (1966) *Acta Neuropathol.* **7**:149–161. Autoradiographische Untersuchung über die Beteiligung von Gliazellen an der axonalen Reaktion im Facilialiskern der Ratte.

Krigman, M. R., and E. L. Hogan. (1976) *Brain Res.* **107**:239–255. Undernutrition in the developing rat: Effect upon myelination.

Krishnan, N., and M. Singer. (1973) *J. Anat.* **136**:1–14. Penetration of peroxidase into peripheral nerve fibers.

Kristensson, K. (1975) Retrograde axonal transport of protein tracers. In *The Use of Axonal Transport for Studies of Neuronal Connectivity* (W. M. Cowan and M. Cuénod, eds.), Elsevier, Amsterdam.

Kristensson, K., and Y. Olsson. (1971) *Brain Res.* **29**:363–365. Retrograde axonal transport of protein.

Kristensson, K.; and Y. Olsson. (1973) *Acta Neuropathol.* **23**:43–47. Uptake and retrograde axonal transport of protein tracers in hypoglossal neurons.

Kristensson, K., and Y. Olsson. (1974) *Brain Res.* **79**:101–109. Retrograde transport of horseradish peroxidase in transected axons. I. Time relationships between transport and induction of chromatolysis.

Kristensson, K., Y. Olsson, and J. Sjöstrand. (1971) *Brain Res.* **32**:399–406. Axonal uptake and retrograde transport of exogenous proteins in the hypoglossal nerve.

Kristensson, K., B. Ghetti, and H. M. Wiśniewski. (1974) *Brain Res.* **69**:189–201. Study on the propagation of *Herpes simplex* virus (type 2) into the brain after intraocular injection.

Kruger, L., and D. S. Maxwell. (1966) *Am. J. Anat.* **118**:411–435. Electron microscopy of oligodendrocytes in normal rat cerebrum.

Kruger, L., and D. S. Maxwell. (1967) *J. Comp. Neur.* **129**:115–142. Comparative fine structure of vertebrate neuroglia: teleosts and reptiles.

Krüger, P., and P. G. Günther. (1955) *Z. Ges. Anat.* **118**:313–323 Fasern mit "Fibrillenstruktur" und Fasern mit "Felderstruktur" in der quergestreiften skeletmuskulatur der Saüger und des Menschen.

Kruska, D. (1970*a*) *Z. Anat. Entwicklungsgesch.* **131**:291–324. Vergleichend cytoarchitektonische Untersuchungen an Gehirnen von Wild- und Hauschweinen.

Kruska, D. (1970*b*) *Z. Säugetierk.* **35**:214–238. Über die Evolution des Gehirns in der Ordnung Artiodactyla Owen, 1848, insbesondere der Teilordnung Suina Gray, 1868.

Kruska, D. (1972) *Z. Anat. Entwicklungsgesch.* **138**:265–282. Volumenvergleich optischer Hirnzentren bei Wild- und Hausschweinen.

Kruska, D., and M. Röhrs. (1974) *Z. Anat. Entwicklungsgesch.* **144**:61–73. Comparative–quantitative investigations on brains of feral pigs from the Galapagos Islands and of European domestic pigs.

Kruska, D., and H. Stephan. (1973) *Acta Anat.* **84**:387–415. Volumenvergleich allokortikaler Hirnzentren bei Wild- und Hausschweinen.

Kuffler, D. P., and K. J. Muller. (1974) *J. Neurobiol.* **5**:331–348. The properties and connections of supernumerary sensory and motor nerve cells in the central nervous system of an abnormal leech.

Kuffler, S. W., and J. G. Nicholls. (1966*a*) *Persp. Biol. Med.* **9**:69–76. How do materials exchange between blood and nerve cells in the brain?

Kuffler, S. W., and J. G. Nicholls. (1966*b*) *Ergeb. Physiol.* **57**:1–90. The physiology of neuroglial cells.

Kuffler, S. W., and J. G. Nicholls. (1976) *From Neuron to Brain,* Sinauer, Sunderland, Mass.

Kuffler, S. W., J. G. Nicholls, and R. K. Orkand. (1966) *J. Neurophysiol.* **29**:768–787. Physiological properties of glial cells in the central nervous system of amphibia.

Kuhlenbeck, H. (1954) *Confin. Neurol.* **14**:329–342. Some histologic age changes in the rat's brain and their relationship to comparable changes in the human brain.

Kuhlenbeck, H. (1967) *The Central Nervous System of Vertebrates,* Vol. 1: *Propaedeutics to Comparative Neurology,* Academic Press, New York.

Kuhlenkampf, H. (1952) *Z. Anat. Entwicklungsgesch.* **116**:304–312. Das Verhalten der Neuroglia in den Vorderhörnen des Rückenmarkes der weissen Maus unter dem Reiz physiologischer Tätigkeit.

Kuhlman, R. E., and O. H. Lowry. (1956) *J. Neurochem.* **1**:173–180. Quantitative histochemical changes during the development of the rat cerebral cortex.

Kumé, M., and K. Dan. (1968) *Invertebrate Embryology,* Nolit, Belgrade, 605 pp.

Kuno, M., and R. Llinás. (1970) *J. Physiol. (London)* **210**:807–821. Enhancement of synaptic transmission by dendritic potentials in chromatolyzed motoneurones of the cat.

Kuno, M., Y. Miyata, and E. J. Muñoz-Martinez. (1974*a*) *J. Physiol. (London)* **240**:725–739. Differential reaction of fast and slow α-motoneurons to axotomy.

Kuno, M., Y. Miyata, and E. J. Muñoz-Martinez. (1974*b*) *J. Physiol. (London)* **242**:273–288. Properties of fast and slow alpha motoneurones following motor reinnervation.

Kupfer, C., and P. Palmer. (1964) *Exp. Neurol.* **9**:400–409. Lateral geniculate nucleus: histological and cytochemical changes following afferent denervation and visual deprivation.

Lahousse, E. (1888) *Arch. Biol. (Liège)* **8**:43–110. Recherches sur l'ontogenèse du cervelet.

Lamb, A. H. (1974) *Brain Res.* **67**:527–530. The timing of the earliest motor innervation in the hind limb bud in the *Xenopus* tadpole.

Lamb, A. H. (1976) *Dev. Biol.* **54**:82–99. The projection patterns of the ventral horn to the hind limb during development.

Landis, S. C. (1973) *Brain Res.* **61**:175–189. Granule cell heterotopia in normal and nervous mutant mice of the BALB/c-strain.

Landmesser, L. (1971) *J. Physiol. (London)* **213**:707–725. Contractile and electrical responses of vagus-innervated frog sartorius muscle.

Landmesser, L. (1972) *J. Physiol. (London)* **220**:243–256. Pharmacological properties, cholinesterase activity and anatomy of nerve–muscle junctions in vagus-innervated frog sartorius.

Landmesser, L., and D. G. Morris. (1975) *J. Physiol. (London)* **249**:301–326. The development of functional innervation in the hind limb of the chick embryo.

Landmesser, L., and G. Pilar. (1970) *J. Physiol. (London)* **211**:203–216. Selective reinnervation of two cell populations in the adult pigeon ciliary ganglion.

Landmesser, L., and G. Pilar. (1972) *J. Physiol. (London)* **222**:691–713. The onset and development of transmission in the chick ciliary ganglion.

Landmesser, L., and G. Pilar. (1974) *J. Physiol. (London)* **241**:737–749. Synaptic transmission and cell death during normal ganglionic development.

Landmesser, L., and G. Pilar. (1976) *J. Cell Biol.* **68**:357–374. Fate of ganglionic synapses and ganglion cell axons during normal and induced cell death.

Landon, D. N. (1972*a*) *J. Anat.* **111**:512–513P. The fine structure of developing muscle spindles in the rat.

Landon, D. N. (1972*b*) *J. Neurocytol.* **1**:189–210. The fine structure of the equatorial regions of developing spindles in the rat.

Landsteiner, K. (1899) *Centr. Bakt. Orig.* **25**:546–549. Zur Kenntnis der Specifisch auf Blutkörperchen wirkenden Sera.

Landsteiner, K. (1936) *The Specificity of Serological Reactions,* Thomas, Springfield, Ill. (Reprint, 1962, Dover, New York.)

Landström, H., T. Caspersson, and G. Wohlfart. (1941) *Z. Mikrosk. Anat. Forsch.* **49**:534–548. Über den Nucleotidumsätz der Nervenzelle.

Landström, U., and S. Lövtrup. (1975) *J. Embryol. Exp. Morphol.* **33**:879–895. On the determination of the dorso-ventral polarity in *Xenopus laevis* embryos.

Langley, J. N. (1895) *J. Physiol. (London)* **18**:280–284. Note on regeneration of pre-ganglionic fibres of the sympathetic.

Langley, J. N. (1897) *J. Physiol. (London)* **22**:215–230. On the regeneration of pre-ganglionic and post-ganglionic visceral nerve fibres.

Langley, J. N. (1898) *J. Physiol. (London)* **23**:240–270. On the union of cranial autonomic (visceral) fibres with the nerve cells of the superior cervical ganglion.

Langley, J. N., and H. K. Anderson. (1904*a*) *J. Physiol. (London)* **30**:439–442. On the union of the fifth cervical nerve with the superior cervical ganglion.

Langley, J. N., and H. K. Anderson. (1904*b*) *J. Physiol. (London)* **31**:365–391. The union of different kinds of nerve fibres.

Langman, J., and C. Haden. (1970) *J. Comp. Neurol.* **138**:419–432. Formation and migration of neuroblasts in the spinal cord of the chick embryo.

Langman, J., and M. Shimada. (1971) *Am. J. Anat.* **132**:355–374. Cerebral cortex of the mouse after prenatal chemical insult.

Langman, J., and G. W. Welch. (1967) *J. Comp. Neurol.* **131**:15–26. Excess vitamin A and development of the cerebral cortex.

Langman, J., R. Guerrant, and B. Freeman. (1966) *J. Comp. Neurol.* **127**:399–412. Behavior of neuroepithelial cells.

Langworthy, O. R. (1928*a*) *J. Comp. Neurol.* **46**:201–248. The behavior of pouch-young opossums correlated with the myelinization of tracts in the nervous system.

Langworthy, O. R. (1928*b*) *Contrib. Embryol. Carnegie Inst.* **20**:127–172. A correlated study of the development of reflex activity in fetal and young kittens and the myelinization of tracts in the nervous system.

Langworthy, O. R. (1929) *Contrib. Embryol. Carnegie Inst.* **20**:127–172. A correlated study of the development of reflex activity in fetal and young kittens and the myelinization of tracts in the nervous system.

Langworthy, O. R. (1930) *Contrib. Embryol. Carnegie Inst.* **21:**37–52. Medullated tracts in the brain stem of a seven month human fetus.

Langworthy, O. R. (1933) *Contrib. Embryol. Carnegie Inst.* **24:**1–58. Development of behavior patterns and myelinization of the nervous system in the human fetus and infant.

Lapham, L. W. (1962) *Am. J. Pathol.* **41:**1–21. Cytologic and cytochemical studies of neuroglia. I. A Study of the problem of amitosis in reactive protoplasmic astrocytes.

Lapham, L. W. (1968) *Science* **159:**310–312. Tetraploid DNA content of Purkinje neurons of human cerebellar cortex.

Lapham, L. W., and M. A. Johnstone. (1963) *Arch. Neurol. (Chicago)* **9:**194–202. Cytologic and cytochemical studies of neuroglia. II. The occurrence of two DNA classes among glial nuclei in the Purkinje cell layer of normal adult human cerebellar cortex.

Laron, Z., A. Pertzelan, S. Mannheimer, J. Coldman, and S. Guttman. (1966) *Acta Endocrinol.* **53:**687–692. Lack of placental transfer of human growth hormone.

Larrabee, M. G. (1969) *Prog. Brain Res.* **31:**95–110. Metabolic effects of nerve impulses and nerve-growth factor in sympathetic ganglion.

Larramendi, L. M. H. (1969) Analysis of synaptogenesis in the cerebellum of the mouse, pp. 803–843. In *Neurobiology of Cerebellar Evolution and Development* (R. Llinás, ed.), A.M.A. Education and Research Foundation, Chicago.

Larsell, O. (1923) *J. Comp. Neurol.* **36:**89–112. The cerebellum of the frog.

Larsell, O. (1925) *J. Comp. Neurol.* **39:**249–289. The development of the cerebellum in the frog (*Hyla regilla*) in relation to the vestibular and lateral-line systems.

Larsell, O. (1929) *J. Comp. Neurol.* **48:**331–353. The effect of experimental excision of one eye on the development of the optic lobe and opticus layer in larvae of the tree frog (*Hyla regilla*).

Larsell, O. (1931) *J. Exp. Zool.* **58:**1–20. The effect of experimental excision of one eye on the development of the optic lobe and opticus layer in larvae of the tree frog (*Hyla regilla*). II. The effect on cell size and differentiation of cell processes.

Larsell, O. (1947) *J. Comp. Neurol.* **87:**85–129. The development of cerebellum in man in relation to its comparative anatomy.

Larsell, O. (1967) *The Comparative Anatomy and Histology of the Cerebellum from Myxinoids through Birds,* Minnesota University Press, Minneapolis.

Lasek, R. J. (1970) *Int. Rev. Neurobiol.* **13:**289–324. Protein transport in neurons.

Lasek, R. J. (1975) *Fed. Proc.* **34:**1603–1611. Axonal transport and the use of intracellular markers in neuroanatomical investigations.

Lasek, R. J., and B. S. Joseph. (1967) *Anat. Rec.* **157:**275–276. Radioautography as a neuroanatomical tracing method.

Lasek, R. J., H. Gainer, and R. J. Przybylski. (1974) *Proc. Natl. Acad. Sci. U.S.A.* **71:**1188–1192. Transfer of newly synthesized proteins from Schwann cells to the squid giant axon.

Lash, J., S. Holtzer, and H. Holtzer. (1957) *Exp. Cell Res.* **13:**292–303. An experimental analysis of the development of the spinal column. VI. Aspects of cartilage induction.

Lasher, R., and R. D. Cahn. (1969) *Dev. Biol.* **19:**415–435. The effect of 5-bromodeoxyuridine on the differentiation of chondrocytes *in vitro.*

Lashley, K. S. (1937) *Arch. Neurol. Psychiat.* **38:**371–387. Functional determinants of cerebral localization.

Laskey, R. A., and J. B. Gurdon. (1970) *Nature* **228:**1332–1334. Genetic content of adult somatic cells tested by nuclear transplantation from cultured cells.

Lassek, A. M., and J. H. Perry. (1944) *J. Comp. Neurol.* **81:**270–284. Retrograde degeneration: Effect of hemisections on the axons of the fasciculus gracilis and cuneatus in the newborn cat.

Lauder, J. M., and F. E. Bloom. (1974) *J. Comp. Neurol.* **155:**469–482. Ontogeny of monoamine neurons in the locus coeruleus, raphe nuclei and substantia nigra of the rat. I. Cell differentiation.

Lauder, J. M., and F. E. Bloom. (1975) *J. Comp. Neurol.* **163:**25 1–264. Ontogeny of monoamine neurons in the locus coeruleus, raphe nuclei and substantia nigra of the rat. II. Synaptogenesis.

LaVail, J. H. (1975) *Fed. Proc.* **34:**1618–1624. The retrograde transport method.

LaVail, J. H., and W. M. Cowan. (1971*a*) *Brain Res.* **28:**391–419. The development of the chick optic tectum. I. Normal morphology and cytoarchitectonic development.

LaVail, J. H., and W. M. Cowan. (1971*b*) *Brain Res.* **28:**421–441. The development of the chick optic tectum. II. Autoradiographic studies.

LaVail, J. H., and M. M. LaVail. (1972) *Science* **176:**1416–1417. Retrograde axonal transport in the central nervous system.

LaVail, J. H., and M. M. LaVail. (1974) *J. Comp. Neurol.* **157:**303–358. The retrograde intraaxonal transport of horseradish peroxidase in the chick visual system: A light and electron microscopic study.

LaVail, J. H., K. R. Winston, and A. Tish. (1973) *Brain Res.* **58:**470–477. A method based on retrograde intraaxonal transport of protein for identification of cell bodies of origin of axons terminating within the CNS.

Lavelle, A. (1951) *J. Comp. Neurol.* **94:**453–473. Nucleolar changes and development of Nissl substance in the cerebral cortex of fetal guinea pigs.

Lavelle, A. (1956) *J. Comp. Neurol.* **104:**175–206. Nucleolar and Nissl substance development in nerve cells.

Lavelle, A. (1973) *Prog. Brain Res.* **40:**161–166. Levels of maturation and reactions to injury during neuronal development.

Lavelle, A., and F. W. Lavelle. (1958) *J. Exp. Zool.* **137:**285–316. The nucleolar apparatus and neuronal reactivity to injury during development.

Lawson, S. H., K. W. Caddy, and T. J. Biscoe. (1974) *Cell Tiss. Res.* **153:**399–413. Development of rat dorsal root ganglion neurones. Studies of cell birthdays and changes in mean cell diameter.

Lázár, G. (1973) *J. Anat.* **116:**347–355. The development of the optic tectum in *Xenopus laevis:* A Golgi study.

Lázár, G., and G. Székely. (1967) *J. Hirnforsch.* **9:**329–344. Golgi studies on the optic center of the frog.

Lázár, G., and G. Székely. (1969) *Brain Res.* **16:**1–14. Distribution of optic terminals in the different optic centers of the frog.

LeDouarin, N. (1973) *Dev. Biol.* **30:**217–222. A biological cell labelling technique and its use in experimental embryology.

LeDouarin, N. M., and M.-A. Teillet. (1973) *J. Embryol. Exp. Morphol.* **30:**31–48. The migration of neural crest cells to the wall of the digestive tract in avian embryo.

LeDouarin, N. M., and M.-A. M. Teillet. (1974) *Dev. Biol.* **41:**162–184. Experimental analysis of the migration and differentiation of neuroblasts of the autonomic nervous system and of neurectodermal mesenchymal derivatives, using a biological cell marking technique.

Leghissa, S. (1951) *Bol. Zool.* **18:**355–365. A proposito dello svillupo del tetto ottico nei Teleostei (*Salmo fario*).

Leghissa, S. (1955) *Z. Anat. Entwicklungsgesch.* **118:**427–463. La struttura microscopica e la citoarchitettonica del tetto ottico dei pesci teleostei.

Leghissa, S. (1957) *Arch. Sci. Biol.* **12:**601–628. Il differenziamento ontogenetico ed istogenetico del tetto ottico nell'embrione di pollo.

Leghissa, S. (1959) *Atti Accad. Sci. Bologna* **6:**56–75. Studio sperimentale sul differenziamento dei neuroni del tetto ottico di gallus. I. Esperienze de asportazione della vesicola ottica.

Leghissa, S. (1962) *Arch. Ital. Anat. Embriol.* **67:**343–413. L'evoluzione del tetto ottico nei bassi vertebrati.

Legrand, J. (1967*a*) *Arch. Anat. Microsc. Morphol. Exp.* **56:**205–244. Analyse de l'action morphogénétique des hormones thyroïdiennes sur le cervelet du jeune Rat.

Legrand, J. (1967*b*) *Arch. Anat. Microsc. Morphol. Exp.* **56:**291–307. Variations, en fonction de l'âge, de la résponse du cervelet à l'action morphogénétique de la thyroide chez le Rat.

Legrand, T. (1963) *Arch. Anat. Microsc. Morphol. Exp.* **52:**205-214. Maturation du cervelet et deficience thyroidienne données chronologiques.

Legrand, T., A. Kriegel, and A. Jost. (1961) *Arch. Anat. Microsc. Morphol. Exp.* **50:**507–519. Deficience thyroidienne et maturation du cervelet chez le rat blanc.

Le Gros Clark, W. E. (1945) *Essays on Growth and Form,* pp. 1–22 (W. E. Le Gros Clark and P. B. Medawar, eds.), Oxford University Press, London.

Lehmann, H. (1959) Die Nervenfaser, pp. 515–701. In *Handbuch der Mikroskopischen Anatomie des Menschen,* Vol. 4, Part 3 (W. Bargmann, ed.), Springer-Verlag, Berlin.

Lenhossék, M. V. (1895) *Arch. Mikrosc. Anat.* **46:**345–369. Centrosom und sphäre in den Spinalganglienzellen des Frosches.

Lenneberg, E. H. (1967) *Biological Foundations of Language,* Wiley, New York, 489 pp.

Lenneberg, E. H. (1975) The concept of language differentiation, pp. 17–33. In *Foundations of Language Development,* Vol. 1 (E. H. Lenneberg and E. Lenneberg, eds.), UNESCO and Academic Press, Paris and New York.

Lentz, R. D., and L. W. Lapham. (1969) *J. Neurochem.* **16**:379–384. A quantitative cytochemical study of the DNA content of neurons of rat cerebellar cortex.

Lentz, R. D., and L. W. Lapham. (1970) *J. Neuropathol. Exp. Neurol.* **29**:43–56. Postnatal development of tetraploid DNA content in rat Purkinje cells: A quantitative cytochemical study.

Letinsky, M. S. (1974) *Dev. Biol.* **40**:129–153. The development of nerve–muscle junctions in *Rana catesbeiana* tadpoles.

Letinsky, M. S., K. H. Fischbeck, and U. J. McMahan. (1976) *J. Neurocytol.* **5**:691–718. Precision of reinnervation of original postsynaptic sites in frog muscle after a nerve crush.

Letourneau, P. C. (1975*a*) *Dev. Biol.* **44**:77–91. Possible roles for cell-to-substratum adhesion in neuronal morphogenesis.

Letourneau, P. C. (1975*b*) *Dev. Biol.* **44**:92–101. Cell-to-substratum adhesion and guidance of axonal elongation.

Lettvin, J. Y., H. R. Maturana, W. S. McCulloch, and W. H. Pitts. (1959) *Proc. Inst. Radio Engr. N.Y.* **47**:1940–1951. What the frog's eye tells the frog's brain.

Lettvin, J. Y., H. R. Maturana, W. H. Pitts, and W. S. McCulloch. (1961) Two remarks on the visual system of the frog, pp. 757–776. In *Sensory Communication* (W. A. Rosenblith, ed.), MIT Press, Cambridge, Mass.

LeVay, S., D. H. Hubel, and T. N. Wiesel. (1975) *J. Comp. Neurol.* **159**:559–576. The pattern of ocular dominance columns in macaque visual cortex revealed by a reduced silver stain.

Leventhal, A. G., and H. V. B. Hirsch, (1975) *Science* **190**:902–904. Cortical effect of early selective exposure to diagonal lines.

Levi, G., and H. Meyer. (1945) *J. Exp. Zool.* **99**:141–181. Reactive, regressive and regenerative processes of neurons, cultivated *in vitro* and injured with a micromanipulator.

Levi-Montalcini, R. (1949) *J. Comp. Neurol.* **91**:209–242. The development of the acoustico-vestibular centers in the chick embryo in the absence of the afferent root fibers and of descending fiber tracts.

Levi-Montalcini, R. (1950) *J. Morphol.* **86**:253–283. The origin and development of the visceral system in the spinal cord of the chick embryo.

Levi-Montalcini, R. (1952) *Ann. N.Y. Acad. Sci.* **55**:330–343. Effects of mouse tumor transplantation on the nervous system.

Levi-Montalcini, R. (1964*a*) *Prog. Brain Res.* **4**:1–29. Events in the developing nervous system.

Levi-Montalcini, R. (1964*b*) Growth and differentiation in the nervous system. pp. 261–295. In *The Nature of Biological Diversity* (J. M. Allen, ed.), McGraw-Hill, New York.

Levi-Montalcini, R. (1964*c*) *Ann. N.Y. Acad. Sci.* **118**:149–168. The nerve growth factor.

Levi-Montalcini, R. (1965) *Arch. Biol. (Liège)* **76**:387–414. Morphological and metabolic effects of the nerve growth factor.

Levi-Montalcini, R. (1966) *Harvey Lect.* **60**:217–259. The nerve growth factor: its mode of action on sensory and sympathetic nerve cells.

Levi-Montalcini, R. (1972) The morphological effects of immunosympathectomy, pp. 55–77. In *Immunosympathectomy* (G. Steiner and E. Schonbaum, eds.), Elsevier, New York.

Levi-Montalcini, R., and P. U. Angeletti. (1963) *Dev. Biol.* **7**:653–659. Essential role of the nerve growth factor in the survival and maintenance of dissociated sensory and sympathetic nerve cells *in vitro*.

Levi-Montalcini, R., and P. U. Angeletti. (1966) *Pharmacol. Rev.* **18**:619–628. Immunosympathectomy.

Levi-Montalcini, R., and P. U. Angeletti. (1968) *Physiol. Rev.* **48**:534–569. Nerve growth factor.

Levi-Montalcini, R., and B. Booker. (1960*a*) *Proc. Natl. Acad. Sci. U.S.A.* **42**:373–384. Excessive growth of the sympathetic ganglia evoked by a protein isolated from mouse salivary glands.

Levi-Montalcini, R., and B. Booker. (1960*b*) *Proc. Natl. Acad. Sci. U.S.A.* **42**:384–391. Destruction of the sympathetic ganglia in mammals by an antiserum to the nerve-growth promoting factor.

Levi-Montalcini, R., and S. Cohen. (1956) *Proc. Natl. Acad. Sci. U.S.A.* **42**:695–699. *In-vitro* and *in-vivo* effects of a nerve growth stimulating agent isolated from snake venom.

Levi-Montalcini, R., and S. Cohen. (1960) *Ann. N.Y. Acad. Sci.* **85**:324–341. Effects of the extract of the mouse salivary glands on the sympathetic system of mammals.

Levi-Montalcini, R., and V. Hamburger. (1951) *J. Exp. Zool.* **116**:321–362. Selective growth-stimulating effects of mouse sarcoma on the sensory and sympathetic nervous system of the chick embryo.

Levi-Montalcini, R., and V. Hamburger. (1953) *J. Exp. Zool.* **123**:233–288. A diffusible agent of mouse sarcoma producing hyperplasia of sympathetic ganglia and hyperneurotization of the chick embryo.

Levi-Montalcini, R., and G. Levi. (1943) *Arch. Biol. (Liège)* **54**:183–206. Recherches quantitatives sur la marche du processus de différenciation des neurones dans les ganglions spinaux de l'embryon de poulet.

Levi-Montalcini, R., H. Meyer, and V. Hamburger. (1954) *Cancer Res.* **14:**49–57. *In-vitro* experiments on the effects of mouse Sarcoma 180 and 37 on the spinal and sympathetic ganglia of the chick embryo.

Levi-Montalcini, R., F. Caramia, S. A. Luse, and P. U. Angeletti. (1968) *Brain Res.* **8:**347–362. *In vitro* effects of the nerve growth factor on the fine structure of the sensory nerve cells.

Levi-Montalcini, R., F. Caramia, and P. U. Angeletti. (1969) *Brain Res.* **12:**54–73. Alterations in the fine structure of nucleoli in sympathetic neurons following NGF-antiserum treatment.

Levine, R. (1975) *J. Exp. Zool.* **192:**363–380. Regeneration of the retina in the adult newt, *Triturus cristatus,* following surgical division of the eye by a limbal incision.

Levine, R., and J. R. Cronly-Dillon. (1974) *Brain Res.* **68:**319–329. Specification of regenerating retinal ganglion cells in the adult newt, *Triturus cristatus.*

Levine, R., and M. Jacobson. (1974) *Exp. Neurol.* **43:**527–538. Deployment of optic nerve fibers is determined by positional markers in the frog's tectum.

Levine, R., and M. Jacobson, (1975) *Brain Res.* **98:**172–176. Discontinuous mapping of retina onto tectum innervated by both eyes.

Levine, S., and R. F. Mullins. (1966) *Science* **152:**1585–1592. Hormonal influence on brain organization in infant rats.

Levinthal, C., and R. Ware. (1972) *Nature* **236:**207–210. Three dimensional reconstruction from serial sections.

Lewis, J. H., (1975) *J. Embryol. Exp. Morphol.* **33:**419–434. Fate maps and the pattern of cell division: A calculation for the chick wing-bud.

Lewis, J. H., D. Summerbell, and L. Wolpert. (1972) *Nature* **239:**276–279. Chimaeras and cell lineage in development.

Lewis, P. D. (1968*a*) *Exp. Neurol.* **20:**203–207. A quantitative study of cell proliferation in the subependymal layer of the adult rat brain.

Lewis, P. D. (1968*b*) *Nature* **217:**974–975. Mitotic activity in the primate subependymal layer and the genesis of gliomas.

Lewis, P. D. (1968*c*) *Brain* **91:**721–736. The fate of subependymal cell in the adult brain, with a note on the origin of microglia.

Lewis, P. D. (1968*d*) *Exp. Neurol.* **20:**208–214. Radiosensitivity of the subependymal cell layer of the adult rat brain.

Lewis, P. D. (1975) *Neuropathol. Appl. Neurobiol.* **1:**21–29. Cell death in the germinal layers of the postnatal rat brain.

Lewis, P. D., and M. Lai. (1974) *Brain Res.* **77:**520–525. Cell generation in the subependymal layer of the rat brain during the early postnatal period.

Lewis, P. D., A. J. Patel, A. L. Johnson, and R. Balázs. (1976) *Brain Res.* **104:**49–62. Effect of thyroid deficiency on cell acquisition in the postnatal rat brain: A quantitative histological study.

Lewis, V. G., J. Money, and R. Epstein. (1968) *Johns Hopkins Med. J.* **122:**192–195. Concordance of verbal and nonverbal ability in the adrenogenital syndrome.

Lewis, W. H. (1910) *Anat. Rec.* **4:**191–200. Localization and regeneration in the neural plate of amphibian embryos.

Lewis, W. H. (1931) *Bull. Johns Hopkins Hosp.* **49:**17–26, Pinocytosis.

Lewis, W. H., and M. R. Lewis (1912) *Anat. Rec.* **6:**7–31. The cultivation of sympathetic nerves from the intestine of chick embryos in saline solutions.

Liao, S. (1975) *Int. Rev. Cytol.* **41:**87–172. Cellular receptors and mechanisms of action of steroid hormones.

Lieberburg, I., and B. S. McEwen. (1975) *Brain Res.* **85:**165–170. Estradiol-17β: A metabolite of testosterone recovered in cell nuclei from limbic areas of neonatal rat brains.

Lieberman, A. R. (1968) *J. Anat. (London)* **104:**49–54. Absence of ultrastructural changes in ganglionic neurons after supranodose vagotomy.

Lieberman, A. R. (1969) *J. Anat. (London)* **104:**309–325. Light and electron microscope observations on the Golgi apparatus of normal and axotomised primary sensory neurons.

Lieberman, A. R. (1971) The axon reaction: A review of the principle features of perikaryal response to axon injury, pp. 49–124. In *International Review of Neurobiology,* Vol. 14 (C. C. Pfeiffer and J. R. Smythies, eds.), Academic Press, New York.

Lieberman, A. R. (1974) Some factors affecting retrograde neuronal responses to axonal lesions, pp. 71–105. In *Essays on the Nervous System* (R. Bellairs and E. G. Gray, eds.), Clarendon, Oxford.

Lilien, J. (1968) *Dev. Biol.* **17:**657–678. Specific enhancement of cell aggregation *in vitro.*

Lindsay, H. A., and M. L. Barr. (1955) *J. Anat. (London)* **89:**47–63. Further observations on the behaviour of nuclear structures during depletion and restoration of Nissl substance.

Linell, E. A., and M. I. Tom. (1931) *Anat. Rec. Suppl.* **48:**27. The postnatal development of the oligodendroglia cell in the brain of the white rat and the possible role of this cell in myelogenesis.

Ling, E. A., J. A. Paterson, A. Privat, S. Mori, and C. P. Leblond. (1973) *J. Comp. Neurol.* **149:**43–72. Investigation of glial cells in semithin sections. I. Identification of glial cells in the brain of young rats.

Linville, G. P., and T. H. Shepard. (1972) *Nature New Biol.* **236:**246–247. Neural tube closure defects caused by cytochalasin B.

Liu, C. N., and W. W. Chambers. (1958) *Arch. Neurol. Psychiat.* **79:**46–61. Intraspinal sprouting of dorsal root axons.

Liu, C. N., and C. Y. Liu. (1971) *Anat. Rec.* **169:**369. Role of afferents in maintenance of dendritic morphology.

Liu, H.-C., and R. B. Maneely. (1968) *Acta Anat.* **71:**249–267. The development of motor end-plates in the embryonic and regenerative tail of *Hemidactylus bowringi* (Gray).

Livingston, W. K. (1947) *J. Neurosurg.* **4:**140–145. Evidence of active invasion of denervated areas by sensory fibers from neighboring nerves in man.

Llinás, R., D. E. Hillman, and W. Precht. (1973) *J. Neurobiol.* **4:**69–94. Neuronal circuit reorganization in mammalian agranular cerebellar cortex.

Loeb, L. (1902) *Arch. Entw.-Mech. Organ.* **13:**487–506. Ueber das Wachstum des Epithels.

Loeb, L., and M. S. Fleisher. (1917) *J. Med. Res.* **37:**75–99. On the factors which determine the movements of tissues in culture media.

Loeser, J. D., R. J. Lemire, and E. C. Alvord, Jr. (1972) *Anat. Rec.* **173:**109–114. The development of the folia in the human cerebellar vermis.

Loewenstein, W. R. (1968*a*) *Persp. Biol. Med.* **11:**260–272. Some reflections on growth and differentiation.

Loewenstein, W. R. (1968*b*) *Dev. Biol. Suppl.* **2:**151–183. Communication through cell junctions: Implications in growth control and differentiation.

Loewenstein, W. (1970) *Sci. Am.* **222:**78–86. Intercellular communication.

Loewenstein, W. R. (1973) *Fed. Proc.* **32:**60–64. Membrane junctions in growth and differentiation.

Loewenstein, W. R. (1975) Permeable junctions: Permeability, formation, and genetic aspects, pp. 419–436. In *The Nervous System,* Vol. 1 (D. B. Tower, ed.), Raven Press, New York.

Lömo, T., and J. Rosenthal. (1972) *J. Physiol. (London)* **221:**493–513. Control of ACh sensitivity by muscle activity in the rat.

Longo, A. M., and E. E. Penhoet. (1974) *Proc. Natl. Acad. Sci. U.S.A.* **71:**2347–2349. Nerve growth factor in rat glioma cells.

Lopresti, V., E. R. Macagno, and C. Levinthal. (1973) *Proc. Natl. Acad. Sci. U.S.A.* **70:**433–437. Structure and development of neuronal connections in isogenic organisms: Cellular interactions in the development of the optic lamina of *Daphnia.*

Lopresti, V., E. R. Macagno, and C. Levinthal. (1974) *Proc. Natl. Acad. Sci. U.S.A.* **71:**1098–1102. Structure and development of neuronal connections in isogenic organisms: Transient gap junctions between growing optic axons and lamina neuroblasts.

Lorenté de Nó, R. (1933*a*) *Laryngoscope* **43:**327–350. Anatomy of the eighth nerve. III. General plan of structure of the primary cochlear nuclei.

Lorenté de Nó, R. (1933*b*) *J. Psychol. Neurol. (Leipzig)* **45:**381–438. Studies on the structure of the cerebral cortex.

Lovejoy, A. (1936) *The Great Chain of Being.* Harvard Univ. Press.

Lubińska, L. (1958) *Nature* **181:**957–958. "Intercalated" internodes in nerve fibers.

Lubińska, L. (1961) *Exp. Cell Res. Suppl.* **8:**74–90. Sedentary and migratory states of Schwann cells.

Lubińska, L. (1964) *Prog. Brain Res.* **13:**1–66. Axoplasmic streaming in regenerating and in normal nerve fibers.

Lubińska, L., and S. Niemierko. (1971) *Brain Res.* **27:**329–342. Velocity and intensity of bidirectional migration of acetylcholinesterase in transected nerves.

Lubińska, L., and M. Olekiewicz. (1950) *Acta Biol. Exp. (Warsaw)* **15:**125–145. The rate of regeneration of amphibian peripheral nerves at different temperatures.

Luco, C. F., and J. V. Luco. (1971) *J. Neurophysiol.* **34:**1066–1071. Sympathetic effects on fibrillary activity of denervated striated muscles.

Luco, J. V., and C. Eyzaguirre. (1955) *J. Neurophysiol* **18:**65–73. Fibrillation and hypersensitivity to ACh in denervated muscle: Effect of length of degenerating nerve fibers.

Ludueña, M. A., and N. K. Wessells. (1973) *Dev. Biol.* **30:**427–440. Cell locomotion, nerve elongation, and microfilaments.

Ludueña, R. F., and D. O. Woodward. (1975) *Ann. N.Y. Acad. Sci.* **253:**272–283. α- and β-Tubulin: Separation and partial sequence analysis.

Ludwig, W. (1932) *Das Rechts-Links-Problem im Tierreich und beim Menschen: Mit einem Anhang: Rechts-Links-Merkmale der Pflanzen.* Julius Springer, Berlin. (Reprinted, 1970, Springer-Verlag, Berlin.)

Lumsden, C. E. (1968) Nervous tissue in culture, pp. 67–142. In *The Structure and Function of Nervous Tissue,* Vol. 1 (G. Bourne, ed.), Academic Press, New York.

Lumsden, C. E., and C. M. Pomerat. (1951) *Exp. Cell Res.* **2:**103–114. Normal oligodendrocytes in tissue culture.

Lunau, H. (1956) *Anat. Anz.* **62:**673–698. Vergleichend-metrische Untersuchungen am Allocortex von Wild- und Hausschweinen.

Lund, E. J. (1923) *Botan. Gaz.* **76:**288–301. Electrical control of organic polarity in the egg of *Fucus.*

Lund, E. J. (1947) *Bioelectric Fields and Growth,* University of Texas Press, Austin.

Lund, R. D., and J. S. Lund. (1973) *Exp. Neurol.* **40:**377–390. Reorganization of the retinotectal pathway in rats after neonatal retinal lesions.

Lund, R. D., T. J. Cunningham, and J. S. Lund. (1973) *Brain Behav. Evol.* **8:**51–72. Modified optic projections after unilateral eye removal in young rats.

Lund, R. K. (1975) *Exp. Eye Res.* **21:**193–203. Variations in the laterality of the central projections of retinal ganglion cells.

Luse, S. A. (1956) *J. Biophys. Biochim. Cytol.* **2:**777–784. Formation of myelin in the central nervous system of mice and rats, as studied with the electron microscope.

Luse, S. A. (1958) *Lab. Invest.* **7:**401–417. Ultrastructure of reactive and neoplastic astrocytes.

Luse, S. A. (1960) *Anat. Rec.* **138:**461–492. The ultrastructure of normal and abnormal oligodendroglia.

Lynch, G., S. Deadwyler, and C. Cotman. (1973*a*) *Science* **180:**1364–1366. Postlesion axonal growth produces permanent functional connections.

Lynch, G., B. Stanfield, and C. W. Cotman. (1973*b*) *Brain Res.* **59:**155–168. Developmental differences in post-lesion axonal growth in the hippocampus.

Lynch, G., S. Mosko, T. Parks, and C. Cotman. (1973*c*) *Brain Res.* **50:**174–178. Relocation and hyperdevelopment of the dentate gyrus commissural system after entorhinal lesions in immature rats.

Lynch, G., B. Stanfield, T. Parks, and C. W. Cotman. (1974) *Brain Res.* **69:**1–11. Evidence for selective postlesion axonal growth in the dentate gyrus of the rat.

Lyser, K. M. (1964) *Dev. Biol.,* **10:**433–466. Early differentiation of motor neuroblast in the chick embryo as studied by electron microscopy.

Lyser, K. M. (1966) *J. Embryol. Exp. Morphol.* **16:**497–517. The development of the chick embryo diencephalon and mesencephalon during the initial phases of neuroblast differentiation.

Lyser, K. M. (1968*a*) *Dev. Biol.* **17:**117–142. Early differentiation of motor neuroblasts in the chick embryo as studied by electron microscopy. II. Microtubules and neurofilaments.

Lyser, K. M. (1968*b*) *J. Embryol. Exp. Morphol.* **20:**343–354. An electron-microscope study of centrioles in differentiating motor neuroblasts.

Lyser, K. M. (1971) *Tiss. Cell* **3:**395–404. Microtubules and filaments in developing axons and optic stalk cells.

Macagno, E. R., V. Lopresti, and C. Levinthal. (1973) *Proc. Natl. Acad. Sci. U.S.A.* **70:**57–61. Structure and development of neuronal connections in isogenic organisms: Variations and similarities in the optic system of *Daphnia magna.*

MacInnis, A. J., W. M. Bethel, and E. M. Cornford. (1974) *Nature* **248:**361–363. Identification of chemicals of snail origin that attract *Schistosoma mansoni* miracidia.

Maekawa, T., and J. Tsuchiya. (1968) *Exp. Cell Res.* **53:**55–64. A method for the direct estimation of the length of G1, S and G2 phase.

Magini, G. (1888) *Arch. Ital. Biol.* **9:**59–60. Sur la neuroglie et les cellules nerveuses cérébrales chez les foetus.

Majno, G., and M. L. Karnofsky. (1958) *J. Exp. Med.* **107:**475–496. A biochemical and morphologic study of myelination and demyelination. I. Lipid biosynthesis *in vitro* by normal nervous tissue.

Malhotra, S. K. (1960) *Quart. J. Microsc. Sci.* **101:**75–93. The cytoplasmic inclusions of the neurones of crustacea.

Malhotra, S. K., and A. van Harreveld. (1966) *J. Anat. (London)* **100:**99–110. Distribution of extracellular material in central white matter.

Mall, F. (1893) *J. Morphol.* **8:**415–432. Histogenesis of the retina in *Amblystoma* and *Necturus.*

Malzacher, P. (1968) *Z. Morphol. Oekol. Tiere* **62:**103–161. Die Embryogenese des Gehirns pauro-metaboler Insekten. Untersuchungen an *Carausius morosus* und *Periplaneta americana.*

Manchot, E. (1929) *Arch. Entw.-Mech. Organ.* **116:**689–708. Abgrenzung des Augenmaterials und andere Teilbezirke in der Medullarplatte; die Teilbewegungen Während der Auffaltung.

Mangold, O. (1931) *Ergeb. Biol.* **7:**193–403. Das Determinationsprobleme III. Das Wirbeltierauge in der Entwicklung und Regeneration.

Mangold, O. (1933) *Naturwissen* **21:**394–397. Isolationsversuche zur Analyse der Entwicklung bestimmter Kopforgane.

Mann, D. M. A., and P. O. Yates. (1973*a*) *J. Neurol. Sci.* **18:** 183–196. Polyploidy in the human nervous system. Part 1. The DNA content of neurones and glia of the cerebellum.

Mann, D. M. A., and P. O. Yates. (1973*b*) *J. Neurol. Sci.* **18:**197–205. Polyploidy in the human nervous system. Part 2. Studies of the glial cell populations of the Purkinje cell layer of the human cerebellum.

Mann, W. S., and B. Salafsky. (1970) *J. Physiol. (London)* **208:**33–47. Enzymic and physiological studies on normal and disused developing fast and slow cat muscle.

Mannen, H. (1965) *Arch. Ital. Biol.* **103:**197–219. Arborizations dendritiques. Étude topographique et quantitative dans le noyau vestibulaire du chat.

Mannen, H. (1966) *J. Comp. Neurol.* **126:**75–90. Contributions to the quantitative study of the nervous tissue. A new method for measurement of the volume and surface area of neurons.

Manuelidis, L., and M. Bornstein. (1970) *Z. Zellforsch. Mikrosk. Anat.* **106:**189–199. ^{125}I-labelled thyroid hormones in cultured mammalian nerve tissue.

Manuelidis, L., and E. E. Manuelidis. (1974) *Exp. Neurol.* **43:**192–206. On the DNA content of cerebellar Purkinje cells *in vivo* and *in vitro.*

March, B. (1935) *Some Technical Terms of Chinese Painting,* American Council of Learned Societies, Studies in Chinese and Related Civilizations, No. 2. Baltimore.

Marchase, R. B. (1976) Biochemical investigations of retinotectal adhesive specificity. Ph.D. thesis, Johns Hopkins University.

Marchase, R. B., A. J. Barbera, and S. Roth. (1975) A molecular approach to retinotectal specificity, pp. 315–327. In *Cell Patterning,* Ciba Foundation Symposium 29, Elsevier, New York.

Marchisio, P. C. (1969) *J. Neurochem.* **16:**665–671. Choline acetyltransferase (ChAc) activity in developing chick optic centres and the effects of monolateral removal of retina at an early embryonic stage and at hatching.

Marchisio, P. C., and J. Sjöstrand. (1972) *J. Neurocytol.* **I:**101–108. Radioautographic evidence for protein transport along the optic pathway of early chick embryos.

Marchisio, P. C., J. Sjöstrand, M. Aglietta, and J. -O. Karlsson. (1973) *Brain Res.* **63:**273–284. The development of axonal transport of proteins and glycoproteins in the optic pathway of chick embryos.

Mareš, V., and Z. Lodin. (1970) *Brain Res.* **23:**343–352. The cellular kinetics of the developing mouse cerebellum. II. The function of the external granular layer in the process of gyrification.

Mareš, V., Z. Lodin, and J. Šrajer. (1970) *Brain Res.* **23:**323–342. The cellular kinetics of the developing mouse cerebellum. I. The generation cycle, growth fraction and rate of proliferation of the external granular layer.

Mareš, V., Z. Lodin, and J. Sacha. (1973) *Brain Res.* **53:**273–289. A cytochemical and autoradiographic study of nuclear DNA in mouse Purkinje cells.

Mareš, V., B. Schultze, and W. Maurer. (1974) *J. Cell Biol.* **63:**665–674. Stability of DNA in Purkinje cell nuclei of the mouse.

Margolis, F. L. (1969) *J. Neurochem.* **16:**447–456. DNA and DNA-polymerase activity in chicken brain regions during ontogeny.

Marin-Padilla, M. (1970*a*) *Brain Res.* **23:**167–183. Prenatal and early postnatal ontogenesis of the human motor cortex: A Golgi study. I. The sequential development of the cortical layers.

Marin-Padilla, M. (1970*b*) *Brain Res.* **23:**185–191. Prenatal and early postnatal ontogenesis of the human motor cortex: A Golgi Study. II. The basket-pyramidal system.

Marin-Padilla, M. (1971) *Z. Anat. Entwicklungsgesch.* **134:**117–145. Early prenatal ontogenesis of the cerebral cortex (neocortex) of the cat *(Felis domestica)*: A Golgi study.

Marin-Padilla, M. (1972) *Z. Anat. Entwicklungsgesch.* **136:**125–142. Prenatal ontogenetic history of the principal neurons of the neocortex of the cat *(Felis domestica)*. A Golgi study. II. Developmental differences and their significances.

Mark, R. F. (1965) *Exp. Neurol.* **12**:292–302. Fin movements after regeneration of neuromuscular connections: an investigation of myotypic specificity.

Mark. R. F. (1969) *Brain Res.* **14**:245–254. Matching muscles and motoneurones. A review of some experiments on motor nerve regeneration.

Mark, R. F. (1974*a*) *Br. Med. Bull.* **30**:122–126. Selective innervation of muscle.

Mark, R. F. (1974*b*) *Memory and Nerve Cell Connections,* Clarendon, Oxford.

Mark, R. F. (1975) Topography and topology in functional recovery of regenerated sensory and motor systems, pp. 289–307. In *Cell Patterning,* Ciba Foundation Symposium 29, Elsevier, New York.

Mark, R. F., G. von Campenhausen, and D. J. Lischinsky. (1966) *Exp. Neurol.* **16**:438–499. Nerve–muscle relations in salamander: Possible relevance to nerve regeneration and muscle specificity.

Mark, R. F., L. R. Marotte, and J. R. Johnstone. (1970) *Science* **170**:193–194. Reinnervated eye muscles do not respond to impulses in foreign nerves.

Mark, R. J., and J. Feldman. (1972) *Invest. Ophthalmol.* **11**:402–410. Binocular interaction in the development of optokinetic reflexes in tadpoles of *Xenopus laevis.*

Marko, P., and M. Cuénod. (1973) *Brain Res.* **62**:419–423. Contribution of the nerve cell body to renewal of axonal and synaptic glycoproteins in the pigeon visual system.

Marler, P. (1971) *Am. Sci.* **58**:669–673. Birdsong and speech development: Could there be parallels?

Marotte, L. R., and R. F. Mark. (1970*a*) *Brain Res.* **19**:41–51. The mechanism of selective reinnervation of fish eye muscle. I. Evidence from muscle function during recovery.

Marotte, L. R. and R. F. Mark. (1970*b*) *Brain Res.* **19**:53–62. The mechanism of selective reinnervation of fish eye muscle. II. Electron microscopy of nerve endings.

Marsh, G., and H. W. Beams. (1946*a*) *Anat. Rec.* **94**:370. Orientation of chick nerve fibers by direct electric currents.

Marsh, G., and H. W. Beams. (1946*b*) *J. Cell. Comp. Physiol.* **27**:139–157. *In vitro* control of growing chick nerve fibers by applied electric currents.

Martin, A. H. (1967) *Nature* **216**:1133–1134. Significance of mitotic spindle fibre orientation in the neural tube.

Martin, A. H., and J. Langman. (1965) *J. Embryol. Exp. Morphol.* **14**:23–35. The development of the spinal cord examined by autoradiography.

Martin, H. P. (1970) *Am. J. Dis. Child.* **119**:128–131. Microcephaly and mental retardation.

Martin, J. R., and H. deF. Webster. (1973) *Dev. Biol.* **32**:417–431. Mitotic Schwann cells in developing nerve: Their changes in shape, fine structure, and axon relationships.

Martínez-Palomo, A. (1970) *Int. Rev. Cytol.* **29**:29–76. The surface coats of animal cells.

Marty, R., and J. Scherrer. (1964) *Prog. Brain Res.* **4**:222–234. Critères de maturation des systèmes afférents corticaux.

Maruyama, S., and A. N. D'Agostino. (1967) *Neurology* **17**:550–558. Cell necrosis in the central nervous system of normal rat fetuses: An electron microscope study.

Maruyama, S., M. Chiga, and A. N. D'Agostino. (1968) *J. Neuropathol. Exp. Neurol.* **27**:96–107. Selective necrosis in the fetal rat central nervous system produced by 5-fluoro-2′-deoxyuridine: A morphologic study.

Mathers, L. H., K. L. Chow, P. D. Spear, and P. Grobstein. (1974) *Exp. Brain Res.* **19**:20–35. Ontogenesis of receptive fields in the rabbit striate cortex.

Matsumoto, S. G., and R. K. Murphey. (1977) *J. Physiol. (London)* **268**:533–548. Sensory deprivation during development decreases the responsiveness of cricket giant interneurones.

Matsumoto, T. (1920) *Bull. Johns Hopkins Hosp.* **30**:91–93. The granules, vacuoles and mitochondria in the sympathetic nerve fibers cultivated *in vitro.*

Mattanza, G. G. (1973) *Acta Anat.* **85**:206–215. Significance of embryonic cell necrosis in the forebrain. II. Histochemical studies in the mouse.

Matthews, M. A. (1968) *Anat. Rec.* **161**:337–352. An electron microscopic study of the relationship between axon diameter and the initiation of myelin production in the peripheral nervous system.

Matthews, M. A. (1974) *Cell Tiss. Res.* **148**:477–491. Microglia and reactive "M" cells of degenerating central nervous system: Does similar morphology and function imply a common origin?

Matthews, M. R., and V. H. Nelson. (1975) *J. Physiol. (London)* **245**:91–135. Detachment of structurally intact nerve endings from chromatolytic neurones of rat superior cervical ganglion during the depression of synaptic transmission induced by postganglionic axotomy.

Matthews, M. R., and G. Raisman. (1972) *Proc. Roy. Soc. London (Biol.)* **181**:43–79. A light and electron microscopic study of the cellular response to axonal injury in the superior cervical ganglion of the rat.

Matthews, M. R., W. M. Cowan, and T. P. S. Powell. (1960) *J. Anat. (London)* **94**:145–169. Transneuronal cell degeneration in the lateral geniculate nucleus of the macaque monkey.

Matthews, S. A., and S. R. Detwiler (1926) *J. Exp. Zool.* **45**:279–292. The reactions of *Amblystoma* embryos following prolonged treatment with chloretone.

Maturana, H. R. (1959) *Nature* **183**:1406. Number of fibers in the optic nerve and the number of ganglion cells in the retina of anurans.

Maturana, H. R. (1960) *J. Biophys. Biochem. Cytol.* **7**:107–120. The fine anatomy of the optic nerve of anurans—An electron microscope study.

Maturana, H. R., J. Y. Lettvin, W. S. McCulloch, and W. H. Pitts. (1959) *Science* **130**:1709–1710. Evidence that cut optic nerve fibers in a frog regenerate to their proper places in the tectum.

Maturana, H. R., J. Y. Lettvin, W. S. McCulloch, and W. H. Pitts. (1960) *J. Gen. Physiol. Suppl.* **43**:129–175. Anatomy and physiology of vision in the frog *(Rana pipiens)*.

Mauro, A. (1961) *J. Biophys. Biochem. Cytol.* **9**:493–495. Satellite cells of skeletal muscle fibers.

Max, S. R., and E. X. Albuquerque. (1975) *Exp. Neurol.* **49**:852–857. Neurotrophic regulation of acetylcholinesterase in regenerating skeletal muscle.

Maxwell, D. S., and L. Kruger. (1965) *Exp. Neurol.* **12**:33–54. Small blood vessels and the origin of phagocytes in the rat cerebral cortex following heavy particle irradiation.

Maxwell, D. S., and L. Kruger. (1966) *Am. J. Anat.* **118**:437–460. The reactive oligodendrocyte. An electron microscopic study of cerebral cortex following alpha particle irradiation.

May, M. K., and T. J. Biscoe. (1973) *Brain Res.* **53**:181–186. Preliminary observations on synaptic development in the foetal rat spinal cord.

May, R. M. 1925) *J. Exp. Zool.* **42**:371–410. The relation of nerves to degenerating and regenerating taste buds.

May, R. M. (1927*a*) *Proc. Natl. Acad. Sci. U.S.A.* **13**:372–374. Modification of nerve centers due to the transplantation of the eye and olfactory organ in anuran embryos.

May, R. M. (1927*b*) *Arch. Biol. (Liège)* **37**:336–396. Modifications des centres nerveux dues à la transplantation de l'oeil et de l'organe olfactif chez les embryon d'Anoures.

May, R. M. (1930) *Bull. Biol. Liège.* **64**:355–387. Répercussions de la greffe de moelle sur le système nerveux chez l'embryon de l'anoure, *Discoglossus pictus* Otth.

May, R. M. (1933) *Bull. Biol. Liège* **67**:327–349. Réactions neurogéniques de la moelle à la greffe en surnombre, ou à l'ablation d'une ébauche de patte postérieure chez l'embryon de l'anoure, *Discoglossus pictus* Otth.

May, R. M., and S. R. Detwiler. (1925) *J. Exp. Zool.* **43**:83–103. The relation of transplanted eyes to developing nerve centers.

Maynard, D. M. (1965) *J. Exp. Biol.* **43**:79–106. The occurrence and functional characteristics of heteromorph antennules in an experimental population of spiny lobsters, *Panulirus argus*.

Maynard, D. M., and M. J. Cohen. (1965) *J. Exp. Biol.* **43**:55–78. The function of a heteromorph antennule in a spiny lobster, *Panulirus argus*.

Mayr, E. (1970) *Populations, Species and Evolution*, Harvard University Press, Cambridge, Mass.

McBride, W. G. (1974) *Teratology* **10**:283–292. Fetal nerve cell degeneration produced by thalidomide in rabbits.

McCarthy, K. D., and L. M. Partlow. (1976*a*) *Brain Res.* **114**:391–414. Preparation of pure neuronal and non-neuronal cultures from embryonic chick sympathetic ganglia: A new method based on both differential cell adhesiveness and the formation of homotypic neuronal aggregates.

McCarthy, K. D., and L. M. Partlow. (1976*b*) *Brain Res.* **114**:415–426. Neuronal stimulation of [^{3}H]thymidine incorporation by primary cultures of highly purified non-neuronal cells.

McConnell, C. H. (1933) *Quart. J. Microsc. Sci.* **75**:495–509. Development of the ectodermal nerve net in the buds of hydra.

McCouch, G. P., G. M. Austin, C. -N. Liu, and C. Y. Liu. (1958) *J. Neurophysiol.* **21**:205–216. Sprouting as a cause of spasticity.

McCutcheon, M. (1946) *Physiol. Rev.* **26**:319–336. Chemotaxis in leukocytes.

McDonald, W. I. (1974) *Br. Med. Bull.* **30**:186–189. Remyelination in relation to clinical lesions of the central nervous system.

McEwen, B. S., and D. W. Pfaff. (1970) *Brain Res.* **21**:1–16. Factors influencing sex hormone uptake by rat brain regions. I. Effects of neonatal treatment, hypophysectomy, and competing steroids on estradiol uptake.

McEwen, B. S., G. Wallach, and C. Magnus. (1974) *Brain Res.* **70**:321–334. Corticosterone binding to hippocampus: Immediate and delayed influences of the absence of adrenal secretion.

McEwen, B. S., L. Plapinger, C. Chaptal, J. Gerlach, and G. Wallach. (1975) *Brain Res.* **96:**400–406. Role of fetoneonatal estrogen binding proteins in the association of estrogen with neonatal brain cell nuclear receptors.

McEwen, B. S., I. Lieberburg, N. Maclusky, and L. Plapinger. (1976) *Ann. Biol. Anim. Biochem. Biophys.* **16:**471–478. Interactions of testosterone and estradiol with the neonatal rat brain: Protective mechanism and possible relationship to sexual differentiation.

McIlwain, H. (1959) *Biochemistry and the Central Nervous System,* 2nd ed., Little, Brown, Boston.

McIntyre, A. K., and G. Robinson. (1958) *Proc. Otago. Univ. Med. School* **36:**25. Stability of spinal reflex patterns.

McKeehan, M. S. (1966) *Anat. Rec.* **154:**705–712. The mitotic pattern in the neural tube of *Amblystoma maculatum.*

McKeown, T., and R. G. Record. (1952) *J. Endocrinol.* **8:**386–401. Observations on foetal growth in multiple pregnancy in man.

McLachlan, E. M. (1974) *J. Physiol. (London)* **237:**217–242. The formation of synapses in mammalian sympathetic ganglia reinnervated with preganglionic or somatic nerves.

McLaughlin, B. J., J. G. Wood, K. Saito, E. Roberts, and J. -Y. Wu. (1975) *Brain Res.* **85:**355–371. The fine structural localization of glutamate decarboxylase in developing axonal processes and presynaptic terminals of rodent cerebellum.

McLoughlin, C. B. (1968) Interaction of epidermis with various types of foreign mesenchyme, pp. 244–251. In *Epithelial-Mesenchymal Interactions* (R. Fleischmajer and R. Billingham, eds.), Williams and Wilkins, Baltimore.

McMahon, D. (1973) *Proc. Natl. Acad. Sci. U.S.A.* **70:**2396–2400. A cell contact model for cellular position determination in development.

McMahon, D. (1974) *Science* **185:**1012–1021. Chemical messengers in development: A hypothesis.

McMahon, T. (1973) *Science* **179:**1201–1204. Size and shape in biology.

McMorris, F. A., and F. H. Ruddle. (1974) *Dev. Biol.* **39:**226–246. Expression of neuronal phenotypes in neuroblastoma cell hybrids.

McMorris, F. A., A. R. Kolber, B. W. Moore, and A. S. Perumal. (1974) *J. Cell. Physiol.* **84:**473–480. Expression of the neuron-specific protein, 14-3-2, and steroid sulfatase in neuroblastoma cell hybrids.

McMurray, V. (1954) *J. Exp. Zool.* **125:**247–263. The development of the optic lobes in *Xenopus laevis:* The effect of repeated crushing of the optic nerve.

McPhedran, A. M., R. B. Wuerker, and E. Henneman. (1965) *J. Neurophysiol.* **28:**71–84. Properties of motor units in a homogeneous red muscle (soleus of the cat).

McPherson, A., and J. Tokunaga. (1967) *J. Physiol. (London)* **188:**121–129. The effects of cross-innervation on the myoglobin concentration of tonic and phasic muscles.

Meek, E. S., and J. F. A. Harbison. (1967) *J. Anat. (London)* **101:**487–489. Nuclear area and deoxyribonucleic acid content in human liver cell nuclei.

Meier, C. (1976) *Brain Res.* **104:**21–32. Some observations on early myelination in the human spinal cord, light and electron microscope study.

Meier, G., and W. G. Hoag. (1962) *J. Neuropathol.-Exp. Neurol.* **21:**649–654. The neuropathology of "reeler," a neuromuscular mutation in mice.

Meier, H., and A. D. MacPike. (1970) *Exp. Brain Res.* **10:**512–525. A neurological mutation *(msd)* of the mouse causing a deficiency of myelin synthesis.

Meinertzhagen, I. A. (1972) *Brain Res.* **41:**39–49. Erroneous projection of retinula axons beneath a dislocation in the retinal equator of *Calliphora.*

Meinertzhagen, I. A. (1975) The development of neuronal connection patterns in the visual system of insects, pp. 265–283. In *Cell Patterning,* Ciba Foundation Symposium 29, Elsevier, New York.

Meinhardt, H., and A. Gierer. (1974) *J. Cell Sci.* **15:**321–346. Applications of a theory of biological pattern formation based on lateral inhibition.

Meller, K., and R. Haupt. (1967) *Z. Zellforsch. Mikrosk. Anat. Abt. Histochem.* **76:**260–277. Die Feinstruktur der Neuro-, Glio- and Ependymoblasten von Hühnerembryonen in der Gewebekultur.

Meller, K., W. Breipohl, and P. Glees. (1968*a*) *Z. Zellforsch. Mikrosk. Anat. Abt. Histochem.* **86:**171–183. The cytology of the developing molecular layer of mouse motor cortex: An electron microscopical and Golgi impregnation study.

Meller, K., W. Breipohl, and P. Glees. (1968*b*) *Z. Zellforsch. Mikrosk. Anat. Abt. Histochem.* **92:**217–231. Synaptic organization of the molecular and outer granular layer in the motor cortex in the white mouse during postnatal development: A Golgi and electron-microscopical study.

Mendell, L. M., and E. Henneman. (1968) *Science* **160:**96–98. Terminals of single la fibers: Distribution within a pool of 300 homonymous motor neurons.

Mendell, L. M., and E. Henneman. (1971) *J. Neurophysiol.* **24:**171–187. Terminals of single Ia fibers: Location, density, and distribution within a pool of 300 homonymous motoneurons.

Mendell, L. M., and J. G. Scott. (1975) *Exp. Brain Res.* **22:**221–234. The effect of peripheral nerve cross-union on connections of single Ia fibers to motoneurons.

Mendell, L. M., J. B. Munson, and J. G. Scott. (1974) *Brain Res.* **73:**338–342. Connectivity changes of 1a efferents on axotomized motoneurons.

Merrill, E. G., and P. D. Wall. (1972) *J. Physiol. (London)* **226:**825–846. Factors forming the edge of a receptive field: The presence of relatively ineffective afferent terminals.

Messier, B., C. P. Leblond, and I. Smart. (1958) *Exp. Cell Res.* **14:**224–226. Presence of DNA synthesis and mitosis in the brain of young adult mice.

Messier, P. E., and C. Auclair. (1973) *J. Embryol. Exp. Morphol.* **30:**661–671. Inhibition of nuclear migration in the absence of microtubules in the chick embryo.

Messier, P. E., and C. Auclair. (1974) *Dev. Biol.* **36:**218–223. Effect of cytochalasin B on interkinetic nuclear migration in the chick embryo.

Messier, P. E., and C. Auclair. (1975) *J. Embryol. Exp. Morphol.* **34:**339–354. Neurulation et migration nucléaire intercinétique chez des embryons de poulet.

Merrell, R., and L. Glaser. (1973) *Proc. Natl. Acad. Sci. U.S.A.* **70:**2794–2798. Specific recognition of plasma membranes by embryonic cells.

Metuzals, J. (1969) *J. Cell. Biol.* **43:**480–505. Configuration of a filamentous network in the axoplasm of the squid.

Meyer, R. L., and R. W. Sperry. (1973) *Exp. Neurol.* **40:**525–539. Tests for neuroplasticity in the anuran retinotectal system.

Miale, I. L., and R. L. Sidman. (1961) *Exp. Neurol.* **4:**277–296. An autoradiographic analysis of histogenesis in the mouse cerebellum.

Miani, N., A. Di Girolamo, and M. Girolamo. (1966) *J. Neurochem.* **13:**755–759. Sedimentation characteristics of axonal RNA in rabbit.

Michetti, F., N. Miami, G. De Renzis, A. Caniglia, and S. Correr. (1974) *J. Neurochem.* **22:**239–244. Nuclear localization of S-100 protein.

Milburn, A. (1973*a*) *J. Cell. Sci.* **12:**175–195. The early development of muscle spindles in the rat.

Milburn, A. (1973*b*) The development of the muscle spindle in the rat. Ph.D. thesis, Durham University.

Milburn, N. S., and D. R. Bentley. (1971) *J. Insect Physiol.* **17:**607–623. On the dendritic topology and activation of cockroach giant interneurons.

Miledi, R. (1960*a*) *J. Physiol. (London)* **151:**1–23. The acetylcholine sensitivity of frog muscle fibres after complete or partial denervation.

Miledi, R. (1960*b*) *J. Physiol. (London)* **151:**24–30. Junctional and extra-junctional acetylcholine receptors in skeletal muscle fibres.

Miledi, R. (1962) *Nature* **193:**281–282. Induced innervation of end plate free muscle segments.

Miledi, R. (1963) *Nature* **199:**1191–1192. Formation of extra nerve–muscle junctions in innervated muscle.

Miledi, R., and P. Orkand. (1966) *Nature* **209:**717–718. Effect of a "fast" nerve on "slow" muscle fibres in the frog.

Miledi, R., and C. R. Slater. (1970) *J. Physiol. (London)* **207:**507–528. On the degeneration of rat neuromuscular junctions after nerve section.

Miledi, R., and E. Stefani. (1969) *Nature* **222:**569–571. Nonselective re-innervation of slow and fast muscle fibres in the rat.

Miledi, R., E. Stefani, and J. Zelená. (1968) *Nature* **220:**497–498. Neural control of acetylcholine-sensitivity in rat muscle fibres.

Millar, J., A. I. Basbaum, and P. D. Wall. (1976) *Exp. Neurol.* **50:**658–672. Restructuring of the somatotopic map and appearance of abnormal neuronal activity in the gracile nucleus after partial deafferentation.

Miller, R. L. (1966) *J. Exp. Zool.* **161:**23–44. Chemotaxis during fertilization in the hybrid *Campanularia.*

Miller, R. L., and C. J. Brokaw. (1970) *J. Exp. Biol.* **52:**699–706. Chemotactic turning behavior of *Tubularia* spermatozoa.

Miner, N. (1956) *J. Comp. Neurol.* **105:**161–170. Integumental specification of sensory fibers in the development of cutaneous local sign.

Minkowski, M. (1920) *Schweiz. Arch. Neurol. Psychiat.* **6:**201–252; **7:**268–303. Über den Verlauf, die Endigung und die zentrale Repräsentation von gekreutzten und ungekreutzten Sehnervenfasern bei einigen Säugetieren und beim Menschen.

Mintz, B. (1971) *Symp. Soc. Exp. Biol.* **25:**345–370. Clonal basis of mammalian differentation.

Mintz, B., and S. Sanyal. (1970) *Genetics (Suppl.)* **64:**43–44. Clonal origin of the mouse visual retina mapped from genetically mosaic eyes.

Mintz, B., and L. S. Stone. (1934) *Proc. Soc. Exp. Biol. Med.* **31:**1080–1082. Transplantation of taste organs in adult *Triturus viridescens.*

Misantone, L. J., and D. J. Stelzner. (1974) *Exp. Neurol.* **45:**364–376. Behavioral manifestations of competition of retinal endings for sites in doubly innervated frog optic tectum.

Mistretta, C. M. (1972) Topographical and histological study of the developing rat tongue, palate and taste buds, pp. 163–187. In *Third Symposium on Oral Sensation and Perception: The Mouth of the Infant* (J. F. Bosma, ed.), Thomas, Springfield, Ill.

Mitra, N. L. (1955) *J. Anat. (London)* **89:**467–483. Quantitative analysis of cell types in mammalian neocortex.

Mize, R. R., and E. H. Murphy. (1973) *Science* **180:**320–323. Selective visual experience fails to modify receptive field properties of rabbit striate cortex neurons.

Mizel, S. B., and J. R. Bamburg. (1976) *Dev. Biol.* **49:**20–28. Studies on the action of nerve growth factor.

Mizel, S. B., and L. Wilson. (1972) *Biochemistry* **11:**2573–2578. Nucleoside transport in mammalian cells: Inhibition by colchicine.

Model, P. G., M. B. Bornstein, S. M. Crain, and G. D. Pappas. (1971) *J. Cell Biol.* **49:**362–371. An electron microscopic study of the development of synapses in cultured fetal mouse cerebrum continuously exposed to xylocaine.

Möller, A. (1950) *Zool. Jahrb. Abt. Allgem. Zool. Physiol. Tiere* **62:**138–182. Die Struktur des Auges bei Urodelen verschiedener Körpergrösse.

Molliver, M. E., and H. Van der Loos. (1970) *Ergeb. Anat. Ent. Gesch.* **42:**7–53. The ontogenesis of cortical circuitry: The spatial distribution of synapses in somesthetic cortex of newborn dog.

Molliver, M. E., I. Kostović, and H. Van der Loos. (1973) *Brain Res.* **50:**403–407. The development of synapses in the cerebral cortex of the human fetus.

Monagle, R. D., and H. Brody. (1974) *J. Comp. Neurol.* **155:**61–66. The affects of age upon the main nucleus of the inferior olive in the human.

Monard, D., F. Solomon, M. Rentsch, and R. Gysin. (1973) *Proc. Natl. Acad. Sci. U.S.A.* **70:**1894–1897. Glia-induced morphological differentiation in neuroblastoma cells (glial–neuronal interactions).

Monard, D., K. Stockel, R. Goodman, and H. Thoenen. (1975) *Nature* **258:**444–445. Distinction between nerve growth factor and glial factor.

Money, J. (1971) *Impact Sci. Soc.* **22:**285–290. Prenatal hormones and intelligence: A possible relationship.

Money, J., and A. A. Ehrhardt. (1972) *Man and Woman, Boy and Girl,* Johns Hopkins University Press, Baltimore.

Money, J., and V. Lewis. (1966) *Bull. Johns Hopkins Hosp.* **118:**365–373. IQ, genetics and accelerated growth: Adrenogenital syndrome.

Monro, A. (Primus) (1732) *The Anatomy of the Human Bones, to Which Are Added an Anatomical Treatise of the Nerves,* W. Monro, Edinburgh.

Montgomery, A. (1972) A study of the effects of disuse upon the isometric characteristics of fast twitch and slow twitch mammalian skeletal muscle. Ph.D. thesis, University of Bristol.

Moor, H., K. Pfenninger, and K. Akert. (1969) *Science* **164:**1405–1407. Synaptic vesicles in electron micrographs of freeze-etched nerve terminals.

Moore, B. W. (1972) *Int. Rev. Neurobiol.* **15:**215–225. Chemistry and biology of two proteins, S-100 and 14-3-2, specific to the nervous system.

Moore, B. W., and V. J. Perez. (1968) Specific acidic proteins of the nervous system, pp. 343–360. In *Physiological and Biochemical Aspects of Nervous Integration* (F. D. Carlson, ed.), Prentice-Hall, Englewood Cliffs, N.J.

Moore, R. Y., A. Björklund, and U. Stenevi. (1971) *Brain Res.* **33:**13–35. Plastic changes in the adrenergic innervation of the rat septal area in response to denervation.

Moore, R. Y., A. Björklund, and U. Stenevi. (1973) Growth and plasticity of adrenergic neurons, pp. 961–977. In *The Neurosciences: Third Study Program* (F. O. Schmitt, ed.), MIT Press, Cambridge, Mass.

Moran, D. T., and J. C. Rowley, III. (1974) *Brain Res.* **74:**373–377. Cytoplasmic order in an invertebrate neuron.

Morest, D. K. (1968) *Z. Anat. Entwicklungsgesch.* **127:**201–220. The growth of synaptic endings in the mammalian brain: A study of the calyces of the trapezoid body.

Morest, D. K. (1969*a*) *Z. Anat. Entwicklungsgesch.* **128:**271–289. The differentiation of cerebral dendrites: a study of the postmigratory neuroblast in the medial trapezoid body.

Morest, D. K. (1969*b*) *Z. Anat. Entwicklungsgesch.* **128:**290–317. The growth of dendrites in the mammalian brain.

Morest, D. K. (1970*a*) *Z. Anat. Entwicklungsgesch.* **130:**265–305. A study of neurogenesis in the forebrain of opossum pouch young.

Morest, D. K. (1970*b*) *Z. Anat. Entwicklungsgesch.* **131:** 45–67. The pattern of neurogenesis in the retina of the cat.

Morest, D. K. (1971) *Z. Anat. Entwicklungsgesch.* **133:**216–246. Dendrodendritic synapses of cells that have axons: The fine structure of the Golgi type II cell in the medial geniculate body of the cat.

Morgan, M. J., J. M. O'Donnell, and R. F. Oliver. (1973) *J. Comp. Neurol.* **149:**203–214. Development of left–right asymmetry in the habenular nuclei of Rana temporaria.

Morgan, T. H. (1905) *J. Exp. Zool.* **2:**495–506. Polarity considered as a phenomenon of gradation of materials.

Mori, S., and C. P. Leblond (1969) *J. Comp. Neurol.* **135:**57–80. Identification of microglia in light and electron microscopy.

Morrell, J. I., D. B. Kelley, and D. W. Pfaff. (1975) Sex steroid binding in the brains of vertebrates, pp. 230–256. In *Brain–Endocrine Interaction II: The Ventricular System* (K. M. Knigge and D. E. Scott, eds.), Karger, Basel.

Morris, V. B. (1973) *J. Comp. Neurol.* **151:**323–330. Time differences in the formation of the receptor types in the developing chick retina.

Morris, V. B. (1975) *J. Comp. Neurol.* **164:**95–104. Non-randomness in the sequential formation of principal cones in small areas of the developing chick retina.

Morrison, L. R. (1932) *Arch. Neurol. Psychiat. (Chicago)* **28:**204–205. Role of oligodendroglia in myelogenesis.

Moscona, A. A. (1962) *J. Cell Comp. Physiol.* (Suppl. 1) **60:**65–80. Analysis of cell recombinations in experimental synthesis of tissues *in vitro.*

Moscona, A. A. (1968) *Dev. Biol.* **18:**250–277. Cell aggregation properties of specific cell-ligands and their role in the formation of multicellular systems.

Moscona, A. A. (1974) Surface specification of embryonic cells: Lectin receptors, cell recognition and specific ligands, pp. 69–99. In *The Cell Surface in Development* (A. A. Moscona, ed.), Wiley, New York.

Mottet, K. (1952) *J. Comp. Neurol.* **96:**519–553. The effect of removal of somatopleur on the development of motor and sensory neurons in the spinal cord and ganglia.

Mottet, K., and D. H. Barron. (1954) *Yale J. Biol. Med.* **26:**275–284. Some effects of the peripheral field on the cytochemical differentiation of neurons.

Moulton, J. M., A. Jurand, and H. Fox. (1968) *J. Embryol. Exp. Morphol.* **19:**415–431. A cytological study of Mauthner's cells in *Xenopus laevis* and *Rana temporaria* during metamorphosis.

Mountcastle, V. B. (1957) *J. Neurophysiol.* **20:**408–434. Modality and topographic properties of single neurons of cat's somatic sensory cortex.

Mountcastle, V. B. (1974) Neural mechanisms in somesthesia, pp. 307–347. In *Medical Physiology,* Vol. 1 (V. B. Mountcastle, ed.), Mosby, St. Louis.

Moussa, T. A. (1955–1956) *Cellule* **57:**321–334. An experimental study of the effect of axon sectioning on the cytoplasmic components of the corresponding neurones.

Moyer, E. K., and B. F. Kaliszewski. (1958) *Anat. Rec.* **131:**681–699. The number of nerve fibers in motor spinal nerve roots of young, mature and aged cats.

Mugnaini, E. (1966) *Anat. Rec.* **154:**391. Ultrastructural aspects of cerebellar morphology in the chick embryo.

Mugnaini, E. (1969) Ultrastructural studies on the cerebellar histogenesis. II. Maturation of nerve cell populations and establishment of synaptic connections in the cerebellar cortex of the chick, pp. 749–782. In *Neurobiology of Cerebellar Evolution and Development* (R. Llinás, ed.), A.M.A. Education and Research Foundation, Chicago.

Mugnaini, E. (1970) *Brain Res.* **17:**169–179. The relation between cytogenesis and the formation of different types of synaptic contact.

Mugnaini, E., and P. F. Forströnen. (1967) *Z. Zellforsch. Mikrosk. Anat. Abt. Histochem.* **77:**115–143. Ultrastructural studies on the cerebellar histogenesis. I. Differentiation of granule cells and development of *glomeruli* in the chick embryo.

Mugnaini, E., and F. Walberg. (1964) *Ergeb. Anat. Entw.-Gersch.* **37:**193–236. Ultrastructure of neuroglia.

Müller, E., and S. Ingvar. (1923) *Arch. Mikrosk. Anat.* **99:**650–671. Über den Ursprung des Sympathicus beim Hühnchen.

Mumenthaler, E., and W. K. Engel. (1961) *Acta Anat.* **47:**274–299. Cytological localization of cholinesterase in developing chick embryo skeletal muscle.

Mungai, J. M. (1967) *J. Anat. (London)* **101:**403–418. Dendritic patterns in the somatic sensory cortex of the cat.

Munro, M., and F. H. C. Crick. (1971) *Symp. Soc. Exp. Biol.* **25:**439–453. The time needed to set up a gradient: Detailed calculations.

Muntz, W. R. A. (1962*a*) *J. Neurophysiol.* **25:**699–711. Microelectrode recordings from the diencephalon of the frog, *(Rana pipiens)* and a blue-sensitive system.

Muntz, W. R. A. (1962*b*) *J. Neurophysiol.* **25:**712–720. Effectiveness of different colors of light in releasing the positive phototactic behavior of frogs, and a possible function of the retinal projection to the diencephalon.

Murphy, C., and C. Tokunaga. (1970) *J. Exp. Zool.* **175:**197–220. Cell lineage in the dorsal mesothoracic disc of *Drosophila.*

Murphy, R. A., N. J. Pantazis, B. G. W. Arnason, and M. Young. (1975) *Proc. Natl. Acad. Sci. U.S.A.* **72:**1895–1898. Secretion of a nerve growth factor by mouse neuroblastoma cells in culture.

Murray, C. D. (1926*a*) *J. Gen. Physiol.* **9:**835–841. The physiological principle of minimum work applied to the angle of branching of arteries.

Murray, C. D. (1926*b*) *Proc. Natl. Acad. Sci. U.S.A.* **12:**207–214. The physiological principle of minimum work. I. The vascular system and the cost of blood volume.

Murray, H. M., and B. E. Walker. (1973) *Exp. Neurol.* **41:**290–302. Comparative study of astrocytes and mononuclear leukocytes reacting to brain trauma in mice.

Murray, M. (1968) *Exp. Neurol.* **20:**460–468. Effects of dehydration on the rate of proliferation of hypothalamic neuroglia cells.

Murray, M., and M. E. Goldberger. (1974) *J. Comp. Neurol.* **158:**19–36. Restitution of function and collateral sprouting in the cat spinal cord: The partially hemisected animal.

Murray, M. R., and H. H. Benitez. (1967) *Science* **155:**1021–1024. Deuterium oxide: direct action on sympathetic ganglia isolated in culture.

Murray, M. R., and H. H. Benitez. (1968) Action of heavy water (D_2O) on growth and development of isolated nervous tissues, pp. 148–178. In *Ciba Foundation Symposium on Growth of the Nervous System* (G. E. W. Wolstenholme and M. O'Connor, eds.), Little, Brown, Boston.

Muthukkaruppan, V. (1966) *J. Exp. Zool.* **159:**269–288. Inductive tissue interaction in the development of the mouse lens *in vitro.*

Myslivecek, J. (1968) *Brain Res.* **10:**418–430. The development of the response to light flash in the visual cortex of the dog.

Naftolin, F., K. J. Ryan, and Z. Petro. (1971*a*) *J. Clin. Endocrinol.* **33:**368–370. Aromatization of androstenedione by the diencephalon.

Naftolin, F., K. J. Ryan, and Z. Petro. (1971*b*) *J. Endocrinol.* **51:**797–796. Aromatization of androstenedione by limbic system tissue from human foetuses.

Naftolin, F., K. J. Ryan, and Z. Petro. (1972) *Endocrinology* **90:**295–298. Aromatization of androstenedione by the anterior hypothalamus of adult male and female rats.

Nageotte, M. J. (1907) Cited in Ramón y Cajal (1928) *Degeneration and Regeneration in the Nervous System,* p. 429.

Nakai, J. (1956) *Am. J. Anat.* **99:**81–130. Dissociated dorsal root ganglia in tissue culture.

Nakai, J. (1960) *Z. Zellforsch. Mikrosk. Anat.* **52:**427–449. Studies on the mechanism determining the course of nerve fibres in tissue culture. II. The mechanism of fasciculation.

Nakai, J. (1965) *Tex. Rep. Biol. Med.* **23:** *Suppl.* **1,** 371–375. Tridimensional nerve formation *in vitro.*

Nakai, J. (1969) *J. Exp. Zool.* **170:**85–106. The development of neuromuscular junctions in cultures of chick embryo tissue.

Nakai, J., and Y. Kawasaki. (1959) *Z. Zellforsch. Mikrosk. Anat.* **51:**108–122. Studies on the mechanism determining the course of nerve fibers in tissue culture. I. The reaction of the growth cone to various obstructions.

Nakajima, S. (1965) *J. Comp. Neurol.* **125:**193–205. Selectivity in fasciculation of nerve fibres *in vitro.*

Nakazawa, S. (1959) *Naturwissenschaften* **46**:333–334. General mechanism of the polarity determination in some fucoid eggs.

Nass, M. M. K. (1969) *Science* **165**:25–35. Mitochondrial DNA: Advances, problems and goals.

Nathanson, N., G. A. Cole, and H. Van der Loos. (1969) *Brain Res.* **15**:532–536. Heterotopic cerebellar granule cells following administration of cyclophosphamide to suckling rats.

Nawar, G. (1956) *Am. J. Anat.* **99**:473–506. Experimental analysis of the origin of the autonomic ganglia in the chick embryo.

Neder, R. (1959) *Zool. Jahrb. Abt. Anat. Ontog. Tiere* **77**:411–464. Allometrisches Wachstum von Hirnteilen bei drei verschieden grossen Schafenarten.

Needham, J. (1942) *Biochemistry and Morphogenesis*, Cambridge University Press, London, 758 pp.

Nicholas, J. S. (1924) *J. Exp. Zool.* **39**:27–41. Ventral and dorsal implantations of the limb bud in *Amblystoma punctatum.*

Nicholas, J. S. (1930*a*) *Anat. Rec.* **45**:234. Movements in transplanted limbs innervated by eye muscle nerves.

Nicholas, J. S. (1933) *J. Comp. Neurol.* **57**:253–283. The correlation of movement and nerve supply in transplanted limbs of *Amblystoma.*

Nicholas, J. S. (1957) *Proc. Natl. Acad. Sci. U.S.A.* **43**:542–545. Results of inversion of neural plate material.

Nicolls, J. G., and Baylor. (1968) *J. Neurophysiol.* **31**:740–756. Specific modalities and receptive fields of sensory neurons in CNS of the leech.

Nicholson, J. L., and J. Altman. (1972) *Brain Res.* **44**:13–23. The effects of early hypo- and hyperthyroidism on the development of rat cerebellar cortex. I. Cell proliferation and differentiation.

Nieuwenhuys, R. (1964) *Prog. Brain Res.* **25**:1–93. Comparative anatomy of the cerebellum.

Nieuwkoop, P. D. (1952) *J. Exp. Zool.* **120**:1–130. Activation and organization of the amphibian central nervous system.

Nieuwkoop, P. D. (1955) *Proc. Koninkl. Ned. Adak. Wetenschap.* **58**:219–239, 356–370. Origin and establishment of organization patterns in embryonic fields during early development in amphibians and birds especially in the nervous system and its substrate.

Nieuwkoop, P. D. (1962) *Acta Biotheoret.* **16**:57–68. The "organization centre," I. Induction and determination.

Nieuwkoop, P. D. (1967*a*) *Acta Biotheoret.* **17**:151–177. The "organization centre," II. Field phenomena, their origin and significance.

Nieuwkoop, P. D. (1967*b*) *Acta Biotheoret.* **17**:178–194. The "organization centre," III. Segregation and pattern formation in morphogenetic fields.

Nieuwkoop, P. D. (1973) *Adv. Morphol.* **10**:1–39. The "organization center" of the amphibian embryo: Its origin, spatial organization, and morphogenetic action.

Nieuwkoop, P. D., and J. Faber. (1956) *Normal Table of Xenopus laevis (Daudin)*, North-Holland, Amsterdam.

Niklowitz, W., and I. J. Bak. (1965) *Z. Zellforsch. Mikrosk. Anat.* **66**:529–547. Elektronenmikroskopische Untersuchungen am Ammonshorn.

Nissl, F. (1892) *Allgem. Z. Psychiat.* **48**:197–198. Über die Veränderungen der Ganglienzellen am Facialiskern des Kaninchens nach Ausreissung der Nerven.

Nissl, F. (1894) *Neurol. Zentralbl.* **13**:676–688. Ueber die sogenannten Granula der Nervenzellen.

Noback, C. R., and M. L. Moss. (1956) *J. Comp. Neurol.* **105**:539–551. Differential growth of the human brain.

Noback, C. R., and D. P. Purpura. (1961) *J. Comp. Neurol.* **117**:291–308. Postnatal ontogenesis of neurons in cat neocortex.

Noble, R. G. (1973) *Horm. Behav.* **4**:45–52. The effects of castration at different intervals after birth on the copulatory behavior of male hamsters *(Mesocricetus auratus)*.

Noetzel, H., and J. Rox. (1964) *Acta Neuropathol.* **3**:326–342. Autoradiographische Untersuchungen über Zellteilung und Zellentwicklung im Gehirn der erwachsenen Maus und der erwachsenen Rhesus-affen nach Injektion von radioaktivem Thymidin.

Nolte, A. (1953) *Zool. Jahrb. Abt. Allgem. Zool. Physiol. Tiere* **64**:538–594. Die Abhängigkeit des Proportionierung und Cytoarchitektonik des Gehirns von der Körpergrösse bei Urodelen.

Nordlander, R. H., and J. S. Edwards. (1968*a*) *Nature* **218**:780–781. Morphological cell death in the post-embryonic development of the insect optic lobes.

Nordlander, R. H., and J. S. Edwards. (1968*b*) *J. Morphol.* **126**:67–94. Morphology of the larval and adult brains of the monarch butterfly, *Danaus plexippus plexippus,* L.

Nordlander, R. H., and J. S. Edwards. (1969) *Arch. Entw.-Mech. Organ.* **162**:197–217. Postembryonic brain development in the monarch butterfly, *Danaus plexippus plexippus,* L. I. Cellular events during brain morphogenesis.

Nordling, S., H. Mietinen, J. Wartiovaara, and L. Saxén. (1971) *J. Embryol. Exp. Morphol.* **26:**231–252. Transmission and spread of embryonic induction. I. Temporal relationships in transfilter induction of kidney tubules *in vitro.*

Norman, R. M. (1963) Malformations of the nervous system, birth injury and diseases of early life, pp. 324–382. In *Greenfield's Neuropathology,* 2nd ed., Williams and Wilkins, Baltimore.

Norman, R. M. (1966) *Dev. Med. Child Neurol.* **8:**170–177. Neuropathological findings in trisomies 13-15 and 17-18 with special reference to the cerebellum.

Nornes, H. O., and G. D. Das. (1974) *Brain Res.* **73:**121–138. Temporal pattern of neurogenesis in spinal cord of Rat. I. An autoradiographic study—time and sites of origin and migration and settling patterns of neuroblasts.

Norr, S. C. (1973) *Dev. Biol.* **34:**16–38. *In vitro* analysis of sympathetic neuron differentiation from chick neural crest cells.

Norr, S. C., and S. Varon. (1975) *Neurobiology* **5:**101–118. Dynamic, temperature-sensitive association of ^{125}I-nerve growth factor *in vitro* with ganglionic and non-ganglionic cells from embryonic chick.

Nörstrom, A., H. -A. Hansson and J. Sjöstrand (1971). *Z. Zellforsch. Mikrosk. Anat.* **113:**271–293. Effects of colchicine on axonal transport and ultrastructure of the hypothalamoneurohypophyseal system of the rat.

Norton, W. T. (1976) Formation, structure, and biochemistry of myelin, pp. 74–99. In *Basic Neurochemistry,* 2nd ed. (G. J. Siegel, R. W. Albers, R. Katzman, and B. W. Agranoff, eds.), Little, Brown, Boston.

Norton, W. T., and S. E. Poduslo. (1970) *Science* **167:**1144–1146. Neuronal soma and whole neuroglia of rat brain: A new isolation technique.

Norton, W. T., and S. E. Poduslo. (1973) *J. Neurochem.* **21:**759–773. Myelination in rat brain: Changes in myelin composition during brain maturation.

Nottebohm, F. (1969) *Ibis* **111:**386–387. The "critical period" for song learning.

Nottebohm, F. (1970) *Science* **167:**950–956. Ontogeny of bird song.

Nováková, V., J. Pilny, W. Sandritter, and G. Kiefer. (1968) Changes in nucleic acids of the central nervous system neuron in the postnatal ontogenesis of the rat, pp. 285–289. In *Ontogenesis of the Brain* (L. Jílek and S. Trojan, eds.), Charles University Press, Prague.

Nowakowski, R. S., and P. Rakic. (1974) *Cell Tiss. Kinet.* **7:**189–194. Clearance rate of exogenous ^{3}H-thymidine from the plasma of Rhesus monkeys.

Nurnberger, J. I., and M. W. Gordon. (1957) The cell density of neural tissues: Direct counting method and possible applications as a biologic referent, pp. 100–128. In *Progress in Neurobiology* (H. Waelsch, ed.), Hoeber, New York.

Nussbaum, J. L., N. Neskovic, and P. Mandel. (1971) *J. Neurochem.* **18:**1529–1543. The fatty acid composition of phospholipids and glycolipids in Jimpy mouse brain.

Nyholm, M., S. Saxén, S. Toivonen, and T. Vainio. (1962) *Exp. Cell Res.* **28:**209–212. Electron microscopy of trans-filter neural induction.

Oakley, B. (1967) *J. Physiol. (London)* **188:**353–371. Altered temperature and taste responses from cross-regenerated sensory nerves in the rat's tongue.

Oakley, B. (1970) *Acta Physiol. Scand.* **79:**88–94. Reformation of taste buds by crossed sensory nerves in the rat's tongue.

Oakley, B. (1974*a*) *Brain Res.* **75:**85–96. On the specification of taste neurons in the rat tongue.

Oakley, B. (1974*b*) Problems in the development of taste receptor properties and synaptic connections, pp. 319–329. In *Transduction Mechanisms in Taste* (T. M. Pointer, ed.), Retrieval, Ltd., London.

Obersteiner, H. (1883) *Biol. Zentralbl.* **3:**145–155. Der feinere Bau der Kleinhirnrinde beim Menschen und bei Tieren.

Ochs, S. (1971*a*) *J. Neurobiol.* **2:**331–345. Characteristics and a model for fast axoplasmic transport in nerve.

Ochs, S. (1971*b*) *Proc. Natl. Acad. Sci. U.S.A.* **68:**1279–1282. Local supply of energy to the fast axoplasmic transport mechanism.

Ochs, S. (1972*a*) *Science* **176:**252–260. Fast transport of materials in mammalian nerve fibers.

Ochs, S. (1972*b*) *J. Physiol. (London)* **227:**627–645. Rate of fast axoplasmic transport in mammalian nerve fibres.

Ochs, S. (1973) *Prog. Brain Res.* **40:**349–362. Effect of maturation and aging on the rate of fast axoplasmic transport in mammalian nerve.

Ochs, S., and D. Hollingsworth. (1971) *J. Neurochem.* **18:**107–114. Dependence of fast axoplasmic transport in nerve on oxidative metabolism.

Ochs, S., and C. Smith. (1971) *Fed. Proc.* **30:**665. Effect of temperature and rate of stimulation on fast axoplasmic transport in mammalian nerve fibers.

Ochs, S., and C. Smith. (1975) *J. Neurobiol.* **6:**85–102. Low temperature slowing and cold-block of fast axoplasmic transport in mammalian nerves *in vitro.*

O'Connor, T. M., and C. R. Wyttenbach. (1974) *J. Cell Biol.* **60:**448–459. Cell death in the embryonic chick spinal cord.

Ogawa, F. (1934) *Sci. Rep. Tohoku Univ. Fourth Ser.* **8:**345–368. The number of ganglion cells and nerve fibers in the nervous system of the earthworm.

Ogawa, F. (1939) *Sci. Rep. Tohoku Univ. Fourth Ser.* **13:**395–488. The nervous system of earthworm *(Pheretima communissima)* in different ages.

Oger, J., B. G. W. Arnason, N. Pantazis, J. Lehrich, and M. Young. (1974) *Proc. Natl. Acad. Sci. U.S.A.* **71:**1554–1558. Synthesis of nerve growth factor by L and 3T3 cells in culture.

Oja, S. S. (1966) *Ann. Acad. Sci. Fenn. Ser. A. V.* **125:**1–67. Postnatal changes in the concentration of nucleic acids, nucleotides and amino acids in the rat brain.

O'Leary, J. L. (1941) *J. Comp. Neurol.* **75:**131–164. Structure of the area striata of the cat.

O'Leary, J. L., J. Inukai, and J. M. Smith. (1971) *J. Comp. Neurol.* **142:**377–391. Histogenesis of the cerebellar climbing fiber in the rat.

Olmsted, J. B., G. B. Witman, K. Carlson, and J. L. Rosenbaum. (1974) *Proc. Natl. Acad. Sci. U.S.A.* **68:**2273–2277. Comparison of the microtubule proteins of neuroblastoma cells, brain, and *Chlamydomonas* flagella.

Olmsted, J. M. D. (1920*a*) *J. Comp. Neurol.* **31:**465–468. The nerve as a formative influence in the development of taste-buds.

Olmsted, J. M. D. (1920*b*) *J. Exp. Zool.* **31:**369–401. The results of cutting the seventh cranial nerve in *Ameiurus nebulosus* (Lesueur).

Olmsted, J. M. D. (1925) *J. Comp. Neurol.* **33:**149–154. Effects of cutting the lingual nerve of the dog.

Olney, J. W. (1968) *Invest. Ophthalmol.* **7:**250–268. An electron microscopic study of synapse formation, receptor outer segment development, and other aspects of developing mouse retina.

Olson, C. B., and C. P. Swett, Jr. (1966) *J. Comp. Neurol.* **128:**475–497. A functional and histochemical characterization of motor units in a heterogeneous muscle (flexor digitorum longus) of the cat.

Olson, C. B., and C. P. Swett, Jr. (1969) *Arch. Neurol. (Chicago)* **20:**263–270. Speed of contraction of skeletal muscle. The effect of hypoactivity and hyperactivity.

Olson, C. R., and R. D. Freeman. (1975) *J. Neurophysiol.* **38:**26–32. Progressive changes in kitten striate cortex during monocular vision.

Olson, L., and T. Malmfors. (1970) *Acta Physiol. Scand. (Suppl.)* **348:**1–112. Growth characteristics of adrenergic nerves in the adult rat. Fluorescence, histochemical and ^{3}H-noradrenaline uptake studies using tissue transplantation to the anterior chamber of the eye.

Olsson, Y., and J. Sjöstrand. (1969) *Exp. Neurol.* **23:**102–112. Origin of macrophages in Wallerian degeneration of peripheral nerves demonstrated autoradiographically.

O'Malley, B. W. (1969) *Trans. N.Y. Acad. Sci.* **31:**478–503. Hormonal regulation of nucleic acid and protein synthesis.

O'Malley, B. W., and A. R. Means. (1974) *Science* **183:**610–620. Female steroid hormones and target cell nuclei.

Opalski, A. (1933) *Z. Ges. Neurol. Psychiat.* **149:**221–254. Ueber lokale Unterschiede im Bau der Ventrikelwände beim Menschen.

Oppenheimer, J. M. (1936) *J. Exp. Zool.* **72:**409–437. Transplantation experiments on developing teleosts (*Fundulus* and *Perca*).

Oppenheimer, J. M. (1941) *J. Comp. Neurol.* **74:**131–167. The anatomical relationships of abnormally located Mauthner's cells in Fundulus embryos.

Oppenheimer, J. M. (1942) *J. Comp. Neurol.* **77:**577–587. The decussation of Mauthner's fibers in *Fundulus* embryos.

Oppenheimer, J. M. (1966) *Bull. Hist. Med.* **40:**525–543. Ross Harrison's contributions to experimental embryology.

O'Rahilly, R., and E. Gardner. (1971) *Z. Anat. Entwicklungsgesch.* **134:**1–12. The timing and sequence of events in the development of the human nervous system during the embryonic period proper.

Ostberg, A. J. C., G. Raisman, P. M. Field, L. L. Iverson, and R. E. Zigmond. (1976) *Brain Res.* **107:**445–470. A quantitative comparison of the formation of synapses in the rat superior cervical sympathetic ganglion by its own and foreign nerve fibers.

Ostertag, B. (1956) Missbildungen, Grundzüge der Entwicklung und Fehlentwicklung: Die Formbestimmenden Faktoren, p. 283. In *Handbuch der speziellen pathologischen Anatomie und Histologie,* Vol. 12, Part 4: *Nervensystem* (O. Lubarsch, F. Henke, and R. Rössle, eds.), Springer-Verlag, Berlin.

Otsuka, N. (1962) *Z. Zellforsch. Mikrosk. Anat. Abt. Histochem.* **58:**33–50. Histologischentwicklungsgeschichtliche Untersuchungen an Mauthnerschen Zellen von Fischen.

Otsuka, N. (1964) *Z. Zellforsch. Mikrosk. Anat. Abt. Histochem.* **62:**61–71. Weitere vergleichendanatomische Untersuchungen an Mauthnerschen Zellen von Fischen.

Otto, K. B., and W. Lierse. (1970) *Acta Anat.* **77:**25–36. Die Kapillarisierung verschiedener Teile des menschlichen Gehirns in der Fetalperiode und in den ersten Lebensjahren.

Packard, A., and V. Albergoni. (1970) *J. Exp. Biol.* **52:**539–552. Relative growth, nucleic acid content and cell numbers of the brain in *Octopus vulgaris* (Lamarck).

Paillard, J. (1960) The patterning of skilled movements, pp. 1679–1708. In *Handbook of Physiology, Neurophysiology,* Vol. III (J. Field, H. W. Magoun, and V. E. Hall, eds.), American Physiology Society, Washington, D.C.

Pakkenberg, H. (1967) *J. Comp. Neurol.* **128:**17–20. The number of nerve cells in the cerebral cortex of man.

Palay, S. L. (1958*a*) An electron microscopical study of neuroglia, pp. 24–49. In *Biology of Neuroglia* (W. F. Windle, ed.), Thomas, Springfield, Ill.

Palay, S. L. (1958*b*) *Exp. Cell Res. Suppl.* **5:**275–293. The morphology of synapses in the central nervous system.

Palay, S. L. (1961) *Anat. Rec.* **139:**262. Structural peculiarities of the neurosecretory cells in the preoptic nucleus of the goldfish, *Carassius auratus.*

Palay, S. L., and G. E. Palade. (1955) *J. Biophys. Biochem. Cytol.* **1:**69–88. The fine structure of neurons.

Palay, S. L., C. Sotelo, A. Peters, and P.M. Orkand. (1968) *J. Cell Biol.* **38:**193–201. The axon hillock and the initial segment.

Palka, J., and J. S. Edwards. (1974) *Proc. Roy. Soc. London (Biol.)* **185:**105–121. The cerci and abdominal giant fibers of the house cricket, *Acheta domesticus.* II. Regeneration and effects of chronic deprivation.

Palkovits, M., P. Magyar, and J. Szentágothai. (1971) *Brain Res.* **32:**1–13. Quantitative histological analysis of the cerebellar cortex in the cat. I. Number and arrangement in space of the Purkinje cells.

Pandazis, G. (1930) *Z. Morphol. Oekol. Tiere* **18:**114–169. Über die relative verschiedene Ausbildung der Gehirnzentren bei biologisch verschiedenen Ameisenarten.

Pannese, E. (1963*a*) *Z. Zellforsch. Mikrosk. Anat.* **60:**711–740. Investigations on the ultrastructural changes of the spinal ganglion neurons in the course of axon regeneration and cell hypertrophy. I. Changes during axon regeneration.

Pannese, E. (1963*b*) *Z. Zellforsch. Mikrosk. Anat.* **61:**561–586. Investigations on the ultrastructural changes of the spinal ganglion neurons in the course of axon regeneration and cell hypertrophy. II. Changes during cell hypertrophy and comparison between the ultrastructure of nerve cells of the same type under different functional conditions.

Pannese, E. (1968) *J. Comp. Neurol.* **132:**331–364. Developmental changes of the endoplasmic reticulum and ribosomes in nerve cells of the spinal ganglia of the domestic fowl.

Pannese, E. (1969) *J. Comp. Neurol.* **135:**381–422. Electron microscopical study on the development of the satellite cell sheath in spinal ganglia.

Pannese, E. (1974) *Adv. Anat. Embryol. Cell Biol.* **47:**6–97. The histogenesis of the spinal ganglia.

Pannese, E., L. Luciano, S. Iurato, and E. Reale. (1971) *J. Ultrastruct. Res.* **36:**46–67. Cholinesterase activity in spinal ganglia neuroblasts: A histochemical study at the electron microscope.

Panov, A. A. (1960) *Dokl. Akad. Nauk SSR* **132:**689–692. Origin of neuroblasts, neurilemma cells and neuroglia in the brain of the larva of *Antheraea pernyi* Guer. (In Russian.)

Panov, A. A. (1962) *Dokl. Akad. Nauk SSR Biol. Sci. Sect. (Transl.)* **145:**904–907. The nature of cell reproduction in the central nervous system of the house cricket. (*G. domesticus,* Orthoptera, Insecta).

Pappas, G. D., and D. P. Purpura. (1961) *Exp. Neurol.* **4:**507–530. Fine structure of dendrites in the superficial neocortical neuropil.

Paravicini, U., K. Stoeckel, and H. Thoenen. (1975) *Brain Res.* **84:**279–291. Biological importance of retrograde axonal transport of nerve growth factor in adrenergic neurons.

Parker, G. H. (1932) *Am. Nat.* **66:**147–158. On the trophic impulse so-called, its rate and nature.

Parker, G. H., and V. L. Paine. (1934) *Am. J. Anat.* **54:**1–25. Progressive nerve degeneration and its rate in the lateral-line nerve of the catfish.

Parks, T. N., and E. W. Rubel. (1975) *J. Comp. Neurol.* **164:**435–448. Organization and development of the brain stem auditory nuclei of the chicken: Organization of projections from n. magnocellularis to n. laminaris.

Parnavelas, J. G., A. Globus, and P. Kaups. (1973) *Exp. Neurol.* **40:**742–747. Continuous illumination from birth affects spine density of neurons in the visual cortex of the rat.

Parnavelas, J. G., G. Lynch, N. Brecha, C. W. Cotman, and A. Globus (1974) *Nature* **248:**71–73. Spine loss and regrowth in hippocampus following deafferentation.

Partlow, L. M., and M. G. Larrabee. (1969) *Fed. Proc.* **28:**886. Metabolic effects of nerve growth factor on chick sympathetic ganglia *in vitro.* Inhibitory effects of actinomycin-D and cycloheximide.

Partlow, L. M., and M. G. Larrabee. (1971) *J. Neurochem.* **18:**2101–2118. Effects of a nerve-growth factor, embryo age and metabolic inhibitors on growth of fibres and on synthesis of ribonucleic acid and protein in embryonic sympathetic ganglia.

Partlow, L. M., C. D. Ross, R. Motwani, and D. V. McDougal, Jr. (1972) *J. Gen. Physiol.* **60:**388–405. Transport of axonal emzymes in surviving segments of frog sciatic nerve.

Pasquini, J. M., B. Kaplun, C. A. Garcia Argiz, and C. J. Gomez. (1967) *Brain Res.* **6:**621–634. Hormonal regulation of brain development. 1. The effect of neonatal thyroidectomy upon nucleic acids, protein and two enzymes in developing cerebral cortex and cerebellum of the rat.

Pasquini, P. (1927) *Boll. Ist. Zool. Univ. Roma* **5:**1–83. Ricerche di embriologia sperimentale sui trapianti omeoplastici della vescicola ottica primaria in *Pleurodeles waltli.*

Pasternak, J. F., and T. A. Woolsey. (1975) *J. Comp. Neurol.* **160:**291–306. The number, size and spatial distribution of neurons in lamina IV of the mouse SmI neocortex.

Patel, A. J., A. Rabié, P. D. Lewis, and R. Balázs. (1976) *Brain Res.* **104:**33–48. Effect of thyroid deficiency on postnatal cell formation in the rat brain: A biochemical investigation.

Pearl, R. (1905) *Biometrika* **4:**13–104. Variation and correlation in brain weight.

Pearson, K. G., and Bradley, A. B. (1972) *Brain Res.* **47:**492–496. Specific regeneration of excitatory motor neurons to leg muscles in the cockroach.

Pease, D. C. (1964) *Histological Techniques for Electron Microscopy,* Academic Press, New York.

Pease, D. C., and T. A. Quilliam. (1957) *J. Biophys. Biochem. Cytol.* **3:**331–342. Electron microscopy of the Pacinian corpuscle.

Peck, C. K., and C. Blakemore. (1975) *Exp. Brain Res.* **22:**57–68. Modification of single neurons in the kitten's visual cortex after brief periods of monocular visual experience.

Pei, Y. F., and J. A. G. Rhodin. (1970) *Anat. Rec.* **168:**105–126. The prenatal development of the mouse eye.

Penfield, W. (1920) *Brain* **43:**290–305. Alterations of the Golgi apparatus in nerve cells.

Penfield, W. (1924) *Brain* **47:**430–452. Oligodendroglia and its relation to classical neuroglia.

Penfield, W. (1928) Neuroglia and microglia. The interstitial tissue of the central nervous system, pp. 1032–1067. In *Special Cytology,* Vol. II (E. V. Cowdry, ed.), Hoeber, New York.

Penfield, W. (1932) Neuroglia: normal and pathological, pp. 423–479. In *Cytology and Cellular Pathology of the Nervous System,* Vol. II (W. Penfield, ed.), Hoeber, New York.

Penfield, W., and W. Cone. (1929) Neuroglia and microglia (the metallic methods). In *Handbook of Microscopical Technique* (C. E. McClung, ed.), Hoeber, New York.

Peng, H. B., and L. F. Jaffe. (1976) *Dev. Biol.* **53:**277–284. Polarization of fucoid eggs by steady electrical fields.

Perdrau, J. R. (1937) *Brain* **6:**204–210. The axis cylinder as a pathway for dyes and salts in solution with observations on the node of Ranvier in the rabbit.

Perri, T. (1956) *Arch. Zool. Ital.* **41:**369–410. Ricerche sulla correlazioni tra midollo spinale, gangli spinali ed arti negli Anfibi annuri: Esperienze d'asportazione di un abbozzo d'arto in *Bufo Vulgaris.*

Perry, R. P. (1966) *Nat. Cancer Inst. Monogr.* **23:**527–545. On ribosome biogenesis.

Pesetsky, I. (1960) *Anat. Rec.* **136:**257. Maintenance and regression of Mauthner's neuron in larval *Rana pipiens.*

Pesetsky, I. (1962) *Gen. Comp. Endocrinol.* **2:**229–235. The throxine-stimulated enlargement of Mauthner's neuron in anurans.

Pesetsky, I. (1966) *Z. Zellforsch. Mikrosk. Anat.* **75:**138–145. The role of the thyroid in the development of Mauthner's neuron: A karyometric study in thyroidectomized anuran larvae.

Pesetsky, I., and J. J. Kollros. (1956) *Exp. Cell Res.* **11:**477–482. A comparison of the influence of locally applied thyroxine upon Mauthner's cell and adjacent neurons.

Pessacq, T. P., and N. J. Reissenweber. (1972) *Acta Anat.* **8:**1–12. Structural aspects of vasculogenesis in the central nervous system. I. Postnatal development of the capillary blood vessels.

Pestronk, A., D. B. Drachman, and J. W. Griffin. (1976*a*) *Nature* **260:**352–353. Effect of muscle disuse on acetylcholine receptors.

Pestronk, A., D. B. Drachman, and J. W. Griffin. (1976*b*) *Nature* **264:**787–789. Effect of botulinum toxin on trophic regulation of acetylcholine receptors.

Peterfi, T., and St. C. Williams. (1933) *Arch. Exp. Zellforsch.* **14:**210–254. Elektrische Reizversuche an gezüchten Gewebezellen. I. Versuche an Nervenzellen.

Peters, A. (1960) *J. Biochem. Biophys. Cytol.* **8:**431–446. The formation and structure of myelin sheaths in the central nervous system.

Peters, A. (1964*a*) *J. Anat. (London)* **98:**125–134. Observations on the connections between myelin sheaths and glial cells in the optic nerve of young rats.

Peters, A. (1964*b*) *J. Cell Biol.* **20:**281–296. Further observations on the structure of myelin sheaths in the central nervous system.

Peters, A. (1966) *Quart. J. Exp. Physiol.* **51:**229–236. The node of Ranvier in the central nervous system.

Peters, A., and A. R. Muir. (1959) *Quart. J. Exp. Physiol.* **44:**117–130. The relationship between axons and Schwann cells during development of peripheral nerves in the rat.

Peters, A., and J. E. Vaughn. (1967) *J. Cell Biol.* **32:**113–119. Microtubules and filaments in the axons and astrocytes of early postnatal rat optic nerve.

Peters, A., S. L. Palay, and H. DeF. Webster. (1970) *The Fine Structure of the Nervous System,* Harper and Row, New York.

Peters, H. G., and H. Bademan. (1963) *J. Anat. (London)* **97:**111–117. The form and growth of stellate cells in the cortex of the guinea-pig.

Peters, V. B., and L. B. Flexner. (1950) *Am. J. Anat.* **86:**133–161. Biochemical and physiological differentiation during morphogenesis. VII. Quantitative morphologic studies on the developing cerebral cortex of the fetal guinea pig.

Petersen, H. (1923) *Ergeb. Anat. Entw.-Gersch.* **24:**327–347. Berichte über Entwicklungsmechanik. I. Entwicklungsmechanik des Auges.

Peterson, E. R., and S. M. Crain. (1968) *Anat. Rec.* **160:**408–409. Re-innervation of denervated mammalian skeletal muscle *in vitro.*

Peterson, E. R., and M. R. Murray. (1955) *Am. J. Anat.* **96:**319–355. Myelin sheath formation in cultures of avian spinal ganglia.

Peterson, J. A., J. J. Bray, and L. Austin. (1968) *J. Neurochem.* **15:**741–745. An autoradiographic study of the flow of protein and RNA along peripheral nerve.

Peterson, R. P., R. M. Hurwitz, and R. Lindsay. (1967) *Exp. Brain Res.* **4:**138–145. Migration of axonal protein: Absence of a protein concentration gradient and effect of inhibition of protein synthesis.

Pettigrew, J. D. (1974*a*) *Ann. N.Y. Acad. Sci.* **228:**393–405. The effects of selective visual experience on stimulus trigger features of kitten cortical neurons.

Pettigrew, J. D. (1974*b*) *J. Physiol. (London)* **237:**49–74. The effect of visual experience on the development of stimulus specificity by kitten cortical neurones.

Pettigrew, J. D., and M. Konishi. (1976) *The Owl and the Pussycat, Neurosci. Abstr.* **II**(2):1130.

Peyronnard, J. -M., L. C. Terry, and A. Aguayo. (1975) *Arch. Neurol.* **32:**36–38. Schwann cell internuclear distances in developing rat unmyelinated nerve fibers.

Pfaff, D. W. (1968*a*) *Experientia* **24:**958–959. Autoradiographic localization of testosterone-^{3}H in the female rat brain and estradiol-^{3}H in the male rat brain.

Pfaff, D. W. (1968*b*) *Science* **161:**1355–1356. Autoradiographic localization of radioactivity in rat brain after injection of tritiated sex hormones.

Pfaff, D. W. (1968*c*) *Endocrinology* **82:**1149–1155. Uptake of ^{3}H-estradiol by the female rat brain. An autoradiographic study.

Pfaff, D., and M. Keiner. (1973) *J. Comp. Neurol.* **151:**121–158. Atlas of estradiol-concentrating cells in the central nervous system of the female rat.

Pfaff, D. W., J. L. Gerlach, B. S. McEwen, M. Ferin, P. Carmel, and E. A. Zimmerman. (1976) *J. Comp. Neurol.* **170:**279–294. Autoradiographic localization of hormone-concentrating cells in the brain of the female rhesus monkey.

Pfeffer, W. (1884) *Untersuch. Bot. Inst. Tübingen* **1:**397–500. Locomotorische Richtungsbewegungen durch chemische Reize.

Pflugfelder, O. (1952) *Roux Arch. Entw.-Mech.* **145:**549–560. Weitere volumetrische Untersuchungen über die Wirkung der Augenextirpation und der Dunkelhaltung auf das Mesencephalon und die Pseudobranchien von Fischer.

Pflugfelder, O. (1958) *Entwicklungsphysiologie der Insekten,* 2d ed., Geest and Portig, Leipzig, 490 pp.

Phelps, C. H. (1972) *Z. Zellforsch. Mikrosk. Anat.* **128:**555–563. The development of glio-vascular relationships in the rat spinal cord.

Phemister, R. D., and S. Young. (1968) *J. Comp. Neurol.* **134:**243–254. The postnatal development of the canine cerebellar cortex.

Phillips, D. E. (1973) *Z. Zellforsch. Mikrosk. Anat.* **140:**145–167. An electron microscopic study of macroglia and microglia in the lateral funiculus of the developing spinal cord in the fetal monkey.

Piatt, J. (1939) *J. Morphol.* **65:**155–185. A study of nerve-muscle specificity in the forelimb of *Triturus pyrrogaster.*

Piatt, J. (1940) *J. Exp. Zool.* **85:**211–241. Nerve-muscle specificity in *Amblystoma,* studied by means of heterotopic cord grafts.

Piatt, J. (1941) *J. Exp. Zool.* **86:**77–85. Grafting of limbs in place of the eye in *Amblystoma.*

Piatt, J. (1942) *J. Exp. Zool.* **91:**79–101. Transplantation of aneurogenic forelimbs in *Amblystoma punctatum.*

Piatt, J. (1943) *J. Comp. Neurol.* **79:**165–183. The course and decussation of ectopic Mauthner's fibers in *Amblystoma punctatum.*

Piatt, J. (1944) *J. Comp. Neurol.* **80:**335–353. Experiments on the decussation and course of Mauthner's fibers in *Amblystoma punctatum.*

Piatt, J. (1945) *J. Comp. Neurol.* **82:**35–54. Origin of the mesencephalic V root in *Amblystoma.*

Piatt, J. (1946) *J. Exp. Zool.* **102:**109. The influence of the peripheral field on the development of the mesencephalic V nucleus in *Amblystoma.*

Piatt, J. (1947) *J. Comp. Neurol.* **86:**199–236. A study of the factors controlling the differentiation of Mauthner's cell in *Amblystoma.*

Piatt, J. (1948) *Biol. Rev.* **23:**1–45. Form and casuality in neurogenesis.

Piatt, J. (1949) *J. Comp. Neurol.* **90:**47–93. A study of the development of fiber tracts in the brain of *Amblystoma* after excision or inversion of the embryonic di-mesencephalic region.

Piatt, J. (1951) *J. Comp. Neurol.* **94:**105–121. An experimental approach to the problem of pallial differentiation.

Piatt, J. (1952) *J. Exp. Zool.* **120:**247–285. Transplantation of aneurogenic forelimbs in place of the hindlimb in *Amblystoma.*

Piatt, J. (1955) *J. Exp. Zool.* **129:**177–207. Regeneration of the spinal cord in the salamander.

Piatt, J. (1957*a*) *J. Exp. Zool.* **134:**103–125. Studies on the problem of nerve pattern. II. Innervation of the intact forelimb by different parts of the central nervous system in *Amblystoma.*

Piatt, J. (1957*b*) *J. Exp. Zool.* **136:**229–247. Studies on the problem of nerve pattern. III. Innervation of the regenerated forelimb in *Amblystoma.*

Piatt, J. (1969) *Devp. Biol.* **19:**608–616. The influence of VIIth and VIIIth cranial nerve roots upon the differentiation of Mauthner's cell in *Amblystoma.*

Picken, L. (1956) *Nature* **178:**1162–1165. The fate of Wilhelm His.

Piddington, R. (1967) *Dev. Biol.* **16:**168–188. Hormonal effects on the development of glutamine synthetase in the embryonic chick retina.

Piddington, R. (1970) *J. Embryol. Exp. Morph.* **23:**729–737. Steroid control of the normal development of glutamine synthetase in the embryonic chick retina.

Pilar, G., and L. Landmesser. (1972) *Science* **177:**1116–1118. Axotomy mimicked by localized colchicine application.

Pilbeam, D., and S. J. Gould. (1974) *Science* **186:**892–901. Size and scaling in human evolution.

Pitman, R. M., C. D. Tweedle, and M. J. Cohen. (1972) *Science* **176:**412–414. Branching of central neurons: Intracellular cobalt injection for light and electron microscopy.

Pitot, H. C., and M. D. Yatvin. (1973) *Physiol. Rev.* **53:**228–325. Interrelationships of mammalian hormones and enzyme levels *in vivo.*

Plapinger, L., and B . S. McEwen. (1973) *Endocrinology* **93:**1119–1128. Ontogeny of estradiol-binding sites in rat brain. I. Appearance of presumptive adult receptors in cytosol and nuclei.

Plapinger, L., B. S. McEwen, and L. E. Clemens. (1973) *Endocrinology* **93:**1129–1139. Ontogeny of estradiol-binding sites in rat brain. II. Characteristics of a neonatal binding macromolecule.

Polacek, P. (1966) *Acta Fac. Med. Univ. Brun.* **23:**1–107. Receptors of the joints.

Poliakov, G. I. (1953) *Arkh. Anat. Gistol. Embriol.* **30(5):**48–63. Fine structural characteristics of man's cortex and functional interrelations among neurons (in Russian).

Poliakov, G. I. (1956) *Zhurn. Vyssh. Nerv. Delat. imeni I.P. Pavlova* **6:**461–478. The ratio of main types of neurons in man's cerebral cortex (in Russian).

Poliakov, G. I. (1959) Progressive neuron differentiation of the human cerebral cortex in onthogenesis, pp. 37–38. In *Razvitic Tsentral'noi Nervnoi Systemy (Development of the Central Nervous System)* (S. A. Sarkisov and N. S. Preobrazhenskaya, eds.), Medgiz, Moscow.

Poliakov, G. I. (1961) *J. Comp. Neurol.* **117:**197–212. Some results of research into the development of the neuronal structure of the cortical ends of the analyzers in man.

Poliakov, G. I. (1965) Development of the cerebral neocortex during the first half of intrauterine life, pp. 22–52. In *Development of the Child's Brain* (S. A. Sarkisov, ed.), Meditsina, Leningrad (in Russian).

Pollack, E. D. (1969) *Anat. Rec.* **163:**111–120. Normal development of the lateral motor column in the brachial cord in *Rana pipiens.*

Pomeranz, B. (1972) *Exp. Neurol.* **34:**187–199. Metamorphosis of frog vision: Changes in ganglion cell physiology and anatomy.

Pomeranz, B., and S. H. Chung. (1970) *Science* **170:**983–984. Dendritic-tree anatomy codes form-vision physiology in tadpole retina.

Pomerat, C. M. (1961) *Int. Rev. Cytol.* **11:**307–339. Cinematology, indispensible tool for cytology.

Popper, K. R. (1962) *Conjectures and Refutations: The Growth of Scientific Knowledge,* Basic Books, New York.

Poritsky, R. L., and M. Singer. (1963) *J. Exp. Zool.* **153:**211–218. The fate of taste buds in tongue transplants to the orbit in the urodele *Triturus.*

Porter, K. R. (1966) Cytoplasmic microtubules and their functions, pp. 308–345. In *Ciba Foundation Symposium: Principles of Biomolecular Organization* (G. E. W. Wolstenholme and M. O'Connor, eds.), Little, Brown, Boston.

Porter, K. R., and M. B. Bowers. (1963) *J. Cell Biol.* **19:**56A–57A. A study of chromatolysis in motor neurons of the frog *Rana pipiens.*

Potter, D. D., E. J. Furshpan, and E. S. Lennox. (1966) *Proc. Natl. Acad. Sci. U.S.A.* **55:**328–336. Connections between cells of the developing squid as revealed by electrophysiological methods.

Potter, H. D. (1969) *J. Comp. Neurol.* **136:**203–232. Structural characteristics of cell and fiber populations in the optic tectum of the frog *(Rana catesbiana).*

Potter, H. D. (1972) *J. Comp. Neurol.* **144:**269–284. Terminal arborizations of retinotectal axons.

Potter, V. R., W. C. Schneider, and G. J. Leibl. (1945) *Cancer Res.* **5:**21–24. Enzyme changes during growth and differentiation in the tissues of the newborn rat.

Poulson, D. F. (1950) Histogenesis, organogenesis, and differentiation in the embryo of *Drosophila melanogaster* Meigen, pp. 168–274. In *Biology of Drosphila* (M. Demerec, ed.), Wiley, New York.

Powell, T. P. S., and S. D. Erulkar. (1962) *J. Anat.* **91:**249–268. Transneuronal cell degeneration in the auditory relay nuclei of the cat.

Powell, T. P. S., and V. B. Mountcastle. (1959) *Bull. Johns Hopkins Hosp.* **105:**133–162. Some aspects of the functional organization of the cortex of the postcentral gyrus of the monkey: A correlation of findings, obtained in single unit analysis, with cytoarchitecture.

Power, M. E. (1952) *J. Morphol.* **91:**389–411. A quantitative study of the growth of the central nervous system of a holometabolous insect, *Drosophila melanogaster.*

Prasad, K. N., and A. W. Hsie. (1971) *Nature New Biol.* **233:**141–142. Morphologic differentiation of mouse neuroblastoma cells induced in vitro by dibutyryl adenosine 3′:5′-cyclic monophosphate.

Prensky, A. L., S. Carr, and H. W. Moser. (1968) *Arch. Neurol. (Chicago)* **19:**522–558. Development of myelin in inherited disorders of amino acid metabolism.

Prescott, D. M. (1964) *Natl. Cancer Inst. Monogr.* **14:**57–72. Comments on the cell life cycle.

Prestige, M. C. (1965) *J. Embryol. Exp. Morphol.* **13:**63–72. Cell turnover in the spinal ganglia of *Xenopus laevis* tadpoles.

Prestige, M. C. (1967*a*) *J. Embryol. Exp. Morphol.* **17:**453–471. The control of cell number in the lumbar spinal ganglia during the development of *Xenopus laevis* tadpoles.

Prestige, M. C. (1967*b*) *J. Embryol. Exp. Morphol.* **18:**359–387. The control of cell number in the lumbar ventral horns during the development of *Xenopus laevis* tadpoles.

Prestige, M. C. (1970) Differentiation, degeneration and the role of the periphery: Quantitative considerations, pp. 73–82. In *The Neurosciences: Second Study Program* (F. O. Schmitt, ed.), Rockefeller University Press, New York.

Prestige, M. C. (1973) *Brain Res.* **59:**400–404. Gradients in time of origin of tadpole motoneurons.

Prestige, M. C. (1974) *Br. Med. Bull.* **30:**107–111. Axon and cell numbers in the developing nervous system.

Prestige, M. C., and D. J. Willshaw. (1975) *Proc. Roy. Soc. London Ser. B* **190:**77–98. On a role for competition in the formation of patterned neural connexions.

Prestige, M. C., and M. A. Wilson. (1974) *J. Embryol. Exp. Morphol.* **32:**819–833. A quantitative study of the growth and development of *Xenopus laevis* tadpoles.

Preyer, W. T. (1885) *Specielle Physiologie des Embryo,* L. Fernau, Grieben, Leipzig. (Embryonic motility and sensitivity, translated by C. E. Coghill and W. K. Legner, *Monogr. Soc. Res. Child Develop.* **2:**1–115, 1937.)

Price, D. L. (1972) *J. Neuropathol. Exp. Neurol.* **31:**267–277. The response of amphibian glial cells to axonal transection.

Price, M. T. (1974) *Brain Res.* **77:**497–501. The effects of colchicine and lumichochicine on the rapid phase of axonal transport in the rabbit visual system.

Privat, A. (1975) *Int. Rev. Cytol.* **40:**281–323. Postnatal gliogenesis in the mammalian brain.

Privat, A., and M. J. Drian. (1976) *J. Comp. Neurol.* **166:**201–244. Postnatal maturation of rat Purkinje cells cultivated in the absence of two afferent systems: An ultrastructural study.

Privat, A., and C. P. Leblond. (1972) *J. Comp. Neurol.* **146:**277–302. The subependymal layer and neighboring region in the brain of the young rat.

Puck, T. T., and J. Steffen. (1963) *Biophys. J.* **3:**379–397. Life cycle analysis of mammalian cells. A method for localizing metabolic events within the life cycle, and its application to the action of colcemide and sublethal doses of X-irradiation.

Purpura, D. P., R. J. Shofer, E. M. Housepian, and C. R. Noback. (1964) *Progr. Brain Res.* **4:**187–221. Comparative ontogenesis of structure-function relations in cerebral and cerebellar cortex.

Purves, D. (1976) *J. Physiol. (London)* **261:**453–475. Competitive and non-competitive re-innervation of mammalian sympathetic neurones by native and foreign fibers.

Puszkin, S., S. Berl, E. Puszkin, and D. D. Clarke. (1968) *Science* **161:**170–171. Actomyosin-like protein isolated from mammalian brain.

Puszkin, S., W. J. Nicklas, and S. Berl. (1972) *J. Neurochem.* **19:**1319–1333. Actomyosin-like protein in brain: Subcellular distribution.

Pysh, J. J. (1969) *Am. J. Anat.* **124:**411–430. The development of the extracellular space in neonatal rat inferior colliculus: An electron microscopic study.

Pysh, J. J. (1970) *Brain Res.* **18:**325–342. Mitochondrial changes in rat inferior colliculus during postnatal development: An electron microscopic study.

Quilliam, T. A. (1962) *Anat. Rec.* **142:**322. Growth, degrowth and regrowth in the Herbst corpuscle.

Raaf, J., and J. W. Kernohan. (1944) *Am. J. Anat.* **75:**151–172. A study of the external granular layer in the cerebellum.

Rabié, A., and J. Legrand. (1973) *Brain Res.* **61:**267–278. Effects of thyroid hormone and undernourishment on the amount of synaptosomal fraction in the cerebellum of the young rat.

Race, J., Jr. (1961) *Gen. Comp. Endocrinol.* **1:**322–331. Thyroid hormone control of development of lateral motor column cells in the lumbo-sacral cord in hypophysectomized *Rana pipiens.*

Race, J., Jr., and R. J. Terry. (1965) *Anat. Rec.* **152:**99–106. Further studies on the development of the lateral motor column in Anuran larvae. I. Normal development in *Rana temporaria.*

Radinsky, L. (1967) *Science* **155:**836–838. Relative brain size: A new measure.

Raedler, A., and J. Sievers. (1976) *Anat. Embryol.* **149:**173–181. Light and electron microscopical studies on specific cells of the marginal zone in the developing rat cerebral cortex.

Rager, G. (1976*a*) *Proc. Roy. Soc. London Biol.* **192:**331–352. Morphogenesis and physiogenesis of the retino-tectal connection in the chicken. I. The retinal ganglion cells and their axons.

Rager, G. (1976*b*) *Proc. Roy. Soc. London Biol.* **192:**353–370. Morphogenesis and physiogenesis of the retino-tectal connection in the chicken. II. The retino-tectal synapse.

Rager, G., and U. Rager. (1976) *Exp. Brain Res.* **25:**551–553. Generation and degeneration of retinal ganglion cells in the chicken.

Raine, C. S., S. E. Poduslo, and W. T. Norton. (1971) *Brain Res.* **27:**11–24. The ultrastructure of purified preparations of neurons and glial cells.

Raisman, G. (1969) *Brain Res.* **14:**25–48. Neuronal plasticity in the septal nuclei of the adult rat.

Raisman, G., and P. M. Field. (1973*a*) *Brain Res.* **54:**1–29. Sexual dimorphism in the neuropil of the preoptic area of the rat and its dependence on neonatal androgen.

Raisman, G., and P. M. Field. (1973*b*) *Brain Res.* **50:**241–264. A quantitative investigation of the development of collateral reinnervation after partial deafferentation of the septal nuclei.

Rakic, P. (1971*a*) *Brain Res.* **33:**471–476. Guidance of neurons migrating to the fetal monkey neocortex.

Rakic, P. (1971*b*) *J. Comp. Neurol.* **141:**283–312. Neuron-glia relationship during granule cell migration in developing cerebellar cortex: A Golgi and electronmicroscopic study in *Macacus rhesus.*

Rakic, P. (1972*a*) *J. Comp. Neurol.* **145:**61–84. Mode of cell migration to the superficial layers of fetal monkey neocortex.

Rakic, P. (1972*b*) *J. Comp. Neurol.* **146:**335–354. Extrinsic cytological determinants of basket and stellate cell dendritic pattern in the cerebellar molecular layer.

Rakic, P. (1973) *J. Comp. Neurol.* **147:**523–546. Kinetics of proliferation and latency between final cell division and onset of differentiation of cerebellar stellate and basket neurons.

Rakic, P. (1974) *Science* **183:**425–427. Neurons in rhesus monkey visual cortex: Systematic relation between time of origin and eventual disposition.

Rakic, P. (1975*a*) *Birth Defects* **11:**95–129. Cell migration and neuronal ectopias in the brain.

Rakic, P. (1975*b*) *Cold Spring Harbor Symp. Quant. Biol.* **40:**333–346. Synaptic specificity in the cerebellar cortex: Study of anomalous circuits induced by single gene mutations in mice.

Rakic, P. (1976) *Nature* **261:**467–471. Prenatal genesis of connections subserving ocular dominance in the Rhesus monkey.

Rakic, P. (1977) *Phil. Trans. Roy. Soc. London. Ser. B.* **278:**245–260. Prenatal development of the visual system in rhesus monkey.

Rakic, P., and R. L. Sidman. (1968) *J. Neuropathol. Exp. Neurol.* **27:**246–276. Supravital DNA synthesis in the developing human and mouse brain.

Rakic, P., and R. L. Sidman (1969) *Z. Anat. Entwicklungsgesch.* **129:**53–82. Telencephalic origin of pulvinar neurons in the fetal human brain.

Rakic, P., and R. L. Sidman. (1970) *J. Comp. Neurol.* **139:**473–500. Histogenesis of cortical layers in human cerebellum, particularly the lamina dissecans.

Rakic, P., and R. L. Sidman. (1972) *J. Neuropathol. Exp. Neurol.* **31:**192. Synaptic organization of displaced and disoriented cerebellar cortical neurons in reeler mice.

Rakic, P., and R. L. Sidman. (1973*a*) *J. Comp. Neurol.* **152:**103–132. Sequence and developmental abnormalities leading to granule cell deficit in cerebellar cortex of weaver mutant mice.

Rakic, P., and R. L. Sidman. (1973*b*) *J. Comp. Neurol.* **152:**133–162. Organization of cerebellar cortex secondary to deficit of granule cells in weaver mutant mice.

Rakic, P., and R. L. Sidman. (1973*c*) *Proc. Natl. Acad. Sci. U.S.A.* **70:**240–244. Weaver mutant mouse cerebellum: Defective neuronal migration secondary to abnormality of Bergmann glia.

Rakic, P., L. J. Stensaas, E. P. Sayre, and R. L. Sidman. (1974) *Nature* **250:**31–34. Computer-aided three-dimensional reconstruction and quantitative analysis of cells from serial electron microscopic montages of foetal monkey brain.

Ralston, H. J., and K. L. Chow. (1973) *J. Comp. Neurol.* **147:**321–350. Synaptic reorganization in the degenerating lateral geniculate nucleus of the rabbit.

Ramón y Cajal, S. (1890*a*) *Int. Monatschr. Anat. Physiol. (Leipzig)* **7:**12–31. A propos de certains éléments bipolaires du cervelet avec quelques détails nouveaux sur l'évolution des fibres cérébelleuses.

Ramón y Cajal, S. (1890*b*) *Int. Monatschr. Anat. Physiol. (Leipzig))* **7:**447–468. Sur les fibres nerveuses de la couche granuleuse du cervelet et sur l'évolution des éléments cérébelleux.

Ramón y Cajal, S. (1890*c*) *Anat. Anz.* **5:**111–119; 609–613; 631–639. Sur l'origine et les ramifications des fibres nerveuses de la moelle embryonaire.

Ramón y Cajal, S. (1891) *Cellule* **7:**125–176. Sur la structure de l'écorce cérébrale de quelques mammifères.

Ramón y Cajal, S. (1894) *Die Retina der Wirbelthiere,* Bergmann-Verlag, Wiesbaden.

Ramón y Cajal, S. (1895) *Revista de Medicina y Cirurgía prácticas,* Madrid. Algunas conjecturas sobre el mechanismo anatómico de la asociatión, ideación, atención.

Ramón y Cajal, S. (1897) *Rev. Trim. Micrograf.* **2:**105–127. Las células de cilindro-eje corto de la capa molecular del cerebro.

Ramón y Cajal, S. (1906) *Studien über die Hirnrinde des Menschen: H.5, Vergleichende Strukturbeschreibung und Histogenesis der Hirnrinde,* J. A. Barth, Leipzig.

Ramón y Cajal, S. (1908) *Anat. Anz.* **23:**1–25; 65–87. Nouvelles observationes sur l'évolution des neuroblasts avec quelques remarques sur l'hypothése neurogénétique de Hensen-Held, p. 71. In *Studies in Vertebrate Neurogenesis* (L. Guth, trans.), Thomas, Springfield, Ill.

Ramón y Cajal, S. (1909–1911) *Histologie du Systeme Nerveux de l'Homme et des Vertébrés,* 2 vols. (L. Azoulay, trans.). (Reprinted by Instituto Ramón y Cajal del C.S.I.C., Madrid, 1952–1955.)

Ramón y Cajal, S. (1910) *Trabajos Lab. Invest. Biol. Univ. Madrid* **8:**63–134. Algunas observaciones favorables á la hipótesis neurotrópica.

Ramón y Cajal, S. (1913) *Trabajos Lab. Invest. Biol. Univ. Madrid* **11:**255–315. Sobre un nuevo proceder de impregnación de la neuroglia y sus resultados en los centros nerviosos del hombre y animales.

Ramón y Cajal, S. (1917) Recollections of my life (H. Craigie, trans.). In *Memoirs of the American Philosophical Society,* Vol. 8, Philadelphia, 1937.

Ramón y Cajal, S. (1919) *Trabajos Lab. Invest. Biol. Univ. Madrid* **17:**181–228. Acción neurotrópica de los epitelios (Algunas detalles sobre el mechanismo genético de las ramificaciones nerviosas intraepiteliales, sensitivas y sensoriales), pp. 149–200. In *Studies on Vertebrate Neurogenesis* (L. Guth, trans.), Thomas, Springfield, Ill., 1960).

Ramón y Cajal, S. (1925) *Trabajos Lab. Invest. Biol. Univ. Madrid* **23:**245–254. Quelques remarques sur les plaques motrices de la langue des mammifères.

Ramón y Cajal, S. (1928) *Degeneration and Regeneration of the Nervous System* (R. M. May, trans.), Hafner, New York, 1959.

Ramón y Cajal, S. (1929*a*) Étude sur la neurogenèse de quelques vertébrés (L. Guth, trans. *Studies on Vertebrate Neurogenesis*) Thomas, Springfield, Ill., 1960.

Ramón y Cajal, S. (1929*b*) *Trabajos Lab. Invest. Biol. Univ. Madr.* **26:**107–130. Considérations critiques sur le rôle trophiques des dendrites et leurs prétendues relations vasculaires.

Ramón y Cajal, S. (1933) *Arch. Neurobiol.* **13:**217–291; 579–646. ¿Neuronismo o reticularismo? Las pruebas objectivas de la unidad anatómica, de las celulas nerviosas. [Neuron theory or reticular theory? Objective evidence of the anatomical unity of nerve cells (M. U. Purkiss and C. A. Fox, trans.), Instituto Ramón y Cajal, Madrid, 1954.]

Ramón y Cajal, S. (1952) *Trabajos Inst. Cajal. Invest. Biol.* **44:**1–8, originally published in *Trabajos Lab. Invest. Biol. Univ. Madrid* **1:**1–8. (1901) Significación probable de las células nerviosas de cilindro-eje corto.

Ramón y Cajal, S., and D. Sánchez. (1915) *Trabajos Lab. Invest. Biol. Univ. Madrid* **13:**1–64. Contribución al conocimiento de los centros nerviosos de los insectos.

Ramón-Moliner, E. (1958) *J. Comp. Neurol.* **110:**157–171. A study of neuroglia: The problem of transitional forms.

Ramón-Moliner, E. (1962) *J. Comp. Neurol.* **119:**211–227. An attempt at classifying nerve cells on the basis of their dendritic patterns.

Ramón-Moliner, E. (1968) The morphology of dendrites, pp. 205–267. In *The Structure and Function of Nervous Tissue,* Vol. 1 (G. H. Bourne, ed.), Academic Press, New York.

Ranke, O. (1910) *Beitr. Pathol. Anat. Allg. Pathol.* **47:**51–125. Beiträge zur Kenntnis der normalen und pathologischen Hirnrindenbildung.

Ranson, S. W. (1906) *J. Comp. Neurol.* **16:**265–293. Retrograde degeneration in the spinal nerves.

Ranson, S. W. (1912) *J. Comp. Neurol.* **22:**487–537. Degeneration and regeneration of nerve fibers.

Rapoport, A., and J. Stempak. (1968) *Anat. Rec.* **161:**361–376. Ultrastructure of the ventral horn cell in the albino rat.

Ratner A., and N. J. Adamo. (1971) *Neuroendocrinology* **8:**26–35. Arcuate nucleus region in androgen-sterilized female rats: Ultrastructural observations.

Rauber, A. (1886a) *Arch. Mikrosk. Anat.* **26:**622–644. Die Kerntheilungsfiguren im Medullarrohr der Wirbeltiere.

Rauber, A. (1886b) *Zool. Anz.* **9:**159–164. Über die Mitosen des Medullarrohres.

Raven, C. P. (1936) *Arch. Entw.-Mech. Organ.* **134:**122–146. Zur Entwicklung der Ganglienleiste. V. Differenzierung des Rumpfganglienleistenmaterials.

Raven, C. P. (1937) *J. Comp. Neurol.* **67:**221–240. Experiments on the origin of the sheath cells and sympathetic neuroblasts in amphibia.

Raynaud, J. P., C. Mercier-Bodard, and C. Baulieu. (1971) *Steroids* **18:**767–788. Rat estradiol binding plasma protein.

Rebière, A., and J. Legrand. (1970) *Brain Res.* **22:**299–312. Absence d'effets marqués de l'hormone hypophysaire de croissance sur la maturation histologique du cortex cérébelleux chez le jeune rat normal ou hypothyroïdien.

Rebière, A., and J. Legrand. (1972*a*) *C. R. Acad. Sci. (D) (Paris)* **274:**3581–3584. Donnees quantitatives sur la synaptogenèse dans le cervelet du rat normal et rendu hypothroïdien par le propylthiouracile.

Rebière, A., and J. Legrand. (1972*b*) *Arch. Anat. Microsc. Morphol. Exp.* **61:**105–126. Effets comparés de las sous alimentation, de l'hypothyroïdisme sur la maturation de la zone moléculaire du cortex cérébelleux chez le jeune Rat.

Reddy, D. R., W. J. Davis, R. B. Ohlander, and D. J. Bihary. (1973) Computer analysis of neuronal structure, pp. 227–253. In *Intracellular Staining in Neurobiology* (S. B. Kater and C. Nicholson, eds.), Springer-Verlag, New York.

Reddy, V. V. R., F. Naftolin, and K. J. Ryan. (1974) *Endocrinology* **94:**117–121. Conversion of androstenedione to estrone by neural tissues from fetal and neonatal rats.

Redfern, P. A. (1970) *J. Physiol. London* **209:**701–709. Neuromuscular transmission in new-born rats.

Rees, R. P., M. P. Bunge, and R. P. Bunge. (1976) *J. Cell Biol.* **68:**240–263. Morphological changes in the neuritic growth cone and target neuron during synaptic junction development in culture.

Reichenbach, H. (1951) *The Rise of Scientific Philosophy,* University of Calif. Press, Berkeley.

Rensch, B. (1958) *Naturwissenschaften* **45:**145–154, 175–180. Die Abhängigkeit der Struktur und der Leistungen tierischer Gehirne von ihrer Grösse.

Rensch, B., and A. Nolte. (1949*a*) *Z. Vergleich. Physiol.* **31:**696–710. Über die Funktion auf den Rücken transplantierter Augen.

Rensch, B., and A. Nolte. (1949*b*) *Verhandl. Deutsch. Zool. (Mainz)* **34:**208–215. Über die Funktion auf den Rücken transplantierter Augen, 2 Mitteilung.

Resko, J. A., R. W. Goy, and C. H. Phoenix. (1967) *Endocrinology* **80:**490–498. Uptake and distribution of exogenous testosterone-1-2-^{3}H in neural and genital tissues of the castrate guinea pig.

Retzius, G. (1893) *Biol. Untersuch.* **5:**1–9. Die Cajal'schen zellen des Grosshirnrinde beim Menschen und bei Saugetieren.

Retzius, G. (1894) *Biol. Untersuch.* **6:**29–37. Weitere beitrage zur Kenntniss der Cajal'schen Zellen der Grosshirnrinde des Menschen.

Revel, J. P., and S. Ito. (1967) The surface components of cells, pp. 211–234. In *The Specificity of Cell Surfaces* (B. D. Davis and L. Warren, eds.), Prentice-Hall, Englewood Cliffs, N.J.

Rexed, B. (1944) *Acta Psychiat. Neurol. Scand. Suppl.* **33:**1–206. Contributions to the knowledge of postnatal development of the peripheral nervous system in man.

Rexed, B., and U. Rexed. (1951) *Br. J. Ophthalmol.* **35:**38–49. Degeneration and regeneration of corneal nerve fibers.

Reynolds, W. A. (1963) *J. Exp. Zool.* **153:**237–250. The effects of thyroxine upon the initial formation of the lateral motor column and differentiation of motor neurons in *Rana pipiens.*

Reynolds, W. A. (1966) *Gen. Comp. Endocrinol.* **6:**453–465. Mitotic activity in the lumbosacral spinal cord of *Rana pipiens* larvae after throxine or thiourea treatment.

Rezai, Z., and C. H. Yoon. (1972) *Dev. Biol.* **29:**17–26. Abnormal rate of granule cell migration in the cerebellum of "weaver" mutant mice.

Rhodin, J. A. (1963) *An Atlas of Ultrastructure,* Saunders, Philadelphia.

Rice, R. L., and H. Van der Loos. (1977) *J. Comp. Neurol.* **171:**545–560. Development of the barrels and barrel field in the somatosensory cortex of the mouse.

Richards, F. F., W. H. Konigsberg, R. W. Rosenstein, and J. M. Varga. (1975) *Science* **187:**130–136. On the specificity of antibodies.

Richman, D. P., R. M. Stewart, and V. S. Caviness, Jr. (1973) *Neurology (Minneapolis)* **23:**413 (abstr.). Microgyria, lissencephaly and neuron migration to the cerbral cortex: An architectonic approach.

Richman, D. P., R. M. Stewart, H. W. Hutchinson, and V. S. Caviness, Jr. (1975) *Science* **189:**18–21. Mechanical model of brain convolutional development.

Ridge, R. M. A. P. (1967) *Quart. J. Exp. Physiol.* **52:**293–304. The differentiation of conduction velocities of slow twitch and fast twitch muscle motor innervation in kittens and cats.

Riese, W. (1956) *J. Nerv. Ment. Dis.* **124:**125–134. The sources of Jacksonian neurology.

Riese, W., and G. E. Arrington (1963) *Bull. Hist. Med.* **37:**179–183. The history of Johannes Müller's doctrine of specific nerve energies of the senses: original and later versions.

Rieske, E. (1969) *Z. Zellforsch. Mikrosk. Anat. Abt. Histochem.* **95:**546–567. Einfluss eines spezifischen Nerven wachstumsfaktors (NGF) auf Zellkulturen des Ganglion trigeminale.

Riley, D. A., and E. F. Allin. (1973) *Exp. Neurol.* **40:**391–413. The effects of inactivity, programmed stimulation, and denervation on the histochemistry of skeletal muscle fiber types.

Roach, F. C. (1945) *J. Exp. Zool.* **99:**53–77. Differentiation of the central nervous system after axial reversals of the medullary plate of *Amblystoma.*

Roback, H. N., and H. J. Scherrer. (1935) *Virchows Arch. Pathol. Anat. Physiol. Klin. Med.* **294:**365–413. Über die feinere Morphologie des frühkindlichen Hirnes unter besonderer Berücksichtigung der Gliaentwicklung.

Robain, O. (1970) *J. Neurol. Sci.* **11:**445–461. Gliogenèse post-natale chex le lapin.

Robbins, E., and N. K. Gonatas. (1964*a*) *J. Cell Biol.* **21:**429–463. Ultrastructure of a mammalian cell during the mitotic cycle.

Robbins, E., and N. K. Gonatas. (1964*b*) *J. Histochem. Cytochem.* **12:**704. Histochemical and ultrastructural studies on HeLa cell cultures exposed to spindle inhibitors with special reference to the interphase cell.

Robbins, N. (1967*a*) *Exp. Neurol.* **17**:364–380. The role of the nerve in maintenance of frog taste buds.

Robbins, N. (1967*b*) *J. Physiol. (London)* **192**:493–504. Peripheral modification of sensory nerve responses after cross-regeneration.

Robbins, N., and T. Yonezawa. (1971) *Science* **172**:395–398. Developing neuromuscular junctions: First signs of chemical transmission during formation in tissue culture.

Robertson, J. D. (1955) *J. Biophys. Biochem. Cytol.* **1**:271–278. The ultrastructure of adult vertebrate peripheral myelinated fibers in relation to myelinogenesis.

Rogers, K. T. (1957) *Anat. Rec.* **127**:97–107. Early development of the optic nerve in the chick.

Rogers, L. A., and W. M. Cowan. (1973) *J. Comp. Neurol.* **147**:291–319. The development of the mesencephalic nucleus of the trigeminal nerve in the chick.

Rogers, W. M. (1934) *Proc. Natl. Acad. Sci. U.S.A.* **20**:247–249. Heterotopic spinal cord grafts in salamander embryos.

Röhrs, M. (1955) *Zool. Anz.* **155**:53–69. Vergleichende Untersuchungen an Wild- und Hauskatzen.

Roisen, F. J., R. A. Murphy, and W. G. Braden. (1972*a*) *J. Neurobiol.* **4**:347–368. Neurite development *in vitro.* I. The effects of adenosine 3′5′-cyclic monophosphate (cyclic AMP).

Roisen, F. J., R. A. Murphy, M. E. Pichichero, and W. G. Braden. (1972*b*) *Science* **175**:73–74. Cyclic adenosine monophosphate stimulation of axonal elongation.

Roisen, F. J., W. G. Braden, and J. Friedman. (1975) *Ann. N.Y. Acad. Sci.* **253**:545–561. Neurite development *in vitro.* III. The effects of several derivatives of cyclic AMP, colchicine, and colcemid.

Romanes, G. J. (1941) *J. Anat. (London)* **76**:112–130. The development and significance of the cell columns in the ventral horn of the cervical and upper thoracic spinal cord of the rabbit.

Romanes, G. J. (1946) *J. Anat. (London)* **80**:117–131. Motor localization and the effects of nerve injury on the ventral horn cells of the spinal cord.

Romanes, G. J. (1947) *J. Anat. (London)* **81**:64–81. The prenatal medullation of the sheep's nervous system.

Romanul, F. C. A. (1964) *Arch. Neurol.* **11**:355–368. Enzymes in muscle. I. Histochemical studies of enzymes in individual muscle fibers.

Romanul, F. C. A., and E. L. Hogan. (1965) *Arch. Neurol.* **13**:263–273. Enzymatic changes in denervated muscle. I. Histochemical studies.

Romanul, F. C. A., and J. P. van der Meulen. (1967) *Arch. Neurol.* **17**:387–402. Slow and fast muscle after cross innervation.

Roncalli, L. (1970) *Monitore Zool. Ital. N.S.* **4**:81–98. The brachial plexus and the wing nerve pattern during early developmental phases in chicken embryo.

Ronnevi, L. -O., and S. Conradi. (1974) *Brain Res.* **80**:335–359. Ultrastructural evidence for spontaneous elimination of synaptic terminals on spinal motoneurons in the kitten.

Roofe, P. G. (1947) *Science* **105**:180–181. Role of the axis cylinder in transport of tetanus toxin.

Rose, G. H., and D. B. Lindsley. (1968) *J. Neurophysiol.* **31**:607–623. Development of visually evoked potentials in kittens: Specific and nonspecific responses.

Rosen, J., D. Stein, and N. Butters. (1971) *Science* **173**:353–356. Recovery of function after serial ablation of prefrontal cortex in rhesus monkey.

Rosenbluth, J. (1963) *Z. Zellforsch. Mikrosk. Anat.* **60**:213–236. The visceral ganglion of *Aplysia californica.*

Rosenbluth, J., and S. L. Wissig. (1964) *J. Cell Biol.* **23**:307–325. The distribution of exogenous ferritin in toad spinal ganglia and the mechanism of its uptake by neurons.

Roth, H. (1950) *Rev. Suisse Zool.* **57**:621–686. Die entwicklung xenoplastischer Neuralchimaeren.

Roux, W. (1881) *Der Kampf der Theile im Organismus,* Wilhelm Engelmann Verlag, Leipzig, 244 pp.

Rovainen, C. M. (1967*a*) *J. Neurophysiol.* **30**:1000–1023. Physiological and anatomical studies on large neurons of central nervous system of the sea lamprey *(Petromyzon marinus)*. I. Muller and Mauthner cells.

Rovainen, C. M. (1967*b*) *J. Neurophysiol.* **30**:1024–1042. Physiological and anatomical studies on large neurons of central nervous system of the sea lamprey *(Petromyzon marinus)*. II. Dorsal cells and giant interneurons.

Rowe, M. H., and J. Stone. (1976) *Exp. Brain Res.* **25**:339–357. Conduction velocity groupings among axons of cat retinal ganglion cells, and their relationship to retinal topography.

Rubel, E. W. (1971) *J. Comp. Neurol.* **143**:447–480. A comparison of somatotopic organization in sensory neocortex of newborn kittens and adult cats.

Rubel, E. W., and T. M. Parks. (1975) *J. Comp. Neurol.* **164**:411–434. Organization and development of brain stem auditory nuclei of the chicken: Tonotopic organization of n. magnocellularis and n. laminaris.

Rubel, E. W., D. J. Smith, and L. C. Miller. (1976) *J. Comp. Neurol.* **166:**469–490. Organization and development of brain stem auditory nuclei of the chicken: Ontogeny of n. magnocellularis and n. laminaris.

Rubinstein, H. S. (1936) *J. Comp. Neurol.* **64:**469–496. The effect of the growth hormone upon the brain and brain weight–body weight relations.

Rugh, R., and J. Wolff. (1955*a*) *Proc. Soc. Exp. Biol. Med.* **89:**248–253. Resilience of the fetal eye following radiation insult.

Rugh, R., and J. Wolff. (1955*b*) *Arch. Opthalmol. (Chicago)* **54:**351–359. Reparation of the fetal eye following radiation insult.

Ruiz-Marcos, A., and F. Valverde. (1969) *Exp. Brain Res.* **8:**284–294. The temporal evolution of the distribution of dendritic spines on the visual cortex of normal and dark raised mice.

Rushton, W. A. H. (1951) *J. Physiol. (London)* **115:**101–122. A theory of the effects of fibre size in medullated nerve.

Russel, D. A., and J. O. W. Bland. (1933) *J. Pathol. Bacteriol.* **36:**273–283. A study of gliomas by the method of tissue culture.

Russell, E. S. (1916) *Form and Function: A Contribution to the History of Animal Morphology,* John Murray, London.

Rustioni, A., and I. Molenaar. (1975) *Exp. Brain Res.* **23:**1–13. Dorsal column nuclei afferents in the lateral funiculus of the cat: Distribution pattern and absence of sprouting after chronic deafferentation.

Rustioni, A., and C. Sotelo. (1974) *Brain Res.* **73:**527–533. Some effects of chronic deafferentation on the ultrastructure of the nucleus gracilis of the cat.

Ryser, H. J. P. (1968) *Science* **159:**390–396. Uptake of protein by mammalian cells: An underdeveloped area.

Ryugo, D. K., R. Ryugo, and H. P. Killackey. (1975) *Brain Res.* **96:**82–87. Changes in pyramidal cell spine density consequent to vibrissae removal in the newborn rat.

Sabatini, M. T., A. P. de Iraldi, and E. de Robertis. (1965) *Exp. Neurol.* **12:**370–383. Early effects of antiserum against the nerve growth factor on fine structure of sympathetic neurons.

Sacher, G. A. (1959) Relation of life span to brain weight in mammals, pp. 115–133. In *The Lifespan of Animals,* CIBA Foundation Colloquia on Aging, Vol. 5 (G. E. W. Wolstenholme and M. O'Connor, eds.), Churchill, London.

Sacher, G. A., and E. F. Staffeldt. (1974) *Am. Nat.* **108:**593–615. Relation of gestation time to brain weight for placental mammals: Implications for the theory of vertebrate growth.

Saetersdal, T. A. S. (1956) *Univ. Bergen Arbok Naturvitenskap. Rekke* **3:**1–53. On the ontogenesis of the avian cerebellum. Part II. Measurements of the cortical layers.

Saetersdal, T. A. S. (1958) *Univ. Bergen Arbok Naturvitenskap. Rekke* **10:**1–20. A critical review of quantitative mitotic recordings in animal tissues with special reference to the central nervous system.

Saetersdal, T. A. S. (1959) *Univ. Bergen Arbok Naturvitenskap. Rekke* **4:**1–39. On the ontogenesis of the avian cerebellum. Part IV. Mitotic activity in the external granular layer with a summary of certain aspects of cortical development.

Sahota, T. S., and J. S. Edwards. (1969) *J. Insect Physiol.* **15:**1367–1373. Development of grafted supernumerary legs in the house cricket, *Acheta domesticus.*

Sakia, F. B. (1965) *J. Comp. Neurol.* **124:**189–202. Post-natal growth of neuroglia cells and blood vessels of the cervical spinal cord of the albino mouse.

Salmons, S., and F. A. Sretér. (1976) *Nature* **263:**30–34. Significance of impulse activity in the transformation of skeletal muscle type.

Salmons, S., and G. Vrbová. (1969) *J. Physiol. (London)* **201:**535–549. The influence of activity on some contractile characteristics of mammalian fast and slow muscles.

Salpeter, M. M. (1966) General area of autoradiography at the the electron microscope level, pp. 229–253. In *Methods in Cell Physiology* (D. M. Prescott, ed.), Academic Press, New York.

Salpeter, M. M., L. Bachmann, and E. E. Salpeter. (1969) *J. Cell Biol.* **41:**1–32. Resolution in electron microscope radioautography.

Salpeter, M. M., G. C. Budd, and S. Mattimoe. (1974) *J. Histochem. Biochem.* **2:**217–222. Resolution in autoradiography using semithin sections.

Samaha, F. J., L. Guth, and R. W. Albers (1970) *Exp. Neurol.* **26:**120–125. Phenotypic differences between actomyosin ATPase of the three fiber types of mammalian skeletal muscle.

Samorajski, T., R. L. Friede, and P. R. Reimer. (1970) *J. Neuropathol. Exp. Neurol.* **29:**507–523. Hypomyelination in the quaking mouse: A model for the analysis of disturbed myelin formation.

Samson, F. E., Jr., W. M. Balfour, and R. J. Jacobs. (1960) *Am. J. Physiol.* **199:**693–696. Mitochondrial changes in developing rat brain.

Samsonova, V. G. (1965) *Pavlov. J. Higher Nervous Activity* (English trans.) **15:**491–499. Functional organization of neurons of different types in the visual center of frogs.

Samuels, L. D., and W. E. Kisielski. (1963) *Radiat. Res.* **18:**620–632. Toxicological studies of tritiated thymidine.

Sanders, F. K. (1948) *Proc. Roy. Soc. (London) Ser. B* **135:**323–357. The thickness of the myelin sheaths of normal and regenerating peripheral nerve fibers.

Sanders, F. K., and D. Whitteridge. (1946) *J. Physiol. (London)* **105:**152–174. Conduction velocity and myelin thickness in regenerating nerve fibers.

Sanders, F. K., and J. Z. Young. (1946) *J. Exp. Biol.* **22:**203–212. The influence of peripheral connexion on the diameter of regenerating nerve fibers.

Sanderson, K. J., R. W. Guillery, and R. M. Shackelford. (1974) *J. Comp. Neurol.* **154:**225–248. Congenitally abnormal visual pathways in mink *(Mustela vision)* with reduced retinal pigment.

Sandritter, W., V. Nováková, J. Pilny, and G. Kiefer. (1967) *Z. Zelforsch. Mikrosk. Anat.* **80:**145–152. Cytophotometrische Messungen des Nukleinsäure- und Proteingehaltes von Ganglienzellen der Ratte während der postnatalen Entwicklung und im Alter.

Sanides, F. (1969) *Ann. N.Y. Acad. Sci.* **167:**404–423. Comparative architectonics of the neocortex of mammals and their evolutionary interpretation.

Santen, R. J., and B. W. Agranoff. (1963) *Biochim. Biophys. Acta* **72:**251–262. Studies on the estimation of deoxyribonucleic acid and ribonucleic acid in rat brain.

Sara, V. R., and L. Lazarus. (1974) *Nature* **250:**257–258. Prenatal action of growth hormone on brain and behaviour.

Sara, V. R., L. Lazaus, M. C. Stuart, and T. King. (1974) *Science* **186:**446–447. Fetal brain growth: Selective action by growth hormone.

Sarkisov, S. A., and N. S. Preobrazhenskaya (eds.). (1959) *Razvitic Tsentral'noi Nervnoi Systemy* (Development of the Central Nervous System), Medgiz, Moscow.

Sauer, F. C. (1935*a*) *J. Comp. Neurol.* **62:**377–405. Mitosis in the neural tube.

Sauer, F. C. (1935*b*) *J. Comp. Neurol.* **63:**13–23. The cellular structure of the neural tube.

Sauer, F. C. (1936) *J. Morphol.* **60:**1–11. The interkinetic migration of embryonic epithelial nuclei.

Sauer, F. C. (1937) *J. Morphol.* **61:**563–579. Some factors in the morphogenesis of vertebrate embryonic epithelium.

Sauer, M. E., and A. C. Chittenden. (1959) *Exp. Cell Res.* **16:**1–6. Deoxyribonucleic acid content of cell nuclei in the neural tube of the chick embryo: Evidence for intermitotic migration of nuclei.

Sauer, M. E., and B. E. Walker. (1959) *Proc. Soc. Exp. Biol. Med.* **101:**557–560. Radiographic study of interkinetic nuclear migration in the neural tube.

Saunders, J. W., Jr. (1966) *Science* **154:**604–612. Death in embryonic systems.

Saunders, J. W., Jr., and J. F. Fallon. (1966) Cell death in morphogenesis, pp. 289–314. In *Major Problems in Developmental Biology* (M. Locke, ed.), Academic Press, New York.

Saunders, J. W., Jr., and M. T. Gasseling. (1968) Ectodermal–mesenchymal interactions, pp. 78. In *Epithelial–Mesenchymal Interactions* (R. Fleischmajer and R. E. Billingham, eds.), Williams and Wilkins, Baltimore.

Saxén, L. (1954) *Ann. Acad. Sci. Fenn. Ser. A.IV* **23:**1–93. The development of the visual cells: Embryological and physiological investigations of *Amphibia.*

Saxén, L. (1961) *Dev. Biol.* **3:**140–152. Transfilter neural induction of amphibian ectoderm.

Saxén, L., and S. Toivonen. (1961) *J. Embryol. Exp. Morphol.* **9:**514–533. The two-gradient hypothesis in primary induction: The combined effect of two types of inductors mixed in different ratios.

Saxén, L., and S. Toivonen. (1962) *Primary Embryonic Induction,* Logos, London.

Saxén, L., E. Lehtonen, M. Karkinen-Jääskeläinen, S. Nordling, and J. Wartiovaara. (1976) *Nature* **259:**662–663. Are morphogenetic tissue interactions mediated by transmissible signal substances or through cell contacts?

Saxod, R. (1967) *Arch. Anat. Microsc. Morphol. Exp.* **56:**153–166. Histogenése des corpuscules sensoriels cutanés chez le poulet et le canard.

Saxod, R. (1970*a*) *J. Ultrastruct. Res.* **32:**477–496. Etude au microscope électronique de l'histogenése du corpuscule sensoriel cutané de Grandry chez le canard.

Saxod, R. (1970*b*) *J. Ultrastruct. Res.* **33:**463–492. Etude au microscope électronique de l'histogenése du corpuscule sensoriel cutané de Herbst chez le canard.

Saxod, R. (1971) *C. R. Acad. Sci. (D) Paris* **273**:89–91. Embryologie expérimentale: Sur l'origine des différentes catégories cellulaires du corpuscle de Herbst.

Saxod, R. (1972*a*) *J. Embryol. Exp. Morphol.* **27**:277–300. Rôle du nerf et du territoire cutané dans le développement des corpuscules de Herbst et de Grandry.

Saxod, R. (1972*b*) *J. Embryol. Exp. Morphol.* **27**:585–601. Interactions morphogènes au course de l'histogenèse du corpuscule de Herbst, étudiées á l'aide de transplantations hètérochrones.

Saxod, R. (1973*a*) *Dev. Biol.* **32**:167–178. Developmental origin of the Herbst cutaneous sensory corpuscle: Experimental analysis using cellular markers.

Saxod, R. (1973*b*) *Tiss. Cell* **5**:269–280. Les organites périnucléaires du corpuscle sensoriel cutané de Grandry: Organisation ultrastructurale et formation.

Saxod, R. (1978) Development of cutaneous sensory receptors in birds. In *Handbook of Sensory Physiology,* Vol. IX: *Development of Sensory Systems* (M. Jacobson, ed.), Springer-Verlag, New York.

Saxod, R., and P. Sengel. (1968) *C. R. Acad. Sci. (Paris)* **267**:1149–1152. Sur les conditions de la différenciation des corpuscules sensoriels cutanés le Poulet et le Canard.

Scalia, F., and K. Fite. (1974) *J. Comp. Neurol.* **158**:455–478. A retinotopic analysis of the central connections of the optic nerve in the frog.

Scalia, F., H. Knapp, M. Halpern, and W. Riss. (1968) *Brain Behav. Evol.* **1**:324–353. New observations on the retinal projection in the frog.

Schadé, J. P. (1959) *Growth* **23**:159–168. Differential growth of nerve cells in cerebral cortex.

Schadé, J. P., and C. F. Baxter. (1960) *Exp. Neurol* **2**:158–178. Changes during growth in the volume and surface area of cortical neurons in the rabbit.

Schadé, J. P., and V. V. Groeningen. (1961) *Acta Anat.* **47**:79–111. Structural organization of the human cerebral cortex.

Schadé, J. P., K. Meeter, and W. B. van Groeningen. (1962) *Acta Morphol. Neerl. Scand.* **5**:37–48. Maturational aspects of the dendrites in the human cerebral cortex.

Schaper, A. (1894*a*) *Anat. Anz.* **9**:489–501. Die morphologische und histologische Entwicklung des Kleinhirns der Teleostier.

Schaper, A. (1894*b*) *Morphol. Jahrb.* **21**:625–708. Die morphologische und histologische Entwicklung des Kleinhirns der Teleostier.

Schaper, A. (1895) *Anat. Anz.* **10**:422–426. Einige kritische Bemerkungen zu Lugaro's Aufsatz; Ueber die Histogenese der Körner der Kleinhirnrinde.

Schaper, A. (1897*a*) *Arch. Entw.-Mech. Organ.* **5**:81–132. Die frühesten Differenzierungsvorgänge im Centralnervensystem.

Schaper, A. (1897*b*) *Science* **5**:430–431. The earliest differentiation in the central nervous system of vertebrates.

Schapiro, S., K. Vukovich, and A. Globus. (1973) *Exp. Neurol* **40**:286–296. Effects of neonatal thyroxine and hydrocortisone administration on the development of dendritic spines in the visual cortex of rats.

Scharf, J.-H. (1951) *Morphol. Jahrb.* **91**:187–252. Die markhaltigen Ganglienzellen und ihre Beziehung zu den myelogenetischen Theorien.

Scharf, J.-H., and R. Blume. (1964) *Z. Zellforsch. Mikrosk. Anat.* **62**:454–467. Quantitativ morphologische Befunde zur Hypothese des Mitochondrientransportes im Neuron.

Scheibel, M. E., T. L. Davies, and A. B. Scheibel. (1973) *Exp. Neurol.* **38**:301–310. Maturation of reticular dentrites: Loss of spines and development of bundles.

Scherrer, J., R. Verley, and L. Garner. (1968) Time, flow and velocity in early life, pp. 303–309. In *Ontogenesis of the Brain* (L. Tilek and S. Trojan, eds.), Charles University, Prague.

Schiff, J., and W. R. Loewenstein. (1972) *Science* **177**:712–715. Development of a receptor on a foreign nerve fiber in a Pacinian corpuscle.

Schjeide, O. A., R. I. S. Lin, and J. de Vallis. (1968) *Radiat. Res.* **33**:107–128. Molecular composition of myelin synthesized subsequent to irradiation.

Schleifenbaum, C. (1973) *Z. Anat. Entichlungsgesch.* **141**:179–205. Untersuchungen zur postnatalen Ontogenese des Gehirns von Grosspudeln und Wölfen.

Schmatolla, E. (1972) *J. Embryol. Exp. Morphol.* **27**:555–576. Dependence of tectal neuron differentiation on optic innervation in teleost fish.

Schmidtke, J., M. T. Zenzes, H. Dittes, and W. Engel. (1975) *Nature* **254**:426–427. Regulation of cell size in fish of tetraploid origin.

Schmidt-Nielson, K. (1970) *Fed. Proc.* **29**:1524–1532. Energy metabolism, body size and problems of scaling.

Schmidt-Nielsen, K. (1975) *J. Exp. Zool.* **194:**287–308. Scaling in biology: The consequences of size.

Schmitt, F. O. (1968) *Proc. Natl. Acad. Sci. U.S.A.* **60:**1092–1101. Fibrous proteins—Neuronal organelles.

Schmitt, F. O., P. Dev, and B. H. Smith. (1976) *Science* **193:**114–120. Electrotonic processing of information by brain cells.

Schneider, G. E. (1970) *Brain Behav. Evol.* **3:**295–323. Mechanisms of functional recovery following lesions of visual cortex or superior colliculus in neonatal and adult hamsters.

Schneider, G. E. (1973) *Brain Behav. Evol.* **8:**73–109. Early lesions of superior colliculus: Factors affecting the formation of abnormal retinal projections.

Schneider, H. R. (1968) *J. Comp. Neurol.* **133:**411–428. Some findings concerning the relationship between ontogenesis and cytoarchitecture of the primate brain.

Schnepp, G., P. Schnepp, and G. Spaan. (1971) *Z. Zellforsch. Mikrosk. Anat.* **119:**77–98. Faseranalytische Untersuchungen an peripheren Nerven bei Tieren verschiedener Grösse. I. Fasergesamtzahl Faserkaliber und Nervenleitungsgeschwindigkeit.

Schnepp, P., and G. Schnepp. (1971) *Z. Zellforsch. Mikrosk. Anat.* **119:**99–114. Faseranalytische Untersuchungen an peripheran Nerven bei Tieren verschiedener Grösse. II. Verhältnis Axondurchmesser, Gesamtdurchmesser und Internodallänge.

Schonback, J., K. H. Hu, and R. L. Friede. (1968) *J. Comp. Neurol.* **134:**21–38. Cellular and chemical changes during myelination: Histologic, autoradiorgraphic, histochemical and biochemical data on myelination in the pyramidal tract and corpus callosum of rat.

Schroeder, T. E. (1969) *Biol. Bull.* **137:**413–414. The role of "contractile ring" filaments in dividing *Arbacia egg.*

Schroeder, T. E. (1970) *J. Embryol. Exp. Morphol.* **23:**427–462. Neurulation in *Xenopus laevis:* An analysis and model based upon light and electron microscopy.

Schroeder, T. E. (1972) *Proc. Natl. Acad. Sci. U.S.A.* **70:**1688–1692. Actin in dividing cells: Contractile ring filaments bind heavy meromysin.

Schubert, P., and G. W. Kreutzberg. (1974) *Brain Res.* **76:**526–530. Axonal transport of adenosine and uridine derivatives and transfer to postsynaptic neurons.

Schubert, P., H. D. Lux, and G. W. Kreutzberg. (1971) *Acta Neuropathol. (Suppl.) (Berl.)* **5:**179–186. Single cell isotope injection technique, a tool for studying axonal and dendritic transport.

Schucker, F. (1972) *Exp. Neurol.* **36:**59–78. Effects of NGF-antiserum in sympathetic neurons during early postnatal development.

Schultz, R. L. (1964) *J. Comp. Neurol.* **122:**281–296. Macroglial identification in electron microscopy.

Schultz, R. L., E. A. Maynard, and D. C. Pease. (1957) *Am. J. Anat.* **100:**369–407. Electron microscopy of neurons and neuroglia of cerebral cortex and corpus callosum.

Schultze, B., B. Nowak, and W. Maurer. (1974) *J. Comp. Neurol.* **158:**207–218. Cycle times of the neural epithelial cells of various types of neuron in the rat: An autoradiographic study.

Schultz, C. (1951) *Zool. Jahrb. Abt. Allgem. Zool. Physiol.* **63:**64–106. Die relative Grösse cytoarchitektonischer Einheiten im Grosshirn der weissen Ratte, weissen Maus und Zwergmaus.

Schumacher, U. (1963) *J. Hirnforsch.* **6:**137–163. Quantitative Untersuchungen an Gehirnen mitteleuropäischer Musteliden.

Schwind, J. L. (1931) *J. Exp. Zool.* **59:** 265–295. Heteroplastic experiments on the limb and shoulder girdle of Amblystoma.

Scott, J. P., J. M. Stewart, and V. J. DeGhett. (1974) *Dev. Psychobiol.* **7:**489–513. Critical periods in the organization of systems.

Scott, M. Y. (1977) *Exp. Neurol.* **54:**579–590. Behavioral tests of compression of retinotectal projection after partial tectal ablation in goldfish.

Scott, S. A. (1975) *Science* **189:**644–646. Persistence of foreign innervation on reinnervated goldfish extraocular muscles.

Scott, T. M. (1974) *J. Embryol. Exp. Morphol.* **31:**409–414. The development of the retino-tectal projection in *Xenopus laevis:* An autoradiographic and degeneration study.

Scott, T. M., and G. Lázár. (1976) *J. Anat.* **121:**485–496. An investigation into the hypothesis of shifting neuronal relationships during development.

Scrimshaw, N. S., and J. E. Gordon (eds.). (1968) *Malnutrition, Learning and Behavior,* MIT Press, Cambridge, Mass.

Sechrist, J. W. (1969) *Am. J. Anat.* **124:**117–134. Neurocytogenesis. I. Neurofibrils, neurofilaments, and the terminal mitotic cycle.

Sechrist, J. W., and A. Lavelle. (1966) *Am. Zool.* **6:**530–531. Neurofilaments and initial neuroblast differentiation.

Sedlaček, J. (1967) *Physiol. Bohemoslav.* **16**:531–537. Development of optic evoked potentials in chick embryos.

Segal. S. J., and D. C. Johnson, (1959) *Arch. Anat. Microsc.* **48**:261–265. Inductive influence of steroid hormones on neural growth.

Seiger, Å., and L. Olson. (1973) *Z. Anat. Entwicklungsgesch.* **140**:281–318. Late prenatal ontogeny of central monoamine neurons in the rat: Fluorescence histochemical observations.

Seil, F. J., and R. M. Herndon. (1970) *J. Cell Biol.* **45**:212–220. Cerebellar granule cells *in vitro:* A light and electron microscope study.

Sellinger, O. Z., and J. M. Azcurra. (1970) *Trans. Am. Neurochem.* **1**:22. Separation of neuronal and glial cell fractions.

Sellinger, O. Z., and P. D. Petiet. (1973) *Exp. Neurol.* **38**: 370–385. Horseradish peroxidase uptake *in vivo* by neuronal and glial lysosomes.

Senglaub, K. (1959) *Morphol. Jahrb.* **100**:11–62. Vergleichende metrische und morphologische Untersuchungen an Organen und am Kleinhirn von Wild-, Gefangenschafts- und Hausenten.

Severinghaus, A. E. (1930) *J. Comp. Neurol.* **51**:237–270. Cellular proliferation in heterotopic spinal-cord grafts.

Shackney, S. E. (1974) *J. Theor. Biol.* **44**:49–90. A cytokinetic model for heterogeneous mammalian cell populations. II. Tritiated thymidine studies: The per cent labeled mitosis (PLM) curve.

Shafiq, S. A. (1970) Satellite cells and fiber nuclei in muscle regeneration, pp. 122–132. In *Regeneration of Striated Muscle and Myogenesis* (A. Mauro, S. A. Shafiq, and A. T. Milhorat, eds.), Excerpta Medica, Amsterdam.

Shantha, T. R., and G. H. Bourne. (1968) The perineural epithelium—A new concept, pp. 379–459. In *The Structure and Function of Nervous Tissue,* Vol. 1 (G. Bourne, ed.), Academic Press, New York.

Shapiro, S., and K. R. Vukovich. (1970) *Science* **167**:292–294. Early experience effects upon cortical dentrites: A proposed model for development.

Shariff, G. A. (1953) *J. Comp. Neurol.* **98**:381–400. Cell counts in the primate cerebral cortex.

Sharma, S. C. (1972*a*) *Exp. Neurol.* **34**:171–182. Reformation of retinotectal projections after various tectal ablations in adult goldfish.

Sharma, S. C. (1972*b*) *Exp. Neurol.* **35**:358–365. Restoration of the visual projection following tectal lesions in goldfish.

Sharma, S. C. (1972*c*) *Brain Res.* **39**:213–223. The retinal projections in the goldfish: An experimental study.

Sharma, S. C. (1972*d*) *Proc. Natl. Acad. Sci. U.S.A.* **69**:2637–2639. Redistribution of visual projections in altered optic tecta of adult goldfish.

Sharma, S. C., and R. M. Gaze. (1971) *Arch. Ital. Biol.* **109**:357–366. The retinotopic organization of visual responses from tectal reimplants in adult goldfish.

Sharma, S. C., and J. C. Hollyfield. (1974) *J. Comp. Neurol.* **155**:395–408. Specification of retinal central connections in *Rana pipiens* before the appearance of the first post-mitotic ganglion cells.

Shaw, C., U. Yinon, and E. Auerbach. (1974) *Exp. Neurol.* **45**:42–49. Diminution of evoked neuronal activity in the visual cortex of pattern deprived rats.

Shear, C. R., and G. Goldspink. (1971) *J. Morphol.* **135**:351–360. Structural and physiological changes associated with the growth of avian fast and slow muscle.

Shepherd, G. M. (1972) *Yale J. Biol. Med.* **45**:584–599. The neuron doctrine: A revision of functional concepts.

Sheridan, J. D. (1966) *J. Cell Biol.* **31**:C1-5. Electrophysiological study of special connections between cells in the early chick embryo.

Sheridan, J. D. (1968) *J. Cell Biol.* **37**:650–659. Electrophysiological evidence for low-resistance intercellular junctions in the early chick embryo.

Sheridan, J. D. (1973) *Am. Zool.* **13**:1119–1128. Functional evaluation of low resistance junctions: Influence of cell shape and size.

Sherk, H., and M. P. Stryker. (1976) *J. Neurophysiol.* **39**:63–70. Quantitative study of cortical orientation selectivity in visually inexperienced kittens.

Sherman, S. M., and K. J. Sanderson. (1972) *Brain Res.* **37**:126–131. Binocular interaction on cells of the dorsal lateral geniculate nucleus of visually-deprived cats.

Sherman, S. M., and J. Stone. (1973) *Brain Res.* **60**:224–230. Physiological normality of the retina in visually deprived cats.

Sherman, S. M., and J. R. Wilson. (1975) *J. Comp. Neurol.* **161**:183–196. Behavioral and morphological evidence for binocular competition in the postnatal development of the dog's visual system.

Sherman, S. M., K.-P. Hoffmann, and J. Stone (1972) *J. Neurophysiol.* **35:**532–541. Loss of a specific cell type from dorsal lateral geniculate nucleus in visually deprived cats.

Sherman, S. M., R. W. Guillery, J. H. Kaas, and R. J., Sanderson (1974) *J. Comp. Neurol.* **158:**1–18. Behavioral, electrophysiological and morphological studies of binocular competition in the development of the geniculo-cortical pathways of cats.

Sherman, S. M., J. R. Wilson, and R. W. Guillery. (1975) *Brain Res.* **100:**441–444. Evidence that binocular competition affects the postnatal development of Y-cells in the cat's lateral geniculate nucleus.

Shieh, P. (1951) *J. Exp. Zool.* **117:**359–395. The neoformation of cells of preganglionic type in the cervical spinal cord of the chick embryo following its transplantation to the thoracic level.

Shimada, M., and J. Langman. (1970) *Am. J. Anat.* **129:**247–260. Repair of the external granular layer after postnatal treatment with 5-fluorodeoxyuridine.

Shimada, M., and T. Nakamura. (1973) *Exp. Neurol.* **41**:163–173. Time of neuron origin in mouse hypothalamic nuclei.

Shlaer, R. (1971) *Science* **173:**638–641. Shifts in binocular disparity causes compensating changes in the cortical structure of kittens.

Sholl, D. A. (1953) *J. Anat. (London)* **87:**387–406. Dendritic organization in the neurons of the visual and motor cortices of the cat.

Sholl, D. A. (1955) *J. Anat. (London)* **89:**571–572. The surface area of cortical neurons.

Sholl, D. A. (1956*a*) *The Organization of the Cerebral Cortex,* Methuen, London.

Sholl, D. A. (1956*b*) *Prog. Neurobiol.* **2:**324–333. The measurable parameters of the cerebral cortex and their significance in its organization.

Shorey, M. L. (1909) *J. Exp. Zool.* **7:**25–64. The effect of the destruction of peripheral areas on the differentiation of the neuroblasts.

Shumway, W. (1940) *Anat. Rec.* **78:**139–147. Stages in the normal development of *Rana pipiens.* I. External forms.

Shumway, W. (1942) *Anat. Rec.* **83:**309–315. Stages in the normal development of *Rana pipiens.* II. Identification of the stages from sectioned material.

Sidman, R. L. (1961) Histogenesis of the mouse retina studied with tritiated thymidine, pp. 487–505. In *The Structure of the Eye* (G. K. Smelser, ed.), Academic Press, New York.

Sidman, R. L. (1968) Development of interneuronal connections in brains of mutant mice. pp. 163–193. In *Physiological and Biochemical Aspects of Nervous Integration* (F. D. Carlson ed.). Prentice-Hall, Englewood Cliffs, N.J.

Sidman, R. L. (1970) Autoradiographic methods and principles for study of the nervous system with thymidine-H^3. In *Contemporary Research Techniques of Neuroanatomy* (S. O. E. Ebbesson and W. J. Nauta, eds.), Springer-Verlag, New York.

Sidman, R. L. (1972) Cell interactions in developing mammalian central nervous system, pp. 1–13. In *Cell Interactions,* Proceedings of the Third Lepetit Colloquium (L. G. Silvestri, ed.), North-Holland, Amsterdam.

Sidman, R. L. (1974) Cell–cell recognition in the central nervous system, pp. 743–758. In *The Neurosciences: Third Study Program* (F. O. Schmitt and F. G. Worden, eds.), MIT Press, Cambridge, Mass.

Sidman, R. L., and M. C. Green. (1970) "Nervous," a new mutant mouse with cerebellar disease. In *Symposium of the Centre National de la Recherche Scientifique,* Orleans-la-Source, France.

Sidman, R. L., and P. Rakic. (1973) *Brain Res.* **62:**1–35. Neuronal migration, with special reference to developing human brain: A review.

Sidman, R. L., I. L. Miale, and N. Feder. (1959) *Exp. Neurol.* **1:**322–333. Cell proliferation and migration in the primitive ependymal zone: An autoradiographic study of histogenesis in the nervous system.

Sidman, R. L., P. W. Lane, and M. M. Dickie. (1962) *Science* **137:**610–611. Staggerer, a new mutation in the mouse affecting the cerebellum.

Sidman, R. L., M. N. Dickie, and S. H. Appel. (1964) *Science* **144:**309–311. Mutant mice (quaking and jimpy) with deficient myelination in the central nervous system.

Sidman, R. L., M. C. Green, and S. H. Appel. (1965) *Catalog of the Neurological Mutants of the Mouse,* Harvard University Press, Cambridge, Mass., 82 pp.

Siegers, M. P., J. C. Schaer, H. Hirsiger, and R. Schindler. (1974) *J. Cell Biol.* **62:**305–315. Determination of rates of DNA synthesis in cultured mammalian cell populations.

Sillito, A. M. (1975*a*) *J. Physiol. (London)* **250:**287–304. The effectiveness of bicuculline as an antagonist of GABA and visually evoked inhibition in the cat's striate cortex.

Sillito, A. M. (1975*b*) *J. Physiol. (London)* **250:**305–329. The contribution of inhibitory mechanisms to the receptive field properties of neurones in the striate cortex of the cat.

Silver, J. (1978) Cell death during development of the nervous system. In *Handbook of Sensory Physiology,* Vol. IX: *Development of Sensory Systems* (M. Jacobson, ed.), Springer-Verlag, New York.

Silver, J., and A. F. Hughes. (1973) *J. Morphol.* **140:**159–170. The role of cell death during morphogenesis of the mammalian eye.

Silver, M. L. (1942) *J. Comp. Neurol.* **77:**1–39. The motoneurons of the spinal cord of the frog.

Simmler, G. M. (1949) *J. Exp. Zool.* **110:**247–257. The effects of wing bud extirpation on the brachial sympathetic ganglia of the chick embryo.

Simpson, I., B. Rose, and W. R. Loewenstein. (1977) *Science* **195:**294–296. Size limit of molecules permeating the junctional membrane channels.

Simpson, S. A., and J. Z. Young. (1945) *J. Anat. (London)* **79:**48–65. Regeneration of fibre diameter after cross-unions of visceral and somatic nerves.

Sims, R. T. (1961) *J. Embryol. Exp. Morphol.* **9:**32–41. The blood vessels of the developing spinal cord of *Xenopus laevis.*

Singer, M. (1952) *Quart. Rev. Biol.* **27:**169–200. The influence of the nerve in regeneration of the amphibian extremity.

Singer, M. (1965) A theory of the trophic nervous control of amphibian limb regeneration, including a re-valuation of quantitative nerve requirement, pp. 20–32. In *Regeneration in Animals and Related Problems* (V. Kiortsis and H. A. L. Trampusch, eds.), North-Holland, Amsterdam.

Singer, M. (1968) Penetration of labelled amino acids into the peripheral nerve fibre from surrounding body fluids, pp. 200–215. In *Ciba Foundation Symposium on Growth of the Nervous System* (G. E. W. Wolstenholme and M. O'Connor, eds.), Churchill, London.

Singer, M., and M. R. Green. (1968) *J. Morphol.* **124:**321–344. Autoradiographic studies of uridine incorporation in peripheral nerve of the newt, *Triturus.*

Singer, M., and M. M. Salpeter. (1966) *Nature* **210:**1225–1227. Transport of tritium-labelled l-histidine through the Schwann and myelin sheaths into the axon of peripheral nerves.

Singer, W., F. Tretter, and M. Cynader. (1975) *J. Neurophysiol.* **38:**1080–1098. Organization of cat striate cortex: A correlation of receptive-field properties with afferent and efferent connections.

Sinha, A. K., and S. P. R. Rose. (1971) *Brain Res.* **33:**205–217. Bulk separation of neurones and glia: A comparison of techniques.

Sisken, B. F., and S. D. Smith. (1975) *J. Embryol. Exp. Morphol.* **33:**29–41. The effects of minute directed electrical currents on cultured chick embryo trigeminal ganglia.

Sjöstrand, J. (1965) *Z. Zellforsch. Mikrosk. Anat. Abt. Histochem.* **68:**481–493. Proliferative changes in glial cells during nerve regeneration.

Sjöstrand, J. (1966*a*) *Acta Physiol. Scand. Suppl. 270* **67:**1–17. Glial cells in the hypoglossal nucleus of the rabbit during nerve regeneration.

Sjöstrand, J. (1966*b*) *Acta Physiol. Scand. Suppl. 270* **67:**19–43. Morphological changes in glial cells during nerve regeneration.

Sjöstrand, J. (1971) *Exp. Neurol.* **30:**178–189. Neuroglial proliferation in the hypoglossal nucleus after nerve injury.

Sjöstrand, J., and M. Frizell. (1975) *Brain Res.* **85:**325–330. Retrograde axonal transport of rapidly migrating proteins in peripheral nerves.

Sjöstrand, J., and J.-O. Karlsson. (1969) *J. Neurochem.* **16:**833–844. Axoplasmic transport in the optic nerve and tract of the rabbit: A biochemical and radioautographic study.

Sjöstrand, J., M. Frizell, and P.-O. Hasselgren. (1970) *J. Neurochem.* **17:**1563–1570. Effects of colchicine on axonal transport in peripheral nerves.

Skarf, B. (1973) *Brain Res.* **51:**352–357. Development of binocular single units in the optic tectum of frogs raised with disparate stimulation to the eyes.

Skarf, B., and M. Jacobson. (1974) *Exp. Neurol.* **42:**669–686. Development of binocularly-driven single units in frogs raised with asymmetrical visual stimulation.

Skeels, H. M. (1966) *Monogr. Soc. Res. Child Dev.* **31 (3):** Serial No. 105. Adult status of children with contrasting early life experiences: A follow-up study.

Sklar, J. H., and R. K. Hunt. (1973) *Proc. Natl. Acad. Sci. U.S.A.* **70:**3684–3688. The acquisition of specificity in cutaneous sensory neurons: A reconsideration of the integumental specification hypothesis.

Skoff, R. P., and V. Hamburger. (1974) *J. Comp. Neurol.* **153:**107–148. Fine structure of dendritic and axonal growth cones in embryonic chick spinal cord.

Sládeček, F. (1952) *Acta Soc. Zool. Bohemoslav.* **16:**322–333. Regulative tendencies of the central nervous system during embryogenesis of the axolotl (*Amblystoma mexicanum* Cope). I. Regulation after inversion of the medio-lateral axes of the medullary plate.

Sládeček, F. (1955) *Acta Soc. Zool. Bohemoslav.* **19:**138-149. Regulative tendencies of the central nervous system during embryogenesis of the axolotl (*Amblystoma mexicanum* Cope). II. Regulation after simultaneous inversion of anteroposterior and medio-lateral axes of medullary plate.

Slavkin, H. C. (1972) Intercellular communication during odontogenesis, pp. 165–199. In *Developmental Aspects of Oral Biology* (H. C. Slavkin and L. A. Bavetta, eds.), Academic Press, New York.

Smart, I. (1961) *J. Comp. Neurol.* **116:**325–347. The subependymal layer of the mouse brain and its cell production as shown by radioautography after thymidine-H^3 injection.

Smart, I., and C. P. Leblond. (1961) *J. Comp. Neurol.* **116:**349–367. Evidence for division and transformation fo neuroglia cells in the mouse brain as derived from radioautography after injection of thymidine-H^3.

Smart, I. H. M. (1976) *J. Anat.* **121:**71–84. A pilot study of cell production by the ganglionic eminences of the developing mouse brain.

Smit, G. J., and E. J. Colon. (1969) *Brain Res.* **13:**485–510. Quantitative analysis of the cerebral cortex. 1. Aselectivity of the Golgi-Cox staining technique.

Smith, A. A., and F. W. Hui. (1971) *Pharmacologist* **13:**235. Familial dysautonomia: A neurotransmitter disease.

Smith, A. A., A. Farbman, and J. Dancis. (1965*a*) *Science* **147**:1040–1041. Absence of taste bud papillae in familial dysautonomia.

Smith, A. A., J. I. Hirsch, and J. Dancis. (1965*b*) *Pediatrics* **36:**225–230. Responses to infused methacholine in familial dysautonomia.

Smith, D. E. (1974) *Brain Res.* **74:**119–130. The effect of deafferentiation on the postnatal development of Clarke's nucleus in the kitten—A Golgi study.

Smith, D. S. (1970) *J. Cell Biol.* **47:**195a–196a. Bridges between vesicles and axoplasmic microtubules.

Smith, R. S., and W. K. Ovalle. (1972) Structure and function of intrafusal muscle fibres, pp. 147–227. In *Muscle Biology,* Vol. 1 (R. G. Cassens, ed.), Marcel Dekker, New York.

Smith, U. (1971) *Phil. Trans. Roy. Soc. London (Biol. Sci.)* **261:**391–394. Uptake of ferritin into neuroscretory terminals.

Snider, R. S., and M. Perez del Cerro. (1967) *Exp. Neurol.* **17:**466–480. Drug-induced dendritic sprouts on Purkinje cells in the adult cerebellum.

Snow, M. H. L. (1975) *J. Embryol. Exp. Morphol.* **34:**707–721. Embryonic development of tetraploid mice during the second half of gestation.

Söderholm, U. (1965) *Acta Physiol. Scand. Suppl.* **65:**256. Histochemical localization of esterases, phosphatases and tetrazolium reductases in the motor neurons of the spinal cord of the rat and the effect of nerve division.

Södersten, P. (1973) *Horm. Behav.* **4:**1–17. Increased mounting behavior in the female rat following a single neonatal injection of testosterone propionate.

Soga, K., and Y. Takahashi. (1975) *Nature* **256:**233–234. Differences in transcription of unique DNA sequences between neuronal and glial cells.

Soga, K., and Y. Takahashi. (1976) *J. Neurochem.* **26:**89–94. Transcription of repeated and unique DNA sequences in brain nuclei.

Sohal, G. S. (1976) *Exp. Neurol.* **51:**684–698. An experimental study of cell death in the developing trochlear nucleus.

Sohal, G. S., and C. H. Narayanan. (1974) *Brain Res.* **77:**243–255. The development of the isthmo-optic nucleus in the duck *(Anas platyrhynchos)*. I. Changes in cell number and cell size during normal development.

Sohal, G. S., and C. H. Narayanan. (1975) *Exp. Neurol.* **46:**521–533. Effects of optic primordium removal on the development of the isthmo-optic nucleus in the duck *(Anas platyrhynchos).*

Solandt, D. Y., C. Partridge, and J. Hunter. (1943) *J. Neurophysiol.* **6:**17–22. The effects of skeletal fixation on skeletal muscle.

Sosula, L., and P. H. Glow. (1970) *J. Comp. Neurol.* **141:**427–452. Increase in number of synapses in the inner plexiform layer of light deprived rat retinae: Quantitative electron microscopy.

Sotelo, C. (1975) *Brain Res.* **94:**19–44. Anatomical physiological and biochemical studies of the cerebellum from mutant mice. II. Morphological study of cerebellar cortical neurons and circuits in the weaver mouse.

Sotelo, C., and J.-P. Changeux. (1974*a*) *Brain Res.* **67:**519–526. Transsynaptic degeneration "en cascade" in the cerebellar cortex of staggerer mutant mice.

Sotelo, C, and J. P. Changeux. (1974*b*) *Brain Res.* **77:**484–491. Bergmann fibers and granular cell migration in the cerebellum of homozygous weaver mutant mouse.

Sotelo, C., and S. L. Palay. (1971) *Lab. Invest.* **25:**653–671. Altered axons and axon terminals in the lateral vestibular nucleus of the rat: Possible example of axonal remodeling.

Sotelo, C., and D. Riche. (1974) *Anat. Embryol.* **146:**209–218. The smooth endoplasmic reticulum and the retrograde and fast orthograde transport of horseradish peroxidase in the nigro-neostriato-nigral loop.

Špacek, J., J. Pářizek, and A. R. Lieberman. (1973) *J. Neurocytol.* **2:**407–428. Golgi cells, granule cells and synaptic glomeruli in the molecular layer of the rabbit cerebellar cortex.

Speidel, C. C. (1932) *J. Exp. Zool.* **61:**279–331. Studies of living nerves. I. The movements of individual sheath cells and nerve sprouts correlated with the process of myelin sheath formation in amphibian larvae.

Speidel, C. C. (1933) *Am. J. Anat.* **52:**1–79. Studies of living nerves. II. Activities of ameboid growth cones, sheath cells, and myelin segments, as revealed by prolonged observation of individual nerve fibers in frog tadpoles.

Speidel, C. C. (1935*a*) *J. Comp. Neurol.* **61:**1–82. Studies on living nerves. III. Phenomena of nerve irritation, recovery, degeneration and repair.

Speidel, C. C. (1935*b*) *Biol. Bull.* **68:**140–161. Studies of living nerves. IV. Growth, regeneration, and myelination of the peripheral nerves in salamanders.

Spiedel, C. C. (1941) *Harvey Lect.* **36:**126–158. Adjustments of nerve endings.

Speidel, C. C. (1942) *J. Comp. Neurol.* **76:**57–69. Studies of living nerves. VII. Growth adjustments of cutaneous terminal arborizations.

Speidel, C. C. (1948) *Am. J. Anat.* **82:**227–320. Correlated studies of sense organs and nerves of the lateral line in living frog tadpoles. II. The trophic influence of specific nerve supply as revealed by prolonged observations of denervated and reinnervated organs.

Speidel, C. C. (1964) *Int. Rev. Cytol.* **16:**173–231. *In vivo* studies of myelinated nerve fibers.

Spemann, H. (1906) *Verhandl. Deut. Ges. Zool.* **16:**195–202. Über eine neue Methode der embryonalen Transplantation.

Spemann, H. (1912) *Zool. Jahrb. Suppl. 15* **3:**1–48. Über die Entwicklung umgedrehter Hirnteile bei Amphibienenbryonen.

Spemann, H. (1938) *Embryonic Development and Induction,* Yale University Press, New Haven. (English transl. of Spemann, 1936, *Experimentelle Beiträge zu einer Theorie der Entwicklung,* Springer-Verlag, Berlin.)

Sperry, R. W. (1940) *J. Comp. Neurol.* **73:**379–404. The functional results of muscle transposition in the hindlimbs of the rat.

Sperry, R. W. (1941) *J. Comp. Neurol.* **75:**1–19. The effect of crossing nerves to antagonistic muscles in the hindlimb of the rat.

Sperry, R. W. (1942) *J. Comp. Neurol.* **76:**283–321. Transplantation of motor nerves and muscles in the forelimb of the rat.

Sperry, R. W. (1943) *J. Comp. Neurol.* **79:**33–55. Visuomotor coordination in the newt *(Triturus viridescens)* after regeneration of the optic nerves.

Sperry, R. W. (1944) *J. Neurophysiol.* **7:**57–69. Optic nerve regeneration with return of vision in anurans.

Sperry, R. W. (1945*a*) *Quart. Rev. Biol.* **20:**311–369. The problem of central nervous reorganization after nerve regeneration and muscle transposition.

Sperry, R. W. (1945*b*) *J. Neurophysiol.* **8:**15–28. Restoration of vision after uncrossing of optic nerves and after contralateral transposition of the eye.

Sperry, R. W. (1947) *Arch. Neurol. Psychiat. (Chicago)* **58:**452–473. Effect of crossing nerves to antagonistic limb muscles in the monkey.

Sperry, R. W. (1948) *Anat. Rec.* **102:**63–75. Orderly patterning of synaptic associations in regeneration of intracentral fiber tracts mediating visuomotor coordination.

Sperry, R. W. (1950*a*) Neuronal specificity, pp. 232–239. In *Genetic Neurology* (P. Weiss, ed.), University of Chicago Press, Chicago.

Sperry, R. W. (1950*b*) *J. Comp. Neurol.* **93:**277–287. Myotypic specificity in teleost motoneurons.

Sperry, R. W. (1951*a*) Mechanisms of neural maturation. pp. 236–280. In *Handbook of Experimental Psychology* (S. S. Stevens ed.), Wiley, New York.

Sperry, R. W. (1951*b*) *Growth Symp.* **10:**63–87. Regulative factors in the orderly growth of neural circuits.

Sperry, R. W. (1963) *Proc. Natl. Acad. Sci. U.S.A.* **50:**703–710. Chemoaffinity in the orderly growth of nerve fiber patterns and connections.

Sperry, R. W. (1965) Embryogenesis of behavioral nerve nets, pp. 161–186. In *Organogenesis,* (R. L. DeHaan and H. Urspring, eds.), Holt, Rinehart and Winston, New York.

Sperry, R. W. (1966) Selective communication in nerve nets: impulse specificity vs. connection specificity, pp. 213–219. In *Neuroscience Research Symposium Summaries,* Vol. 1 (F. O. Schmitt and T. Melnechuk, eds.), MIT Press, Cambridge, Mass.

Sperry, R. W. (1968) *Dev. Biol. Suppl.* **2:**306–327. Plasticity of neural maturation.

Sperry, R. W., and H. L. Arora. (1965) *J. Embryol. Exp. Morphol.* **14:**307–317. Selectivity in regeneration of the oculomotor nerve in the cichlid fish *Astronotus ocellatus.*

Sperry, R. W., and N. Deupree. (1956) *J. Comp. Neurol.* **106:**143–158. Functional recovery following alterations in nerve–muscle connections of fishes.

Sperry, R. W., and N. Miner. (1949) *J. Comp. Neurol.* **90:**403–423. Formation within sensory nucleus V of synaptic associations mediating cutaneous localization.

Spratt, N. T. (1952) *J. Exp. Zool.* **120:**109–130. Localization of the prospective neural plate in the early chick blastoderm.

Stahl, W. R. (1962) *Science* **137**:205–212. Similarity and dimensional methods in biology.

Stahl, W. R. (1970) *Physiological Similarity and Modeling: The Application of Dimensional Analysis and Physical Similarity Theory to Mammalian Physiology.* Appleton-Century-Crofts, New York.

Stanfield, B., and W. M. Cowan. (1976) *Brian Res.* **104:**129–136. Evidence for a change in the retino-hypothalamic projection in the rat following early removal of one eye.

Starre-van der Molen, L. G. (1974) *Cell Tiss. Res.* **151:**219–230. Embryogenesis of *calliphora* erythrocephala Meigen. IV. Cell death in the central nervous system during late embryogenesis.

Stasný, F., J. Fröhlich, and J. Svoboda. (1968) Development of some essential components in different parts of the chick embryo brain, pp. 37-50. In *Ontogenesis of the Brain* (L. Jílek and S. Trojan, eds.), Charles University Press, Prague.

Stebbins, G. L. (1973) *Brookhaven Symp. Biol.* **25:**227–243. Evolution of morphogenetic patterns.

Stefanelli, A. (1950) Studies on the development of Mauthner's cell, pp. 161–165. In *Genetic Neurology* (P. Weiss, ed.), University of Chicago Press, Chicago.

Stefanelli, A. (1951) *Quart. Rev. Biol.* **26:**17–34. The Mautherian apparatus in the Ichthyopsida; Its nature and function and correlated problems of histogenesis.

Stefanowska, M. (1898) *Trav. Lab. Physiol. Inst. Solvay* **2:**1–44. Évolution des cellules nerveuses corticales chez le souris aprés le naissance.

Stein, D. G., J. J. Rosen, J. Graziadei, D. Mishkin, and J. J. Brink. (1969) *Science* **166:**528–529. Central nervous system: Recovery of function.

Stein, J. M., and H. A. Padykula. (1962) *Am. J. Anat.* **110:**103–124. Histochemical classification of individual skeletal muscle fibers of the rat.

Steinbach, J. H., A. J. Harris, J. Patrick, D. Schubert, and S. Heinemann. (1973) *J. Gen. Physiol.* **62:**255–270. Nerve-muscle interaction *in vitro.*

Steinberg, M. S. (1962*a*) *Proc. Natl. Acad. Sci. U.S.A.* **48:**1577–1582. On the mechanism of tissue reconstruction by dissociated cells, I. Population kinetics, differential adhesiveness and the absence of directed migration.

Steinberg, M. S. (1962*b*) *Proc. Natl. Acad. Sci. U.S.A.* **48:**1769–1776. On the mechanism of tissue reconstruction by dissociated cells. III. Free energy relations and the reorganization of fused, heteronomic tissue fragments.

Steinberg, M. S. (1963) *Science* **141:**401–408. Reconstruction of tissues by dissociated cells.

Steinberg, M. S. (1964) The problem of adhesive selectivity in cellular interactions, pp. 321–366. In *Cellular Membranes in Development* (M. Locke, ed.), Academic Press, New York.

Steinberg, M. S. (1970) *J. Exp. Zool.* **73:**395–434. Does differential adhesion govern self-assembly processes in histogenesis? Equilibrium configurations and the emergence of a hierarchy among populations of embryonic cells.

Steinberger, W. W., and E. M. Smith. (1968) *Arch. Phys. Med. Rehabil.* **49:**573–577. Maintenance of denervated rabbit muscle with direct electrostimulation.

Steindler, A. (1916) *Am. J. Orthopedic Surg.* **14:**707–719. Direct neurotization of paralyzed muscles, further study of the question of direct nerve implantation.

Stenevi, U., A. Björklund, and R. Y. Moore. (1973) *Brain Behav. Evol.* **8:**110–134. Morphological plasticity of central adrenergic neurons.

Stenevi, U., B. Bjerre, A. Bjorklund, and W. Mobley (1974) *Brain Res.* **69:**217–234. Effects of localized intracerebral injections of nerve growth factor on the regenerative growth of lesioned central noradrenergic neurones.

Stensaas, L. J. (1967*a*) *J. Comp. Neurol.* **129:**59–70. The development of hippocampal and dorsolateral pallial regions of the cerebral hemisphere in fetal rabbits I. Fifteen millimeter stage, spongioblast morphology.

Stensaas, L. J. (1967*b*) *J. Comp. Neurol.* **129:**71–84. The development of hippocampal and dorsolateral pallial regions of the cerebral hemisphere in fetal rabbits II. Twenty millimeter stage, neuroblast morphology.

Stensaas, L. J., and W. H. Reichert. (1971) *Z. Zellforsch. Mikrosk. Anat.* **119:**147–163. Round and amoeboid microglial cells in the neonatal rabbit brain.

Stensaas, L. J., and S. S. Stensaas. (1971) *Brain Res.* **31:**67–84. Light and electron microscopy of motoneurons and neuropile in the amphibian spinal cord.

Stephan, H. (1951) *Zool. Jahrb. Abt. Anat. Ontog. Tiere* **71:**487–586. Vergleichende Untersuchungen über den Feinbau des Hirnes von Wild- und Haustieren. I. Studien am Schwein und Schaf.

Stephens. L. B. (1965) *Am. Zool.* **5:**222–223. The influence of thyroxine upon Rohon-Beard cells of *Rana pipiens* larvae.

Stern, C. (1956*a*) *Cold Spring Harbor Symp. Quant. Biol.* **21:**375–382. Genetic mechanisms on the localized initiation of differentiation.

Stern, C. (1956*b*) *Arch. Entw.-Mech. Organ.* **149:**1–25. The genetic control of developmental competence and morphogenetic tissue interactions in genetic mosaics.

Stern, C. (1968) *Genetic Mosaics and Other Essays,* Harvard University Press, Boston.

Stevens, A. R. (1966) High resolution autoradiography, pp. 255–310. In *Methods in Cell Physiology* (D. M. Prescott, ed.), Academic Press, New York.

Steward, O., C. W. Cotman, and G. S. Lynch. (1974) *Exp. Brain Res.* **20:**45–66. Growth of a new fiber projection in the brain of adult rats: Re-innervation of the dentate gyrus by the contralateral entorhinal cortex following ipsilateral entorhinal lesions.

Steward, O., W. F. White, C. E. Cotman, and G. Lynch. (1976) *Exp. Brain Res.* **26:**423–441. Potentiation of excitatory synaptic transmission in the normal and in the reinnervated dentate gyrus of the rat.

Stewart. J. A. (1975) *Dev. Biol.* **44:**178–186. Contribution of a change in mRNA half-life to the accumulation of the tissue-specific S-100 protein during postnatal development of the mouse brain.

Stewart, J. A., and M. I. Urban. (1972) *Dev. Biol.* **29:**372–384. The postnatal accumulation of S-100 protein in mouse central nervous system: Modulation of protein synthesis and degradation.

Stewart, R. M., D. P. Richman, and V. S. Caviness, Jr. (1975) *Acta Neuropathol. (Berl.)* **31:**1–12. Lissencephaly and pachygyria: An architectonic and topographical analysis.

Stirewalt, W. S., I. G. Wool, and P. Cavicchi. (1967) *Proc. Natl. Acad. Sci. U.S.A.* **57:**1885–1892. The relation of RNA and protein synthesis to the sedimentation of muscle ribosomes: effect of diabetes and insulin.

Stoch, M. B., and P. M. Smythe. (1963) *Arch. Dis. Child.* **38:**546–552. Does undernutrition during infancy inhibit brain growth and subsequent intellectual development?

Stoch, M. B., and P. M. Smythe. (1967) *S. Afr. Med. J.* **41:**1027–1030. The effect of undernutrition during infancy on subsequent brain growth and intellectual development.

Stoch, M. B., and P. M. Smythe. (1976) *Arch. Dis. Child.* **51:**327–336. 15-year developmental study on effects of severe undernutrition during infancy on subsequent physical growth and intellectual functioning.

Stockdale, F. E., and H. Holtzer. (1961) *Exp. Cell Res.* **24:**508–520. DNA synthesis and myogenesis.

Stoeckel, K., and H. Thoenen. (1975) *Brain Res.* **85:**337–341. Retrograde axonal transport of nerve growth factor: Specificity and biological importance.

Stoeckel, K., U. Paravincini, and H. Thoenen. (1974) *Brain Res.* **76:**413–421. Specificity of the retrograde axonal transport of nerve growth factor.

Stoeckel, K., M. Schwab, and H. Thoenen. (1975) *Brain Res.* **89:**1–14. Specificity of retrograde transport of nerve growth factor (NGF) in sensory neurons: A biochemical and morphological study.

Stoeckel, K., G. Guroff, M. Schwab, and H. Thoenen. (1976) *Brain Res.* **109:**271–284. The significance of retrograde axonal transport for the accumulation of systemically administered nerve growth factor (NGF) in the rat superior cervical ganglion.

Stone, J., and B. Dreher. (1973) *J. Neurophysiol.* **36:**551–567. Projection of X- and Y-cells of the cat's lateral geniculate nucleus to areas 17 and 18 of visual cortex.

Stone, J., and Y. Fukuda. (1974*a*) *J. Neurophysiol.* **37:**722–748. Properties of cat retinal ganglion cells: A comparison of W-cells with X- and Y-cells.

Stone, J., and Y. Fukuda. (1974*b*) *J. Comp. Neurol.* **155:**377–394. The naso-temporal division of the cat's retina re-examined in terms of Y-, X- and W-cells.

Stone, L. S. (1929) *Arch. Entw.-Mech. Organ.* **118:**41–77. Experiments showing the role of migrating neural crest (mesectoderm) in the formation of the head skeleton and loose connective tissue in *Rana palustris.*

Stone, L. S. (1930) *J. Exp. Zool.* **55:**193–261. Heteroplastic transplantation of eyes between the larvae of two species of *Amblystoma.*

Stone, L. S. (1933) *Proc. Soc. Exp. Biol. Med.* **30:**1256–1257. Independence of taste organs with respect to their nerve fibers demonstrated in living salamanders.

Stone, L. S. (1940) *J. Exp. Zool.* **83:**481–506. The origin and development of taste organs in salamanders observed in the living condition.

Stone, L. S. (1941) *Trans. N.Y. Acad. Sci.* **3:**208–212. Transplantation of the vertebrate eye and return of vision.

Stone, L. S. (1944) *Proc. Soc. Exp. Biol. Med.* **57:**13–14. Functional polarization in retinal development and its reestablishment in regenerated retinae of rotated eyes.

Stone, L. S. (1948) *Ann. N.Y. Acad. Sci.* **49:**856–865. Functional polarization in developing and regenerating retinae of transplanted eyes.

Stone, L. S. (1953) *Arch. Ophthalmol. (Chicago)* **49:**28–35. Normal and reversed vision in transplanted eyes.

Stone, L. S. (1960) *J. Exp. Zool.* **145:**85–93. Polarization of the retina and development of vision.

Stone, L. S. (1963) *J. Exp. Zool.* **153:**57–67. Vision in eyes of several species of adult newts transplanted to adult *Triturus viridescens.*

Stone, L. S. (1964) *Invest. Ophthalmol.* **3:**555–565. Return of vision in eyes exchanged between *Amblystoma punctatum* and the cave salamander, *Typhlotriton spelaeus.*

Stone, L. S., and C. H. Cole. (1943) *Yale J. Biol. Med.* **15:**735–754. Grafted eyes of young and old salamanders *(Amblystoma punctatum)* showing return of vison.

Stone, L. S., and F. S. Ellison. (1940) *Proc. Soc. Biol. Med.* **45:**181–182. Exchange of eyes between adult hosts of *Amblystoma punctatum* and *Triturus viridescens.*

Stone, L. S., and L. S. Farthing. (1942) *J. Exp. Zool.* **91:**265–285. Return of vision four times in the same adult salamander eye *(Triturus viridescens)* repeatedly transplanted.

Stone, L. S., and J. S. Zaur. (1940) *J. Exp. Zool.* **85:**243–270. Reimplantation and transplantation of adult eyes in the salamander *(Triturus viridescens)* with return of vision.

Stott, D. H. (1960) *Br. J Educ. Psychol.* **30:**95–102. Interaction of heredity and environment in regard to "measured intelligence."

Stough, H. B. (1930) *J. Comp. Neurol.* **50:**17–229. Polarization of the giant nerve fibers of the earthworm.

Straus, W. L. (1939) *Anat. Rec. Suppl. 2* **73:**50–55. Changes in the structure of skeletal muscle at the time of its first visible contraction in living rat embryos.

Straus, W. L. (1946) *Biol. Rev.* **21:**75–91. The concept of nerve–muscle specificity.

Straus, W. L., and G. Weddell. (1940) *J. Neurophsiol.* **3:**358–369. Nature of the first visible contractions of the forelimb musculature in rat foetuses.

Straznicky, K. (1963) *Acta Biol. Acad. Sci. Hung.* **14:**143–155. Function of heterotopic spinal cord segments investigated in the chick.

Straznicky, K. (1967) *Acta Biol. Acad. Sci. Hung.* **18:**437–448. The development of the innervation and the musculature of wings innervated by thoracic nerves.

Straznicky, K. (1973) *J. Embryol. Exp. Morphol.* **29:**397–409. The formation of the optic fibre projection after partial tectal removal in *Xenopus.*

Straznicky, K., and R. M. Gaze. (1971) *J. Embryol. Exp. Morphol.* **26:**67–79. The growth of the retina in *Xenopus laevis:* An autoradiographic study.

Straznicky, K., and R. M. Gaze. (1972) *J. Embryol. Exp. Morphol.* **28:**87–115. The development of the tectum in *Xenopus laevis:* An autoradiographic study.

Straznicky, K., and G. Székely. (1967) *Acta Biol. Acad. Sci. Hung.* **18:**449–456. Functional adaptation of thoracic spinal cord segments in the newt.

Straznicky, K., and D. Tay. (1977) *J. Embryol. Exp. Morphol.* Retinal growth in double dorsal and double ventral eyes in *Xenopus.*

Straznicky, K., R. M. Gaze, and M. J. Keating. (1971) *J. Embryol. Exp. Morphol.* **26:**523–542. The retinotectal projections after uncrossing the optic chiasma in *Xenopus* with one compound eye.

Straznicky, K., R. M. Gaze, and M. J. Keating. (1974) *J. Embryol. Exp. Morphol.* **31:**123–137. The retinotectal projection from a double-ventral compound eye in *Xenopus laevis.*

Stretton, A. O. W., and E. A. Kravitz. (1968) *Science* **162:**132–134. Neuronal geometry: Determination with a technique of intracellular dye injection.

Strong, L. H. (1961) *Acta Anat.* **44:**80–108. The first appearance of vessels within the spinal cord of the mammal: Their developing patterns as far as partial formation of the dorsal septum.

Stryker, M. P., and H. Sherk. (1975) *Science* **190:**904–905. Modification of cortical orientation selectivity in the cat by restricted visual experience: A reexamination.

Stryker, M. P., H. V. B. Hirsch, H. Sherk, and A. G. Leventhal. (1976) Orientation selectivity in cat visual cortex following selective orientation deprivation using goggles. Paper presented at ARVO, Sarasota, Florida.

Stultz, W. A. (1942) *Anat. Rec.* **82:**450. Alterations in the spinal cord of *Amblystoma* following changes in the peripheral field.

Stumpf, H. F. (1966*a*) *Nature* **212:**430–431. Mechanism by which cells estimate their location within the body.

Stumpf, H. F. (1966*b*) *J. Insect Physiol.* **12:**601–617. Über Gefälleabhangige Bildungen des Insektensegmentes.

Stumpf, H. F. (1968) *J. Exp. Biol.* **49:**49–60. Further studies on gradient-dependent diversification in the pupal cuticle of *Galleria mellonella.*

Stumpf, W. E. (1971*a*) *Am. Zool.* **11:**725–739. Autoradiographic techniques and the localization of estrogen, androgen, and glucocorticoid in the pituitary and brain.

Stumpf, W. E. (1971*b*) *J. Neuro-Visceral Relations Suppl.* **10:**51–64. Probable sites for estrogen receptors in brain and pituitary.

Sturrock, R. R. (1974*a*) *J. Anat.* **117:**17–24. Histogenesis of the anterior limb of the anterior commissure of the mouse brain. I. A quantitative study of changes in the glial population with age.

Sturrock, R. R. (1974*b*) *J. Anat.* **117:**27–35. Histogenesis of the anterior limb of the anterior commissure of the mouse brain. II. A quantitative study of pre and postnatal mitosis.

Stussi, T. (1960) *Arch. Sci Physiol. (Paris)* **14:**261–277. Etudes des localisations motrices du renflement lombaire chez la grenouille.

Sulston, J. E. (1976) *Phil. Trans. Roy. Soc. London Ser. B* **275:**287–297. Post-embryonic development in the ventral cord of *Caenorhabditis elegans.*

Sumi, S. M. (1970) *Brain* **93:**821–830. Brain malformation in the trisomy 18 syndrome.

Summerbell, D., and J. H. Lewis. (1975) *J. Embryol. Exp. Morphol.* **33:**621–643. Time, place and positional value in the chick limb-bud.

Sumner, B. E. H. (1975) *Exp. Neurol.* **46:**605–615. A quantitative analysis of the response of presynaptic boutons to postsynaptic motor neuron axotomy.

Sumner, B. E. H. (19760 *Exp. Brain Res.* **26:**141–150. Quantitative ultrastructural observations on the inhibited recovery of the hypoglossal nucleus from the axotomy response when regeneration of the hypoglossal nerve is prevented.

Sumner, B. E. H., and F. I. Sutherland. (1973) *J. Neurocytol.* **2:**315–328. Quantitative electron microscopy on the injured hypoglossal nucleus in the rat.

Sumner, B. E. H., and W. E. Watson. (1971) *Nature* **233:**273–275. Retraction and expansion of the dendritic tree of motor neurons of adult rats induced in vivo.

Sunderland, S. (1947) *Arch. Neurol. Psychiat.* **58:**251–295. Rate of regeneration in human peripheral nerves: Analysis of interval between injury and onset of recovery.

Sutherland, E. W. (1972) *Science* **177:**401–408. Studies on the mechanism of hormone action.

Sutton, A. C. (1915) *Am. J. Anat.* **18:**117–144. On the development of the neuro-muscular spindle in the extrinsic eye muscles of the pig.

Suzuki, A., and K. Kuwabara. (1974) *Dev. Growth Differ.* **16:**29–40. Mitotic activity and cell proliferation in primary induction of newt embryo.

Suzuki, A., K. Kuwabara, and Y. Kuwabara. (1975) *Dev. Growth Differ.* **17:**343–353. Temporal relations between extension of archenteron roof and realization of neural induction during gastrulation of newt embryo.

Suzuki, D. T., T. Grigliatti, and R. Williamson. (1971) *Proc. Natl. Acad. Sci. U.S.A.* **68:**890–893. Temperature-sensitive mutations in *Drosophila melanogaster.* VII. A mutation *(para^{ts})* causing reversible adult paralysis.

Swash, M., and K. P. Fox. (1974) *J. Neurol. Sci.* **22:**1–24. The pathology of the human muscle spindle: Effect of denervation.

Swett, F. H. (1927) *J. Exp. Zool.* **47:**385–439. Differentiation of the amphibian limb.

Swett, F. H. (1937) *Quart. Rev. Biol.* **12:**322–339. Determination of limb-axes.

Swett, F. H. (1938) *J. Exp. Zool.* **78:**47–79. Experiments designed to hasten polarization of the dorsoventral limb axis in *Amblystoma punctatum.*

Swift, H. (1950) *Physiol. Zool.* **23:**169–198. The desoxyribose nucleic acid content of animal nuclei.

Szarski, H. (1976) *Int. Rev. Cytol.* **44:**93–111. Cell size and nuclear DNA content in vertebrates.

Székely, G. (1954) *Acta Biol. Acad. Sci. Hung.* **5:**157–167. Zur Ausbildung der lokalen funktionellen Spezifität der Retina.

Székely, G. (1957) *Arch. Entw.-Mech. Organ.* **150:**48–60. Regulationstendenzen in der Ausbildung der 'funktionellen Spezifität" der Retinaanlage bei *Triturus vulgaris.*

Székely, G. (1959*a*) *J. Embryol. Exp. Morphol.* **7:**375–379. The apparent "corneal specificity" of sensory neurons.

Székely, G. (1959*b*) *Acta Biol. Acad. Sci. Hung.* **10:**107–116. Functional specificity of cranial sensory neuroblasts in Urodela.

Székely, G. (1963) *J. Embryol. Exp. Morphol.* **11:**431–444. Functional specificity of spinal cord segments in the control of limb movements.

Székely, G. (1966) *Adv. Morphogenesis* **5:**181–219. Embryonic determination of neural connections.

Székely, G. (1968) Development of limb movements: Embryological physiological and model studies, pp. 77–93. In *Growth of the Nervous System: A Ciba Foundation Symposium* (G. E. W. Wolstenholme and M. O'Connor, eds.), Little, Brown, Boston.

Székely, G. (1971) *Vision Res. Suppl.* **3:**269–279. The mesencephalic and diencephalic optic centres in the frog.

Székely, G. (1973) Anatomy and synaptology of the optic tectum, pp. 1–26. In *Handbook of Sensory Physiology,* Vol. VII/3B (R. Jung, ed.), Springer-Verlag, Berlin.

Székely, G. (1974) Problems of neuronal specificity in the development of some behavior patterns in amphibia pp. 115–150. In *Studies on the Development of Behavior and the Nervous System,* Vol. 2: *Aspects of Neurogenesis* (G. Gottlieb, ed.), Academic Press, New York.

Székely, G., and G. Czéh. (1967) *Acta Physiol. Acad. Sci. Hung.* **32:**3–18. Localization of motoneurones in the limb moving spinal cord segments of *Amblystoma.*

Székely, G., G. Czéh, and G. Vörös. (1969) *Exp. Brain Res.* **9:**53–62. The activity pattern of limb muscles in freely moving normal and deafferented newts.

Székely, G., G. Sétáló, and G. Lázár. (1973) *J. Hirnforsch.* **14:**189–225. Fine structure of the frog's optic tectum: optic fibre termination layers.

Szentágothai, J. (1948) *J. Comp. Neurol.* **88:**207–220. The representation of facial and scalp muscles in the facial nucleus.

Szentágothai, J. (1949) *J. Comp. Neurol.* **90:**111–120. Functional representation in the motor trigeminal nucleus.

Szentágothai, J., and G. Székely. (1956*a*) *Acta Biol. Acad. Sci. Hung.* **6:**215–229. Zum Problem des Kreuzung von Nervenbahnen.

Szentágothai, J., and G. Székely. (1956*b*) *Acta Physiol. Acad. Sci. Hung.* **10:**43–55. Elementary nervous mechanisms underlying optokinetic responses, analysed by contralateral eye grafts in urodele larvae.

Szepsenwol, J. (1947) *Anat. Rec.* **98:**67–85. Electrical excitability and spontaneous activity in explants of skeletal and heart muscles of chick embryos.

Taber Pierce, E. (1966) *J. Comp. Neurol.* **126:**219–239. Histogenesis of the nuclei griseum pontis, corporis pontobulbaris and reticularis tegmenti pontis (Bechterew) in the mouse: An autoradiographic study.

Taber Pierce, E. (1967*a*) *J. Comp. Neurol.* **131:**27–54. Histogenesis of the dorsal and ventral cochlear nuclei in the mouse: An autoradiographic study.

Taber Pierce, E. (1967*b*) *Anat. Rec.* **157:**301. Histogenesis of deep cerebellar nuclei studied autoradiographically with thymidine-H^3 in the mouse.

Taber Pierce, E. (1973) *Prog. Brain Res.* **40:**53–65. Time of origin of neurons in the brain stem of the mouse.

Taxi, J., and C. Sotelo. (1973) *Brain Res.* **62:**431–437. Cytological aspects of the axonal migration of catecholamines and of storage material.

Taylor, A. C. (1943) *Anat. Rec.* **87:**379–413. Development of the innervation pattern in the limb bud of the frog.

Taylor, A. C. (1944) *J. Exp. Zool.* **96:**159–185. Selectivity of nerve fibers from the dorsal and ventral roots in the development of the frog limb.

Taylor, A. C., and J. J. Kollros. (1946) *Anat. Rec.* **94:**7–23. Stages in the normal development of *Rana pipiens* larvae.

Taylor, E. W. (1965) *J. Cell Biol.* **25:**145–160. The mechanism of colchicine inhibition of mitosis. I. Kinetics of inhibition and the binding of H^3-colchicine.

Tello, J. F. (1922*a*) *Trabajos Lab. Invest. Biol. Univ. Madrid* **21:**1–93. Les différenciations neuronales dans l'embryon des poulet pendent les premiers jours de l'incubation.

Tollo, J. F. (1922*b*) *Z. Anat. Entw. Gesch. Organ.* **64:**248–440. Die Entstehung der motorischen und sensiblen Nervenendigungen. I. In dem lokomotorischen system der höheren Wirbeltiere: Muskulare histogenese.

Tello, J. F. (1925) *Trabajos Lab. Invest. Biol. Univ. Madrid* **23** :1–28. Sur la formation des chaines primaires et secondaires du grand sympathique dans l'embryon de poulet.

Tello, J. F. (1932) *Trabajos Lab. Invest. Biol. Univ. Madrid* **28:**1–58. Contribution a la connaissance des terminaisons sensitives dan les organes genitaux externes et de leur développement.

Tennyson, V. M. (1965) *J. Comp. Neurol.* **124:**267–318. Electron microscopic study of the developing neuroblast of the dorsal root ganglia of the rabbit embryo.

Tennyson, V. M. (1970) *J. Cell Biol.* **44:**62–79. The fine structure of the axon and growth cone of the dorsal root neuroblast of the rabbit embryo.

Tennyson, V. M., and G. D. Pappas. (1962) *Z. Zellforsch. Mikrosk. Anat. Abt. Histochem.* **56:**595–618. An electron microscope study of ependymal cells of the fetal, early postnatal and adult rabbit.

Tennyson, V. M., M. Brzin, and P. E. Duffy. (1967) *J. Neuropathol. Exp. Neurol.* **26:**136–137. Cholinesterase localization in the dorsal root ganglion of the rabbit embryo by electron microscopic histochemistry.

Teräväinen, H. (1968) *Z. Zellforsch. Mikrosk. Anat. Abt. Histochem.* **87:**249–265. Development of the myoneural junction in the rat.

Ter Horst, J. (1947) *Arch. Entw.-Mech. Organ.* **143:**275–303. Differenzierungs und Induktionsleistungen verschiedener Abschnitte der Medullarplatte und des Urdarmdaches von Triton im Kombinat.

Terplan, K. L., E. C. Lopez, and H. B. Robinson. (1970) *Am. J. Dis. Child.* **119:**228–235. Histologic structural anomalies in the brain in trisomy 18 syndrome.

Terry, R. J., and J. Gordon, Jr. (1960) *J. Exp. Zool.* **143:**245–257. The effects of unilateral and bilateral enucleation on optic lobe development and pigmentation of the skin in *Rana catesbeiana* larvae.

Tettenborn, U., R. Dofuku, and S. Ohno. (1971) *Nature New Biol.* **234:**37–40. Noninducible phenotypes exhibited by a proportion of female mice heterozygous for the X-linked testicular feminization mutation.

Thesleff, S. (1960) *Physiol. Rev.* **40:**734–752. Effects of motor innervation on the chemical sensitivity of skeletal muscle.

Thoa, N. B., G. F. Wooten, J. Axelrod, and I. J. Kopin. (1972) *Proc. Natl. Acad. Sci. U.S.A.* **69:**520–522. Inhibition of release of dopamine-β-hydroxylase and norepinephrine from sympathetic nerves by colchicine, vinblastine or cytochalasin.

Thoenen, H., P. U. Angeletti, R. Levi-Montalcini, and R. Kettler. (1971) *Proc. Natl. Acad. Sci. U.S.A.* **68:**1598–1602. Selective induction by nerve growth factor of tyrosine hydroxylase and dopamine β-hydroxylase in the rat superior cervical ganglia.

Thoenen, H., A. Saner, R. Kettler, and P. U. Angeletti. (1972) *Brain Res.* **44:**593–602. Nerve growth factor and preganglionic cholinergic nerves: Their relative importance to the development of the terminal adrenergic neuron.

Thom, R. (1975) *Structural Stability and Morphogenesis: An Outline of a General Theory of Models,* W. A. Benjamin, Reading, Mass.

Thomas, G. A. (1948) *J. Anat. (London)* **82:**135–145. Quantitative histology of Wallerian degeneration. II. Nuclear population in two nerves of different fibre spectrum.

Thomas, P. K. (1955) *Proc. Roy. Soc. Biol.* **143:**380–391. Growth changes in myelin sheath of peripheral nerve fibers in fishes.

Thomas, P. K. (1970) *J. Anat. (London)* **106:**463–470. The cellular response to nerve injury. 3. The effect of repeated crush injuries.

Thomas, P. K., and J. Z. Young (1949) *J. Anat. (London)* **83:**336–350. Internode lengths in nerves of fishes.

Thompson, H. (1899) *J. Comp. Neurol.* **9:**113–140. The total number of functional nerve cells in the cerebral cortex of man.

Thorpe, W. H. (1961) *Bird-Song,* Columbia University Press, New York.

Thorpe, W. H., (1964) *Learning and Instinct in Animals,* Methuen, London.

Tiedemann, F. (1816) *Anatomie und Bildungsgeschichte des Gehirns in Foetus des Menschen,* Steinischen Buchhandlung, Nuremberg. (English transl. by W. Bennet, 1823, *The Anatomy of the Foetal Brain,* Carfrae, Edinburgh.)

Tiedemann, H. (1968) *J. Cell. Physiol. Suppl. I.* **72:**129–144. Factors determining embryonic differentiation.

Tiegs, O. W. (1953) *Physiol. Rev.* **33:**90–144. Innervation of voluntary muscle.

Tigges, J., W. B. Spatz, and M. Tigges. (1973) *J. Comp. Neurol.* **148:**481–490. Reciprocal point-to-point connections between parastriate and striate cortex in the squirrel monkey *(Saimiri)*.

Tilney, F. (1933) *Bull. Neurol. Inst. N.Y.* **3:**252–358. Behavior in its relation to the development of the brain. Part II. Correlation between the development of the brain and behavior in the albino rat from embryonic states to maturity.

Tilney, F., and L. Casamajor. (1924) *Arch. Neurol. Psychiat. (Chicago)* **12:**1–6. Myelogeny as applied to the study of behavior.

Tilney, L. G., and M. Mooseker. (1971) *Proc. Natl. Acad. Sci. U.S.A.* **68:**2611–2615. Actin in the brush border of epithelial cells of the chicken intestine.

Tilney, L. G., J. Bryan, D. J. Bush, K. Fujiwara, M. S. Mooseker, D. B. Murphy, and D. H. Snyder. (1973) *J. Cell Biol.* **59:**267–275. Microtubules: evidence for 13 protofilaments.

Tizard, J. (1974) *Br. Med. Bull.* **30:**169–174. Early malnutrition, growth and mental development in man.

Toivonen, S., and S. Saxén. (1955*a*) *Exp. Cell Res. Suppl.* **3:**346–357. The simultaneous inducing action of liver and bone-marrow of the guinea-pig in implantation and explantation experiments with embryos of *Triturus*.

Toivonen, S., and Saxén, L. (1955*b*) *Ann. Acad. Sci. Fenn. Ser. A.* **30:**1–29- Ueber die Induktion des Neuralrohrs bei Trituruskeimen als simultane Leistungs des Leber- und Knochenmarkgewebes vom Meerschweinchen.

Toivonen, S., and L. Saxén. (1968) *Science* **159:**539–540. Morphogenetic interaction of presumptive neural and mesodermal cells mixed in different ratios.

Toivonen, S., D. Tarin, L. Saxén, P. J. Tarin, and J. Wartiovaara. (1975) *Differentiation* **4:**1–7. Transfilter studies on neural induction in the newt.

Toivonen, S., D. Tarin, and S. Saxén. (1976) *Differentiation* **5:**49–55. The transmission of morphogenetic signals from amphibian mesoderm to ectoderm in primary induction.

Tomanek, R. J., and D. L. Lund. (1974) *J. Anat.* **118:**531–541. Degeneration of different types of skeletal muscles fibres. II. Immobilization.

Tonge, D. A. (1974*a*) *J. Physiol. (London)* **236:**22–23P. Reinnervation of skeletal muscle in the mouse.

Tonge, D. A. (1974*b*) *J. Physiol. (London)* **239:**96–97P. Synaptic function in experimental dually innervated muscle in the mouse.

Tonge, D. A. (1974*c*) *J. Physiol. (London)* **241:**141–153. Physiological characteristics of re-innervation of skeletal muscle in the mouse.

Torrey, T. W. (1934) *J. Comp. Neurol.* **59:**203–220. The relation of taste buds to their nerve fibers.

Torrey, T. W. (1936) *J. Comp. Neurol.* **64:**325–336. The relation of nerves to degenerating taste buds.

Torrey, T. W. (1940) *Proc. Natl. Acad. Sci. U.S.A.* **26:**627–634. The influence of nerve fibers upon taste buds during embryonic development.

Torvik, A. E. (1956) *J. Neuropathol. Exp. Neurol.* **15:**119–145. Transneuronal changes in the inferior olive and pontine nuclei in kittens.

Torvik, A. E. (1972) *J. Neuropathol. Exp. Neurol.* **31:**132–146. Phagocytosis of nerve cells during retrograde degeneration.

Torvik, A. E., and A. Heding. (1969) *Acta Neuropathol.* **14:**62–71. Effect of actinomycin D on retrograde nerve cell reaction. Further observations.

Torvik, A. E., and F. Skjörten. (1971*a*) *Acta Neuropathol.* **17:**248–264. Electron microscopic observations on nerve cell regeneration and degeneration after axon lesions. I. Changes in the nerve cell cytoplasm.

Torvik, A. E., and F. Skjörten. (1971*b*) *Acta Neuropathol.* **17:**265–282. Electron microscopic observations on nerve cell regeneration and degeneration after axon lesions. II. Changes in the glial cells.

Torvik, A. E., and F. Skjörten. (1974) *J. Neurocytol.* **3:**87–97. The effect of actinomycin D upon normal neurons and retrograde nerve cell reaction.

Torvik, A. E., and A. J. Söreide. (1972) *J. Neuropathol. Exp. Neurol.* **31:**683–695. Nerve cell regeneration after axon lesions in newborn rabbits: A light and electron microscopic study.

Torvik, A. E., and A. J. Söreide. (1975) *Brain Res.* **95:**519–529. The perineuronal glial reaction after axotomy.

Toschi, G., E. Dore, P. U. Angeletti, R. Levi-Montalcini, and C. H. Dehaën. (1965) *J. Neurochem.* **13:**539–544. Characteristics of labelled RNA from spinal ganglia of chick embryo and the action of a specific growth factor (NGF).

Towe, A. L. (1975) *Brain Behav. Evol.* **11:**16–47. Notes on the hypothesis of columnar organization in somatosensory cerebral cortex.

Tower, S. S. (1932) *Brain* **55:**77–89. Atrophy and degeneration in the muscle spindle.

Tower, S. S. (1937*a*) *J. Comp. Neurol.* **67:**109–131. Function and structure in the chronically isolated lumbo-sacral spinal cord of the dog.

Tower, S. S. (1937*b*) *J. Comp. Neurol.* **67:**241–269. Trophic control of non-nervous tissues by the nervous system: A study of muscle and bone innervated from an isolated and quiescent region of spinal cord.

Townes, P. L., and J. Holtfreter. (1955) *J. Exp. Zool.* **128:**53–120. Directed movements and selective adhesions of embryonic amphibian cells.

Trinkaus, J. P. (1966) Morphogenetic cell movements, pp. 125–176. In *Major Problems in Developmental Biology* (M. Locke, ed.), Academic Press, New York.

Trinkaus, J. P., and M. Gross. (1960) *Exp. Cell Res.* **24:**52–57. The use of triated thymidine for marking migrating cells.

Trujillo-Cenóz, O. (1962) *Z. Zellforsch. Mikrosk. Anat. Abt. Histochem.* **56:**649–682. Some aspects of the structural organization of the arthropod ganglia.

Tsang, Y. (1939) *J. Comp. Neurol.* **70:**1–8. Ventral horn cells and polydactyly in mice.

Tschumi, P. A. (1957) *J. Anat. (London)* **91:**149–173. The growth of the hindlimb bud of *Xenopus laevis* and its dependence upon the epidermis.

Tucker, T. J., and A. Kling. (1967) *Brain Res.* **5:**377–389. Differential effects of early and late lesions of frontal granular cortex in the monkey.

Tumbleson, M. E. (1973) *Growth:* **37:**13–17. Brain weight, as a function of age, in miniature swine.

Tuohimaa, P., and R. Johansson. (1971) *Endocrinology* **88:**1159–1164. Decreased estradiol binding in the uterus and anterior hypothalamus of androgenized female rats.

Tuohimaa, P., and M. Niemi. (1972) *Acta Endocrinol. (Kbh.)* **71:**45–54. *In vitro* uptake of tritiated sex steroids by the hypothalamus of adult male rats treated neonatally with an antiandrogen (cyproterone).

Turing, A. (1952) *Phil. Trans. Roy. Soc. London Ser. B* **237:**37–72. The chemical basis of morphogenesis.

Twitty, V. C. (1932) *J. Exp. Zool.* **61:**333–374. Influence of the eye on the growth of its associated structures, studied by means of heteroplastic transplantation.

Twitty, V. C. (1955) Organogenesis: The eye, pp. 402–414. In *Analysis of Development* (B. H. Willier, P. A. Weiss, and V. Hamburger eds.), Saunders, Philadelphia.

Twitty, V. C., and J. I. Schwind. (1931) *J. Exp. Zool.* **59:**61–86. The growth of eyes and limbs transplanted heteroplastically between two species of *Amblystoma.*

Uchizono, K. (1965) *Nature* **207:**642–643. Characteristics of excitatory and inhibitory synapses in the central nervous system of the cat.

Uchizono, K. (1966) *Jpn. J. Physiol.* **16:**570–575. Excitatory and inhibitory synapses in the cat spinal cord.

Udenfriend, S. (1966) *Harvey Lect.* **60:**57–83. Biosynthesis of the sympathetic neurotransmitter, norepinephrine.

Udin, S. B. (1975) *Neurosci. Abstr.* **1:**799. Retinotectal plasticity after half-tectum ablation in adult frogs.

Udin, S. B. (1976) *Neurosci. Abstr.* **II/(2):**1213. Progressive alterations in optic tract and retinotectal topography during optic nerve regeneration in Rana pipiens.

Ulett, G., Jr., R. S. Dow, and O. Larsell. (1944) *J. Comp. Neurol.* **80:**1–10. The inception of conductivity in the corpus callosum and the cortico-pontocerebellar pathway of young rabbits with reference to myelination.

Uzman, B. G., and E. T. Hedley-Whyte. (1968) *J. Gen. Physiol.* **51:**8S-18S. Myelin: Dynamic or stable?

Uzman, B. G., and G. M. Villegas. (1960) *J. Biophys. Biochim. Cytol.* **7:**761–762. A comparison of nodes of Ranvier in sciatic nerves with nodelike structures in optic nerves of the mouse.

Uzman, L. L. (1960) *J. Comp. Neurol.* **114:**137–148. The histogenesis of the mouse cerebellum as studied by its tritiated thymidine uptake.

Valverde, F. (1967) *Exp. Brain Res.* **3:**337–352. Apical dendritic spines of the visual cortex and light deperivation in the mouse.

Valverde, F. (1968) *Exp. Brain Res.* **5:**274–292. Structural changes in the area striata of the mouse after enucleation.

Valverde, F. (1971) *Brain Res.* **33:**1–11. Rate and extent of recovery from dark rearing in the visual cortex of the mouse.

Valverde, F. (1976) *J. Neurocytol.* **5:**509–529. Aspects of cortical organization related to the geometry of neurons with intracortical axons.

Valverde, F., and M. E. Estéban. (1968) *Brain Res.* **9:**145–148. Peristriate cortex of mouse: Location and the effects of enucleation on the number of dendritic spines.

Valverde, F., and A. Ruiz-Marcos. (1969) *Exp. Brain Res.* **8:**269–383. Dendritic spines in the visual cortex of the mouse: introduction to a mathematical model.

Van Buren, J. M. (1963) *J. Neurol. Neurosurg. Psychiat.* **26:**402–409. Trans-synaptic retrograde degeneration in the visual system of primates.

Van Buren, J. M., and D. A. Maccubin. (1962) *J. Neurosurg.* **19:**811–839. An outline atlas of the human basal ganglia with estimation of anatomical variants.

Van Buskirk, C. (1945) *J. Comp. Neurol.* **82:**303–333. The seventh nerve complex.

Van Campenhout, E. (1930*a*) *Quart. Rev. Biol.* **5:**23–50, 217–234. Historical survey of the development of the sympathetic nervous system.

Van Campenhout, E. (1930*b*) *J. Exp. Zool.* **56:**295–320. Contributions to the problem of the development of the sympathetic nervous system.

Van Campenhout, E. (1931) *Arch. Biol. (Paris)* **42:**479–507. Le développement du système nerveux sympathique chez le poulet.

Van Campenhout, E. (1935) *J. Exp. Zool.* **72:**175–193. Experimental researches on the origin of the acoustic ganglion in amphibian embryos.

Vandenburg, S. G. (1966) *Psychol. Bull.* **66:**327–352. Contributions of twin research to psychology.

Van der Loos, H. (1965) *Bull. Johns Hopkins Hosp.* **117:**228–250. The "improperly" oriented pyramidal cell in the cerebral cortex and its possible bearing on problems of growth and cell orientation.

Van der Loos, H., and T. A. Woolsey. (1973) *Science* **179:**395–398. Somatosensory cortex: Structural alterations following early injury to sense organs.

Van Essen, D., and J. K. S. Jansen. (1977) *J. Comp. Neurol.* **171:**433–454. The specificity of re-innervation by identified sensory and motor neurons in the leech.

Van Essen, D., and J. Kelly. (1973) *Nature* **241:**403–405. Correlation of cell shape and function in the visual cortex of the cat.

Van Harreveld, A. (1945) *Am. J. Physiol.* **144:**477–493. Re-innervation of denervated muscle fibers by adjacent functioning motor units.

Van Harreveld, A. (1947) *Am. J. Physiol.* **150:**670–676. On the mechanism of the "spontaneous" re-innervation in paretic muscle.

Van Harreveld, A. (1972) The extracellular space in the vertebrate central nervous system, pp. 447–511. In *The Structure and Function of Nervous Tissue* (G. H. Bourne, ed.), Academic Press, New York.

Van Harreveld, A., and F. I. Khattab. (1969) *J. Cell Sci.* **4:**437–453. Changes in extracellular space of the mouse cerebral cortex during hydroxyadipaldehyde fixation and osmium tetroxide post-fixation.

Van Harreveld, A., and J. Steiner. (1970) *Anat. Rec.* **166:**117–130. Extracellular space in frozen and ethanol substituted central nervous tissue.

Van Harreveld, A., and J. Trubatch. (1974) *Anat. Rec.* **178:**587–598. Conditions affecting the extracellular space in the frog's forebrain.

Van Harreveld, A., J. Crowell, and S. K. Malhotra. (1965) *J. Cell Biol.* **15:**117–137. A study of extracellular space in central nervous tissue by freeze-substitution.

Van Harreveld, A., H. Collewijn, and S. K. Malhotra. (1966) *Am. J. Physiol.* **210:**251–256. Water, electroytes, and extracellular space in hydrated and dehydrated brains.

Van Sluyters, R. C., and D. L. Stewart. (1974) *Exp. Brain Res.* **19:**196–204. Binocular neurons of the rabbit's visual cortex: Effects of monocular sensory deprivation.

Van Valen, L. (1974) *Am. J. Phys. Anthropol.* **40:**417–424. Brain size and intelligence in man.

Vargas-Lizardi, P., and K. M. Lyser. (1974) *Dev. Bio.*. **38:**220–228. Time of origin of Mauthner's neuron in *Xenopus laevis* embryos.

Varon, S., J. Nomora and E. M. Shooter (1968) *Biochem.* **7:**1296–1303. Reversible dissociation of the mouse nerve growth factor protein into different subunits.

Varon, S., C. Raiborn, and P. A. Burnham. (1974*a*) *Neurobiol.* **4:**231–252. Selective potency of homologous ganglionic non-neuronal cells for the support of dissociated ganglionic neurons in culture.

Varon, S., C. Raiborn, and S. Norr. (1974*b*) *Exp. Cell Res.* **88:**247–256. Association of antibody to nerve growth factor with ganglionic non-neurons (glia) and consequent interference with their neuron-supportive action.

Vaughn, J. E. (1969) *Z. Zellforsch. Mikrosk. Anat. Abt. Histochem.* **94:**293–324. An electron microscopic analysis of gliogenesis in rat optic nerves.

Vaughn, J. E., and A. Peters. (1968) *J. Comp. Neurol.* **133:**269–288. A third neuroglial cell type: An electron microscope study.

Vaughn, J. E., and A. Peters. (1971) The morphology and development of neuroglial cells, pp. 103–140. In *Cellular Aspects of Growth and Differentiation,* UCLA Forum Med. Sci. No. 14 (D. C. Pease, ed.), University of California Press, Los Angeles.

Vaughn, J. E., P. L. Hinds, and R. P. Skoff. (1970) *J. Comp. Neurol.* **140:**175–206. Electron microscopic studies of Wallerian degeneration in rat optic nerves. I. The multipotential glia.

Vaughn, J. E., C. K. Henrikson, and J. A. Grieshaber. (1974) *J. Cell Biol.* **60:**664–672. A quantitative study of synapses on motor neuron dendritic growth cones in developing mouse spinal cord.

Vendrely, R., and C. Vendrely. (1956) *Int. Rev. Cytol.* **5:**171–197. The results of cytophotometry in the study of the deoxyribonucleic acid (DNA) content of the nucleus.

Veneroni, G. (1968) *Anat. Rec.* **160:**503. Formation *de novo* and development of neuromuscular junctions *in vitro.*

Veneroni, G., and M. R. Murray. (1969) *J. Embryol. Exp. Morphol.* **21:**369–382. Formation *de novo* and development of neuromuscular junction *in vitro.*

Verbitskaya, L. B. (1969) Some aspects of the ontogenesis of the cerebellum, pp. 859–874. In *Neurobiology of Cerebellar Evolution and Development* (R. Llinás, ed.), A.M.A. Education and Research Foundations, Chicago.

Vernadakis, A., and D. M. Woodbury. (1965) *Arch. Neurol. (Chicago)* **12:**284–293.- Cellular and extracellular spaces in developing rat brain.

Vernadakis, A., and D. M. Woodbury. (1971) Effects of cortisol on maturation of the central nervous system, pp. 85–97. In *Influence of Hormones on the Nervous System* (D. H. Ford, ed.), Karger, Basel.

Vernon, J. A., and J. Butsch. (1957) *Science* **125:**1033–1034. Effect of tetraploidy on learning and retention in the salamander.

Vertes, M., A. Barnea, H. R. Lindner, and R. J. B. King. (1973) *Adv. Exp. Med. Biol.* **36:**137–173. Studies on androgen and estrogen uptake by rat hypothalamus.

Vignal, W. (1888) *Arch. Physiol. Norm. Pathol. Paris Ser. IV* **2:**311–338. Recherches sur le développement de la substance corticale du cerveau et du cervelet.

Visintini, F., and R. Levi-Montalcini. (1939) *Schweiz. Arch. Neurol. Neurochir. Psychiat.* **43:**381–393. **44:**119–150. Relazione tra differenziazione strutturale e funzionale dei centri e delle vie nervose nell' embrione di pollo.

Vizoso, A. D. (1950) *J. Anat. (London)* **82:**342–353. The relationship between internodal length and growth in human nerves.

Vizoso, A. D., and J. Z. Young. (1948) *J. Anat. (London)* **82:**110–134. Internode length and fiber diameter in developing and regenerating nerves.

Voeller, K., G. D. Pappas, and D. P. Purpura. (1963) *Exp. Neurol.* **7:**107–130. Electron microscope study of development of cat superficial neocortex.

Vogt, W. (1925) *Arch. Entw.-Mech. Organ.* **106:**542–610. Gestaltungsanalyse am Amphibienkeim mit örtlicher Vitalfärbung. I. Methodik und Wirkungsweise der örtlichen Vitalfärbung mit Agar als Farbtäger.

Vogt, W. (1929) *Arch. Entw.-Mech. Organ.* **120:**384–706. Gestaltungsanalyse am Amphibienkeim mit örtliche Vitalfärbung II. Gastrulation und Mesodermbildung bei Urodelen und Anuren.

Volkmann, R. (1893) *Beitr. Pathol. Anat.* **12:**233–332. Über die Regeneration des quergestrieften Muskelgewebes beim Menschen und Säugethier.

Volkmar, F. R., and W. T. Greenough. (1972) *Science* **176:**1445–1447. Rearing complexity affects branching of dendrites in the visual cortex of the rat.

Von Baer, K. E. (1828) *Über Entwickelungsgeschichte der Thiere, Beobachtung und Reflexion,* I. Theil, Gebrüder Bornträger, Königsberg.

Von Bonin, G. (1934) *J. Comp. Neurol.* **59:**1–28. On the size of man's brain, as indicated by skull capacity.

Von Bonin, G. (1937) *J. Gen. Psychol.* **16:**379–389. Brain-weight and body-weight in mammals.

Von Bonin, G. (1963) *The Evolution of the Human Brain,* University of Chicago Press, Chicago.

Von Economo, C. (1926) *Deutsch. Klin. Wochenschr.* **5:**593–595. Ein Koefficient für Organisationshohe der Grosshirnrinde.

Von Economo, C., and G. N. Koskinas. (1925) *Die Cytoarchitektonik der Hirnrinde des erwachsenen Menschen,* Berlin.

Von Gudden, B. A. (1869) *Arch. Psychiat.* **2:**693–723. Experimentaluntersuchungen über das peripherische und centrale Nervensystem.

Von Vintschgau, M. (1880) *Arch. Ges. Physiol.* **23:**1–13. Beobachtungen über die Veränderungen der Schmeckbecher nach Durchschneidung des N. glossopharyngeus.

Von Vintschgau, M., and J. Hönigschmied. (1876) *Arch. Ges. Physiol.* **14:**443–448. Nervus glossopharyngeus und Schmeckbecher.

Von Woellwarth, C. (1950) *Arch. Entw.-Mech. Organ.* **144:**178–256. Experimentelle Untersuchungen über den Situs Inversus der Eingeweide und der Habenula des Zwischenhirns bei Amphibien.

Von Woellwarth, C. (1952) *Arch. Entw.-Mech. Organ.* **145:**582–668. Die Induktionsstufen des Gehirns.

Von Woellwarth, C. (1960) *Arch. Entw.-Mech. Organ.* **152:**602–631. Über das Anlagenmuster und die Kinematik des Ektoderms, im Neural- und Schwanzknospenstadium von *Triturus alpestris.*

Von Woellwarth, C. (1969) *Roux' Arch. Entwicklungsmech. Organ.* **162:**336–340. Auslösung von Situs inversus durch Materialdefekte im lateralen Ektoderm der Gastrula bei *Triturus alpestris.*

Vrbová, G. (1963*a*) *J. Physiol. (London)* **166:**241–250. Changes in the motor reflexes produced by tenotomy.

Vrbová, G. (1963*b*) *J. Physiol. (London)* **169:**513–526. The effect of motoneurone activity on the speed of contraction of striated muscle.

Vrensen, G., and D. de Groot. (1974) *Brain Res.* **78:**263–278. The effect of dark rearing and its recovery on synaptic terminals in the visual cortex of rabbits: A quantitative electron microscopic study.

Wada, J. A., R. Clarke, and A. Hamm. (1975) *Arch. Neurol.* **32:**239–246. Cerebral hemispheric asymmetry in humans.

Waddington, C. H. (1952) *The Epigenetics of Birds,* Cambridge University Press, London.

Waddington, C. H. (1966) Fields and gradients, pp. 105–124. In *Major Problems in Developmental Biology* (M. Locke, ed.), Academic Press, New York.

Waddington, C. H., and M. M. Perry. (1966) *Exp. Cell Res.* **41:**691–693. A note on the mechanisms of cell deformation in the neural folds of amphibia.

Waechter, H. (1953) *Arch. Entw.-Mech. Organ.* **146:**201–274. Die Induktionsfähigkeit der Gehirnplatte bei Urodelen und ihr medianlaterales Gefälle.

Waechter, R. V., and B. Jaensch. (1972) *Brain Res.* **46:**235–250. Generation times of the matrix cells during embryonic brain development: An autoradiographic study in rats.

Wagner, R. P. (1969) *Science* **163:**1026–1031. Genetics and phenogenetics of mitochondria.

Wahn, H. L., L. E. Lightbody, T. T. Tchen, and J. D. Taylor. (1975) *Science* **188:**366–369. Induction of neural differentiation in cultures of amphibian undetermined presumptive epidermis by cyclic AMP derivatives.

Wake, K. (1964) *Arch. Histol. (Japan)* **25:**23–41. Motor endplates in developing duck embryo skeletal muscle: histological structure and histochemical localization of cholinesterase activity.

Walberg, F. (1963) *Exp. Neurol.* **8:**112–124. Role of normal dendrites in removal of degenerating terminal boutons.

Waldeyer, H. W. G. (1891) *Deutsch. Med. Wochenschr.* **17:**1213–1218, 1244–1246, 1267–1269, 1287–1289, 1331–1332, 1352–1356. Über einige neuere Forschungen im Gebiete der Anatomie des Centralnervensystems.

Waldeyer, W. (1865) *Arch. Pathol. Anat. Physiol.* **34:**473–514. Ueber die Veränderungen der quergestreiften Muskeln bei der Entzündung und dem Typhusprozess, sowie über die Regeneration derselben nach Substanzdefecten.

Walker, A. E. (1942) *Arch. Neurol. Psychiat.* **48:**13–29. Lissencephaly.

Walker, B. E. (1960) *Am. J. Anat.* **107:**95–105. Renewal of cell populations in the female mouse.

Walker, C. R., and B. W. Wilson. (1975) *Nature* **256:**215–216. Control of acetylcholinesterase by contractile activity of cultured muscle cells.

Walker, P. A., and J. Money. (1972) *Hormones* **3:**119–128. Prenatal androgenization of females.

Wall, P. D., and M. D. Egger. (1971) *Nature* **232:**542–545. Formation of new connexions in adult rat brains after partial deafferentation.

Wallace, H. (1972) *J. Embryol. Exp. Morphol.* **28:**419–435. The components of regrowing nerves which support the regeneration of irradiated salamander limbs.

Wallace, L. J., and L. M. Partlow. (1976) *Proc. Natl. Acad. Sci. U.S.A.* **73:**4210–4214. α-Adrenergic regulation of secretion of mouse saliva rich in nerve growth factor.

Waller, A. (1851) *Edinburgh Med. Surg. J.* **76:**369–376. Experiments on the section of the glossopharyngeal and hypoglossal nerves of the frog, and observations of the alterations produced thereby in the structure of their primitive fibres.

Waller, A. (1852) *Arch. Anat. Physiol. (Liepzig)* **11:**392–401. Sur la reproduction des nerfs et sur la structure et les fonctions des ganglions spinaux.

Walz, M. A., R. W. Price, and A. L. Notkins. (1974) *Science* **184:**1185–1187. Latent ganglionic infection with herpes simplex virus types 1 and 2: Viral reactivation *in vivo* after neurectomy.

Wand, M., E. Zeuthen, and E. A. Evans. (1967) *Science* **157:**436–438. Tritiated thymidine: Effect of decomposition by self-radiolysis on specificity as a tracer for DNA synthesis.

Wanner, R. A., M. J. Edwards, and R. G. Wright. (1976) *J. Pathol.* **118:**235–244. The effect of hyperthermia on the neuroepithelium of the 21-day guinea-pig foetus: Histologic and ultrastructural study.

Ware, R. W., and V. Lopresti. (1975) *Int. Rev. Cytol.* **40:**325–440. Three-dimensional reconstruction from serial sections.

Warner, A. E. (1970) *J. Physiol. (London)* **210:**150–151P. Electrical connexions between cells at neural stages of the axolotl.

Warner, A. E. (1973) *J. Physiol. (London)* **235:**267–286. The electrical properties of the ectoderm in the amphibian embryo during induction and early development of the nervous system.

Wartiovaara, J., S. Nordling, E. Lehtonen, and L. Saxén. (1974) *J. Embryol. Exp. Morphol.* **31:**667–682. Transfilter induction of kidney tubules: Correlation with cytoplasmic penetration into Nucleopore filters.

Watanabe, I. (1965) *Tohoku J. Exp. Med.* **86:**201–218. Enzyme histochemical study of the motor nerve cells in axonal reaction.

Waterlow, J. C., J. Cravioto, and J. M. L. Stephen. (1960) *Adv. Protein Chem.* **15:**131–238. Protein malnutrition in man.

Watson, J. B. (1903) *Chicago Univ. Contrib Phil.* **4:**90–111. Animal education: An experimental study of the psychical development of the white rat correlated with the growth of its nervous system.

Watson, W. E. (1965) *J. Physiol. (London)* **180:**741–753. An autoradiographic study of the incroporation of nucleic acid precursors by neurones and glia during nerve regeneration.

Watson, W. E. (1968) *J. Physiol. (London)* **196:**655–676. Observations on the nucleolar and total cell body nucleic acid of injured nerve cells.

Watson, W. E. (1969) *J. Physiol. (London)* **202:**611–630. The response of motor neurones to intramuscular injection of botulinum toxin.

Watson, W. E. (1974*a*) *Brain Res.* **65:**317–322. The binding of actinomycin D to the nuclei of axotomised neurons.

Watson, W. E. (1974*b*) *Physiol. Rev.* **54:**245–271. Physiology of neuroglia.

Watson, W. E. (1974*c*) *Br. Med. Bull.* **30:**112–115. Cellular responses to axotomy and to related procedures.

Watterson, R. L., and I. Fowler. (1953) *Anat. Rec.* **117:**773–803. Regulative development in lateral halves of chick neural tubes.

Watterson, R. L., P. Veneziano, and A. Bartha. (1956) *Anat. Rec.* **124:**379. Absence of a true germinal zone in neural tubes of young chick embryos as demonstrated by the colchicine technique.

Waxman, S. G., and M. V. L. Bennett. (1972) *Nature New Biol.* **238:**217–219. Relative conduction velocities of small myelinated and non-myelinated fibres in the central nervous system.

Waxman, S. B., and G. D. Pappas. (1969) *Brain Res.* **14:**240–244. Pinocytosis at postsynaptic membranes: Electron microscopic evidence.

Waxman, S. G., and G. D. Pappas. (1971) *J. Comp. Neurol.* **143:**41–72. An electron microscopic study of synaptic morphology in the oculomotor nuclei of three inframammalian species.

Weber, K., and U. Groeschel–Stewart. (1974) *Proc. Natl. Acad. Sci. U.S.A.* **70:**750–754. Antibody to Myosin: The specific visualization of myosin-containing filaments in nonmuscle cells.

Weber, L., R. Pollack, and T. Bibring. (1975) *Proc. Natl. Acad. Sci. U.S.A.* **72:**459–463. Antibody against tubulin: The specific visualization of cytoplasmic microtubules in tissue culture cells.

Weber, R. (1962) *Experientia* **18:**84–85. Induced metamorphosis in isolated tails of *Xenopus.*

Webster, H. deF. (1971) *J. Cell Biol.* **48:**348–367. The geometry of peripheral myelin sheaths during their formation and growth in rat sciatic nerves.

Webster, H. deF., J. R. Martin, and M. F. O'Connell. (1973) *Dev. Biol.* **32:**401–416. The relationships between interphase Schwann cells and axons before myelination: A quantitative electron microscopic study.

Webster, W., M. Shimada, and J. Langman. (1973) *Am. J. Anat.* **137:**67–85. Effect of fluorodeoxyuridine, colcemid, and bromodeoxyuridine on developing neocortex of the mouse.

Wechsler, W. (1966*a*) *Z. Zellforsch. Mikrosk. Anat.* **74:**232–251. Elektronenmikroskopischer Beitrag zur Histogenese der Weissen Substanz des Rückenmarks von Hühnerembryonen.

Wechsler, W. (1966*b*) *Z. Zellforsch. Mikrosk. Anat.* **74:**401–422. Elektronenmikroskopischer Beitrag zur Nervenzelldifferenzierung und Histogenese der grauen Substanz des Rückenmarks von Hühnerembryonen.

Wechsler, W. (1966*c*) *Z. Zellforsch. Mikrosk. Anat.* **74:**423–442. Elektronenmikroskopischer Beitrag zur Differenzierung des Ependyms am Rückenmark von Hühnerembryonen.

Wechsler, W. (1967) Electron-microscopy of the cytodifferentiation in the developing brain of chick embryos, pp. 213–224. In *Evolution of the Forebrain* (R. Hassler and H. Stephan eds.), Plenum, New York.

Weddell, G., L. Guttmann, and E. Guttmann. (1941) *J. Neurol. Neurosurg. Psychiat.* **4**(N.S.)**:**206–225. The local extension of nerve fibers into denervated areas of skin.

Wegener, K., S. Hollweg, and W. Maurer. (1963) *Naturwissenschaften* **50:**738–739. Autoradiographische Bestimmung der Dauer des DNS-Verdopplung und der Generationszeit bei fetalen Zellen der Ratte.

Wegener, K., S. Hollweg, and W. Maurer. (1964) *Z. Zellforsch. Mikrosk. Anat. Abt. Histochem.* **63:**309–326. Autoradiographische bestimmung der DNS-Verdopplungszeit und anderer Teil-Phasen des Zell-Zyklus bei fetalen Zellarten der Ratte.

Weichsel, M. E., Jr. (1974) *Brain Res.* **78:**455–465. Effect of thyroxine on DNA synthesis and thymidine kinase activity during cerebellar development.

Weinberg, H. J., and P. S. Spencer. (1975) *J. Neurocytol.* **4:**395–418. Studies on the control of myelinogenesis. I. Myelination of regenerating axons after entry into a foreign unmyelinated nerve.

Weinberg, H. J., and P. S. Spencer. (1976) *Brain Res.* **133:**363–378. Studies on the control of myelinogenesis. II. Evidence for neuronal regulation of myelin production.

Weis, P. (1970) *J. Embryol. Exp. Morphol.* **24:**381–392. The *in vitro* effect of the nerve growth factor in chick embryo spinal ganglia—A light microscopic evaluation.

Weis, P. (1971) *J. Comp. Neurol.* **141:**117–132. The *in vitro* effect of the nerve growth factor on chick embryo spinal ganglia: An electron microscopic evaluation.

Weiss, P. (1922) *Ost. Akad. Wiss. Math. Naturwiss. Klin. Abt. 1.* **59:**199–201. Die Funktion transplantierter Amphibienextremitäten.

Weiss, P. (1924) *Arch. Entw.-Mech. Organ.* **102:**635–672. Die Funktion transplantierter Amphibienextremitäten. Aufstellung einer Resonanztheorie der motorischen Nerventätigkeit auf Grund abgestimmter Endorgane.

Weiss, P. (1928*a*) *Naturwissenschaften* **16:**626–636. Eine neue theorie der Nervenfunktion: Nicht durch gesonderte Bahnen, Sondern durch spezifische Formen der Erregung schaltet das Nervensystem mit den Muskein.

Weiss, P. (1928*b*) *Ergeb. Biol.* **3:**1–151. Erregungspezifität und Erregungsresonanz.

Weiss, P. (1929) *Arch. Entw.-Mech. Organ.* **116:**438–554. Erzwingung elementarer Strukturverschiedenheiten am *in vitro* wachsenden Gewebe.

Weiss, P. (1931) *Wien. Klin. Wochschr.* **39:**1–17. Das Resonanzprinzip der Nerventätigkeit.

Weiss, P. (1934) *J. Exp. Zool.* **68:**393–448. *In vitro* esperiments on the factors determining the course of the outgrowing nerve fiber.

Weiss, P. (1935) *J. Comp. Neurol.* **61:**135–174. Experimental innervation of muscles by the central ends of afferent nerves (establishment of one-neuron connection between receptor and effector organ), with functional tests.

Weiss, P. (1936) *Biol. Rev.* **11:**494–531. Selectivity controlling the central–peripheral relations in the nervous system.

Weiss, P. (1937*a*) *J. Comp. Neurol.* **66:**181–209. Further investigations on the phenomenon of homologous response in transplanted amphibian limbs. I. Functional observations.

Weiss, P. (1937*b*) *J. Comp. Neurol.* **66:**481–535. Further experimental investigations on the phenomenon of homologous response in transplanted amphibian limbs. II. Nerve regeneration and the innervation of transplanted limbs.

Weiss, P. (1937*c*) *J. Comp. Neurol.* **66:**537–548. Further experimental investigations on the phenomenon of homologous response in transplanted amphibian limbs. III. Homologous response in the absence of sensory innervation.

Weiss, P. (1937*d*) *J. Comp. Neurol.* **67:**269–315. Further experimental investigations on the phenomenon of homologous response in transplanted amphibian limbs. IV. Reverse locomotion after the interchange of right and left limbs.

Weiss, P. (1939) *Principles of Development,* Holt, New York.

Weiss, P. (1941*a*) *Third Growth Symp.* **5:**163–203. Nerve patterns: The mechanics of nerve growth.

Weiss, P. (1941*b*) *Comp. Psychol. Monogr.* **17:**1–96. Self-differentiation of the basic patterns of coordination.

Weiss, P. (1942) *J. Comp. Neurol.* **77:**131–169. Lid-closure reflex from eyes transplanted to atypical locations in *Triturus torosus:* Evidence of a peripheral origin of sensory specificity.

Weiss, P. (1947) *Yale J. Biol. Med.* **19:**235–278. The problem of specificity in growth and development.

Weiss, P. (1950) *J. Exp. Zool.* **113:**397–461. Deplantation of fragments of nervous system in amphibians. I. Central reorganization and the formation of nerves.

Weiss, P. (1952) *Res. Publ. Assoc. Res. Nerv. Ment. Dis.* **30:**3–23. Central versus peripheral factors in the development of coordination.

Weiss, P. (1955) Nervous system, pp. 346–401. In *Analysis of Development* (B. H. Willier, P. Weiss, and V. Hamburger, eds.), Saunders, Philadelphia.

Weiss, P. (1963) Self-renewal and proximo-distal convection in nerve fibers, pp. 171–183. In *The Effect of Use and Disuse on Neuromuscular Functions* (E. Gutman and P. Hnik, eds.), Czechoslovak Academy of Science, Prague.

Weiss, P. (1964) *Proc. Nat. Acad. Sci. U.S.A.* **52:**1024–1029. The dynamics of the membrane-bound incompressible body: a mechanism of cellular and subcellular motility.

Weiss, P. (1972) *Proc. Natl. Acad. Sci. U.S.A.* **69:**1309–1312. Neuronal dynamics and axonal flow: Axonal peristalsis.

Weiss, P., and G. Andres. (1952) *J. Exp. Zool.* **121:**449–488. Experiments on the fate of embryonic cells (chick) disseminated by the vascular route.

Weiss, P., and M. V. Edds, Jr. (1945) J. Neurophysiol. **8:**173–193. Sensory-motor nerve crosses in the rat.

Weiss, P., and M. V. Edds, Jr. (1946) *Am. J. Physiol.* **145:**587–607. Spontaneous recovery of muscle following partial denervation.

Weiss, P., and H. B. Hiscoe. (1948) *J. Exp. Zool.* **107:**315–396. Experiments on the mechanism of nerve growth.

Wiess, P., and A. Hoag. (1946) *J. Neurophysiol.* **9:**413–418. Competitive reinnervation of rat muscles by their own and foreign nerves.

Weiss, P., and R. Mayr. (1971) *Acta Neuropathol. (Suppl.) (Berl.)* **5:**198–206. Neuronal organelles in neuroplasmic ("axonal") flow. II. Neurotubules.

Weiss, P., and A. Pillai. (1965) *Proc. Natl. Acad. Sci. U.S.A.* **54:**48–56. Convection and fate of mitochondria in nerve fibers: Axonal flow as vehicle.

Weiss, P., and F. Rossetti. (1951) *Proc. Natl. Acad. Sci. U.S.A.,* **37:**540–556. Growth responses of opposite sign among different neuron types exposed to thyroid hormone.

Weiss, P., and A. C. Taylor. (1944) *J. Exp. Zool.* **95:**233–257. Further experimental evidence against "neurotropism" in nerve regeneration.

Weiss, P., M. V. Edds, and M. Cavanaugh. (1945*a*) *Anat. Rec.* **92:**215–233. The effects of terminal connections on the caliber of the nerve fibers.

Weiss, P., H. Wang, A. C. Taylor, and M. V. Edds, Jr. (1945*b*) *Am. J. Physiol.* **143:**521–540. Proximo-distal fluid convection in the endoneurial spaces of peripheral nerves, demonstrated by colored and radioactive (isotope) tracers.

Weiss, P., A. C. Taylor, and P. A. Pillai. (1962) *Science* **136:**330. The nerve fiber as a system in continuous flow: microcinematographic and electron-microscopic demonstrations.

Welker, C. (1973) *Anat. Rec.* **175:**467–468. Organization of somatosensory cerebral neocortex in micrencephalic rat.

Welker, C. (1976) *J. Comp. Neurol.* **166:**173–190. Receptive fields of barrels in the somatosensory neocortex of the rat.

Welker, C., and T. A. Woolsey. (1974) *J. Comp. Neurol.* **158:**437–454. Structure of layer IV in the somatosensory neocortex of the rat; description and comparison with the mouse.

Welker, W. I., and G. B. Campos. (1963) *J. Comp. Neurol.* **120:**19–36. Physiological significance of sulci in somatic sensory cerebral cortex in mammals of the family Procyonidae.

Welker, W. I., and J. I. Johnson. (1975) *Brain Res.* **83:**504–508. Barrels in cerebral cortex altered by receptor disruption in newborn, but not in five-day-old mice (Cricetidae and Muridae).

Welker, W. I., and S. Seidenstein. (1959) *J. Comp. Neurol.* **111:**469–501. Somatic sensory representation in the cerebral cortex of the raccoon *(Procyon lotor).*

Welker, W. I., J. I. Johnson, Jr., and B. H. Pubols, Jr. (1964) *Am. Zool.* **4:**75–94. Some morphological and physiological characteristics of the somatic sensory system in raccoons.

Wendell-Smith, C. P., M. J. Blunt, and F. Baldwin. (1966) *J. Comp. Neurol.* **127:**219–240. The ultrastructural characterization of macroglial cell types.

Wenger, E. L. (1950) *J. Exp. Zool.* **114:**51–85. An experimental analysis of relations between parts of the brachial spinal cord of the embryonic chick.

Went, F. W. (1937) *Science* **86:**127. Salt accumulation and polar transport of plant hormones.

Werner, G. (1970) The topology of the body representation in the somatic afferent pathway. In *The Neurosciences: Second Study Program* (F. O. Schmitt ed.), Rockefeller University Press, New York.

Werner, G., and B. L. Whitsel. (1967) *J. Physiol. (London)* **192:**123–144. The topology of dermatomal projection in the medial lemniscal system.

Werner, G., and B. L. Whitsel. (1968) *J. Neurophysiol.* **31:**856–869. Topology of the body representation in somatosensory area 1 of primates.

Werner, J. K. (1973) *Exp. Neurol.* **41:**214–217. Duration of normal innervation required for complete differentiation of muscle spindles in newborn rats.

Wessells, N. K. (1965) *Dev. Biol.* **12:**121–153. Morphology and proliferation during early feather development.

Wessells, N. K., and K. Roessner. (1965) *Dev. Biol.* **12:**419–433. Nonproliferation in dermal condensations of mouse vibrissae and pelage hairs.

Wessells, N. K., B. S. Spooner, J. F. Ash, M. O. Bradley, M. A. Ludueña, E. L. Taylor, J. T. Wrenn, and K. M. Yamada. (1971*a*) *Science* **171:**135–143. Microfilaments in cellular and developmental processes.

Wessells, N. K., B. S. Spooner, J. F. Ash, M. A. Ludueña, and J. T. Wrenn. (1971*b*) *Science* **173:**356–359. Cytochalasin B: Microfilaments and "contractile" processes.

Weston, J. A. (1963) *Dev. Biol.* **6:**279–310. A radioautographic analysis of the migration and localization of trunk neural crest cells in the chick.

Weston, J. A. (1970) *Adv. Morphogenet.* **8:**41–114. The migration and differentiation of neural crest cells.

Weston, J. A. (1971) *UCLA Forum Med. Sci.* **14:**1–19. Neural crest cell migration and differentiation.

Weston, J. A., and S. L. Butler. (1966) *Dev. Biol.* **14:**246–266. Temporal factors affecting localization of neural crest cells in chicken embryo.

Weyl, H. (1949) *Philosophy of Mathematics and Natural Science,* Princeton University Press, Princeton, N.J.

Whalen, R. E., and W. G. Luttge. (1971*a*) *Horm. Behav.* **2:**117–125. Testosterone, androstenedione, and dihydrotestosterone: Effects of mating behavior of rats.

Whalen, R. E., and G. E. Luttage. (1971*b*) *Endocrinol.* **89:**1320–1322. Perinatal administration of dihydrotestosterone to female rats and the development of reproductive function.

Wheeler, W. M. (1891) *J. Morphol.* **4:**337–343. Neuroblasts in the arthropod's embryo.

Wheeler, W. M. (1893) *J. Morphol.* **8:**1–160. A contribution to insect morphology.

Whitaker, D. M. (1940*a*) *J. Cell. Comp. Physiol.* **15:**173–188. The effects of ultracentrifuging and of pH on the development of Fucus eggs.

Whitaker, D. M. (1940*b*) *Growth Suppl.,* 73–90. Physical factors of growth.

Whitaker, D. M. (1941) *J. Gen. Physiol.* **24:**263–278. The effect of unilateral ultraviolet light on the development of the Fucus egg.

White, E. L. (1948) *J. Exp. Zool.* **108:**439–469. An experimental study of the relationship between the size of the eye and the size of the optic tectum in the brain of the developing teleost, *Fundulus heteroclitus.*

White, E. L., and F. D. Nolan. (1974) *Anat. Rec.* **178:**486. Absence of re-innervation in the chinchilla medial superior olive.

White, J. G., E. Southgate, J. N. Thomson, and S. Brenner. (1976) *Phil. Trans. Roy. Soc. London Ser. B* **275:**327–348. The structure of the ventral nerve cord of *Caenorhabditis elegans.*

Whiting, H. P. (1957) *Quart J. Micros. Sci.* **98:**163–178. Mauthner neurones in young larva lampreys (*Lampetra* spp.)

Whiting, P. W. (1932) *J. Comp. Psychol.* **14:**345–363. Reproductive reactions of sex mosaics of a parasitic wasp *Habrobracon juglandis.*

Whitsel, B. L., L. M. Petrucelli, and G. Werner. (1969) *J. Neurophysiol.* **32:**170–183. Symmetry and connectivity in the map of the body surface in somatosensory area II of primates.

Whitten, J. M. (1969) *Science* **163:**1456–1457. Cell death during early morphogenesis: parallels between insect limb and vertebrate limb development.

Wickelgren, B. G., and P. Sterling. (1969) *J. Neurophysiol.* **32:**16–23. Influence of visual cortex on receptive fields in the superior colliculus of the cat.

Wieman, H. L., and T. C. Nussmann. (1929) *Physiol. Zool.* **2:**99–124. Experimental modification of nerve development in *Amblystoma.*

Wiersma, C. A. G. (1931) *Arch. Neurol. Physiol.* **16**:337–345. An experiment on the "resonance theory" of muscular activity.

Wiersma, C. A. G. (1957) *Acta Physiol. Pharmacol. Neerl.* **6**:135–142. On the number of nerve cells in a crustacean central nervous system.

Wiesel, T. N., and D. H. Hubel. (1963*a*) *J. Neurophysiol.* **26**:978–993. Effects of visual deprivation on morphology and physiology of cells in the cat's lateral geniculate body.

Wiesel, T. N., and D. H. Hubel. (1963*b*) *J. Neurophysiol.* **26**:1003–1017. Single-cell responses in striate cortex of kittens deprived of vision in one eye.

Wiesel, T. N., and D. H. Hubel. (1965) *J. Neurophysiol.* **28**:1029–1040. Comparison of the effects of unilateral and bilateral eye closure on cortical unit responses in kittens.

Wiesel, T. N., and D. H. Hubel. (1974) *J. Comp. Neurol.* **158**:307–318. Ordered arrangement of orientation columns in monkeys lacking visual experience.

Wiesel, T. N., D. H. Hubel, and D. M. K. Lam. (1974) *Brain Res.* **79**:273–279. Autoradiographic demonstration of ocular-dominance columns in the monkey striate cortex by means of trans-neuronal transport.

Wiest, W. D., and J. Hallervorden. (1958) *Deutsch. Z. Nervenheilk.* **178**:224–238. Migrationshemmung in Gross und Kleinhirn.

Wigger, H. (1939) *Z. Morphol. Oekol. Tiere* **36**:1–20. Vergleichende Untersuchungen am Auge von Wild und Hausschwein unter besonderer Berücksichtigung der Retina.

Wiggins, R. C., S. L. Miller, J. A. Benjamins, R. M. Krigman, and P. Morell. (1976) *Brain Res.* **107**:257–273. Myelin synthesis during postnatal nutritional deprivation and subsequent rehabilitation.

Willerman, L., and J. A. Churchill. (1967) *Child Dev.* **38**:623–629. Intelligence and birth weight in identical twins.

Williams, P. L., and S. M. Hall. (1971) *J. Anat.* **108**:397–408. Prolonged *in vivo* observations of normal peripheral nerve fibres and their acute reactions to crush and deliberate trauma.

Willshaw, D. J., and C. Von der Malsburg. (1976) *Proc. Roy. Soc. London (Biol.)* **194**:431–445. How patterned neural connections can be set up by self-organization.

Wilson, D. B. (1972) *Am. J. Anat.* **135**:549–560. Effects of embryonic overgrowth on the avian optic tectum.

Wilson, D. B. (1973) *J. Embryol Exp. Morphol.* **29**:745–751. Chronological changes in the cell cycle of chick neuroepithelial cells.

Wilson, D. B. (1974) *Brain Res.* **69**:41–48. The cell cycle of ventricular cells in the overgrown optic tectum.

Wilson, H. V. (1907) *J. Exp. Zool.* **5**:245–258. On some phenomena of coalescence and regeneration in sponges.

Wilson, J. R., and S. M. Sherman. (1976) *J. Neurophysiol.* **39**:512–533. Receptive-field characteristics of neurons in cat striate cortex: Changes with visual field eccentricity.

Wilson, L., J. Bryan, A. Ruby, and D. Mazia. (1970) *Proc. Natl. Acad. Sci. U.S.A.* **66**:807–814. Precipitation of proteins by vinblastine and calcium ions.

Wilson, L., J. R. Bamburg, S. B. Mizel, L. M. Grisham, and K. M. Creswell. (1974) *Fed. Proc.* **33**:158–166. Interaction of drugs with microtubule proteins.

Wilson, M. A. (1971) *J. Exp. Physiol.* **56**:83–91. Optic nerve fibre counts and retinal ganglion cell counts during development of *Xenopus laevis* (Daudin).

Wilt, F. H., and M. Anderson. (1972) *Dev. Biol.* **28**:443–447. The action of 5-bromodeoxyuridine on differentiation.

Wimer, R. E., C. C. Wimer, J. E. Vaughn, R. P. Barber, B. A. Balvanz, and C. R. Chernow. (1976) *Brain Res.* **118**:219–243. The genetic organization of neuron number in Ammon's horns of house mice.

Windle, W. F., and D. W. Orr. (1934) *J. Comp. Neurol.* **60**:287–307. The development of behavior in chick embryos: Spinal cord structure correlated with early somatic motility.

Windle, W. F., M. W. Fish, and J. E. O'Donnell. (1934) *J. Comp. Neurol.* **59**:139–165. Myelogeny of the cat as related to development of fiber tracts and prenatal behavior patterns.

Windle, W. F., W. L. Minear, M. F. Austin, and D. W. Orr. (1935) *Physiol. Zool.* **8**:156–185. The origin and early development of somatic behavior in the albino rat.

Wine, J. J. (1973) *Exp. Neurol.* **38**:157–169. Invertebrate central neurons: Orthograde degeneration and retrograde changes after axonotomy.

Winick, M. (1967) *J. Pediatr.* **71**:390–395. Cellular growth of the human placenta. III. Intrauterine growth failure.

Winick, M. (1969) *J. Pediatr.* **74**:667–679. Malnutrition and brain development.

Winick, M. (1970*a*) *Pediatr. Clin. N. Am.* **17**:69–78. Cellular growth in intrauterine malnutrition.

Winick, M. (1970*b*) *Exp. Neurol.* **26**:393–400. Cellular growth of cerebrum, cerebellum, and brain stem in normal and marasmic children.

Winick, M., and R. E. Greenberg. (1965*a*) *Nature* **205**:180–181. Chemical control of sensory ganglia during a critical period of development.

Winick, M., and R. E. Greenberg. (1965*b*) *Pediatrics* **35**:221–228. Appearance and localization of a nerve growth-promoting protein during development.

Winick, M., and A. Noble. (1965) *Dev. Biol.* **12**:451–466. Quantitative changes in DNA, RNA and protein during prenatal and postnatal growth in the rat.

Winick, M., and P. Rosso. (1969) *Pediatr. Res.* **3**:181–184. Effects of severe early malnutrition on cellular growth of human brian.

Winick, M., A. Coscia, and A. Noble (1967) *Pediatrics* **39**:248–251. Cellular growth in human placenta. I. Normal placental growth.

Winick, M., P. Rosso, and J. Waterlow. (1970) *Exp. Neurol.* **26**:393–400. Cellular growth of cerebrum, cerebellum, and brain stem in normal and marasmic children.

Wisniewski, H., and R. D. Terry. (1968) *Lab. Invest.* **17**:577–578. Experimental colchicine encephalopathy. I. Induction of neurofibrillary degeneration.

Wisniewski, H., M. L. Shelanski, and R. D. Terry. (1968) *J. Cell Biol.* **38**:224–229. Effects of mitotic spindle inhibitors on neurotubules and neurofilaments in anterior horn cells.

Witelson, S. F., and W. Pallie. (1973) *Brain Res.* **96**:641–646. Left hemisphere specialization for language in the newborn: Neuroanatomical evidence of asymmetry.

Witpaard, J. (1976) Frog's vision: Electrophysiological and developmental aspects. Ph.D. thesis, University of Leiden, Holland.

Witpaard, J., and H. E. D. J. ter Keurs. (1975) *Vision Res.* **15**:1333–1338. A reclassification of retinal ganglion cells in the frog, based upon tectal endings and response properties.

Woerdeman, M. W. (1929) *Arch. Entw.-Mech. Organ.* **116**:220–241. Experimentelle Untersuchungen über Lage und Bau der augenbildenden Bezirke in der Medullarplatte beim Axolotl.

Wohlfarth-Bottermann, K. E. (1964) *Int. Rev. Cytol.* **16**:61–131. Cell structures and their significance for amoeboid movement.

Wohlman, A., and R. D. Allen. (1968) *J. Cell Sci.* **3**:105–114. Structural organization associated with pseudopod extension and contraction during cell locomotion in *Difflugia.*

Wolf, M. K. (1964) *J. Cell Biol.* **22**:259–279. Differentiation of neuronal types and synapses in myelinating cultures of mouse cerebellum.

Wolf, M. K., and M. Dubois-Dalcq. (1970) *J. Comp. Neurol.* **140**:261–280. Anatomy of cultured mouse cerebellum. I. Golgi and electron microscopic demonstrations of granule cells, their afferent and efferent synapses.

Wolf, M. K., and A. B. Holden. (1969) *J. Neuropathol. Exp. Neurol.* **28**:195–213. Tissue culture analysis of the inherited defect of central nervous system myelination in jimpy mice.

Wolpert, L. (1969) *J. Theor. Biol.* **25**:1–47. Positional information and the spatial pattern of cellular differentiation.

Wolpert, L. (1971) *Curr. Top. Dev. Biol.* **6**:183–224. Positional information and pattern formation.

Wolpert, L. (1974) *Lect. Math. Life Sci.* **6**:29–41. Positional information and the development of pattern and form.

Wood, J. C., and N. King. (1971) *Nature* **229**:56–57. Turnover of basic protein of rat brain.

Wood, P. M., and R. P. Bunge. (1975) *Nature* **256**:662–664. Evidence that sensory axons are mitogenic for Schwann cells.

Woodard, J. S. (1960) *J. Comp. Neurol.* **115**:65–73. Origin of the external granule layer of the cerebellar cortex.

Woods, J. E., G. W. De Vries, and R. C. Thommes. (1971) *Gen. Comp. Endocrinol.* **17**:407–415. Ontogenesis of the pituitary-adrenal axis in the chick embryo.

Woodward, D. J., B. J. Hoffer, G. R. Siggins, and F. E. Bloom. (1971) *Brain Res.* **34**:73–97. The ontogenetic development of synaptic junctions, synaptic activation and responsiveness to neurotransmitter substances in rat cerebellar Purkinje cells.

Woodward, D. J., B. J. Hoffer, and J. Altman. (1974) *J. Neurobiol.* **5**:283–304. Physiological and pharmacological properties of Purkinje cells in rat cerebellum degranulated by postnatal x-irradiation.

Woolsey, T. A., and H. Van der Loos. (1970) *Brain Res.* **17**:205–242. The structural organization of layer IV in the somatosensory region (SI) of mouse cerebral cortex: The description of a cortical field composed of discrete cytoarchitectonic units.

Woolsey, T. A., and J. R. Wann. (1976) *J. Comp. Neurol.* **170**:53–66. Areal changes in mouse cortical barrels following vibrissal damage at different postnatal ages.

Woolsey, T. A., C. Welker, and R. H. Schwartz. (1975) *J. Comp. Neurol.* **164**:79–94. Comparative anatomical studies of the SmI face cortex with special reference to the occurrence of "barrels" in layer IV.

Wright, B. A., and J. M. Spink. (1959) *Gerontologia* **3**:277–287. A study of the loss of nerve cells in the central nervous system in relation to age.

Wright, M. R. (1964) *J. Exp. Zool.* **156**:377–390. Taste organs in tongue-to-liver grafts in the newt, *Triturus viridescens.*

Wuerker, R. B., and J. B. Kirkpatrick. (1972) *Int. Rev. Cytol.* **33**:45–75. Neuronal microtubules, neurofilaments, and microfilaments.

Wuerker, R. B., and S. L. Palay. (1969) *Tiss. Cell* **1**:387–402. Neurofilaments and microtubules in anterior horn cells of the rat.

Wuerker, R. B., A. M. McPhedran, and E. Henneman. (1965) *J. Neurophysiol.* **28**:85–99. Properties of motor units in a homogeneous pale muscle (M. gastrocnemius) of the cat.

Xeros, N. (1962) *Nature* **194**:682–683. Deoxyriboside control and synchronization of mitosis.

Yakovlev, P. I., and A.-R. Lecours. (1967) The myelogenetic cycles of regional maturation of the brain, pp. 3–64. In *Regional Development of the Brain in Early Life* (A. Minkowski, ed.), Blackwell, Oxford.

Yamada, K. M., and N. K. Wessells. (1971) *Exp. Cell Res.* **66**:346–352. Axon elongation: Effect of nerve growth factor on microtubule protein.

Yamada, K. M., B. S. Spooner, and N. K. Wessels. (1970) *Proc. Natl. Acad. Sci. U.S.A.* **66**:1206–1212. Axon growth: Roles of microfilaments and microtubules.

Yamada, K. M., B. S. Spooner, and N. K. Wessells. (1971) *J. Cell Biol.* **49**:614–635. Ultrastructure and function of growth cones and axons of cultured nerve cells.

Yamada, T. (1950) *Embryologia* **1**:1–20. Regional differentiation of the isolated ectoderm of the *Triturus gastrula* induced through a protein extract.

Yamada, T. (1958) *Experientia* **14**:81–87. Induction of specific differentiation by samples of proteins and nucleoproteins in the isolated ectoderm of *Triturus* gastrulae.

Yates, R. D. (1961) *J. Exp. Zool.* **147**:167–182. A study of division in chick embryonic ganglia.

Yellin, H. (1967*a*) *Anat. Rec.* **157**:345. Muscle fiber plasticity and the creation of localized motor units.

Yellin, H. (1967*b*) *Exp. Neurol.* **19**:92–103. Neural regulation of enzymes in muscle fibers of red and white muscle.

Yntema, C. L. (1943) *J. Exp. Zool.* **94**:319–349. Deficient efferent innervation of the extremities following removal of neural crest in *Amblystoma.*

Yntema, C. L., and W. S. Hammond. (1945) *J. Exp. Zool.* **100**:237–263. Depletions and abnormalities in the cervical sympathetic system of the chick following extirpation of the neural crest.

Yntema, C. L., and W. S. Hammond. (1947) *Biol. Rev.* **22**:344–359. The development of the autonomic nervous system.

Yolton, L. W. (1923) *Proc. Natl. Acad. Sci. U.S.A.* **9**:383–395. The effects of cutting the giant fibers in the earthworm *Eisenia foetida* (Sav.).

Yonezawa, T., M. B. Bornstein, E. R. Peterson, and M. R. Murray. (1962) *J. Neuropathol. Exp. Neurol.* **21**:479–487. A histochemical study of oxidative enzymes in myelinating cultures of central and peripheral nervous tissue.

Yoon, M. G. (1971) *Exp. Neurol.* **33**:395–411. Reorganization of retinotectal projection following surgical operations on the optic tectum in goldfish.

Yoon, M. G. (1972*a*) *Exp. Neurol.* **37**:451–462. Transposition of the visual projection from the nasal hemiretina onto the foreign rostral zone of the optic tectum in goldfish.

Yoon, M. G. (1972*b*) *Exp. Neurol.* **35**:565–577. Reversibility of the reorganization of retinotectal projection in goldfish.

Yoon, M. G. (1975*a*) *J. Physiol. (London)* **252**:137–158. Readjustment of retinotectal projection following reimplantation of a rotated or inverted tectal tissue in adult goldfish.

Yoon, M. G. (1975*b*) *Cold Spring Harbor Symp. Quant. Biol.* **15**:503–509. Topographic polarity of the optic tectum studied by reimplantation of tectal tissue in adult goldfish.

Yoon, M. G. (1976) *J. Physiol. (London)* **257**:621–643. Progress of topographic regulation of the visual projection in the halved optic tectum of adult goldfish.

Yoon, M. G. (1977) *J. Physiol. (London)* **264**:379–410. Induction of compression in the re-established visual projections on to a rotated tectal reimplant that retains its original topographic polarity within the halved optic tectum of adult goldfish.

Young, D. (1972) *J. Exp. Biol.* **57**:305–316. Specific reinnervation of limbs transplanted between segments in the cockroach, *Periplaneta americana.*

Young, D. (1973) Specificity and regeneration in insect motor neurons, pp. 179–202. In *Developmental Neurobiology of Arthropods* (D. Young, ed.), Cambridge University Press, London.

Young, J. Z. (1932) *Quart. J. Micros. Sci.* **75**:1–49. On the cytology of the neurons of cephalopods.

Young, J. Z. (1942) *Physiol. Rev.* **22**:318–374. The functional repair of nervous tissue.

Young, J. Z. (1944) *Nature* **153**:333. Contraction, turgor and the cytoskeleton of nerve fibers.

Young, J. Z. (1945) The history of the shape of a nerve fiber, pp. 41–94. In *Essays on Growth and Form* (W. E. Le Gros Clark and P. B. Medawar, eds.), Clarendon, Oxford.

Young, J. Z. (1951) *Proc. Roy. Soc. (London) Ser. B* **139**:18–37. Growth and plasticity in the nervous system.

Young, J. Z. (1963) *Proc. Zool. Soc. London* **140**:229–254. The number and sizes of nerve cells in octopus.

Young, J. Z. (1964) *A Model of the Brain,* Clarendon, Oxford.

Young, M., J. Oger, M. H. Blanchard, H. Asdourian, H. Amos, and B. G. W. Arnason. (1975) *Science* **187**:361–362. Secretion of a nerve growth factor by primary chick fibroblast cultures.

Young, R. M. (1970) *Mind, Brain and Adaptation in the Nineteenth Century,* Clarendon, Oxford.

Zacharias, L. R. (1938) *J. Exp. Zool.* **78**:135–157. An analysis of cellular proliferation in grafted segments of embryonic spinal cords.

Zacks, S. I., and A. Saito. (1969) *J. Histochem. Cytochem.* **17**:161–170. Uptake of exogenous horseradish peroxidase by coated vesicles in mouse neuromuscular junctions.

Zagon, I. S. (1975) *Exp. Neurol.* **46**:69–77. Prolonged gestation and cerebellar development in the rat.

Zaimis, E. (1964) *J. Physiol. (London)* **177**:35–36. The immunosympathectomized animal: A valuable tool in physiological and pharmacological research.

Zaimis, E., L. Berk, and B. A. Callingham. (1965) *Nature* **206**:1220–1222. Morphological, biochemical and functional changes in the sympathetic nervous system of rats treated with nerve growth factor-antiserum.

Zalewski, A. A. (1968) *Exp. Neurol.* **22**:40–51. Changes in phosphatase enzymes following denervation of the vallate papilla of the rat.

Zalewski, A. A. (1969*a*) *Exp. Neurol.* **23**:18–28. Role of nerve and epithelium in the regulation of alkaline phosphatase activity in gustatory papillae.

Zalewski, A. A. (1969*b*) *J. Neurobiol.* **1**:123–132. Neurotrophic–hormonal interaction in the regulation of taste buds in the rat's vallate papilla.

Zalewski, A. A. (1969*c*) *Exp. Neurol.* **24**:285–297. Combined effects of testosterone and motor, sensory, or gustatory nerve reinnervation on the regeneration of taste buds.

Zalewski, A. A. (1970*a*) *Exp. Neurol.* **26**:621–629. Regeneration of taste buds in the lingual epithelium after excision of the vallate papilla.

Zalewski, A. A. (1970*b*) *Exp. Neurol.* **29**:462–467. Trophic influence of *in vivo* transplanted sensory neurons on taste buds.

Zalewski, A. A. (1970*c*) *Am. J. Physiol.* **219**:1675–1679. Effects of reinnervation on denervated skeletal muscle by axons of motor, sensory, and sympathetic neurons.

Zalewski, A. A. (1972) *Exp. Neurol.* **35**:519–528. Regeneration of taste buds after transplantation of tongue and ganglia grafts to the anterior chamber of the eye.

Zalewski, A. A. (1973) *Exp. Neurol.* **40**:161–169. Regeneration of taste buds in tongue grafts after reinnervation by neurons in transplanted lumbar sensory ganglia.

Zalewski, A. A. (1974*a*) *Ann. N.Y. Acad. Sci.* **228**:344–349. Neuronal and tissue specifications involved in taste bud formation.

Zalewski, A. A. (1974*b*) *Exp. Neurol.* **45**:189–193. Trophic function of neurons in transplanted neonatal ganglia.

Zamenhof, S. (1941) *Growth* **5**:123–139. Stimulation of the proliferation of neurons by the growth hormone. I. Experiments on tadpoles.

Zamenhof, S. (1942) *Physiol. Zool.* **15**:281–292. Stimulation of cortical-cell proliferation by the growth hormone. III. Experiments on albino rats.

Zamenhof, S. (1976) *Brain Res.* **109**:392–394. Final number of Purkinje and other large cells in the chick cerebellum influenced by incubation temperatures during their proliferation.

Zamenhof, S., and E. Van Marthens. (1971) Hormonal and nutritional aspects of prenatal brain development, pp. 329–359. In *Cellular Aspects of Neural Growth and Differentiation* (D. C. Pease, ed.), University of California Press, Berkeley.

Zamenhof, S., H. Bursztyn, K. Rich, and P. J. Zamenhof. (1964) *J. Neurochem.* **11**:505–509. The determination of deoxyribonucleic acid and of cell number in brain.

Zamenhof, S., J. Mosley, and E. Schuller. (1966) *Science* **152**:1396–1397. Stimulation of the proliferation of cortical neurons by prenatal treatment with growth hormone.

Zamenhof, S., E. van Marthens, and F. L. Margolis. (1968) *Science* **160**:322–323. DNA (cell number) and protein in neonatal brain: Alteration by maternal dietary protein restriction.

Zamenhof, S., L. Grauel, and E. van Marthens. (1971*a*) *Biol. Neonate* **18**:140–145. Study of possible correlations between prenatal brain development and placental weight.

Zamenhof, S., L. Grauel, and E. van Marthens. (1971*b*) *Res. Commun. Chem. Pathol. Pharmacol.* **2**:261–270. The effect of thymidine and 5-bromodeoxyuridine on developing chick embryo brain.

Zamenhof, S., E. van Marthens, and H. Bursztyn. (1971*c*) The effect of hormones on DNA synthesis and cell number in the developing chick and rat brain, pp. 101–119. In *Hormones in Development* (M. Hamburgh and E. J. W. Barrington, eds.), Appleton-Century-Crofts, New York.

Zamenhof, S., E. van Marthens, and L. Grauel. (1971*d*) *J. Nutr.* **9**:1265–1270. DNA (cell number) and protein in neonatal rat brain: Alteration by timing of maternal dietary protein restriction.

Zamenhof, S., E. van Marthens, and L. Grauel. (1971*e*) *Science* **172**:850–851. DNA (cell number) in neonatal brain: Second generation F_2) alteration by maternal (F_0) dietary protein restriction.

Zamenhof, S., E. van Marthens, and L. Grauel. (1971*f*) *Science* **174**:954–955. Prenatal cerebral development: Effect of restricted diet, reversal by growth hormone.

Zander, E., and G. Weddell. (1951) *J. Anat. (London)* **85**:66–99. Observations on the innervation of the cornea.

Zanini, A., P. Angeletti, and R. Levi-Montalcini. (1968) *Proc. Natl. Acad. Sci. U.S.A.* **61**:835–842. Immunochemical properties of the nerve growth factor.

Zecevic, N., and P. Rakic. (1976) *J. Comp. Neurol.* **167**:27–48. Differentiation of Purkinje cells and their relationship to other components of developing cerebellar cortex in man.

Zelená, J. (1957) *J. Embryol. Exp. Morphol.* **5**:283–292. The morphogenetic influence of innervation on the ontogenetic development of muscle spindles.

Zelená, J. (1964) *Prog. Brain Res.* **13**:175–213. Development, degeneration and regeneration of receptor organs.

Zelená, J. (1965) *Cesk. Fysiol.* **14**:377–378. The influence of fusimotor innervation upon the development of muscle spindles.

Zelená, J. (1968) *Z. Zellforsch. Mikrosk. Anat.* **92**:186–196. Bidirectional movements of mitochondria along axons of an isolated nerve segment.

Zelená, J. (1972*a*) *Z. Zellforsch. Mikrosk. Anat.* **124**:217–220. Ribosomes in myelinated axons of dorsal root ganglia.

Zelená, J. (1972*b*) *Folia Morphol. (Praha)* **20**:91–93. Ribosomes in the axoplasm of myelinated nerve fibers.

Zelená, J., and M. Sobotková. (1971) *Physiol. Bohemoslov.* **20**:433–439. Absence of muscle spindles in regenerated muscles of the rat.

Zelená, J., and T. Soukup. (1973) *Z. Zellforsch. Mikrosk. Anat.* **144**:435–452. Development of muscle spindles deprived of fusimotor innervation.

Zelená, J., and T. Soukup. (1974*a*) *Cell Tiss. Res.* **153**:115–136. The differentiation of intrafusal fibre types in rat muscle spindles after motor denervation.

Zelená, J., and T. Soukop. (1974*b*) *Folia Morphol. (Praha)* **22**:268–269. Ultrastructural differentiation of muscle spindles after de-efferentation.

Zelená, J., L. Lubińska, and E. Gutmann. (1968) *Z. Zellforsch. Mikrosk. Anat.* **91**:200–219. Accumulation of organelles at the ends of interrupted axons.

Zeman, F. J., and E. C. Stanbrough. (1969) *J. Nutr.* **99**:274–282. Effect of maternal protein deficiency on cellular development in the fetal rat.

Zenker, W., and E. Hohberg. (1973) *Z. Anat. Entwicklungsgesch.* **139**:163–172. α-Motorische Nervenfaser: Axonquerschnittsfläche von Stammfaser und Endästen.

Zigmond, R. E., F. Nottebohm, and D. W. Pfaff. (1973) *Science* **179**:1005–1007. Androgen-concentrating cells in the midbrain of a songbird.

Zigmond, S. H. (1974) *Nature* **249**:450–452. Mechanisms of sensing chemical gradients by polymorphonuclear leukocytes.

Zukin, S. R., A. B. Young, and S. H. Synder. (1975) *Brain Res.* **83**:525–530. Development of the synaptic glycine receptor in chick embryo spinal cord.

Zwaan, J., P. R. Bryan, Jr., and T. L. Pearce. (1969) *J. Embryol. Exp. Morphol.* **21**:71–83. Interkinetic nuclear migration during the early stages of lens formation in the chicken embryo.

Index

GPSR Compliance
The European Union's (EU) General Product Safety Regulation (GPSR) is a set of rules that requires consumer products to be safe and our obligations to ensure this.

If you have any concerns about our products, you can contact us on

ProductSafety@springernature.com

In case Publisher is established outside the EU, the EU authorized representative is:

Springer Nature Customer Service Center GmbH
Europaplatz 3
69115 Heidelberg, Germany

www.ingramcontent.com/pod-product-compliance
Ingram Content Group UK Ltd.
Pitfield, Milton Keynes, MK11 3LW, UK
UKHW051132260726
13967UKWH00010B/2998
* 9 7 8 1 4 7 5 7 4 9 5 2 6 *